EXERCISE
AND
THE HEART

clinical concepts

Second Edition

EXERCISE AND THE HEART

clinical concepts

Second Edition

VICTOR F. FROELICHER, M.D.

Professor of Medicine
Assistant Chief of Cardiology
University of California at Irvine
Irvine, California
Chief, Cardiology Section
Long Beach Veterans Administration Medical Center
Long Beach, California

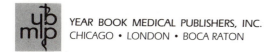

YEAR BOOK MEDICAL PUBLISHERS, INC.
CHICAGO • LONDON • BOCA RATON

Library of Congress Cataloging-in-Publication Data

Froelicher, Victor F.
  Exercise and the heart.

  Rev. ed. of: Exercise testing & training. c1983.
  Includes bibliographies and index.
  1. Exercise tests.   2. Heart function tests.
3. Heart—Diseases—Diagnosis.   4. Radioisotope
scanning.   I. Froelicher, Victor F. Exercise
testing & training.   II. Title.   [DNLM: 1. Exercise
Test—methods.   2. Exercise Therapy—methods.
3. Exertion.   4. Heart Diseases—rehabilitation.
WG 141.5.F9 F926e]
RC683.5.E94F76   1987   616.1'2   86–26693
ISBN 0–8151–3336–7

Sponsoring Editor: Richard J. Lampert
Manager, Copyediting Services: Frances M. Perveiler
Copyeditor: Francis A. Byrne
Director, Editing and Production: James A. Ross

To my father,

who knew I'd be happier in medicine
than in the seminary, in the Air Force, or in astrophysics

and

To Erika

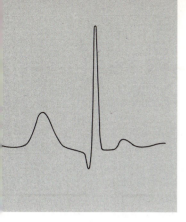

PREFACE

What's new? Surprisingly, a lot! The first edition of this book had 5 chapters, while this edition has 11. In regard to Chapter 7 on screening, three new studies have totally changed my ideas on using the exercise test for screening apparently healthy people. Previous studies, including my USAF studies, used angina as an endpoint. Newer studies using hard cardiac endpoints show exercise testing to cause far more harm than good as a screening test. Only 5 of 100 individuals with ST depression go on to have a cardiac event such as hospital admission, myocardial infarction, or death. The angina reported in previous studies is part of the psychological harm done by telling "well people" they have abnormal tests. The data from CASS also disproves Erikssen's contention that an abnormal test means a bad outcome even if the coronary angiography is normal. Exercise testing "well people" can be beneficial, but those individuals with false positive responses must be carefully managed so as not to do iatrogenic harm.

Detrano's work at Cleveland Clinic shows that Hollenberg's computerized treadmill score must be validated at other centers before it is widely utilized. This is also the case for the ST/HR ratio that Fox in London has not found to be as predictive as the original work from Leeds. Careful review of the 24 follow-up studies of exercise testing post-myocardial infarction (MI) and the application of meta-analysis in Chapter 6 leave much uncertainty as to the prognostic value of post-MI exercise testing.

The new radionuclide chapter (Chapter 8) replaces an optimistic, enthusiastic approach with a more realistic one. The ejection fraction and wall motion responses to exercise are not as specific as once thought and phase analysis of the LV wall did not add anything to wall motion analysis. Detrano's findings with exercise ventriculography using digital subtraction angiography (DSA) confirm the poor predictive accuracy reported with radionuclide ventriculography. Left ventricular volume analysis is far too gross a measurement to have clinical application. Slow washout on thallium scans appears to be largely related to heart rate and so computerized interpretation, which relies on slow washout, does not add much to visual analysis. Perhaps the nuclear cardiology exercise tests will be eventually replaced by exercise echocardiography. Exercise echocardiography will deserve a chapter next edition. PERFEXT was completed and now its results are presented in an expanded chapter on cardiac rehabilitation (Chapter 11).

As the years pass, I become more eccentric and have developed some maxims. First, the testing procedure should be called "exercise testing" not "stress testing" since there are many types of stress. Second, test responses should not be reported as positive or negative or as subjective or objective, but the actual response should be described. Third, exercise capacity should be reported in the MET equivalent of the workload achieved and not in total time. The optimal duration for a test is 8 to 10 minutes and so the protocol should be adjusted to the individual to permit this. Fourth, age adjusted maximal heart rates should not be used to grade effort or to end a test since there is so wide a scatter relative to age.

Who to acknowledge? Many co-workers and friends. Mike Sullivan has performed gas analysis research with me for over 5 years and much of his writing and work are in this book. Mike is now in his third year of medical school at UCI and continues to keep my lab "in order." Eddie Atwood developed the thallium scoring system that much of my work at UCSD was based on. He now directs our catheterization laboratory and is using gas analysis to evaluate patients with atrial fibrillation and other conditions. Bill Pewen came with me from San Diego, and his thesis and work with Kirk Hammond resulted in the prediction of outcome from PERFEXT. Also, Bill leads our microprocessor efforts utilizing electronic spreadsheets for meta-analysis, word processing using outline capabilities, reference management, and data processing for research. Kirk also made significant contributions with our work on maximal heart rate and markers of ischemia. He is now a cardiology fellow at UCSD and plans to continue an academic career. Jon Myers worked with me in San Diego analyzing some of the PERFEXT data and now directs our ventilatory gas exchange exercise testing while working on R wave data and perceived exertion. Dave Jensen managed the PERFEXT analysis and did a particularly fine job with its nuclear medicine aspects—he now works for Seimens on the west coast. Jeff Froning and Mark Olson have helped me understand computer analysis of the exercise ECG and developed a software package for analyzing the exercise ECG on a microprocessor.

Staffan Ahnve, Marios Saavides, Sliman Aboutantoun, Kioshi Watanabe, and Alex Battler were research cardiologists who worked with me at the University of California in San Diego. Their work is cited and they are responsible for some of the figures that appear in this book. Numerous medical students (who are now physicians) worked with me on data and helped with figures used also (particularly Paul Gamble, Mark Roberts, and Gene Robinson). Gary Starr, a resident in rehabilitation medicine at LBVAMC, helped with the review of the prognostic studies of cardiac rehabilitation.

Bill Pewen and I transferred the first edition from a DEC WPS 78 to our Rainbow then from CPM to MSDOS . . . then Lesley Sanderson and Mona Risch did the changes, rewrites and updates . . . and thanks especially to Mona who rechecked all the page proofs.

VICTOR F. FROELICHER, M.D.

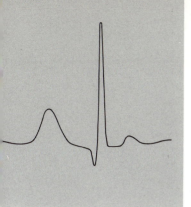

CONTENTS

10. EXERCISE IN THE PREVENTION OF CORONARY HEART DISEASE   386

11. CARDIAC REHABILITATION 423

1 STANDARD EXERCISE TESTING

Exercise, a human being's most common physiologic stress, can bring out cardiac abnormalities not present at rest. For this reason, exercise can be considered the most practical test of cardiac perfusion and function. This chapter presents the methodologies of standard exercise testing as performed in most clinics, hospitals, and doctors' offices.

If the two basic principles of exercise physiology are understood, much confusion can be avoided. The first is a physiologic principle: total body oxygen consumption and myocardial oxygen consumption are distinct in their determinants and in the way they are measured or estimated (Table 1–1). Total body, or ventilatory oxygen consumption (VO_2), is the amount of oxygen that is extracted from inspired air as the body performs work. Accurate measurement of VO_2 requires gas analysis equipment, but it can be estimated from the work load performed because there is relatively small variation in the oxygen cost of a given work load. Maximal VO_2 is equal to maximal cardiac output times maximal arteriovenous oxygen (AV O_2) difference. The maximal AV O_2 difference during exercise has a physiologic limit that cannot be exceeded; hence, if a maximal effort is given, maximal oxygen consumption can be used to estimate maximal cardiac output noninvasively. Since cardiac output is equal to the product of stroke volume and heart rate, it is, of course, related to heart rate. Total body oxygen consumption is best estimated by the aerobic work load performed rather than by total exercise time because the latter is influenced by endurance and muscular strength.

Accurate measurement of myocardial oxygen consumption requires the placement of catheters in a coronary artery and in the coronary venous sinus to measure oxygen content. Its determinants include intramyocardial wall tension (left ventricular pressure times end diastolic volume), contractility, and heart rate. It has been shown that myocardial oxygen consumption is best estimated by the product of heart rate and systolic blood pressure (double product). Angina usually occurs at the same double product rather than at the same work load. When this is not the case, the influence of other factors should be suspected, such as a recent meal or abnormal ambient temperature or coronary artery spasm.

The second principle is one of pathophysiology: considerable interaction

TABLE 1–1.
Two Basic Principles of Exercise Physiology

Myocardial Oxygen Consumption	$\cong$ Heart rate $\times$ systolic blood pressure (determinants include wall tension $\cong$ left ventricular pressure $\times$ volume; contractility; and heart rate)
Ventilatory Oxygen Consumption (VO_2)	$\cong$ External work performed, or cardiac output $\times$ AV O_2 difference*

*AV O_2 difference is approximately 15 to 17 vol% at maximal exercise; therefore, VO_2 MAX is a noninvasive method for estimating cardiac output.

takes place between the exercise test manifestations of abnormalities of myocardial perfusion and function. The ECG response and angina are closely related to myocardial ischemia and coronary artery occlusion while the exercise capacity, systolic blood pressure response, and the heart rate response to exercise can be determined by either myocardial ischemia or dysfunction, as well as by the reactions in the periphery. Exercise-induced ischemia can cause cardiac dysfunction which results in exercise impairment and an abnormal systolic blood pressure response. Often it is difficult to separate the impact of ischemia from the impact of LV dysfunction on exercise responses. This results in an interaction that complicates the interpretation of exercise test findings.

The severity of ischemia or the amount of myocardium in jeopardy is known clinically to be inversely related to the heart rate, blood pressure, and exercise level achieved. Neither resting nor exercise ejection fraction or change in ejection fraction correlate well with measured or estimated maximal ventilatory oxygen consumption even in patients without signs or symptoms of ischemia. Exercise-induced markers of ischemia do not correlate well with each other either. Silent ischemia (i.e., markers of ischemia presenting without angina pectoris) does not appear to affect the exercise capacity in patients with coronary heart disease. Though not conclusive, two clinical radionuclide studies from UCSD by McKirnan and Hammond support this position. They lead to the conclusion that in most middle-aged males with stable coronary heart disease, exercise capacity is limited or controlled by the periphery and not by the heart, unless it is severely impaired.

The response to dynamic muscular exercise consists of a complex series of cardiovascular adjustments designed to (1) see that active muscles receive a blood supply appropriate to their metabolic needs, (2) dissipate the heat generated by active muscles, and (3) maintain the blood supply to the brain and the heart. There is an immediate dilation of the arteries and arterioles in active muscle because of the sudden increase in metabolites. This results in a decrease in systemic vascular resistance proportional to the muscle mass involved. To maintain arterial blood pressure, there is an increase in sympathetic activity. This causes constriction of the resistance vessels in the splanchnic bed and the kidneys. The resistance vessels also constrict in nonworking muscles. The generalized vasoconstriction in inactive tissues as well as the increased venous return result in maintenance of the heart's filling volume and pressure. As cardiac output increases, there is an increase in systemic arterial pressure. The increase in pulmonary blood flow causes a moderate increase in mean pulmonary artery pressure.

The relationship of pressure, flow, and resistance is defined in Ohm's law. This physical law states that resistance is equal to pressure divided by flow. Peripheral resistance increases in the tissues that do not function in the performance of the ongoing exercise and decreases in active muscle. The total result is a decrease in overall systemic resistance. This is explained by the fact that while pressure only increases mildly, flow can increase by as much as five times during dynamic exercise. Since the denominator (flow) increases much more than the numerator (pressure) in the formula for resistance, the result is a decrease in systemic resistance.

As described by Rowell, the regulation of circulation during exercise involves the following adaptations: (1) local—the resistance vessels dilate in the active muscle owing to the products of muscle metabolism. These products disconnect the sympathetic nerves from the muscle vessels so there will not be constriction; (2) mechanical—during upright exercise, the muscle pump returns blood from the legs to the central circulation; (3) nervous—the sympathetic outflow to the heart and systemic blood vessels is increased; the vagal outflow to the heart decreases. This causes tachycardia, increased contractility, and constriction of the resistance vessels in the kidneys and gut. The increased sympathetic outflow is due in part to a central command from the cerebral cortex and to activation of receptors in contracting skeletal muscles. The arterial and cardiopulmonary mechanoreceptors prevent marked fluctuations in arterial pressure from normal values. As exercise continues and body temperature rises, the temperature sensitive cells in the hypothalamus are activated. They inhibit the sympathetic outflow to the skin vessels and stimulate the cholinergic fibers to the sweat glands. This results in dilation of the skin vessels; (4) humoral—if exercise is severe, the cholinergic fibers to the adrenal medulla are activated and epinephrine is released into the blood stream. This further increases the heart rate and myocardial contractility and tightens the constriction of the veins and renal arterial system.

There is a highly predictable relationship between oxygen consumption and the cardiovascular and respiratory responses to exercise. To explain this relationship, six major hypotheses have been advanced. The first is the arterial baroreflex hypothesis, which is based on the idea that vasodilation of active muscle would cause a fall in blood pressure which in turn would trigger a baroreflex and raise heart rate and cardiac output. However, a fall in blood pressure cannot be the stimulus for the exercise response. Second, the central nervous system excitation hypothesis: the outflow of motor impulses could interact with the centers that regulate the cardiovascular responses to exercise. The major problem with this hypothesis is that there is no feedback mechanism to the central nervous system to maintain the delicate relationship between these responses and exercising muscle. The third and fourth hypotheses are based on chemoreflexes in the arterial or central venous systems. However, there is little data to support the idea that changes in PO_2, CO_2, or pH are the mediators. Fifth, the skeletal muscle mechanoreceptors hypothesis: these receptors cannot be involved in the exercise reflex since there is no cardiovascular or respiratory response to muscle vibration which is a potent stimulus to mechanoreceptors, and selective blockade of large mechanoreceptor afferents does not block the exercise response.

The sixth and most logical hypothesis is based on muscle chemoreceptors. According to Rowell, the most current evidence suggests that some sensor within skeletal muscle detects small changes in the local chemical environment and serves to monitor the adequacy of muscle perfusion.

METHODOLOGY

The numerous approaches to the methodology of performing exercise testing pose problems. Should patients be hyperventilated prior to testing or can that cause false positives? (We do not routinely have patients hyperventilate, but if a false positive ECG response is suspected, the patient is asked to hyperventilate with ECG monitoring at another time). Should patients do a cool-down walk, stop abruptly, sit or lie down after testing? (This should depend on the purpose of the test and on the clinical status of the individual tested.) There is little agreement regarding these basic points, but most laboratories consistently agree on safety precautions.

Safety Precautions and Risk.   The safety precautions indicated by the American Heart Association are explicit about the requirements for exercise testing. Everything necessary for cardiopulmonary resuscitation must be available, and regular drills should be performed to make certain that both personnel and equipment are ready for a cardiac emergency. A survey of clinical exercise facilities has shown exercise testing to be a safe procedure with approximately one death and five nonfatal complications per 10,000 tests. However, the literature contains reports of acute infarctions and deaths occurring secondarily to this procedure. Bruce has reported the association of exercise-induced hypotension and ventricular fibrillation. Though the test is remarkably safe, the population referred for this procedure usually is at high risk for coronary events. Shepard has hypothesized the following risk levels for exercise: (1) 3 or 4 times normal in a cross-country foot race; (2) 6 to 12 times normal in a coronary prone population performing unaccustomed exercise; and, (3) as high as 60 times normal when exercise is performed by coronary disease patients in a stressful environment, such as a physician's office. Cobb estimates the risk to be over 100 times in the latter situation and points out the dangers of the recovery period. The risk of exercise testing to coronary artery disease patients cannot be disregarded even with its excellent safety record.

Contraindications.   Table 1–2 lists the absolute and relative contraindications to performing an exercise test. Good clinical judgment

TABLE 1–2.
Absolute and Relative Contraindications to Exercise Testing

ABSOLUTE	RELATIVE*
Acute myocardial infarction or any recent change in the resting electrocardiogram	Any less serious noncardiac disorder
Unstable angina	Ventricular conduction defects
Serious cardiac dysrhythmias	Significant arterial or pulmonary hypertension
Acute pericarditis or myocarditis	Tachydysrhythmias or bradydysrhythmias < serious
Endocarditis	Moderate valvular or myocardial heart diseases
Severe aortic stenosis	Drug effect or electrolyte abnormalities
Severe left ventricular dysfunction	Fixed-rate artificial pacemaker
Acute pulmonary embolus or pulmonary infarction	Left main obstruction or its equivalent
Any acute or serious noncardiac disorder	Psychiatric disease or inability to cooperate
Severe physical handicap	

*Under certain circumstances, relative contraindications can be superseded.

should be foremost in deciding the indications and contraindications for exercise testing. In selected cases with relative contraindications, testing can provide valuable information even if performed submaximally.

Patient Preparation.   Preparations for exercise testing include the following: (1) the patient should be instructed not to eat for two to three hours prior to the test and to come dressed for exercise; (2) a brief history and physical examination should be performed to rule out any contraindications to testing (particularly aortic outflow obstruction); (3) specific questioning should determine if there are any drugs being taken or possible electrolyte abnormalities (medications should be brought along so they can be identified and recorded; there should not be an automatic rule to stop all medications because of life-threatening rebound phenomena, particularly with beta blockers); (4) if the reason for the exercise test is not obvious, the patient should be questioned and the referring physician contacted; (5) a 12-lead electrocardiogram should be obtained. The latter is an important rule, particularly in patients with known heart disease, since an abnormality may prohibit testing. On occasion, a patient referred for a treadmill test will instead be admitted to the coronary care unit. There should be a careful explanation of the testing procedure with its risks and possible complications. The patient should be instructed on how to perform the exercise test, and treadmill walking should be demonstrated.

The Treadmill.   The treadmill should have front and side rails for patients to steady themselves, and some patients may benefit from the helping hand of the person administering the test. It should be calibrated at least monthly. Some models can be greatly affected by the weight of the patient and will not deliver the appropriate work load with heavy patients. The emergency stop button should be readily available to the staff only. A small platform or stepping area at the level of the belt is advisable so that the patient can start off striding the belt and "pedaling" it with one foot until ready to start. Patients should not grasp the front or side rails as this decreases oxygen uptake and work and increases exercise time and ECG muscle artifact. It is helpful to have patients take their hands off the rails, close their fists, and extend one finger touching the rails in order to maintain balance while walking, after they are accustomed to the treadmill. The addition of isometric work should be avoided, but when the patient first steps on the treadmill, it is best to allow grasping the rail as much as is necessary.

Most problems can be avoided by having an experienced physician, nurse, or exercise physiologist stand next to the patient, measuring blood pressure, judging skin temperature, and assessing the patient during the test. The exercise technician should operate the recorder and treadmill, take the appropriate tracings, enter data on a form, and alert the physician to any abnormalities that may have been missed on the monitor scope. If the patient's appearance causes concern, systolic blood pressure drops or plateaus, there are alarming electrocardiographic abnormalities, chest pain occurs and becomes worse than the patient's usual pain, or a patient feels he or she is being harmed in any way, the test should be stopped, even at a submaximal heart rate. In most instances, a symptom-limited maximal test is preferred, but it is usually advisable to stop if 0.2 mV of ST-segment elevation or depression occurs. In some patients estimated to be at high risk because of their clinical history, it may be appropriate to stop at a submaximal level since it is not unusual for severe ST-segment depression, dysrhythmias, or both to occur only after exercise. If the measurement of maximal exercise capacity or other information is needed, it is better to repeat the test later, once the patient has demonstrated a safe performance of a submaximal work load.

Exercise testing should be an extension of the history and physical examination. A physician obtains the most information by being present to talk with, observe, and examine the patient in conjunction with the test. In this way, patient safety and an optimal yield of information are assured. In some instances, such as when asymptomatic men are being screened, research studies are being performed, or a repeat treadmill test is being done on a patient whose condition is stable, a physician need not be present, but should be in close proximity and prepared to respond promptly. The physician's reaction to signs or symptoms should be moderated by the information the patient gives regarding his usual activity. If abnormal findings occur at levels that the patient says he usually performs, then it may not be necessary to stop the test for them. Also, the patient's activity history should help decide on appropriate work loads for testing.

Consent Form. In any procedure with a risk of complications, it is advisable to make certain the patient understands the situation and acknowledges the risks. Some physicians believe that informing patients of the risks involved will often make them overly anxious or discourage them from having a test performed. Because of this and the fact that a signed consent form does not protect a physician from legal action, there has been less insistence on consent forms. If those performing the exercise test carefully explain in detail the possible risks and complications of the test to each patient, a consent form should be superfluous.

Legal Implications of Exercise Testing. The legal implications of performing exercise testing include several considerations. Establishment of physician-patient communication before and after performance of the exercise test should be the first consideration. A test should not be performed without first obtaining the patient's informed consent, in writing or verbal. In the process of obtaining informed consent, the patient should be made aware of the potential risks and benefits of the procedure. A physician may be held responsible in the event of a major untoward effect, even if the test is carefully done, if consent is not first obtained. The argument can be made that the patient would not have undergone the procedure had he or she been made aware of the risks associated with the test. After the test, responsibility rests with the physician for prompt interpretation and consideration of the implications of the test. Communication of these results to the patient is necessary—with advice concerning adjustments in life-style—without delay. It would be of major concern if an untoward event occurred during such a delay. The second consideration should be adherence to proper standards of care during performance of the test. Exercise testing should be carried out only by persons thoroughly trained in its administration and in the prompt recognition of problems that may arise. A physician trained in exercise testing and resuscitation should be readily available during the test to make the judgment to stop the study. Resuscitative equipment should always be available.

Blood Pressure Measurement. Though numerous clever devices have been developed to automate BP measurement during exercise, none can be recommended. The time-proven method of the physician holding the patient's arm straight out with a stethoscope placed over the brachial artery is most effective. The patient's arm should be free of the handrails so that noise is not carried up the arm. It is sometimes helpful to mark the brachial artery. An anesthesiologist's auscultory piece or an electronic microphone can be fastened to the arm. A device that inflates and deflates the cuff on the push of a button can be helpful also. These devices free up the physician and enable more blood pressures to be taken.

Rasmussen et al. compared rest and exercise BP measurements in 27 subjects determined directly by catheterization of the radial artery with simultaneous values obtained indirectly by auscultation of the brachial artery. As work increased, the systolic BP increased, whereas the diastolic BP did not change. Considering all comparisons, direct BP was greater than indirect BP by a mean of 29 mm Hg for systolic BP and 12 mm Hg for diastolic BP. As exercise level increased, the difference between direct and indirect systolic BP decreased whereas the difference between direct and indirect diastolic BP did not change. Both methods have advantages for assessment of BP response to exercise: normality of BP response is best assessed by auscultation, whereas beat-by-beat trends in BP are more accurately defined by the direct method.

Recording Instruments. Many technologic advances in electrocardiographic recorders have taken place. The medical instrumentation industry has promptly complied with specifications set forth by various professional groups. Machines with a high-input impedance ensure that the voltage recorded graphically is equivalent to that on the surface of the body despite the high natural impedance of the skin. There remains some concern about mismatching lead impedances, which can result in distortion. Optically isolated buffer amplifiers have ensured patient safety, and machines with a frequency response from 0 to 100 Hz are commercially available. The 0 Hz lower end is possible because DC coupling is technically feasible. However, only Marquette Electronics makes it commercially available.

Some electrocardiographic equipment has monitoring and diagnostic modes, particularly equipment used in coronary care units. The diagnostic mode follows diagnostic instrument specifications with a frequency response from 0.05 Hz to 100 Hz whereas the monitor mode has a frequency range of 4 Hz to 50 Hz. In the monitor mode, there can be distortion of the electrocardiogram. The monitor mode is available to lessen the effects of electrical interference, motion, and respiration in the ECG and should not be used for exercise testing. The type of distortion is affected by the electrocardiographic waveform that is presented. If the ECG waveform is a tall R-wave without an S-wave, the ST-segment distortion can be different than if there is an R-wave followed by a large S-wave. In general, an inadequate low-frequency response can greatly decrease the Q- and R-wave amplitude and create S-waves. The middle-range frequency response of recorders is important and is particularly affected by stylus overpressure. Alteration of the 25 Hz to 45 Hz frequency response is the most common cause of ST-segment distortion found in tracings with abnormal ST-segments. A simple office test is available for checking the 0.05 to 45 Hz frequency response of a recorder. It consists of recording approximately five seconds of the decay curve of a 1 cm/mV calibration pulse at the standard paper speed of 25 mm/sec. The time between the initial upstroke of this calibration pulse and the point at which the initial signal has decayed to 3.7 mm should be at least 3.2 seconds to meet the 0.05 Hz low-frequency endpoint. In this same recording, the presence of a sharp, square-cornered leading edge at the peak of the pulse reflects the existence of a high-frequency response of at least 45 Hz, because roundness at that junction becomes visually apparent below this frequency. Not all ambulatory monitoring recorders or telemetry equipment meet diagnostic frequency requirements.

Waveform Averaging. Analog and digital averaging techniques have made it possible to average ECG signals to remove noise. There is a need for consumer protection in these areas since most manufacturers do not specify how the use of such procedures modifies an ECG. Signal averaging can distort the ECG signal. These techniques are attractive since they can produce a clean tracing in spite of poor skin preparation. However, the common expression used by computer scientists, "garbage in, garbage out," applies here. The clean-looking ECG signal produced may not be a true representation of the actual waveform and in fact may be dangerously misleading. Also, the instruments that make computer ST-segment measurements cannot be totally reliable since they are based on imperfect algorithms. For instance, the algorithm that measures QRS end at 70 or 80 msec after the peak of the R-wave can hardly be valid, particularly with a changing heart rate.

It is advantageous to have a recorder with a slow paper speed of 5 mm/sec. This speed makes it possible to record all of an exercise test and reduces the likelihood of missing any dysrhythmias. A faster paper speed of 50 mm/sec can be helpful for making accurate ST-segment slope measurements. There are many different types of electrocardiographic paper that can be used. Wax-treated paper is known to retain an electrocardiographic image for 20 years or longer. However, it is pressure sensitive and easily marred. Thermochemical-treated paper is sturdy and resists marring. There are many different types of such paper, and the life expectancy of images recorded on it is usually adequate. There has been at least one instance of this paper losing recorded electrocardiographic images that subsequently resulted in legal action by a hospital against a manufacturer. Ceramic-coated paper is very sturdy and comparable in price; it has a hard finish with a high contrast, which makes it durable and easy to interpret. Untreated paper is the cheapest, but the ink jet and carbon-transfer technique characteristically produces fuzzy images. The ink-jet and carbon-transfer recorders are available with six channels and are expensive, but they do have an excellent upper-frequency response for phonocardiography. The ceramic paper also requires an ink-jet stylus rather than a heat stylus. Ink-jet recorders are said to require more maintenance, but recent models are reliable. Copying can be a problem since blues and reds are poorly copied by some xerographic reproduction machines.

A recent advance has been the availability of thermal head printers. These recorders are amazing in that they can use blank thermal paper and write out the grid as well as the ECG, vector loops, and alpha-numerics. They can record graphs and figures as well as tables and typed reports. They are totally digitally driven and can produce very high resolution records. The paper price is comparable, and these devices will replace all other recording devices since they are reasonably priced and very durable, particularly because no stylus is needed.

Z-fold paper has the advantage over roll paper in that it is easily folded, and the study can be interpreted in a manner similar to paging through a book. Exercise electrocardiograms can be microfilmed on rolls, cartridges, or in fiche cards for storage. They can also be stored in digital or analog format on magnetic media. The latest technology involves optical discs called "WORMS," standing for "write once, read many." These devices can be easily interfaced with microcomputers and can store gigabytes of digital information, equivalent to 100 complete multilead exercise tests.

Exercise Test Modalities.   Three types of exercise can be used to stress the cardiovascular system: isometric, dynamic, and a combination of the two. Isometric exercise, defined as constant muscular contraction without movement (i.e., handgrip), imposes a disproportionate pressure load on the left ventricle relative to the body's ability to supply oxygen. Dynamic

exercise, defined as rhythmic muscular activity resulting in movement, initiates a more appropriate increase in cardiac output and oxygen exchange.
Since a delivered work load can be accurately calibrated and the physiologic
response easily measured, dynamic exercise is preferred for clinical testing.
Using progressive work loads of dynamic exercise, patients with coronary artery disease can be protected from rapidly increasing myocardial oxygen demand. Although bicycling is a dynamic exercise, most individuals are more
likely to give adequate muscular effort on a treadmill because of their greater
familiarity with walking and the specificity of training.

Numerous modalities have been used to provide the dynamic exercise for
exercise testing including steps, escalators, and ladder mills. Today, however,
the bicycle ergometer and the treadmill are the most commonly used dynamic
exercise devices. The bicycle ergometer is usually cheaper, takes up less
space, and makes less noise. Upper body motion usually is reduced, but care
must be taken so that isometric exercise is not performed by the arms. The
work load administered by the simple bicycle ergometers is not well calibrated and is very dependent upon pedaling speed. It is too easy for a patient
to slow pedaling speed during exercise testing and decrease the administered
work load. More expensive electronically braked bicycle ergometers keep the
administered work load at a determined level over a wide range of pedaling
speeds. They are particularly needed for supine exercise testing.

Arm Ergometry.   Balady notes that alternative methods of
exercise testing are needed for patients with vascular, orthopedic, or neurologic conditions who cannot perform leg exercise. To determine the sensitivity of arm exercise in detecting coronary artery disease, they tested 30 patients
with angina pectoris with both arm ergometry and treadmill before coronary
angiography. All patients had at least 70% diameter reduction in one or more
major coronary arteries. Ischemic ST depression (≥ 0.1 mV) or angina occurred more frequently (86%, 26 patients) with leg exercise than with arm
exercise (40%, 12 patients). There was no significant difference in peak rate-
pressure product achieved with either test, although the peak oxygen consumption was greater during leg exercise than during arm exercise (18 versus
13 ml/kg/min). For concordantly positive tests, the oxygen consumption at
onset of ischemia was significantly lower during arm testing than during leg
testing (12 versus 17 ml/kg/min). There was no significant difference in heart
rate during either test at onset ischemia. Thus, arm exercise testing is a reasonable but not equivalent alternative to leg exercise testing in patients who
cannot perform leg exercise.

Supine Versus Erect Exercise Testing.   European cardiologists have favored supine bicycle testing because of safety reasons or because
of their experience with this technique in the cardiac catheterization laboratory. There is a marked difference between the body's response to acute exercise in the supine and erect positions. In normal persons, stroke volume
and end-diastolic volume do not change much during supine bicycle exercise

from volumes obtained at rest, whereas in the erect position, these values increase during mild work and then plateau. In patients with abnormalities, left ventricular filling pressure is more likely to increase during exercise in the supine position than in the erect position. When angina patients perform identical submaximal bicycle work loads in supine and erect positions, heart rate is higher in the supine position. The maximal work load is lower in the supine position, and angina develops at a lower double product. ST-segment depression is often greater in the supine position because of the greater left ventricular volume.

The linear relationship of cardiac output to oxygen uptake during supine bicycle exercise has been demonstrated and has been used to separate heart disease patients from normal persons. Exercise factor, or the increase of cardiac output for an increase in oxygen uptake, is based on studies of normal persons. For every 100-ml increase in oxygen consumption, cardiac output should increase by 500 ml. Left ventricular filling pressure does not increase in proportion to work in normal persons, but very often increases in patients with abnormalities. Radionuclide imaging has shown that the ejection fraction can decrease during exercise in patients with ischemia or LV dysfunction and usually increases in normal persons. Patients with coronary artery disease, however, can have discordance between their disease and ventricular function and can respond normally to exercise.

Bike Versus Treadmill.   In most studies comparing erect bicycle exercise with treadmill exercise, maximal heart rate values have been similar whereas maximal oxygen consumption values were greater during treadmill exercise. However, these studies were based mostly on the performance of athletes and the results would be more comparable if higher pedaling speeds had been used (60 to 90 rpm). Niederberger et al. concluded that bicycle exercise constitutes a greater stress on the cardiovascular system in terms of the double product at any given oxygen uptake than does treadmill exercise. The clinical importance of their findings in relation to patients with cardiovascular disease undergoing exercise testing is that slightly higher maximal oxygen uptakes are achieved with slightly less hemodynamic stress when treadmill exercise is used. Wickes, Oldridge, and coworkers found similar ECG changes with treadmill testing as compared with bicycle testing in coronary patients. Rather than for any medical reason, however, the treadmill is the most commonly used dynamic testing modality in the United States because patients are more familiar with walking than they are with bicycling. They are more likely to give the muscular effort necessary to adequately increase myocardial oxygen demand by walking rather than by bicycling.

Exercise With Intracardiac Catheters.   Exercise testing with intracardiac catheters has significant advantages over alternative diagnostic methods for (1) separation of cardiac from pulmonary dyspnea, (2) separation of left ventricular systolic from diastolic dysfunction, and (3) quantitative evaluation of the clinical significance of valvular disease.

1. *Cardiac Versus Pulmonary Dyspnea.*—Patients with severe chronic obstructive pulmonary disease (COPD) have clinical findings that make the assessment of left ventricular function extremely difficult. Many patients with COPD have left heart disease secondary to coronary artery disease, hypertension, or left-sided valvular disease. In left heart disease, there is a common denominator for cardiac dyspnea: elevation of the left atrial pressure. This leads to elevation of the pulmonary wedge pressure (PWP), which leads to increased pulmonary interstitial fluid, decreased pulmonary compliance, and dyspnea. In contrast, significant elevation of left atrial or PWP is unusual in uncomplicated COPD. Therefore, measurement of rest/exercise wedge pressure allows one to distinguish the pathophysiology of COPD from left heart disease. In the former case, pulmonary artery pressure may rise markedly, but PWP will remain below 20 mm Hg even with maximal supine exercise. In left heart disease, a PWP greater than 25 mm Hg occurs at maximal exercise.

2. *Left Ventricular Systolic Versus Diastolic Dysfunction.*—Left ventricular systolic dysfunction with a resultant increase in LV volume leads to an increase in diastolic filling pressure. The patient with heart failure after MI is the classic example of systolic dysfunction. In hypertrophic cardiomyopathy, systolic, or contractile function can be normal or even supernormal, but a thick noncompliant ventricle that cannot readily fill leads to increased PWP. Diastolic dysfunction is characterized by a normal cardiac output for a given work load, but this output comes at the expense of an elevated filling pressure. The distinction between systolic and diastolic function requires the measurement of cardiac output.

3. *Quantitation of Valvular Disease.*—Patients whose symptoms seem out of proportion to their valvular disease can be assessed. In the case of significant valvular lesions, exercise leads to an increase in PWP. Forward output may be maintained until late in their course. Elevation of exercise PWP at symptom-limited exercise suggests that valve disease rather than concomitant pulmonary disease is the cause of clinical symptoms.

Protocols.   Some standardization of exercise testing is necessary to compare tests among patients and between subsequent tests in the same patient. Unfortunately, there are many different treadmill protocols in use. The most commonly used protocols are progressive, i.e., they are uninterrupted and the work load is increased in stages. Of note are branching protocols that increase grade and speed depending on the patient's heart rate response. In this type of protocol, patients of different functional capacity perform for approximately the same time period so that differences in endurance are minimized. This type of protocol is usually too complicated for clinical use.

Ramp Protocols.   An interesting approach are ramp protocols where work load is continuously increased, gradually causing heart rate to increase in a "ramp" upward. Ramp tests have currently been developed to continually increase work at a predetermined rate throughout an exercise test. Whipp et al. reported on the accuracy and reproducibility of selected aerobic parameters during a ramp test administered on a bicycle ergometer. The advantages to such a test are a constant work rate, decreased exercise time, and accurate determination and possibly estimation of aerobic parameters. This approach allows for a more definite change at anaerobic threshold and lessens the chance of it being simulated by other causes of hyperventilation. It is uncertain what the hemodynamic and ECG responses to a ramp treadmill test are. However, data could be similar to that acquired using incremental testing due to the similar response obtained in these parameters using the original Balke protocol (1% increments every minute) which closely parallels a ramp test. The slope of a given population's regression equation (i.e., 1 MET per minute for coronary artery disease patients) could be used as the predetermined rate of increase for a ramp test. Extrapolating this work rate would produce a range of approximately 5 to 12 minutes of total exercise time with a mean of 8 minutes.

USAFSAM Protocol. When compared with other protocols, the Air Force School of Aerospace Medicine (USAFSAM) or other modification of the Balke-Ware protocol using a constant speed has many advantages. The USAFSAM protocol consists of a constant brisk walking speed (3.3 mph) with 5% increases in grade every three minutes. The constant treadmill speed requires only an initial adaptation in stride, reduces technician adjustment, and produces less electrocardiographic and blood pressure artifact than do protocols using multiple or higher treadmill speeds or a combination of both. This protocol provides a larger number of appropriate work loads for patients and increases in even increments of work load. Speed can be started at 2.0 mph for patients who find 3.3 mph too brisk. For individuals with above-average exercise capacity, it is better to increase the speed rather than the grade after reaching an incline of 25%. It is advisable to individualize any exercise protocol for the type of patient being tested. Three-minute stages are certainly not needed to achieve steady state at a low work load. Performance can be estimated with the oxygen cost of maximal work load achieved rather than in total treadmill time. In this way, performance in different protocols can be compared. After evaluating a number of protocols, this estimation has been found to be as accurate as predicting maximal oxygen uptake from maximal treadmill time.

Figure 1-1 compares the USAFSAM protocol with the Bruce protocol. In stage 4 of the Bruce protocol, an individual can walk or run. Since running is much less efficient, the oxygen cost is greater than if the individual walks. Figure 1-2 indicates the work loads and the estimated oxygen costs of the many different treadmill protocols currently used.

Walking Test. Guyatt et al. point out that bike and treadmill exercise tests can be difficult for many patients with heart failure and may not reflect capacity to undertake day-to-day activities. Also, walking tests have proven useful as measures of outcome for patients with chronic lung disease. To investigate the potential value of the six-minute walk as an objec-

VO₂ ESTIMATION FROM TREADMILL TIME

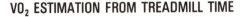

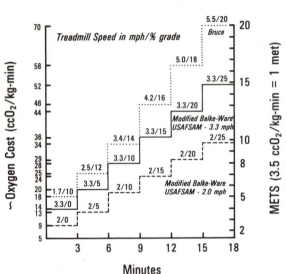

FIG 1–1.
A comparison of the Bruce and USAFSAM treadmill protocols.

tive measure of exercise capacity in patients with chronic heart failure, the test was administered six times over 12 weeks to 18 patients with chronic heart failure and 25 with chronic lung disease. The subjects also underwent bike testing, and their functional status was evaluated by means of conventional measures. The walking test proved highly acceptable to the patients, and reproducible results were achieved after the first two walks. The results correlated with the conventional measures of functional status and exercise capacity.

Submaximal Versus Maximal Exercise Testing. The most commonly used submaximal treadmill test is the graded exercise test of Sheffield and Reeves. They utilize the Bruce protocol, but the test is terminated when the patient reaches 90% of predicted maximal heart rate for age and level of training. Predicted maximal heart rate was determined from a study of normal individuals; in the study, athletically trained subjects had a slightly lower maximal heart rate than did the others. Unfortunately, as in other studies, there is a wide spread of maximal heart rate around the regression line (SD of 12 beats/minute). Thus, the target heart rate is maximal for some subjects, beyond the limits of others, and submaximal for others. This testing procedure has the advantage that patients can be tested in street shoes and clothes and are not usually uncomfortable during it since most patients are not stressed to a maximal effort. However, maximal sensitivity is not obtained and thus exercise capacity cannot be accurately estimated or measured.

A test is considered maximal when the patient appears to give a true maximal effort or when other clinical endpoints are reached. A true maximal exercise test is achieved when measured oxygen uptake reaches a value that will not increase despite an increase in work load. When using submaximal tests,

FUNCTIONAL CLASS	CLINICAL STATUS	O2 COST ML/KG/MIN	METS	BICYCLE ERGOMETER (1 WATT = 60 KPDS) FOR 70 KG BODY WEIGHT, KPDS	BRUCE 3 MIN STAGES MPH / %GR	KATTUS MPH / %GR	BALKE WARE % GRAD AT 3.3 MPH, 1-MIN STAGES	ELLESTAD 3/2/3-MIN STAGES MPH / %GR	USAFSAM 2 OR 3 MIN STAGES MPH / %GR	"SLOW" USAFSAM MPH / %GR	McHENRY MPH / %GR	STANFORD % GRADE AT 3 MPH	STANFORD % GRADE AT 2 MPH	METS
NORMAL AND I (HEALTHY, DEPENDENT ON AGE, ACTIVITY)					5.5 / 20		26 25 24								
		56.0	16		5.0 / 18		23 22	6 / 15							16
		52.5	15			4 / 22	21 20	5 / 15							15
		49.0	14	1500			19		3.3 / 25		3.3 / 21				14
		45.5	13	1350	4.2 / 16	4 / 18	18 17								13
		42.0	12	1200	—		16		3.3 / 20		3.3 / 18	22.5			12
		38.5	11			4 / 14	15 14	5 / 10		2 / 25	3.3 / 15	20.0			11
SEDENTARY HEALTHY		35.0	10	1050	3.4 / 14	4 / 10	13 12	4 / 10	3.3 / 15		3.3 / 12	17.5			10
		31.5	9	900			11			2 / 20	3.3 / 9	15.0			9
		28.0	8	750		3 / 10	10	3 / 10	3.3 / 10	2 / 15	3.3 / 6	12.5			8
		24.5	7		2.5 / 12	2 / 10	9 8			2 / 10		10.0	17.5		7
LIMITED		21.0	6	600	1.7 / 10		7 6		3.3 / 5	2 / 5		7.5	14		6
II		17.5	5	450	1.7 / 5		5	1.7 / 10			2.0 / 3	5.0	10.5		5
III		14.0	4	300	1.7 / 0		4 3		3.3 / 0	2 / 0		2.5	7		4
	SYMPTOMATIC	10.5	3				2					0.0	3.5		3
		7.0	2	150			1		2.0 / 0						2
IV		3.5	1												1

TREADMILL PROTOCOLS

FIG 1-2.
The oxygen cost per stage for most of the commonly used treadmill protocols.

there exists a paradox that the most vulnerable patients are stressed to a relatively greater extent whereas the less impaired are limited by submaximal target heart rates. A submaximal test is clinically indicated in patients in the immediate period post-MI and in patients with dangerous dysrhythmias. In the latter group, even if dysrhythmias are overridden during exercise, they can occur in the postexercise period.

Borg Scale.   Rather than use heart rate to clinically determine the intensity of exercise, it is preferable to use either the 6 to 20 Borg scale or his later, nonlinear 1 to 10 scale of perceived exertion (Table 1–3). The 6 to 20 scale was developed by noting that young men could approximate their exercise heart rate if a scale ranging from 60 to 200 was aligned with labels of very, very light for 60 to very very hard for 200. One zero was dropped and the scale was used for all ages. Because sensory perception of pain or exertion is nonlinear, Borg developed the 1 to 10 scale (Table 1–4).

Skin Preparation.   Proper skin preparation is essential for the performance of an exercise test. During exercise, because noise increases with the square of resistance, it is extremely important to lower the resistance at the skin-electrode interface and thereby improve the signal-to-noise ratio. It is often difficult to make technicians consistently prepare the skin properly because doing so may cause the patient discomfort and minor skin irritation. The performance of an exercise test with an electrocardiographic signal that cannot be continuously monitored and accurately interpreted because of artifact is worthless and can even be dangerous.

The general areas for electrode placement are cleansed with an alcohol-saturated gauze pad, then the exact areas for electrode application are marked with a felt-tip pen. The mark serves as a guide for removal of enough of the superficial layer of skin. The electrodes are placed using anatomic landmarks

TABLE 1–3.
The Linear 6 to 20 Borg Scale of Perceived Exertion or
Pain

6	
7	Very, very light
8	
9	Very light
10	
11	Fairly light
12	
13	Somewhat hard
14	
15	Hard
16	
17	Very hard
18	
19	Very, very hard
20	

TABLE 1–4.
The Nonlinear 1 to 10 Borg Scale
of Perceived Exertion or Pain

0	Nothing at all	
0,5	Extremely light	(Just noticeable)
1	Very light	
2	Light	(Weak)
3	Moderate	
4	Somewhat heavy	
5	Heavy	(Strong)
6		
7	Very heavy	
8		
9		
10	Extremely heavy	(Almost max)
●	Maximal	

that are found with the patient supine. Some individuals with loose skin can have a considerable shift of electrode positions when they assume an upright position. The next step is to somewhat remove the superficial layer of skin either with a handheld drill or by light abrasion with fine-grain emery paper. Skin resistance should be reduced to 5,000 ohms or less, which can be verified prior to the exercise test with an inexpensive AC impedance meter driven at 10 Hz. Do not use a DC meter since it can polarize the electrodes. Each electrode is tested against a common electrode with the ohm meter, and when 5,000 ohms or less is not achieved, the electrode must be removed and skin preparation repeated. This maneuver saves time by obviating the need to interrupt a test due to noisy tracings.

Electrodes and Cables. The only suitable electrodes are constructed with a metal interface that is sunken to create a column that can be filled with either an electrolyte solution or a saturated sponge. These fluid column electrodes markedly decrease motion artifact as compared with those with direct metal-to-skin contact. There are many disposable electrodes that perform excellently. Silver plate or silver-silver chloride crystal pellets are the best electrode materials. Platinum is too expensive and the frequently used German silver is actually an alloy. If electrodes of different types of metals are used together, an offset voltage can be generated that makes it impossible to record an electrocardiogram. The disposable electrodes have the advantages of quick application and no need for cleansing for reuse. They are more expensive to use than nondisposable electrodes, however, and they require a wire connection on the electrode that may induce motion artifact. The better nondisposable electrodes can be used for over 100 tests. Breakdown usually occurs in the wire connection as it goes through the electrode housing. This problem can be reduced if the electrodes are not removed by pulling the connecting wire. An electrode that has an abrasive center that is spun by an applicator after the electrode is attached to the skin called Quickprep is available from Quinton Instrument Co. This approach does not require skin preparation. A clever feature of the applicator is a built-in impedance meter that stops it from spinning when the necessary impedance is achieved.

Developing suitable connecting cables between the electrodes and the recorder has been a problem in gathering exercise ECG data. The earliest versions of these cables were subject to wire-continuity problems, frequent failures, and motion artifact; they were improperly shielded and utilized inadequate connectors. Shielding of the electrode wires and cables is especially important in metropolitan areas or near high-voltage x-ray equipment. Several commercial companies have concentrated on solving these problems, and now there are exercise cables available that are constructed to avoid this. Buffer amplifiers carried by the patient are no longer advantageous. Some systems have utilized A to D converters in the patient junction box. Digital signals are relatively impervious to noise, and so the patient cable can be unshielded and very light.

Lead Systems.   Electrodes have been placed in a variety of ways and in many different lead systems. This situation has complicated making comparisons of the ST-segment response to exercise. The four major exercise electrocardiographic lead systems are the bipolar, the Mason-Likar 12-lead, a simulation of Wilson's central terminal, and the three-dimensional (orthogonal or nonorthogonal systems).

Bipolar lead systems have been used because of the relatively short time required for placement, the relative freedom from motion artifact, and the ease with which noise problems can be located. Figure 1–3 illustrates electrode placement for most of the bipolar lead systems. The usual positive reference is an electrode placed the same as the positive reference for V5. The negative reference for V5 is Wilson's central terminal, which consists of connecting

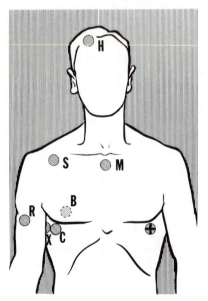

FIG 1–3.
The common bipolar ECG leads used during exercise testing.

the limb electrodes-right arm (RA), left arm (LA), and left leg (LL). The only other notable bipolar lead system is the roving bipolar lead, which was introduced by McHenry. In this sytem, beginning with a CC5 placement, the electrodes are moved around to obtain the maximal R wave with a small S wave. McHenry feels that this type of left ventricular waveform is the most sensitive for ST-segment changes.

The problem with comparing the results of ST-segment analysis if different leads are used has been demonstrated by a computer analysis study. ST-segment depression and slope measurements were made on signals gathered simultaneously from CC5, CM5, and V5. A common positive reference electrode was used. CM5 consistently had a more negative J junction and a more positive slope than did V5 and CC5. V5 and CC5 were essentially identical on the basis of standard analysis, but differed statistically when computer measurements were compared. This difference in the leads most likely explains why investigators using CM5 have reported an inadequate ST slope to be as serious as horizontal depression.

Vector Leads.   There are a number of three-dimensional or vectorcardiographic lead systems that can be used during exercise. The corrected Frank lead system has the advantage that the electrical activity of the heart is orthogonally represented in the three derived signals. The relative ease of placement of only seven electrodes required for the Frank system has made it the most popular orthogonal lead system. Care should be taken so that the X and Z electrodes are placed as described by Frank in his original paper, at the fifth intercostal space level at the sternum. The vectorcardiographic approach makes it possible to evaluate the spatial changes of the ST-segment vector.The Frank X is a left precordial lead but is about 25% smaller in amplitude to V5 because of the Frank network resistance, which is an attempt to electrically move the heart to the center of the chest. However, ST-segment criteria have not been adjusted for this fact. When using both the 12-lead and Frank systems, several electrodes can be shared. V4 and V6 are I and A, LF can also be F, and in this way, 14 electrodes can be used to obtain both systems.

The Dalhousie square is a simple way to assist with the proper and reproducible placement of the Frank electrodes and of the Wilson precordial electrodes. It is a simple right-angle device that is held to the chest. Proper placement is necessary for the application of ECG/VCG interpretive criteria. Reproducible placement is essential to assess serial changes.

MASON-LIKAR ELECTRODE PLACEMENT

Since a 12-lead ECG could not be obtained accurately during exercise with electrodes placed on the wrists and ankles, Mason and Likar suggested that adhesive electrodes be placed at the base of the limbs for exercise testing. In addition to providing a noise-free exercise tracing, their modified placement apparently showed no differences in electrocardiographic configuration when

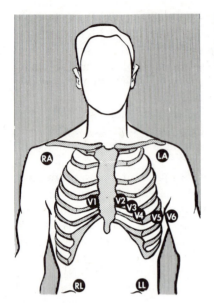

FIG 1–4.
The Mason-Likar simulated standard 12-lead
ECG electrode placement for exercise testing.

compared to the standard limb lead placement. However, this has been disputed by others who have found that the Mason-Likar placement causes amplitude changes and axis shifts when compared to standard placement. Since this could lead to diagnostic changes, it has been recommended that the modified exercise electrode placement not be used for recording a resting ECG. The preexercise test ECG has been further complicated by the recommendation that it should be obtained standing since that is the position maintained during exercise. This is worsened by the common practice of moving the limb electrodes onto the chest in order to minimize motion artifact.

It is clinically important to obtain an accurate preexercise ECG since it should be compared to previous tracings in order to see if any changes have occurred or to use it as a baseline tracing. Our hypothesis was that much of the confusion regarding distortion of the preexercise ECG has been due to misplacement of limb electrodes medially on the torso and by obtaining the ECG in the standing position. Therefore, we compared 12-lead ECGs utilizing the standard limb placement (electrodes on wrists and ankles) to two modified exercise placements in the same patients. We have also compared supine to standing ECGs in these patients.

Figure 1–4 illustrates the Mason-Likar torso-mounted limb lead system. The conventional ankle and wrist electrodes are replaced by electrodes mounted on the torso at the base of the limbs. In this way, the artifact introduced by movement of the limbs is avoided. The standard precordial leads use Wilson's central terminal as their negative reference, which is formed by connecting the right arm, left arm, and left leg. This triangular configuration around the heart results in a zero voltage reference through the cardiac cycle. The use of Wilson's central terminal for the precordial leads (V leads) requires the negative reference to be a combination of three additional electrodes rather than the single electrode used as the negative reference for bipolar leads. Simulation of Wilson's central terminal by other combinations of electrodes has not been validated, and therefore such alternate configurations should be avoided.

The UCSD Electrode Placement.   Prior to exercise testing, we (Gamble et al) studied 104 male patients with stable coronary heart disease. Included were 30 men with ECG criteria for an inferior MI, 13 with anterior MI, 5 with diagnostic Q-waves in multiple locations, 6 with right bundle branch block (3 with diagnostic Q-waves), 33 with other abnormalities, and 17 with normal ECGs. Just prior to a treadmill test, each patient had 12-lead ECGs recorded with lead placements as illustrated in Figure 1–5. The four electrode placements include placement 1—the standard limb lead electrode placement on the wrists and ankles, supine ("standard"); placement 2—arm electrodes placed medially on the torso, 2 cm below the midpoint of the clavicle and leg electrodes below the umbilicus ("misplaced"); placement 3—the "correct" Mason-Likar placement with the arm electrodes placed at the base of the shoulders against the deltoid border 2 cm below the clavicle, and the leg electrodes the same as placement 2 with the patient supine ("exercise-supine"); and, placement 4—the same as placement 3 except with the patient standing ("exercise-standing"). Also, the Frank X, Y, Z leads were recorded at the same time as the exercise-supine and exercise-standing ECGs.

The tracings were read by two blinded observers looking for definite diagnostic changes that might be clinically important (including "new" Q-waves in aVL or III), and other obvious changes. Q-waves were considered diagnostic if 25% or greater of the amplitude of the following R-wave and 40 msec or longer in duration. Visual analysis of each of the 104 patients' four ECGs was performed independently and in concensus by two observers. The tracings were interpreted separately and then compared to the standard limb lead ECG looking for "serial" changes in the other three tracings.

Differences between the standard limb lead ECG and the other ECGs were grouped into three categories: (1) diagnostic changes; (2) important changes;

FIG 1–5.
Electrode placement for the UCSD study of the effects of limb lead placement and standing on the routine ECG.

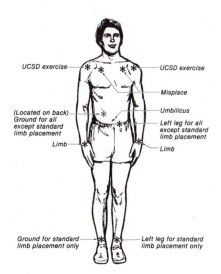

TABLE 1–5.

Differences Noted by Standard Visual Interpretation Between Exercise-Test Electrode Placements and Standard Supine Electrocardiogram*

	MISPLACED	EXERCISE-STANDING	EXERCISE-SUPINE
Diagnostic changes	6	12	3
Important changes	19	12	7
Other obvious changes	3	6	0
Total changes	28	30	10

*See the text for an explanation of the changes.

and (3) other obvious changes (Table 1–5). The category "diagnostic changes" contained tracings whose waveforms had changed by altering the lead placement or by standing such that the diagnosis was different than the supine limb lead ECG. In all cases except one, the change in diagnosis was either the loss or appearance of an inferior infarct. The one exception was a standing tracing that the change in position had caused an anterior infarct pattern to disappear. The "exercise standing" placement had a total of 12 diagnostic changes: seven where a new diagnosis of inferior infarct was made, four where an inferior infarct diagnosis was lost, and the above exception of losing an anterior infarct diagnosis. The "misplaced" electrode placement had six diagnostic changes: one where the criteria for an inferior infarct was reached and five where it was lost. The "supine exercise" placement had three diagnostic changes, all showing a loss of the criteria for an inferior infarct compared to the standard ECG.

The category "important changes" consisted of changes that may be clinically important but do not of themselves alter the electrocardiographic diagnosis. Such changes included significant Q-waves in III or aVL alone, ST and T-wave changes such as flipped or flattened T-waves or ST depression, and one instance of a Q-wave appearing in V6. The "misplaced exercise" placement had 19 important changes: eight where a new Q-wave appeared in aVL, seven where a Q-wave in only III disappeared, one where a Q-wave appeared in III, one where a Q-wave appeared in V6, and one where an additional Q-wave appeared in II. The "exercise-standing" placement had 12 important changes: five where a Q in III disappeared, three where a Q in III appeared, two ST or T-wave changes and one where a Q appeared in aVL. The "exercise-supine" placement has seven important changes: four where a Q in III disappeared, one where it appeared, and two where a Q in aVL appeared. Figure 1–6 illustrates the changes seen in three patients; in the bottom two tracings, changes only occurred in the limb leads.

QRS frontal plane axis means, standard deviation, and differences analyzed by computer for the four electrode placements are given in Table 1–6. When compared to the standard electrode placement, "misplaced" showed an average of 26 degrees of deviation to the right (p <.01), "supine-exercise" showed an average of 9 degrees rightward deviation (not significant) and "standing-

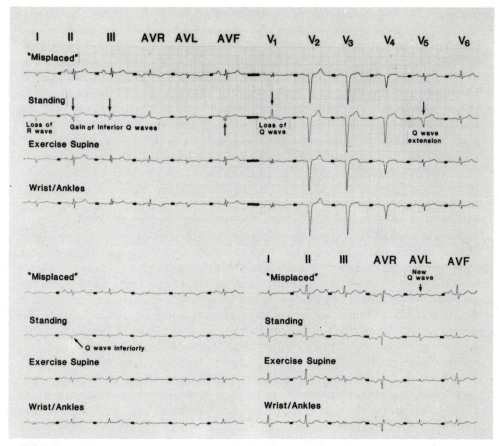

FIG 1–6.
Examples of the artifact seen in the preexercise test 12-lead ECG study.

TABLE 1–6.
Computer Analysis of QRS Axis Measured in Frontal Plane Presented as Mean Values, Standard Deviation, Mean of the Differences and Standard Deviation of Difference*

	STANDARD	SUPINE-EXERCISE	MISPLACED	STANDING-EXERCISE
Mean	18	27	44	18
Standard deviation	43	48	48	53
Mean difference		9	26	−3
Standard deviation of the differences		36	41	48
Significant difference		NS	p<0.01	NS

*The differences are presented as modified ECG measurements minus standard limb electrode placement measurements. Only the "misplaced" electrode placement measurements were significantly different from standard electrode placement measurements.

exercise" showed an average of 3 degrees of deviation to the left (not significant). "Standing-exercise" showed the greatest amount of variability with a standard deviation of +53 degrees.

Measurements were compared between supine and standing in Frank leads X, Y, and Z to assess the affect of position. There was a decrease in Q-wave amplitude and duration in Z upon standing. R-wave amplitude decreased in Y and increased in Z with standing. S-wave amplitude increased in Y on standing. There was no statistically significant difference in the mean frontal plane axis. There were also no differences in T-wave amplitudes or J junction.

Kleiner et al. compared ECGs gathered on 75 patients using the standard wrist and ankle placement to the Mason-Likar placement. Of the 75 patients, 50 had a rightward axis shift of 30 degrees or more on the modified ECG compared to the standard. In addition, 11 of these patients had a rightward shift in axis on their modified ECG that resulted in Q-wave and T-wave inversion in lead aVL, without prior history or MI by ECG. Seventeen patients had diagnostic criteria for an old inferior MI, and 7 (41%) had these criteria erased by the rightward axis shift on the modified placement. In eight patients with diagnostic criteria for anterior infarction, there was no change with the modified placement. They cautioned that the modified exercise placement of Mason and Likar should not be considered interchangeable with the standard electrodes placement. However, it was not stated where the shoulder electrodes were placed or if the modified ECG was recorded supine or standing.

Rautaharju et al. compared ECGs gathered with standard wrist and ankle electrodes to the Mason-Likar modification. They studied 68 healthy adult male subjects at rest in the supine position and made computer measurements of QRS axis and waveform amplitudes and durations. The modified exercise placement produced an average of 16 degrees shift of the mean QRS axis rightward toward a more vertical position. This shift resulted in an increase of the R-wave amplitude in leads II, III, and aVF and a decrease in leads I and aVL. P and T-wave amplitude changes corresponded to axis shifts similar to those observed for the R-wave. They also noted significant changes in the ST slope with an increase in leads II, III, and aVF and a decrease in aVL in the modified placement compared to the standard. The foot electrode placement did not alter supine tracings as long as they were positioned below the umbilicus. They cautioned against the use of the Mason-Likar placement for routine ECGs.

Diamond et al. studied 11 patients using the standard placement followed by modified limb lead placement and came to a different conclusion. They also measured maximum amplitudes in leads V1 and V6 and compared the measurements in two consecutive standard ECGs. They found minor variations using the two placements, which were random and did not alter the diagnostic interpretation. They concluded that the changes were equivalent to the variation seen in two consecutive standard ECGs taken on the same patient.

The preexercise ECG is further complicated by positional differences when it is recorded. Shapiro et al. studied the differences between supine and sitting Frank lead vectorcardiograms in 59 adult male patients with suspected coronary artery disease. They observed that QRS spatial and R-wave amplitudes in Z were significantly higher and R-wave amplitudes in lead Y lower for sitting than for supine positions. They concluded that the preexercise ECG should be obtained pretest with the patient in the same position as that maintained during exercise. However, other studies have also shown differences between ECGs taken supine and sitting or standing. Sigler studied 100 patients and found a tendency for the QRS electrical axis to shift to the left for abnormal tracings and to the right for normal tracings when changing from supine to standing. Dougherty correlated changes in the frontal plane QRS axis with changes in heart position measured with a chest x-ray brought about by moving from supine to standing. He found that every degree of positional heart change caused a three-degree shift in QRS frontal axis throughout the normal range in the same direction. A higher prevalence of false positive polarcardiographic criteria for MI was found standing than supine by Bruce et al. in 72 normal men and women.

Another complicating factor is the effect of respiration on inferior Q-waves. Because it was suggested that inspiration caused a Q in III to diminish or disappear in normal subjects and to persist among patients with inferior MI, Mimbs et al. studied the effect of respiration on the Q in III in normals and patients with documented inferior MI. They found that the Q in III decreased on inspiration in 82% of the patients with recent MI and in 44% of patients with prior infarction. In eight normals with a Q in III, only one showed a decrease in amplitude and the rest showed no change. They concluded that the effect of inspiration on the ECG was variable although they did not report specific amplitude changes.

As part of a thorough study of 194 patients, Riekkinen and Rautaharju analyzed the effects of respiration and sitting up on the vectorcardiogram. Because of the great variability of the changes, rarely with any significant differences in the means, they reported the percent of patients who increased or decreased specific values beyond an arbitrary threshold. The changes with deep inspiration were much more prominent than deep expiration. With inspiration, 35% of their patients had a posterior shift in the horizontal plane and 8% had an anterior shift; 45% had a rightward shift in the frontal plane and 3% had a leftward shift. R-wave amplitude in Z decreased a mean of 0.5 mV, Q-wave amplitude decreased, and the QRS-T angle increased. During sitting, R-wave amplitude increased in Z, Q-wave amplitude decreased in Y, and the mean QRS maximal spatial magnitude increased. Also with sitting, 26% of their patients had a posterior shift in the horizontal plane and 10% had an anterior shift; 15% had rightward and 10% had leftward shifts in the frontal plane; and 36% had an increase in the QRS-T angle.

The results of the UCSD study clarify much of the confusion regarding the preexercise test electrocardiogram. Misplacement of the Mason-Likar arm leads is common and has even been published as the correct exercise modification. By placing the leads medially, near the mid clavicular line, we have shown that the frontal plane axis shifts rightward on the average of nearly 26 degrees. This shift caused decreased amplitudes in the Q in III, R in I and aVL and increased the Q amplitude in aVL and the R waves in II, III, and aVF. Of clinical importance is what these shifts did to the visual interpretation of the ECG. In five patients, the ECG diagnosis of old inferior infarct was lost. In addition, seven patients lost significant Q-waves in III alone. There were instances of Q-waves gained. Eight patients had new Q's in aVL, one had a new Q in III, one had a new Q in II, one had a new Q in V6, and one patient gained an inferior infarct diagnosis. Though these "serial" changes are merely artifact, produced by electrode misplacement, they could be very misleading. The changes caused by our misplaced electrode arrangement were similar to those reported by Kleiner.

Standing can cause many changes in the visual interpretation of the electrocardiogram including those that would be most alarming, i.e., appearance of new Q-waves (particularly inferiorly). The misplacement of the arm electrodes in the mid clavicular area also causes many clinical changes including the appearance of Q-waves in aVL as well as large axis shifts and amplitude changes. The correct Mason and Likar modification also caused amplitude and duration changes but less clinically important changes. The modified exercise electrode placement should not be used for routine electrocardiography. However, the changes caused by the exercise electrode placement can be kept to a minimum by keeping the arm electrodes off of the chest on the shoulders and by having the patient supine. In this situation, the modified exercise limb lead placement of Mason and Likar can serve well as the reference resting ECG prior to an exercise test.

Relative Sensitivity of Leads.   Robertson and associates reported their results using 12-lead exercise tests in 39 patients with both abnormal exercise tests and abnormal coronary angiograms. Eighteen percent had an abnormal response in leads other than V5. Patients with right coronary artery lesions usually showed ST-segment depression in inferior leads, and patients with left coronary system lesions usually showed ST-segment depression in leads I and aVL and in the chest leads. However, almost a third of the patients showed ST-segment depression in leads other than those anticipated from their angiographic anatomy. Tucker and colleagues reported their results using 12-lead exercise tests in 100 consecutive patients who were also studied with coronary angiography. Forty-eight had abnormal tests, with 30% of the abnormal responses occurring in leads other than V5 (17% in AVF and 13% in other leads). Two false positives occurred in V5 and two in AVF, whereas 16 positives occurred in leads other than V5 or AVF. Of those abnormal in AVF alone, five had lesions in the right coronary or left circumflex artery and two had disease in the left anterior descending artery.

It remains to be demonstrated what the specificity of leads other than V5 eventually will be, but it appears that inferior leads have more false positives and may require different criteria. This apparent lack of specificity may be due to the effect of atrial repolarization in inferior leads, which causes depression of the ST-segment. With adequate experience, atrial repolarization can be recognized as causing ST-segment depression. The end of the PR segment can be seen to be depressed in a curved fashion to the same level that the ST segment begins. Such findings also support the concept of an intercoronary artery steal during exercise; that is, ischemic areas obtain blood flow through collaterals. This phenomenon makes it impossible for ST-segment depression with multilead exercise testing to predict the location of coronary artery occlusions.

Chaitman and colleagues reported the role of multiple-lead electrocardiographic systems and clinical subsets in interpreting treadmill test results. Two hundred men with normal ECGs at rest had a maximal treadmill test using 14 ECG leads and then underwent coronary angiography. This study included standard leads plus three bipolar leads. The prevalence of significant coronary stenosis was 86% in 87 men with typical angina, 65% in 64 men with probable angina, and 28% in 49 men with nonspecific chest pain. The predictive value of ST-segment deviation in any one of 14 leads was 45% in men with nonspecific chest pain versus 70% in men with probable angina, and 55% in men with typical angina. The investigators found multiple-lead not to increase the yield in men with nonspecific chest pain. Recording a single lead such as CM5 was adequate. In men with typical or probable angina, a normal response in 14 leads associated with treadmill work time longer than nine minutes reduced the chance of three-vessel disease to less than 10%. The likelihood of multivessel disease in a patient with an abnormal ST response and a treadmill time equal to or less than three minutes was approximately 90%. In patients with angina, the use of 14 leads increased sensitivity over that of V5 alone from 52% and 65% to 75%. This value was increased even further to 86% by the additional consideration of bipolar leads.

BODY SURFACE MAPPING

Studies in Normal Subjects. The normal repolarization response to exercise using large electrode arrays have been described by Mirvis and by Miller. Mirvis used a 42-electrode left precordial lead system in 15 normal volunteers during supine exercise. Analyses of the exercise isopotential maps revealed a minimum during the early portions of the ST segment located below the standard V3 and V4 chest positions with negative potentials involving most of the precordial region. Isopotential "difference" maps were constructed by subtracting potentials at the beginning of the ST from potentials later in the ST. These maps characterized the direction and magnitude of ST-segment slopes and revealed upsloping ST segments over regions of negative ST potentials.

Miller obtained total thoracic surface exercise maps in 20 normal subjects, recording from 24 electrode sites and deriving the remaining potentials at 150 locations using previously developed mathematical transformations. Isopotential maps during the early ST segment were less negative than those described by Mirvis et al., primarily because of Miller's "zero" reference potential. Miller chose the end of the PR segment in contrast to Mirvis who used the TP segment (which shortens with heart rate increases). Exercise isopotential maps in normals were characterized by a left anterior maximum during ST-T.

Studies of Patients With Coronary Artery Disease.   Fox et al. from London have used simple exercise ECG mapping techniques to detect myocardial ischemia. Using a 16-lead precordial map and visual interpretation of the scalar ECG data, contour maps were drawn for each patient illustrating regions on the precordial surface where significant ST-segment depression was observed. The first study involved 100 patients undergoing coronary angiography for evaluation of chest pain. In that study, the sensitivity of the precordial mapping technique (96%) for diagnosing coronary disease was better than the modified 12-leads (80%), using 0.1 mV horizontal ST-segment depression as abnormal. This improved sensitivity was due to the improved recognition of patients with single-vessel disease. Also of interest was the regional localization of the ischemic ST contours in single-vessel disease. ST-segment depression involving the uppermost horizontal row of electrodes was highly specific for proximal left anterior descending or left-main coronary artery disease. This was done without a loss in specificity (90%).

In a second exercise study involving 200 patients undergoing coronary angiography, Fox et al. again compared the 12-lead ECG to a 16-lead map and found that the standard precordial leads only sampled 41% of the ST-segment depression projected to the front of the chest. In only 7% of patients, however, was the ST-segment depression not apparent in the standard precordial leads. The right-most column of electrodes never recorded ST-segment depression that was not seen in one or more of the remaining 12 electrodes on the precordial surface. The authors concluded that these 12 precordial leads along with the standard limb leads would optimize the detection of ST-segment changes.

Yanowitz at the University of Utah has reported using a 32-lead electrode array to derive torso potential distributions at 192 locations by means of a mathematical transformation. He evaluated this system during exercise testing in 25 patients with documented coronary artery disease. In this study, the distribution of 80 msec ST-segment isoarea contours (ST80 isoarea maps) was plotted and compared to the standard precordial leads. He found that in 25% of patients with ischemic ECG changes the maximal ST change was located at sites distant to the standard leads. In addition, there was some evidence of localization in patients with single-vessel disease.

Simoons and Block recorded exercise body surface maps in 25 normal subjects and 25 patients with coronary disease using a system of 120 thoracic surface electrodes. Evaluation of normal subjects revealed a low-level (less than 90 μV) precordial minimum during early ST followed by the development of a prominent maximum later in the ST-T wave, similar to the observations of Miller. In the coronary patients, exercise maps frequently showed a prolonged negative area in the precordium with varying locations of the minimum. There was no relation between the specific ST isopotential distributions and either the coronary anatomy or the location of thallium scan defects. The maps, however, were more sensitive (84%) in detecting abnormal repolarization patterns in coronary patients as compared to the 12-lead exercise ECG (60%), using an ST-segment minimum of > 90 μV at 60 msec after the J point as the criterion for an abnormal map. None of the normal subjects had negative ST potentials of this magnitude (specificity of 100%).

It is simplistic to consider ST-segment mapping data as quantitative of ischemic myocardium. The physiological mechanisms responsible for ST-segment (and TQ-segment) shifts in ischemic injury are complex and depend upon the shape and location of the ischemic region in relation to the electrode sites on the body surface. Since currents of injury primarily occur at the boundaries between normal and abnormal tissue, cancellation of forces will likely distort the relationships between body surface ST-segment changes and the degree of ischemia. The subendocardial and nontransmural locations of most exercise-induced ischemia make it unreasonable to expect that body surface ECG recordings would reflect the extent, magnitude, and location of the ischemic tissues.

Experimental confirmation of these concerns has been provided by Mirvis et al. Body surface maps were obtained in dogs with previously placed ameroid constrictors around one of the three major coronary arteries. Reversible myocardial ischemia was induced by atrial pacing. Although the location of the ischemic repolarization abnormalities on the maps varied with the particular artery involved, significant spatial overlap was observed so as to preclude any identification of discrete ischemic zones unique to a given arterial lesion. These findings plus the added cost of specialized recorders and more electrodes leave mapping as a research tool without much clinical applicability.

Number of Leads to Record.   Since the question of how many leads need to be recorded during an exercise test has not been resolved, it seems advisable to record as many as economically and practically possible. In patients with normal resting ECGs, a V5 or similar bipolar lead along the long axis of the heart usually is adequate. In patients with ECG evidence of myocardial damage or with a history suggestive of coronary spasm, additional leads are needed. As a minimal approach, it is advisable to record three leads: a V5 type lead, an anterior V2 type lead, and an inferior lead such as AVF; or, Frank X, Y, and Z leads may be used. This approach is also helpful for the detection and identification of dysrhythmias. It is also advisable to be able to record a second three-lead grouping consisting of V4, V5, and V6. Sometimes abnormalities may be seen as borderline in V5 while they will be clearly abnormal in V4 or V6.

Postexercise Period.   If maximal sensitivity is to be achieved with an exercise test, patients should be supine in the postexercise period. It is advisable to record about 10 seconds of electrocardiographic data while the patient is standing motionless but still experiencing near maximal heart rate, and then have him lie down. Some patients must be allowed to lie down immediately to avoid hypotension. Having the patient perform a cool-down walk after the test can delay or eliminate the appearance of ST-segment depression. It also appears to minimize the postexercise peril due to catecholamines and lessen the chance for dysrhythmic events in this high-risk time. This factor is not an important consideration when the test is not being performed for diagnostic purposes. According to the law of LaPlace, increased supine heart volume increases myocardial oxygen consumption. Investigators have reported that this relation enhances ST-segment abnormalities.

Monitoring should continue for six to eight minutes after exercise or until changes stabilize. In the supine position four to five minutes into recovery, approximately 85% of patients with abnormal responses in a large series were abnormal at this time only or in addition to other times. An abnormal response occurring only in the recovery period is not unusual and may be due to reactive hyperemia. All such responses are not false positives, as has been suggested. Experiments confirm mechanical dysfunction and electrophysiologic abnormalities in the ischemic ventricle following exercise. A cool-down walk can be helpful when doing tests on patients with an established diagnosis undergoing testing for other than diagnostic reasons, when testing athletes, or patients with dangerous dysrhythmias.

Indications for Treadmill Test Termination. The absolute and relative indications for termination of an exercise test listed in Table 1–7 have been derived from clinical experience. As before, absolute indications are clear-cut, whereas relative indications can sometimes be disregarded if good clinical judgment is used. Absolute indications include a drop in systolic blood pressure despite an increase in work load, anginal chest pain becoming worse than usual, central nervous system symptoms, signs of poor perfusion (such as pallor, cyanosis, and cold skin), serious dysrhythmias, technical problems with monitoring the patient, patient's request to stop, and marked

TABLE 1–7.
Indications for Termination of an Exercise Test

Absolute Indications
1. Acute MI, or suspicion of an MI
2. Onset of severe angina
3. Drop in SBP with increasing work load accompanied by signs/symptoms
4. Serious dysrhythmias (second or third degree AV block, ventricular tachycardia, or strings of PVCs)
5. Signs of poor perfusion, including pallor, cyanosis, or cold and clammy skin
6. CNS symptoms, including ataxia, vertigo, visual or gait problems, and confusion
7. Technical problems with monitoring any parameters
8. Patient's request

Relative Indications
1. Marked ECG changes from baseline including more than 0.2 mV of horizontal or downsloping ST-segment depression, or 0.2 mV of ST-segment elevation
2. Other ST or QRS changes (excessive junctional depression or new appearance of axis deviation or BBB)
3. Any chest pain that is increasing
4. Marked fatigue and shortness of breath
5. Wheezing
6. Leg cramps or intermittent claudication
7. Hypertensive response (systolic BP > 280 mm Hg; diastolic BP > 120 mm Hg)
8. Less serious dysrhythmias, such as SVT

electrocardiographic changes, e.g., more than 0.3 mV of horizontal or down-sloping ST-segment depression, and 0.2 mV of ST-segment elevation. Relative indications for termination are other worrisome ST or QRS changes such as excessive junctional depression; increasing chest pain; fatigue, shortness of breath, wheezing, leg cramps, or intermittent claudication; worrisome appearance; hypertensive response (systolic pressure greater than 280 mm Hg, diastolic pressure greater than 115 mm Hg), and less serious dysrhythmias including supraventricular tachycardias. In some patients estimated to be precarious by their clinical history, it may be appropriate to stop at a submaximal level since the most severe ST-segment depression or dysrhythmias can occur only after exercise. If more information is required, the test can be repeated later.

SUMMARY

PHYSIOLOGY

Myocardial and ventilatory oxygen consumption have different determinants, and their estimates have different clinical implications during exercise. The ECG response and angina are closely related to myocardial ischemia and coronary artery occlusion while exercise capacity and the SBP and HR responses to exercise can be determined by either myocardial ischemia or dysfunction as well as by the reactions to exercise in the periphery. In most middle-aged men with stable CHD, exercise capacity is limited or controlled by the periphery and not limited by heart disease, except in its severe forms. The relationship between oxygen consumption and the cardiovascular and pulmonary responses to exercise are best explained by sensors in the skeletal muscle that detect changes in the local chemical environment reflecting the adequacy of muscle perfusion.

METHODOLOGY

Utilization of proper methodology is critical to patient safety and to obtaining accurate results. Preparing the patient physically and emotionally for testing is necessary. Skin preparation must cause some discomfort since a layer of the corneum must be removed. The use of specific criteria for exclusion and termination, physician interaction with the patient, and appropriate emergency equipment are essential. In patients with heart disease, a pretest standard ECG is important, and care must be taken with electrode placement to avoid artifact. The changes caused by the exercise electrode placement can be kept to a minimum by keeping the arm electrodes off of the chest on the shoulders and by having the patient supine. In this situation, the modified exercise limb lead placement of Mason and Likar can serve well as the reference resting ECG prior to an exercise test.

Few studies have correctly evaluated the relative yield or sensitivity and specificity of different electrode placements for exercise-induced ST-segment shifts. Studies show that using other leads in addition to V5 will increase the sensitivity, but the specificity is decreased. Vectorcardiographic and body surface mapping lead systems do not appear to offer any advantage over simpler approaches for clinical purposes.

The exercise protocol should be progressive with even steps in grade and with stages long enough to permit a steady state to be reached. With small work load increments, steady state can be reached by one minute in fit subjects performing submaximal exercise. The optimal test length is from 6 to 10 minutes; the protocol work loads should be adjusted to permit this duration. Target HRs based on age prediction should not be used because this is a poor relationship with a wide scatter around many different recommended regression lines. Such HR targets permit only a submaximal effort for some individuals and the consideration of another's maximal response as submaximal. The Borg scales are an excellent means of quantifying an individual's effort. Exercise capacity should not be reported in total time but rather as the VO_2 or MET equivalent of the work load achieved. This permits the comparison of the results of many different exercise testing protocols.

For diagnostic testing, hyperventilation should be avoided prior to testing, and the patient should be placed in the supine position immediately after the treadmill is stopped. A cool-down walk can be used for tests performed for reasons other than diagnosis. The postexercise period is the most dangerous for ventricular tachycardia or fibrillation. This risk can be lessened by allowing a cool-down walk or allowing the patient to sit.

BIBLIOGRAPHY

Alexander J, Holder AR, Wolfson S: Legal implications of exercise testing. *Cardiovasc Med* 1978;1:1137–39.

Ask P, Oberg PA, Odman S, et al: ECG electrodes—A study of electrical and mechanical long-term properties. *Acta Anaesthesiol Scand* 1979;23:189–206.

Atterhog JH, Jonsson B, Samuelsson R: Exercise testing: A prospective study of complication rates. *Am Heart J* 1979;98:572–579.

Balady GJ, Schick EC, Weiner DA, et al: Comparison of determinants of myocardial oxygen consumption during arm and leg exercise in normal persons. *Am J Cardiol* 1986;57:1385–1387.

Balady GJ, Weiner DA, McCabe CH, et al: Value of arm exercise testing in detecting coronary artery disease. *Am J Cardiol* 1985;55:37–39.

Berson A, Haisty R, Pipberger H: Electrode position effects on Frank lead ECGs. *Am Heart J* 1978;95:463–466.

Berson AS, Pipberger HV: Skin-electrode impedance problems in electrocardiography. *Am Heart J* 1968;76:514–525.

Borg G: Perceived exertion as an indicator of somatic stress. *Scand J Rehabil Med* 1970; 2–3:92–98.

Borg G, Holmgren A, Lindblad I: Quantitative evaluation of chest pain. *Acta Med Scand* 1981;644:43–45.

Brown BG, Lee AB, Bolson EL, et al: Reflex constriction of significant coronary stenosis as a mechanism contributing to ischemic left ventricular dysfunction during isometric exercise. *Circulation* 1984;70:18–24.

Bruce RA: Methods of exercise testing step test, bicycle, treadmill, isometrics. *AM J Cardiol* 1974;33:715–720.

Bruce RA, Detry JM, Early K, et al: Polarcardiographic responses to maximal exercise in healthy young adults. *Am Heart J* 1972;83:206–212.

Channer KS, James MA, Papouchado, et al: Anxiety and depression in patients with chest pain referred for exercise testing. *Lancet* 1985;2:820–823.

Clements IP, Offord KP, Baron DW, et al: Cardiovascular hemodynamics of bicycle and handgrip exercise in normal subjects before and after administration of propranolol. *Mayo Clin Proc* 1984;59:604–611.

Council Scientific Affairs of the AMA: Indications and contraindications for exercise testing. *JAMA* 1981;246:1015–1018.

Dempsey JA, Vidruk EH, Mitchell GS: Pulmonary control systems in exercise: Update. *Fed Proc* 1985;44:2260–2270.

Diamond D, Griffith DH, Greenberg ML, et al: Torso mounted electrocardiographic electrodes for routine clinical electrocardiography. *J Electrocardiol* 1979;12:403–406.

Dougherty JD: Change in the frontal QRS axis with changes in the anatomic positions of the heart. *J Electrocardiol* 1970;3:299–311.

Erikssen J, Jervell J, Forfang K: Blood pressure responses to bicycle exercise testing in apparently healthy middle-aged men. *Cardiology* 1980;66:56–63.

Fink LI, Wilson JR, Ferraro N: Exercise ventilation and pulmonary artery wedge pressure in chronic stable congestive heart failure. *Am J Cardiol* 1986;57:249–253.

Foster C, Dymond DS, Anholm JD, et al: Effect of exercise protocol on the left ventricular response to exercise. *Am J Cardiol* 1983;51:859–864.

Foster C, Pollock ML, Rod JL, et al: Evaluation of functional capacity during exercise radionuclide angiography. *Cardiology* 1983;70:85–93.

Fox KM, England D, Jonathan A, et al: Precordial surface mapping of the exercise ECG. *Br J Hosp Med* 1982:291–299.

Fox KM, Selwyn AP, Shillingford JP: A method for precordial surface mapping of the exercise electrocardiogram. *Br Heart J* 1978;40:1339–1343.

Froelicher VF, Wolthius R, Keiser N, et al: A comparison of several bipolar leads to V5. *Chest* 1976;70:611–616.

Gamble P, McManus H, Jensen D, Froelicher V: A comparison of the standard 12-lead electrocardiogram to exercise electrode placements. *Chest* 1984;85:616–622.

Gleim GW, Coplan NL, Nicholas JA: Acute cardiovascular response to exercise. *Bull NY Acad Med* 1986;62:211–218.

Goldman L, Hashimoto B, Cook EF, et al: Comparative reproducibility and validity of systems for assessing cardiovascular functional class: Advantages of a new specific activity scale. *Circulation* 1981;64:1227–1234.

Gordon NF, Kruger PE, VanRensburg JP, et al: Effect of B-adrenoceptor blockage on thermoregulation during prolonged exercise. *J Appl Physiol* 1985;58:899–906.

Gutman RA, Alexander ER, Li YB, et al: Delay of ST depression after maximal exercise by walking for two minutes. *Circulation* 1970;42:229–233.

Gutmann MC, Squires RW, Pollock ML, et al: Perceived exertion-heart rate relationship during exercise testing and training in cardiac patients. *J Cardiac Rehabil* 1981;1:52–59.

Guyatt GH, Sullivan MJ, Thompson PJ, et al: The six-minute walk: A new measure of exercise capacity in patients with chronic heart failure. *Can Med Assoc J* 1985;132:919–923.

Guyton AC: The relationship of cardiac output and arterial pressure control. *Circulation* 1981;64:1079–1088.

Hakki AH, Iskandrian AD: Determinants of exercise capacity in patients with coronary artery disease: Clinical implications. *J Cardiopulmonary Rehabil* 1985;5:341–348.

Herbert WG, Herbert DL: A window of legal vulnerability? *Optimal Health* 1985:22–25.

Hietanen E: Cardiovascular responses to static exercise. *Scand J Work Environ Health* 1984;10:397–402.

Higginbotham MB, Morris KG, Williams RS, et al: Physiologic basis for the age-related decline in aerobic work capacity. *Am J Cardiol* 1986;57:1374–1379.

Higginbotham MB, Morris KG, Williams RS, et al: Regulation of stroke volume during submaximal and maximal upright exercise in normal man. *Circ Res* 1986;58:281–291.

Hossack KF, Gros BW, Ritterman JB, et al: Evaluation of automated blood pressure measurements during exercise testing. *Am Heart J* 1982;104:1032–1038.

Jawad I, Kinhal V, Boudoulas H: Respiratory arrest after treadmill exercise testing. *Respiratory Arrest* 1984;75:241–248.

Kleiner JP, Nelson WP, Boland MJ: The 12-lead electrocardiogram in exercise testing. *Arch Intern Med* 1978;138:1572–1573.

Kristensson BE, Arnman K, Ryden L: The hemodynamic importance of atrioventricular synchrony and rate increase at rest and during exercise. *Eur Heart J* 1985;6:773–778.

Ladimer I: Professional liability in exercise testing for cardiac performance. *Am J Cardiol* 1972;30:753–756.

Lam J, Chaitman BR: Diagnostic choice of exercise ECG lead systems in the routine clinical assessment of patients with chest pain. *Prac Cardiol* 1983;9:72–80.

Lintgen AB: Death from myocardial infarction after exercise test with normal results. *JAMA* 1976;235:837–863.

Loke J: *Clinics in Chest Medicine.* Philadelphia, WB Saunders Co, 1984, pp 1–210.

Longhurst JC: Arterial baroreceptors in health and disease. *Cardiovasc Rev Rep* 1982;3: 271–300.

Lyle AM: Further observations on the deep Q3 of the electrocardiogram. *Am Heart J* 1944;28:199–206.

Marton KI, Tul V, Sox HC: Modifying test-ordering behavior in the outpatient medical clinic: A controlled trial of two educational interventions. *Arch Intern Med* 1985;145:816–821.

Mason RE, Liker I: A new system of multiple-lead exercise electrocardiography. *Am Heart J* 1966;71:196–205.

McGregor M, Sniderman A: On pulmonary vascular resistance: The need for more precise definition. *Am J Cardiol* 1985;55:217–221.

McHenry PL: Risks of graded exercise testing. *Am J Cardiol* 1977;39:935–937.

McPherson DD, Horacek M, Sutherland DJ, et al: Exercise electrocardiographic mapping in normal subjects. *J Electrocardiol* 1985;18:351–360.

Miller WT, Spach MS, Warren RB: Total body surface potential mapping during exercise: QRS-T-wave changes in normal young adults. *Circulation* 1980;62:632.

Mimbs JW, deMello V, Roberts R: The effect of respiration on normal and abnormal Q-waves. *Am Heart J* 1977;94:579–584.

Mirvis DM, Keller FW, Cox JW, et al: Left precordial isopotential mapping during supine exercise. *Circulation* 1977;56:245.

Mirvis DM, Wilson JL, Ramanathan KB: Effects of experimental myocardial infarction on the ST-segment response to tachycardia. *J Am Coll Cardiol* 1985;6:665–673.

Montoye HJ, Ayen T, Nagle F, et al: The oxygen requirement for horizontal and grade walking on a motor-driven treadmill. *Med Sci Sports Exerc* 1985;17:640–645.

Niederberger M, Detry JM: A symposium on exercise and old age. *Eur Heart J* 1984;5: 1–123.

Niederberger M, Gaul G: Use of flow-directed catheters for assessment of left ventricular function during exercise: Methods, risks, and meaning for cardiac rehabilitation. *J Cardiac Rehabil* 1983;3:780–787.

Niederberger M, Bruce RA, Kusumi F, Whitkanack S: Disparities in ventilatory and circulatory responses to bicycle and treadmill exercise. *Br Heart J* 1974;36:377.

Perski A, Tzankoff SP, Engel BT: Central control of cardiovascular adjustments to exercise. *J Appl Physiol* 1985;58:431–435.

Pollock ML, Foster C, Schmidt D, et al: Comparative analysis of physiologic responses to three different maximal graded exercise test protocols in healthy women. *Am Heart J* 1982;103:363–373.

Ragg KE, Murray TF, Karbonit LM, et al: Errors in predicting functional capacity from a treadmill exercise stress test. *Am Heart J* 1980;100:581–583.

Rasmussen PH, Staats BA, Driscoll DJ, et al: Direct and indirect blood pressure during exercise. *Chest* 1985;87:743–748.

Rautaharju PM, Prineas RJ, Crow RS, et al: The effect of modified limb positions on electrocardiographic wave amplitudes. *J Electrocardiol* 1980;13:109–114.

Riekkinen H, Rautaharju P: Body position, electrode level, and respiration effects on the Frank lead electrocardiogram. *Circulation* 1976;57:40–45.

Rochmis P, Blackburn H: Exercise tests: A survey of procedures, safety, and litigation experience in approximately 170,000 tests. *JAMA* 1971;217:1061–1066.

Rothe CF: Physiology of venous return: An unappreciated boost to the heart. *Arch Intern Med* 1986;146:977–982.

Rowell LB: What signals govern the cardiovascular responses to exercise? *Med Sci Sports Exerc* 1980;12:307–315.

Saltin B, Rowell LB: Functional adaptations to physical activity and inactivity. *Fed Proc* 1980;39:1506–1513.

Schrager BR, Ellestad M: The importance of blood pressure measurement during exercise testing. *Cardiovas Rev Rep* 1983;4:381–394.

Shapiro W, Berson AS, Pipberger HV: Differences between supine and sitting Frank-lead electrocardiograms. *J Electrocardiol* 1976;9:303–308.

Shaw JG, Johnson EC, Voyles WF, et al: Noninvasive Doppler determination of cardiac output during submaximal and peak exercise. *J Appl Physiol* 1985;59:722–731.

Sheffield LT, Haskell W, Heiss G, et al: Safety of exercise testing volunteer subjects: The lipid research clinics' prevalence study experience. *J Cardiac Rehabil* 1982;2:395–400.

Sheldahl LM, Wann LS, Clifford PS, et al: Effect of central hypervolemia on cardiac performance during exercise. *J Appl Physiol* 1984;57:1662–1667.

Shellock FG, Swan HJC, Rubin SA: Muscle and femoral vein temperatures during short-term maximal exercise in heart failure. *J Appl Physiol* 1985;58:400–408.

Shepard RJ: Tests of maximum oxygen uptake—A critical review. *Sports Med* 1984;1:99–124.

Sigler LH: Electrocardiographic changes occurring with alterations of posture from recumbent to standing positions. *Am Heart J* 1938;15:146–152.

Sox HC, Margulies I, Sox CH: Psychologically mediated effects of diagnostic tests. *Ann Intern Med* 1981;95:680–685.

Squires RW, Rod JL, Pollock ML, et al: Effect of propranolol on perceived exertion soon after myocardial revascularization surgery. *Med Sci Sports Exerc* 1982;14:276–280.

Steward RI, Lewis CM: Cardiac output during exercise in patients with COPD. *Chest* 1986;89:199–205.

Strong WB, Miller MD, Striplin M, et al: Blood pressure response to isometric and dynamic exercise in healthy black children. *Am J Dis Child* 1978;132:587–591.

Stuart RJ, Ellestad MH: National survey of exercise stress testing facilities. *Chest* 1980;77:94–97.

Symposium: Exercise testing in the dyspneic patient. *Am Rev Respir Dis* 1984;129:S1–S100.

Symposium: Directions—1985. *Med Sci Sports Exerc* 1985;17:2–44.

Walgenbach SC, Shepherd JT: Role of arterial and cardiopulmonary mechanoreceptors in the regulation of arterial pressure during rest and exercise in conscious dogs. *Mayo Clin Proc* 1984;59:467–475.

Wasserman K: Dyspnea on exertion. *JAMA* 1982;248:2039–2043.

Wickes JR, Oldridge N, et al: Comparison of the electrocardiographic changes induced by maximum exercise testing with treadmill and cycle ergometer. *Circ Res* 1978;57:1066.

Wolthuis R, Froelicher VF, Fischer J, et al: The response of healthy men to maximal treadmill exercise. *Circulation* 1977;55:153–157.

Yanowitz FG, Vincent GM, Lux RL, et al: Application of body surface mapping to exercise testing: S-T80 isoarea maps in patients with coronary artery disease. *Am J Cardiol* 1982;50:1109.

Younes M, Kivinsen G: Respiratory mechanics and breathing pattern during and following maximal exercise. *Respirat Environ Exerc Physiol* 1984;57:1773–1782.

Zeimetz GA, McNeill JF, Hall JR, et al: Quantifiable changes in oxygen uptake, heart rate, and time to target heart rate when hand support is allowed during treadmill exercise. *J Cardiopulmonary Rehabil* 1985;5:525–530.

2 SPECIAL METHODS: COMPUTERIZED EXERCISE ECG ANALYSIS

A digital computer was first used for electrocardiographic analysis by Taback and colleagues in 1959. They pointed out the advantages of digital versus analog data processing, including more precise and more accurate measurements, less distortion in recording, and direct accessibility to digital computer analysis and storage techniques. Other advantages include rapid mathematical manipulation (averaging), avoidance of the drift inherent in analog components, digital algorithm control permitting changing analysis schema with ease (software rather than hardware changes), and no degradation with repetitive playback. Advantages of digital processing that are apparent when outputting data include higher plotting resolution (not real time) and facile repetitive manipulation (plotting with different gains and filters).

The two critical problems posed by exercise ECG testing are (1) reduction of the amount of electrocardiographic data collected during the testing and (2) the elimination of electrical noise and movement artifact associated with exercise. Since the total period of an exercise test can exceed 30 minutes, and many physicians want to analyze all 12 leads during and after testing, the resulting quantity of ECG data and measurements can quickly become excessive. The three-lead vectorcardiographic (VCG) approach would reduce the amount of data, but clinicians still favor the 12-lead electrocardiogram (ECG). The exercise electrocardiogram often includes both random and periodic noise of both high and low frequency that can be due to respiration, muscle artifact, electrical interference, wire continuity, and for electrode-skin contact problems. In addition to reducing noise and facilitating data reduction, computer processing techniques have also demonstrated the potential to make precise and accurate measurements, to separate and capture dysrhythmic beats, to perform spatial analysis, and to apply optimal diagnostic criteria for ischemia.

With the advent of large-scale integrated electronics, microcomputers have been developed to process the exercise ECG, thus eliminating the need for the larger, more expensive digital computers required in the past. Microcomputers can be used to digitize electrocardiographic signals and immediately apply digital techniques while the data are being gathered; that is, on-line and in real time. Earlier approaches to computer processing required that analog data be initially recorded during the test, digitized later, and then subsequently analyzed off-line.

CAUSES OF NOISE

There are many reasons noise appears in the exercise ECG signal that cannot be corrected, even by meticulous skin preparation. Noise is defined here as any electrical signal that is foreign to or that distorts the true electrocardiographic waveform. With this definition of noise, the types of noise that may be present can be due to any combination of line-frequency (60 Hz), muscle, respiration, contact, and/or continuity artifact. Line-frequency noise is generated by the interference of the 60 Hz electrical energy with the electrocardiogram. This noise can be reduced by using shielded patient cables. If despite these precautions this noise is still present, the simplest way to remove it is to design a 60 Hz notch filter and apply it in series with the ECG amplifier. A notch filter removes only the line frequency; that is, it attenuates all frequencies in a narrow band around 60 Hz (Figure 2–1). This noise can also be removed by attentuating all frequencies above 59 Hz, but this method of re-

FIG 2–1.
Example of the effect of a notched filter on 60 Hz interference.

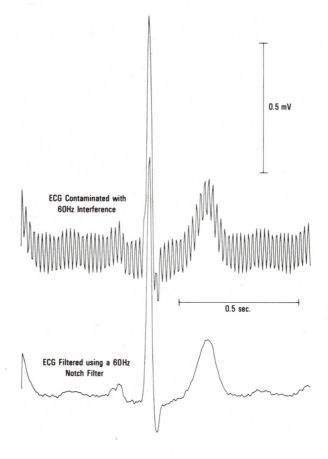

0.5 mV

ECG Contaminated with
60Hz Interference

0.5 sec.

ECG Filtered using a 60Hz
Notch Filter

moving line-frequency noise is not recommended since it causes waveform distortion and results in a system that does not meet American Heart Association specifications. The most obvious manifestation of distortion caused by such filters is a decrease in R-wave amplitude. These problems are reduced if a true notch filter is used.

Muscle noise is generated by the activation of muscle groups and is usually of high frequency. This noise, along with other types of high-frequency noise, can be reduced by signal averaging. Motion noise, another form of high-frequency noise, is caused by the movement of skin and the electrodes that cause a change in the contact resistance. Respiration causes an undulation of the waveform amplitude, and the baseline varies with the respiratory cycle. Baseline wander can be reduced by low-frequency filtering, but this results in distortion of the ST-segment and can cause artifactual ST-segment depression and slope changes. Other baseline removal approaches have been used, including linear interpolation between isoelectric regions, high-order polynomial estimates, and cubic-spline techniques that can each smooth the baseline to various degrees (Figure 2–2). Changes in waveform amplitude with respiration are physiologic and may have clinical significance, but these changes can be modified by signal averaging. This method can cause problems when comparing the average beats between rest and exercise, because the ratio of inspiratory to expiratory beats is greater during exercise than at rest.

Contact noise appears as low-frequency noise or sometimes as step discontinuity baseline drift. It can be caused by either poor skin preparation resulting in high skin impedance, or by air bubble entrapment in the electrode gel. It is reduced by meticulous skin preparation and by rejecting beats that show large baseline drift. Also, by using the median rather than the mean for signal

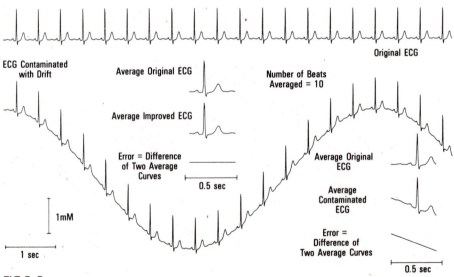

FIG 2–2.
Example of the effect of a cubic spline filter on baseline wander.

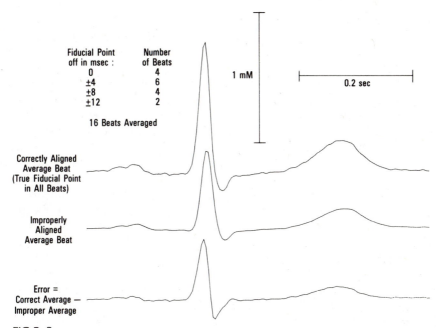

Fiducial Point off in msec :	Number of Beats
0	4
±4	6
±8	4
±12	2

16 Beats Averaged

1 mM

0.2 sec

Correctly Aligned
Average Beat
(True Fiducial Point
in All Beats)

Improperly
Aligned
Average Beat

Error =
Correct Average −
Improper Average

FIG 2–3.
Example of the effect of misalignment of QRS complexes on the resultant averaged wave form.

averaging, this type of drift can be reduced. Continuity noise caused by intermittent breaks in the cables is rarely a problem because of technologic advances in cable construction except when cables are abused or overutilized.

Most of the sources of noise can be effectively reduced by beat averaging. However, two types of artifact that can actually be caused by the signal averaging process are due to (1) the introduction of beats that are morphologically different than others in the average and (2) the misalignment of beats during averaging (Fig 2–3). As the number of beats included in the average increases, the level of noise reduction is greater. Electrocardiographic waveforms change in morphology over time; thus, averaging time and the number of beats to be included in the average has to be compromised.

OUTLINE OF COMPUTER FUNCTIONS

The computer converts the original continuous analog electrocardiographic signal into a discrete, digital signal of voltages sampled at regular fixed intervals that can be easily handled during subsequent computer processing. Provided that the frequency of signal sampling is appropriate, the duration of the sampling window is long enough, and the computer word size is adequate, the resultant digital signal will faithfully describe and reproduce the shape of the original electrocardiographic wave form. The following functions are found in all computerized exercise systems:

1. *Recognition of Electrocardiographic Complexes.*—The ECG complex is detected either on the basis of the largest amplitude, specific frequency components, or the rate of voltage change which is usually greatest during the downslope of the R-wave.
2. *Finding a Fiducial Point or Landmark.*—Serial beats can be accurately time-aligned with reference to a recognizable feature or point in each complex; this alignment point can be the peak of the R-wave, the downslope of the R-wave using rate of voltage change, frequency components, or a maximum correlation.
3. *Choosing the Beats To Be Averaged.*—This process excludes all PVCs, all aberrant beats, and regions of excessive noise by choosing beats that are as similar as possible. This is accomplished by utilizing one or more of four methods such as recognition of R-R interval duration and polarity differences, classification by multivariate cluster analysis, calculation of the area differences, template comparison, and/or maximal cross correlation of complexes.
4. *Averaging the Selected Beats.*—This is accomplished using either the mean or the median approach and results in a single representative ECG cycle with reduced noise; the median has the advantage of being relatively insensitive to the inclusion of PVCs and/or abrupt baseline shifts (Fig 2–4).
5. *Waveform Recognition.*—Once the representative ECG cycle is formed, the algorithms for recognizing the beginning and end of the P-wave, QRS-complex, and T-wave are implemented. These algorithms can recognize the waveform complexes and intervals by one of three ways: (1) the peak of the R-wave or the nadir of the S-wave is located and measurements of the ST-segment amplitude at a fixed time interval beyond this landmark are taken; (2) the onset or offset of a complex can be identified by using time derivatives from a single lead such as V5; and (3) the beginning and end of the ORS-complex can be demarcated by using a variety of mathematical constructs, such as change in spatial velocity. The third approach is the most accurate, but little validation has been done of the various algorithms that have been empirically derived to accomplish this recognition process.

Once the boundaries of the P, QRS, and T-wave components are demarcated, measurements can then be made of the ST-segment. These measurements are made with reference to an isoelectric baseline located within the PR-segment. This can be found using a fixed interval before the Q or R-wave or by various other algorithms that search for a flat region.

COMPUTER PRINCIPLES

The following is an explanation of the principles of computerized exercise ECG signal processing. Figure 2–5 illustrates analog-to-digital conversion. An analog signal can be represented by a continuous signal that varies in amplitude with time. Converting the analog signal into a digital signal requires period sampling at fixed time intervals and converting the amplitudes at any point in time into binary numbers that have a time index or sequence. The digital signal is recorded as a binary number with each bit corresponding to a fixed voltage level determined by the analog-to-digital converter.

The basic computer storage unit is the byte, or word, that has a certain number of bits for a given computer and reflects how large or small an integer can be represented within the computer. Analog-to-digital conversion resolution is determined in part by the word size. Storage unit size affects the resolution by controlling the range of measurements that are possible, according to the formula 2^n minus 1 where n equals the number of bits in the word or

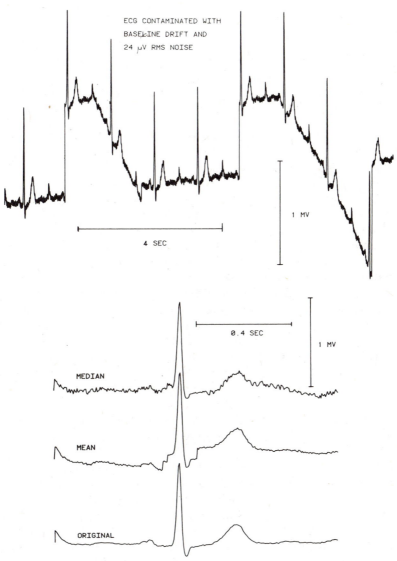

FIG 2–4.
Example of the effect of the median process on electrical discontinuities.

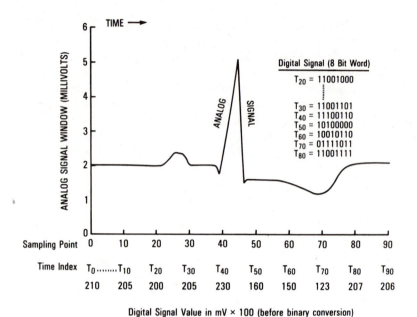

FIG 2–5.
An illustration of the analog to digital process.

byte size being used. An eight-bit digitizer divides the analog input range into 2^8 minus 1, or 255 fixed voltage units in the range -127 to $+127$. In general, the more bits per word, the greater the resolution. Resolution is also dependent on the sampling rate. The greater the sampling rate, the greater the detail of the analog signal that is retained. The more points sampled, however, the more digital data that must be analyzed and stored. The usual sampling rates used for electrocardiography are 250/sec (4 msec increments) or 500/sec (2 msec increments). In addition to sampling rate and word size, signal resolution is also determined by the positive to negative analog input voltage window. The analog window must be large enough to accept the largest possible ECG signal amplitude excursions, but a large window will decrease the resolution for small ECG signals dependent on the number of analog-to-digital bits.

Figure 2–6 illustrates the effects of analog-to-digital converter resolution and input signal range, or window, on the details of the electrocardiogram. The top line is the actual electrocardiogram. The second line shows this ECG signal after being digitized and then being reconstructed as an analog signal. Five-bit resolution of the analog-digital converter loses details but roughly follows the S, R, and T-waves. The three-bit analog-digital convertor distorts the P, S, and T-waves. When only half of the input range of the three-bit convertor is used, the P and T-waves are completely lost and the S-wave considerably distorted roughly equivalent to a two-bit analog-digital converter. The bottom figure shows the effects of sampling rate on the original ECG when reconstructed back as an analog signal. Sampling at 100 samples/sec accurately represents the P, R, S, and T-wave amplitudes but loses some detail. Sampling at 10 samples/sec loses either the P or R-wave and distorts the T-wave. A slight shift of the point in time when digitization begins (a phase shift) greatly effects resolution.

The American Heart Association and others have recommended that eight-bit resolution and 250 samples/sec are minimal digitizing specifications for computer processing of an electrocardiogram. High-frequency information can be lost, but now the industry can deliver instruments with higher resolution. Research indicates the value of higher-frequency components of the ECG and so more rigorous digitizing specifications are necessary.

FIG 2–6.
An illustration of the effect of different sampling rates and word size on signal resolution.

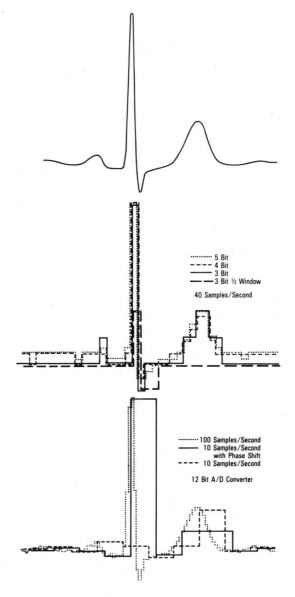

Mathematical Constructs. Mathematical constructs applied by computers to digital electrocardiographic data are used for three purposes: (1) to locate and characterize QRS complexes; (2) to obtain a reference, or fiducial point, in the QRS complex; and (3) to determine the beginning and the end of the P-wave, QRS, and T-wave. The crucial purpose for these constructs, however, is the definition of a reference point to align beats and thus permit averaging. Peak R-wave was first used, but because of the rapid amplitude changes at each peak, different peak regions could be sampled during digitizing and result in misalignment of complexes. The point of most rapid change in electrocardiographic amplitude (dx/dt), which usually occurs in the downslope of the R-wave or in upslope of QS, can be consistently found and has been used.

Particularly for one-lead analysis, the mathematical construct of maximal dx/dt can be a reliable and efficient fiducial point. More recently, investigators have used spatial constructs from three time-coherent leads to achieve alignment. Figure 2–7 illustrates the major spatial mathematical constructs.

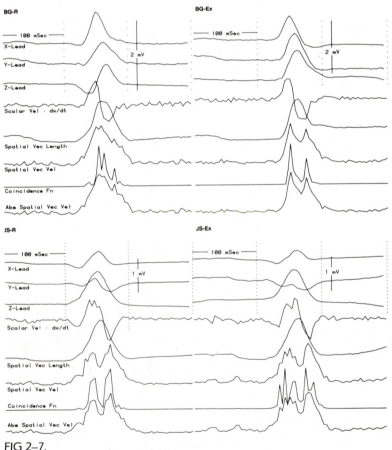

FIG 2–7.
The major mathematical constructs utilized in digital signal processing.

Thresholds set in these mathematical constructs also permit the localization of a waveform's beginning and end. Intuitively, the spatial recognition of the QRS, ST, and T-waves that requires multiple leads would be more accurate than algorithms applied to only one lead. Electrical activity may appear to end in a single lead but continue in a perpendicular direction with later activity seen in another lead.

Averaging is performed after beats are aligned by a fiducial point specified in a mathematical construct derived from the electrocardiogram. After alignment, each time-indexed sample referenced to the fiducial point has an aligned series of values from each beat included in the averaging. These values can then be averaged in two ways. The easiest way is to sum the values of the samples at each aligned point and divide them by the number of beats included in the alignment array yielding the mean. The second approach is to determine the median. The median requires calculation of the 50th percentile or midpoint value at each time-index point. Because of its mathematical characteristics, the median has a greater central tendency and thus is less affected by discrepant values. When the median is used, however, the amount of random noise is not reduced as much as when the mean is used since the mean has a higher signal-to-noise ratio. If a few PVCs or aberrancies are included in beats used to generate an average, the median beat will not be affected, but it will be distorted. Thus, the median beat appears to be a better estimate of the so-called true complex, although it is slightly higher in random noise content. Calculation of median requires larger computer memory and more computing time.

Many researchers have utilized approximately 10 seconds of sampling time rather than a specific number of beats. This sample usually includes sufficient beats for averaging techniques and lessens the chances of physiologic changes occurring and disturbing the average, particularly during exercise.

RESEARCH APPLICATIONS OF COMPUTERS

Several investigators have proposed various computer criteria for detecting ischemia during exercise testing. Some of these are shown in Figure 2–8 and described in Table 2–1. In 1965, Blomqvist reported a computerized quantitative study of the Frank vector leads. He divided the PR, QRS, and ST-T segments into eight subsegments of equal duration (i.e., time-normalized). He found that the maximal information for differentiation of patients with angina pectoris from normals was obtained by measuring the ST amplitude at the time-normalized midpoint (ST4) of the ST-T segment.

In 1966, Bruce and colleagues reported using a computer of average transients to analyze exercise electrocardiographic data gathered from bipolar lead CB5. They reported that in apparently healthy middle-aged men, ST-segment depression with exercise was found to be more prevalent and of greater magnitude than anticipated. In 1969, Hornstein and Bruce reported measuring the ST forces of the Frank leads and bipolar lead CB5 using a computer of averaged transients and a large digital computer. They concluded that a single

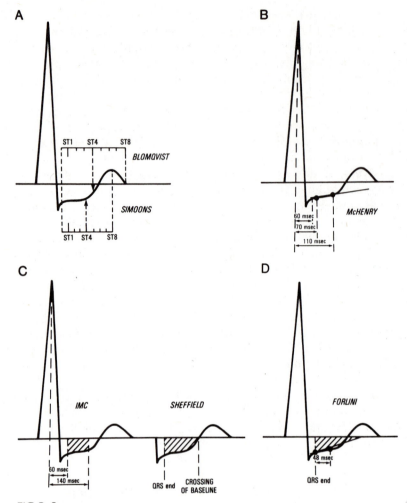

FIG 2–8.
Illustration of some of the computer-derived criteria for myocardial ischemia.

bipolar precordial lead appeared to be as reliable for purposes of classifying electrocardiographic response to maximal exercise as was the three-dimensional Frank lead system. In 1973, Neiderberger and Bruce reported on the spatial ST-T magnitudes at rest and immediately after maximal exercise. They noted that in patients with ischemic heart disease the spatial magnitudes of late ST and T vectors at rest were smaller than those in a normal group. Somewhat contrary to the prior study, they reported that even if the electrocardiogram did not show an ischemic pattern, this spatial trend became more obvious with exercise.

McHenry (at USAFSAM) and colleagues reported results with a computerized exercise electrocardiographic system developed at USAFSAM and later applied at the University of Indiana. In their study, ST-segment amplitude

TABLE 2–1.
Criteria for ST-Depression Abnormalities Seen During or After Exercise Testing

METHOD	CRITERIA FOR ABNORMAL (ISCHEMIA)
Classic ST-Segment Depression	With junctional depression of 0.1 mV (1 mm) or more: exercise-induced ST-segment depression must be flat or downsloping to be abnormal.
Upsloping ST 80	For upsloping ST segment with junctional depression of > 2 mm from the isoelectric baseline: abnormal if ST segment is depressed 2 mm or more at 0.08 sec (80 msec) after J point (QRS end); normal if less depressed at that point.
ST Midpoint (ST$_4$)	Blomqvist divided the ST segment from QRS end until the end of the T wave into eight equal time periods. He found ST$_4$, or the midpoint, to provide the most discrimination between normal and abnormal. Simoons used a midpoint from QRS end until peak of the T-wave, since peak is easier to identify than T-end.
ST index	If ST-segment depression is 1.0 mm or greater and the sum of ST-segment depression in mm plus ST slope in mV/sec equal to or greater than 1.0. (Mean ST depression measured at 60–70 msec after R-wave peak, slope in 40 msec window afterward.)
ST Integral	ST integral greater than -10 μV-sec (1 square mm on electrocardiographic paper at standard speed and calibration = 4 μV-sec). Sheffield originally described measuring the ST integral from the end of the QRS complex to the beginning of the T-wave or where the ST segment crossed the isoelectric line. Commercial systems have implemented this by using the peak of the R wave and measuring the area from 60 to 140 msec after the R wave.
Spatial ST-T Magnitudes	Dower and Bruce analyzed magnitudes and slopes at time-normalized areas of $\sqrt{X^2 + Y^2 + Z^2}$.
ST 60	A range of amplitudes at 60 msec after QRS end for different exercise heart rates with abnormal being measurements outside of a normal band.

was measured over the 10 msec interval of the ST segment, starting at 60 msec after the peak of the R-wave. The slope of the ST-segment was measured from 70 msec to 110 msec beyond the R-wave peak. The PQ, or isoelectric, interval was found by scanning before the R-wave for the 10 msec interval with the least slope (rate of change). If the ST-segment depression was 1.0 mm or greater and if the sum of ST-segment depression in millimeters and ST slope in millivolts-per-second equaled or was less than 1.0 during or immediately after exercise, the response was defined as abnormal. This measurement, called the ST index, was developed by comparing two groups of subjects, one with angina pectoris and the other consisting of age-matched clinically normal people. Used as a criterion for diagnosing coronary disease, they demonstrated a specificity of 83% and sensitivity of 95%.

The magnitude of the ST-segment deviation from the baseline has been expressed by some investigators in terms of the ST area or integral. Sheffield and colleagues measured the area from the end of the QRS to either the beginning of the T-wave or to where the ST segment first crossed the isoelectric baseline. The diagnostic efficacy of this parameter was tested in a group of normal controls and in a group of patients with coronary artery disease. In this study, normals demonstrated a modest increase in ST-integral with increasing heart rate, with the mean integral at maximal heart rate being

-4.3μV (for a reference comparison, 25 mm/second paper speed and gain of one centimeter equals 1 mV, a 1=mm block thus equals 4 μV. Patients with angina pectoris had a mean integral of -15.3 μV and this occurred at significantly lower heart rates. They reported an on-line approach in which V4, V5, V6 and Frank X, Y, and Z leads were digitized at 500 samples per second. They computed the time-voltage integral of the ST-segment beginning at QRS end and continuing until crossing the isoelectric line or until reaching 80 msec after QRS end. This integral expresses the area of ST-segment deviation from the baseline. An ST integral greater than $-$ 10 μV/sec was found to be an abnormal exercise electrocardiographic response, and the normal range was from 0 to $-$ 7.5 μV/sec. By arbitrarily taking -7.5 μV/sec as the cutoff range for normals, Sheffield obtained a sensitivity of 81% and a specificity of 95% on 41 normal and 31 angina patients. The MRFIT recently used -16 μV/ sec as a criterion for abnormal.

Wolf and colleagues reported their computer processing for rest and exercise electrocardiograms in 1972. The diagnostic criteria for exercise-induced ischemia were based on the vector analysis of the ST-T segment waveform according to the Dalhousie code. This code classified the ST-segment into three categories by means of the orientation (W) and the magnitude (D) of the ST-slope vector; the difference vector between $\frac{3}{8}$ and $\frac{1}{8}$ of the ST-segment (ST-3 $-$ ST-1). The orientation of the slope vector was defined as the spatial angle W between the slope vector D and the reference angle (pointing in the direction of the left lower anterior octant). In 123 normal males, increases in ST-slope vector D was found to be in proportion to increases in heart rate during exercise. In 1973, they reported the normal values for Chebyshev waveform polynomials fitted to the ST-segment during exercise.

Simoons and colleagues reported using a PDP-8E computer on-line to process the Frank orthogonal leads. The program, which Simoons wrote largely himself, consisted of four parts: (1) detection of the QRS complex; (2) selection of beats; (3) averaging of selected beats; and (4) waveform analysis. The interactive computer system also controlled the exercise test which allowed the physician and technician to interact with the patient. In trying to decide the optimal criteria for the detection of ischemic heart disease, Simoons compared the computerized criteria of other investigators. These criteria included ST area, ST index, polar coordinates, time-normalized ST-T amplitudes, and Chebyshev polynomials. These criteria were applied to a population of 95 coronary artery disease patients and 129 healthy males. He obtained the best results with ST-segment amplitude at 60 msec after the end of the QRS complex. A range of amplitudes for exercise heart rates was established by considering the response of the normal group. This approach is a logical one since ST-segment depression increases in proportion to heart rate. He obtained a sensitivity of 81% and a specificity of 93% using this new criterion. In comparison, previous computer criteria were not superior to this ST-amplitude measurement adjusted for heart rate.

In 1976, Werner and colleagues published a description of their rest and exercise computerized ECG system. Six Wilson precordial leads (V1-5 and V7) and extremity leads I and II were recorded at rest. A computer algorithm reconstructed leads III, aVL, aVF, and aVR from I and II. Six chest-head leads were processed (CHl-5, CH7). The ST-T segment arbitrarily extended to 400 msec times the square root of 60, divided by the heart rate. The ST-segment was reported by both the amplitude and temporal position of the lowest point in the first two-thirds of the ST-T segment, the amplitude at the J junction, the ST area, and early and late ST-segment slopes. In this study, ST area was calculated from 10 msec after the QRS end to crossing the isoelectric line or to the end of the ST segment. Early and late slopes of the ST segment were defined as the slope of the regression line between 20 to 120 msec and 120 to 180 msec after the end of QRS complex. The T-wave was evaluated according to the Minnesota Code. These investigators believed that their system reduced costs and performed high-quality exercise tests. It also enabled technicians to pay more attention to the patients since much of their job was automated. Werner and colleagues also examined the reliability of their computer program by comparison of ST-segment and T-wave interpretation between their program and two observers. At rest, there was agreement in 75% of the computer observer ST-code comparisons and in 71% of the interobserver ST codes. With exercise, the agreements decreased to 59%, whereas inter observer ST-code agreements decreased to 55%. They have not tested the utility of their approach for diagnosing coronary artery disease.

Sketch and colleagues conducted a study to evaluate the validity and usefulness of the Viagraph, a system made by International Medical Corp. for automated exercise ECG analysis. Here, 107 patients who were referred for evaluation for chest pain underwent a Bruce test and coronary angiography. Patients who had a previous myocardial infarction and those on digitalis were excluded. Twenty-nine patients were considered to have performed submaximal testing because of not reaching 85% of maximal heart rate predicted for age. Lead V5 was continuously sampled at 500 samples/sec, and 16 complexes were averaged sequentially. They measured the ST integral over an interval from 60 to 140 msec after the peak of the R-wave and chose -6 μV as the cutoff point for normals. The system measured and stored the area of depression that was maximal during exercise and in recovery. This area measurement began at 60 msec after the peak of the R-wave and extended for 80 msec. Postexercise areas were more specific, whereas areas measured during exercise were more sensitive. Also, as the criteria for ischemia were lessened, sensitivity increased while specificity decreased; these values varied over the range of ST-area criteria presented. It appeared that automated analysis of the ST area was valid and comparable to visual analysis. They concluded that it should not negate the need for visual confirmation or for the physician's consideration of hemodynamic responses. In the subgroup who performed maximal tests, a nomogram was constructed including duration of exercise and ST area used in predicting severity of disease.

In an attempt to test the diagnostic value of an isolated ST integral, Forlini and colleagues exercise-tested 133 subjects. In this study, there were 62 normals (Group 1), 29 patients with coronary disease and an abnormal visual exercise test (Group 2), and 42 patients with CHD but with normal visual exercise tests (Group 3). Using the isolated ST-integral measurement, Forlini found an overall sensitivity of 85% and a specificity of 90%. In Group 3, 79% of the patients were diagnosed as abnormal despite having normal or nondiagnostic exercise tests as determined by visual criteria. In addition, more than 50% of the patients in Group 2 manifested abnormal isolated ST integrals before development of typical "ischemic" ST changes as detected visually. Also, in more than half of these patients, the isolated ST-integral continued to be abnormal long after the disappearance of classic visual criteria for ischemia.

In 1979, Turner and colleagues reported their findings in 125 consecutive patients who had undergone exercise treadmill tests and coronary angiography. The Quinton model 740 ECG data computer analyzed V5 and calculated ST index. Of the 125 patients studied, 38 had normal coronary arteries and the rest had significant disease. Unfortunately, their results were confounded by consideration of angina in the determination of abnormal results and a vague classification of "inadequate test."

Hollenberg and associates have developed a treadmill score that grades the ST-segment response to exercise by combining the total of all changes in ST amplitude and slope measured during the entire exercise test and throughout recovery. This treadmill score is derived by summing the areas of the time curves that describe the ST-segment amplitude and slope changes in two leads (AVF and V5) and dividing this summed area by the duration of exercise (in minutes) and the percent maximal predicted heart rate achieved during the exercise test (Fig 2–9). These area measurements were obtained using a Marquette CASE I computerized exercise system. They reported that the treadmill exercise score could distinguish patients with three-vessel or left main disease from those with no significant disease.

In their first study, 70 patients who had coronary angiography and 46

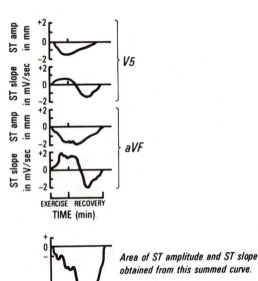

FIG 2–9.
The area measurements made by the CASE I for the Hollenberg scoring system.

healthy volunteers were included. Using the treadmill exercise score shown below, sensitivity and specificity were 85% and 98%, respectively.

Treadmill score =

$$\frac{\text{J-point amplitude and ST-slope curve area score}}{(\text{duration of exercise}) \times (\text{percent predicted maximum HR achieved})}$$

This score includes the following measures of severity: depth of J-point depression, slope, occurrence of depression in relation to heart rate, decreased heart rate response to exercise, and functional capacity. The area under the curves were considered during hyperventilation and when ST-segment abnormalities were present at rest. In their hands, this technique was highly reproducible. Subsequent refinements by this group included validation of adjusting the amplitude of ST depression by R-wave amplitude using a thallium ischemia score. They then applied the modified TES to asymptomatic Army officers and demonstrated a high specificity. This requires further validation because sensitivity was not adequately evaluated, and thallium scores have not accurately quantified ischemia. In addition, Detrano at the Cleveland Clinic, in a large series of patients without prior MI, found visual analysis to outperform the original, uncorrected Hollenberg treadmill exercise score.

Subranmanian and colleagues used the Marguette CASE I to analyze the ST-segment response to exercise in angina patients treated with verapamil. They found a significant improvement in exercise-induced ST-segment depression while their subjects were taking verapamil.

In 1977, Ascoop and colleagues reported on the diagnostic performance of automatic analysis of the exercise ECG studied in 147 patients with coronary angiography. The computer-determined results were compared with visual analyses of the same recordings. Using bicycle ergometry and recording two bipolar thoracic leads, computer processing was performed on the electrocardiograms gathered only during the stage of maximal exercise. A single, averaged beat was obtained, and onset and the offset of the QRS complex were determined using a template method. The ST depressions at 10 and 50 msec after QRS end, ST slope, and ST integral were measured. A group of patients with a mean age of 48 were divided into a learning and testing set. Many of the patients were referred from other hospitals where they had negative exercise tests. Of the 87 patients in the learning set, 57 had abnormal coronary angiograms and 30 essential had no coronary lesions. In the test population of 60 patients, 39 had significant coronary disease while 21 had no angiographic disease. The integral value of 8 μV/sec was similar to a previous value used by Sheffield. Ascoop concluded that the bipolar leads he used were superior to vector leads and that the computer criteria yielded higher sensitivities and specificities than visual analysis.

In 1982, Elamin, Linden, and colleagues reported results with a new exercise test criteria proposed to detect the presence and severity of coronary artery disease. In 206 patients with anginal pain and using recordings from 13 electrocardiographic leads (including CM5), the maximal rate of progression of ST-segment depression relative to increases in heart rate (maximal ST/HR ratio) was measured. Displacement of the ST segment was measured at 80 msec after QRS end. Curves were constructed, relating the values of the ST segment to heart rate during rest and exercise in each of the 13 leads. Rate of development of ST-segment depression with respect to increments in heart rate observed in any one lead was represented as the slope of a computed regression line. The ranges of maximal ST/HR slopes in the 38 patients with no disease, 49 with single-vessel, 75 with double-vessel, and 44 with triple-vessel disease were different from each other, and there was no overlap in the data between the adjacent groups. They claimed they had no false positives, false negatives, or indeterminate results. This procedure requires three hours of analysis time per test by a knowledgeable person but could be computerized.

Thwaites et al. performed a study to determine whether the maximal ST/HR slope using a bicycle ergometer is better than the standard 12-lead analysis using a Bruce treadmill protocol. The maximal ST segment/HR slope was calculated in 81 patients and compared with the results of a standard 12-lead exercise test. In 21 patients (26%), the ST/HR slope could not be calculated. In 60 patients with ST/HR slope values, the extent of the CAD was predicted in 24 patients (40%). The sensitivity and specificity of the ST/HR slope in predicting the presence of CAD in the 60 patients with slope values were 91% and 27%, respectively. The sensitivity and specificity of the usual treadmill test in the 81 patients were 81% and 64%, respectively.

Kligfield et al. compared the exercise ECG with radionuclide ventriculography and coronary angiography in 35 patients with stable angina to assess the value of the ST/heart rate slope. An ST/heart rate slope of 6.0 or more identified three-vessel coronary disease with a sensitivity of 89% and specificity of 88%. The exercise ST/heart rate slope was directly related to the exercise EF, but there was considerable scatter. Somewhat poorer results were obtained when they enlarged their series, and they have demonstrated marked variability in the maximal slope measurement particularly as effected by the rate of heart rate changes and the frequency with which the ST measurements are made. Quyyumi et al. assessed this criteria in 78 patients presenting with chest pain and found the maximum ST segment/heart rate slope had a sensitivity of 90%, but a specificity of only 40%, and was not useful in predicting the extent of coronary disease. This approach appears to have a logical basis to it, but the methods of the Leed's group most likely will have to be replaced by a less cumbersome and laborious measurement schema.

Dower and Bruce have reported that computer derived early postexercise polarcardiographic (PCG) changes in the ST-segment vector distinguish normal subjects from those with myocardial ischemia. Lam et al. prospectively assessed the value of this test in detecting coronary artery disease (CAD) during treadmill exercise in 178 patients within one week of diagnostic coronary angiography. All were free of prior myocardial infarction. The optimal ratio of sensitivity to specificity was 57% and 56% for a discriminate value of 12. The sensitivity and specificity of simultaneously recorded 14-lead ECG data using standard criterion was 71% and 78%, respectively. The computerized

PCG results were not improved by analyzing MS during exercise, or by analyzing the difference in MS between rest and exercise or rest and postexercise. The sensitivity of the PCG for multivessel or left anterior descending CAD was higher than for less severe forms of CAD, but was significantly less sensitive than the 14-lead exercise ECG. Table 2–2 lists the major studies reported evaluating computer criteria for myocardial ischemia.

COMMERCIALIZATION

Computers are being widely utilized as part of commercial exercise testing systems for processing exercise electrocardiograms gathered during clinical testing for three reasons: (1) inexpensive microprocessors can use software for filtering, averaging, and measuring ECG signals that previously could only be performed on larger, more expensive computers; (2) these microprocessors can present and summarize the exercise ECG responses in an attractive series of waveforms along with tables or graphs, and can make a variety of measurements not previously possible or accurate when using standard visual techniques; and, (3) prior research has demonstrated that computerized measurements, particularly of the ST segment, significantly improve both the sensitivity and specificity of exercise testing.

TABLE 2–2.
Angiographic Studies Using Computerized Exercise Electrocardiography for Diagnosis of Coronary Heart Disease

FIRST AUTHOR	NO. IN STUDY	MEAN AGE	COMPUTER CRITERIA FOR ISCHEMIA	STANDARD VISUAL ANALYSIS		COMPUTER ANALYSIS	
				SENSITIVITY (%)	SPECIFICITY (%)	SENSITIVITY (%)	SPECIFICITY (%)
McHenry	86 Patients	50	ST index	68	—	82	95
Sheffield	31 Patients	48	ST integral (using	Not given		81	95
	41 Normals	56	QRS end)				
Sketch	107 Patients	48	ST integral (using R wave on Viagraph)	59	92	58	88
Turner	125 Patients	48	ST index (Quinton analog system)	Not given		82	83
Forlini	71 Patients	53	Isolated ST Integral	Not given		85	90
	62 Normals	44					
Hollenberg	70 Patients	53	Treadmill score	71	82	85	91
	46 Normals	23	(Marquette CASE I)				
Simoons	Initial:						
	52 Patients	21–65	ST 60 with heart rate	50	94	85	91
	86 Normals		considered				
	Test:						
	43 Patients	21–65		51	95	84	88
	43 Normals						
Ascoop	39 Patients	52	0.035 mV 50 msec	28	100	67	95
	21 Normals		Post J jct in CC5				
Detrano	122 Patients	54	0.1 mV 80 msec Post			51	87
	149 Normals		J jct in V5	51	86	50	85
			Hollenberg Score				

In 1977, Marquette Electronics introduced a commercial on-line exercise system using a LSI-11 computer (CASE I). The computer performed test-control functions, signal conditioning, beat averaging, and on-line ST-segment measurements. Instead of simple mean beat averages, a new technique of averaging was introduced in this system. Called *incremental averaging* by the developers, it is a method well-suited to a continuous input with slow changes. In this method of averaging, each digital sample of a new, time aligned QRS complex is compared with its corresponding member in the current average. Alignment is accomplished using frequency components of the QRS complex. Wherever the average is low (or high), it is incremented (or decremented) by a small, fixed amount (3.5 μV) independent of the size of the difference. ST-level and slope measurements were displayed and recorded. These measurements were made from the average cycle, using the onset and offset of QRS determined during initialization. ST-slope measurements were made to correlate with visual impressions by dynamically adjusting the ST-slope interval with heart rate. This system is the only commercial system that actually determines QRS end rather than making ST measurements at a fixed point after the R-wave peak or S-wave nadir. The ST interval for slope measurement was one-eighth of the average RR interval. After sales exceeding 1,000 units world wide, this unit was replaced by the CASE II. Also designed by David Mortara, it added 12-lead analysis, A-to-D signal conversion at the patient junction box, and a remote infrared handheld controller. It has recently been replaced by the CASE 12 that processes 12 leads on-line. This system is extremely flexible due to all programming being contained on a micro floppy and a trim-knob that allows configuration of the screen by the operator.

In 1983, a microprocessor-based commercial system called the Status 1000 was introduced by Quinton Instrument. Analog electrocardiographic data is converted to digital data with a stated resolution of 0.1%. The computer programs used to analyze this digitized information are primarily coded in a structured higher-level language similar to PASCAL that facilitates program modularity and ease of modifications. A few critical fast computations, such as real time waveform averaging, are written in computer assembly language. These assembly language routines are written in modules and incorporated into the basic structure of the higher-level language. The strong point of this system is that the exercise testing protocols and methodology can be easily programmed into the system by the operator. Since then, subsequent models have been released (Q2000 and Q3000) that have improved on their concept. A most admirable outcome has been a lowering of price without a loss in quality. The latest version sells for under $16,000 with a treadmill and utilizes a thermal head printer that can mix graphics and alpha-numerics. Time histograms of all parameters are recorded on a summary report at the end of the test. The three leads from which this information is obtained are selectable.

There are two reasons for utilizing computerized exercise testing systems. First, a computerized system can decrease the time the referring physician must wait for the results of the test. The tests are facilitated by automation of the procedure and by the rapid generation of a final report. Systems using thermal head printers can mix graphics with alpha-numerics, producing a printed report that does not need typing. Secondly, if they meet their promise of improved diagnostic and prognostic information, this could result in more cost effective and higher quality health care. Unfortunately, despite good sales, neither of the two major commercial units has had independent validation of its signal processing or measurement algorithms. Nor have their diagnostic capacities been adequately compared to standard visual techniques.

Though cardiologists agree that computerized analysis simplifies the evaluation of exercise ECG, there has been less agreement as to whether or not accuracy is enhanced. Detrano et al. have produced evidence to refute the results of Sketch and Hollenberg in a large group of patients without prior MI who were referred for angiography to Cleveland Clinic. In their study using the CASE I, neither the algorithm developed by Hollenberg nor the ST index proposed by McHenry were superior to careful visual analysis of ST-segment shifts induced by exercise. Needless to say, this issue is still open to debate, and clinicians should be cautious when trusting commercial microprocessors to analyze exercise tracings.

UCSD-UCI-LBVA REAL TIME ECG SIGNAL PROCESSING

The advancement of digital integrated circuit technology has made it possible to use increasingly sophisticated methods to process exercise ECGs in real time. This section describes a combination of techniques developed by Olson, Froning, and Froelicher for beat classification and temporal alignment, baseline removal, and representative beat extraction which can be incorporated into a microprocessor system. The introduction of ever-faster single-chip general purpose microprocessors makes possible the implementation of increasingly sophisticated algorithms at reasonable cost. As more powerful ECG signal processing techniques become affordable, previously acceptable standards of performance must be reevaluated.

Our signal processing techniques used for the real time processing of exercise ECG were refined over a period of several years in a number of off-line minicomputer testbed systems. These techniques can be applied in a real time microprocessor-based exercise system. Four areas of signal processing for the exercise ECG are described: (1) absolute spatial vector velocity generation, (2) baseline removal, (3) beat classification and temporal alignment, and (4) representative beat extraction.

Absolute Spatial Vector Velocity.   In any approach to the processing of ECG data, a central issue is the choice of the methods to be used for identification and comparison of the various waves and intervals in the ECG signal. Determination of onset and offset of waves should be based on the earliest onset and latest offset seen in any lead. This necessitates the use of a mathematical construct or combination waveform derived from three orthogonal (i.e., statistically independent) leads where electrical activity in all orientations will be represented. There are many mathematical constructs of this type under investigation. Some require the computation of powers of derivatives and/or roots of sums of such terms. These operations can be slow on a microprocessor system and should be avoided if alternatives with satisfactory performance can be found. Two such alternatives are the absolute spatial vector velocity (ASVV) and the coincidence function (CF) as illustrated in Figure 2–7.

The CF suffers the risk of being overly sensitive to extreme noise in one lead because of the multiplicative combination of data; the ASVV shows more robustness in the presence of a single noisy lead. Additionally, the ASVV is computationally less expensive than the CF. Since relative scaling of the ASVV curve values is performed, the division of each term by dt is unnecessary. The approach taken is to use a filtered ASVV curve as the basis for all similarity measures and temporal alignments.

Submitting a low- and high-pass filtered signal derived from one or more ECG leads to a threshold detection algorithm is a standard technique for R-wave detection. The low-pass filter tends to minimize effects of power-line interference and high-frequency muscle noise while the high-pass filter reduces low-frequency baseline drift and wander. There are many different filter cutoff frequencies suggested for R-wave detection filters, indicating some variance in the empirical results seen by investigators in the field. A summary of the filter performance characteristics of several systems is discussed by Thakor et al. In the system described here, the ASVV is used both for detecting the QRS-complex and also for detecting other features of the ECG waveform. These other features have their own inherent power spectra, and the filter cutoff frequencies must be chosen to optimize its use in detecting all of these features.

It was discovered empirically that a greater immunity to noise is preserved by separately filtering the slope calculations from each of the orthogonal leads prior to the nonlinear operation of taking the absolute value of this sum. This is apparent when this approach is contrasted to the results of performing the computationally faster method of first summing the absolute slopes and then filtering only the sums (i.e., the ASVV curve itself). In order to reduce the computational requirements of this multiple-lead filtering operation, the filter was redesigned into a prefilter/equalizer form. The prefilter is a simple moving average (recursive running sum), which does much of the stop-band attenuation at an insignificant cost in processing time. The equalizer is a standard filter designed to act in concert with the prefilter to improve the passband and stopband performance where needed. This optimization resulted in the same filter performance characteristics while using only 60% of the coefficients required for the more conventional approach.

These filtering operations do not disturb the ECG data itself; they are used to generate a derived waveform (the ASVV) which is convenient for internal processing. The ASVV curve is subsequently used to detect R-waves, align beats for fiducial marking, and determine onsets and offsets of the major ECG waveform components. Later measurements on the unfiltered ECG signals from individual, simultaneously recorded leads are made in relation to these detected fiducial points and markers along the ASVV curve.

Baseline Removal. The baseline for the ECG often wanders or drifts in an unpredictable and undesirable manner during exercise. This wander can take several forms such as sharp discontinuities, ramps, or cyclical swings. Such baseline wander can be induced by electrode impedance changes resulting from perspiration, motion, respiration, or other sources. It is easy to imagine the difficulties of making accurate measurements if the undesired baseline drift has several times the power of the desired ECG signal.

A commonly used technique for removing unwanted baseline fluctuations is to pass the ECG signal through a high-pass filter. The low end of the passband of this type of filter is designed to remove much of the baseline wander. Since the clinically relevant portion of the ECG power spectrum often has most of its energy at frequencies above those of the baseline drift, this simple technique can work fairly well and is still popular. However, it can be risky. If this type of filter design attenuates frequencies that are clinically relevant, the diagnostic accuracy of many measurements can be affected.

Another method of dealing with baseline wander takes advantage of an a priori knowledge of the underlying morphology of the ECG signal. The degree of baseline wander present in an individual QRS complex is estimated by measuring the relative levels of the TP segments both before and after the QRS complex. If the amplitude difference between these levels exceeds some threshold, the beat is discarded for further processing. This technique has the advantage of not introducing any distortion into the waveform, and works best for detecting and avoiding QRS complexes that have sharp discontinuities or ramps in their baseline. Unfortunately, this method tends to preferentially select heavily distorted QRS complexes if the baseline wander is of cyclic form since it will accept complexes that begin and end on opposite sides of a cycle or "hump." Such complexes can have surrounding TP segments of nearly identical amplitudes yet have quite a bit of distortion during the "hump." This is analogous to taking the points along a sine-wave located at identical and/or opposite phases in each cycle with the resultant line drawn between these points being flat. Another factor to be considered when this method is applied during exercise is that the TP segment is not a consistent estimator of the ECG baseline at high heart rates displaying TP fusion.

The cubic spline baseline estimate first reported from USAFSAM avoids these problems and also takes advantage of knowledge of the underlying form of the ECG signal. Even at the high heart rates seen in exercise testing, the PR segment is a more consistent estimate of the isoelectric baseline of the ECG than the TP segment (except in certain uncommon ECG abnormalities). To remove the ECG baseline, a cubic spline (minimum energy smooth curve) is passed through all detected PR segments. This spline is then subtracted from the raw ECG curve. The cubic spline as described by Myers et al. was found to be computationally too slow. A reformulation of their original equations resulted in removing several arithmetic operations per point (as suggested by

Krishnan et al.), thus dramatically lowering processing time. The cubic-spline baseline estimate adjusts itself to the data, does not violate AHA frequency response requirements, and can be used to remove enormous amounts of baseline wander.

Of course, removing an estimate of the baseline wander from the signal is not the same as removing the true baseline wander. All baseline compensation methods have theoretical and practical limits, and all are capable of introducing a certain amount of distortion. In the case of the cubic spline, the fundamental limit is the lack of sufficient baseline estimation points to unambiguously specify the form of the baseline wander. In other words, it is likely that the set of PR-segment values and their locations does not contain enough points to satisfy the Nyquist sampling criterion, given the power spectra of the baseline wander. However, the advantages of the cubic-spline method over the other methods considered are manifest, especially its low distortion when removing large amounts of baseline wander. Additionally, the cubic-spline is only one of the signal processing techniques used in our approach, and the final QRS complex extraction procedure is designed to be insensitive to precisely the kinds of problems sometimes seen during the baseline removal stage.

Beat Classification and Alignment. The major increase in signal to noise ratio is achieved by coherent processing of the ECG signal by QRS fiducial alignment and averaging point by point. Thus, a representative ECG complex is extracted from many beats that have been temporarily aligned. It is imperative that only similar beats be used in this extraction process. Distorted complexes, arrhythmic or aberrant complexes, and noise must be excluded. Cross-correlation of segments of the ASVV is used both to determine which template a QRS complex will be assigned to and also to adjust the final temporal alignment point for each classified QRS complex. Previously, other statistical techniques have been used since the high computational cost of cross-correlation was prohibitive. However, cross-correlation is a superior technique to such schemes as area comparison or sum of differences, and is preferred when using current solid state devices.

A threshold detection algorithm applied earlier to the ASVV curve generates several candidate R-waves. Templates are then formed by computing the cross-correlation of 200-msec regions of the ASVV curves containing the candidate QRS complexes. The cross-correlations are computed for alignments at every point from -20 to $+20$ msec of each initial point considered. The point at which the maximum correlation is achieved is then considered to be the final alignment fiducial for the complexes being correlated. Also, a minimum correlation coefficient of $+0.90$ is needed to classify a beat into a template. Choosing the alignment corresponding to the maximum correlation is more accurate than using the threshold-selected alignment and gives increased immunity for the template selection process to noise. A short burst of noise in a critical spot (e.g., near the temporary alignment point selected earlier) may cause the alignment point to be missed, since thresholds use properties of the signal that are local to only a few points. Cross-correlation, on the other hand, uses properties of the signal that are distributed over the entire range being correlated, and thus is more immune to the effects of short bursts of noise which may be present. However, cross-correlation is affected by errors in alignment. Computing the cross-correlation for many alignments in the region increases the probability that the correct final alignment is achieved and the optimal template selected. Since only the QRS complex is used for alignment, T or ST alternans and R-wave alternans are "lost" in the average. Also, this type of cross-correlation procedure is insensitive to amplitude differences, and a resultant correlation coefficient reflects primarily phase differences in the QRS-complex morphologies between the complexes being compared.

Representative Beat Extraction. It is desired to produce, from the set of aligned and similar beats, one ECG complex that is representative of the set. This composite ECG complex should emphasize characteristics of the set, and minimize characteristics that appear only in a few ECG complexes in the set. Thus, such a composite, representative ECG complex would have an increased SNR, largely because most of the noise in the signal should not be aligned consistently between all of the ECG complexes and is effectively "averaged" out.

An arithmetic mean is the linear process that produces the greatest increase in SNR when the noise satisfies several constraints including that it be Gaussian distributed. However, in the case of exercise ECG data, the noise is not distributed in a Gaussian manner, particularly due to the presence of skeletal muscle artifact. In addition, the noise often contains significant transient components that are due to sharp discontinuities in the baseline or the "hump" effect of cyclical baseline swing. Taking a point-by-point mean from set QRS complexes with this type of noise would pass 1/N of the noise level to the representative complex (where N is the number of QRS complexes in the original set).

A process that gives less of an increase in the SNR for Gaussian type noise but is relatively immune to the effects of sharp discontinuities or "humps" is the median. Also, the attenuation of muscle noise by using the median seems adequate for consistent measurements. However, the median is a computationally expensive operation requiring a sorting procedure on each of the representative beat epochs on a point-by-point basis. An algorithm that uses an estimate based on the previous median point index can speed up the sorting for the next point. In most cases, this implementation of the median operation is five times faster than a standard median computation implementation, thus allowing use of this attractive extraction method.

A hybrid method sometimes referred to as a trimmed mean combines some advantages of both of the two methods described above. It computes an arithmetic mean based only on the "center" points surrounding the median point, throwing out several extreme points on both the high and low side. This gives an added increase in SNR compared to the median while retaining some of the immunity to discontinuities and humps. However, one would like to adjust the number of trimmed points based on some estimate of the types of noise in the set of aligned, similar beats. Estimators of discontinuities exist, but are computationally expensive. Estimators of humps would have to qualitatively gauge the nature of the removed baseline wander; it might also be expensive. For these reasons, the median was chosen as our preferred method because it possesses both superior immunity to discontinuities and humps, and because it has adequate attenuation of muscle artifact.

SUMMARY

Though computers can record very clean representative ECG complexes and neatly print a variety of measurements, the algorithms they use are far from perfect and can result in serious differences from the raw signal. Even if computerization of the original raw analog ECG data could be accomplished without distortion, the problem of interpretation still remains. Numerous algorithms have been recommended for obtaining the optimal diagnostic value from the exercise electrocardiogram. These algorithms have been shown to give improved sensitivity and specificity compared to standard visual interpretation. This improvement has usually been documented and substantiated only by the investigator who proposed the new measurement. Simoons has compared four of these suggested computer criteria in the same series of patients with coronary heart disease, and ultimately concluded that his own new algorithm was the best. Detrano compared several computer criteria to visual analysis including the Hollenberg score and found the diagnostic power to be similar; that is, computer analysis offered no improvement in diagnostic power. The physician who uses commercially available computer-aided systems to analyze the results of exercise tests should be aware of the problems and always review the raw analog recordings to see if they are consistent with the processed output. ST measurement points must always be verified.

BIBLIOGRAPHY

Ahnve S: Correction of the QT interval for heart rate: Review of different formulas and the use of Bazett's formula in myocardial infarction. *Am Heart J* 1985;109:568–574.

Ahnve S, Sullivan M, Myers J, et al: Computer analysis of exercise-induced changes in QRS duration in patients with angina pectoris and in normal subjects. *Am Heart J* 1986;111:903.

Angelhed JE, Bjuro TI, Ejdeback J, et al: Computer-aided exercise electrocardiographic testing and coronary arteriography in patients with angina pectoris and with myocardial infarction. *Br Heart J* 1984;52:140–146.

Ascoop CA, Distelbrink CA, De Lang PA: Clinical value of quantitative analysis of ST slope during exercise. *Br Heart J* 1977;39:212–217.

Balcon R, Brooks N, Layton C: Correlation of heart rate/ST slope and coronary angiographic findings. *Br Heart J* 1984;52:304–311.

Beattie JM, Seibert GB, Blomqvist CG: Lead specificity of the maximum ST/heart rate slope response. *Br Heart J* 1984;53:349–357.

Bhargava V, Watanabe K, Froelicher VF: Progress in computer analysis of the exercise ECG. *Am J Cardiol* 1981;47:1143–1151.

Blomqvist G: The Frank lead exercise electrocardiogram. *Acta Med Scand* 1965;178:1–98.

Detrano R, Salcedo E, Leatherman J, et al: Computer-assisted versus unassisted analysis of the exercise electrocardiogram in patients without myocardial infarction. JACC 1986; in press.

Detrano R, Salcedo E, Passalacqua M, et al: Exercise electrocardiographic variables: A critical appraisal. *J Am Coll Cardiol* 1986;8:836–847.

Elamin MS, Boyle R, Kardash MM, et al: Accurate detection of coronary heart disease by new exercise test. *Br Heart J* 1982;48:311–320.

Elamin MS, Mary DASG, Smith DR, et al: Prediction of severity of coronary artery disease using slope of submaximal ST segment/heart rate relationship. *Cardiovasc Res* 1980;14:681–691.

Forlini FJ, Cohn K, Langston ME: ST-segment isolation and quantification as a means of improving diagnostic accuracy in treadmill stress testing. *Am Heart J* 1975;90:431–438.

Fox KM, Dearfield J, Ribero P, et al: Projection of ST-segment changes on to the front of the chest: Practical implications for exercise testing and ambulatory monitoring. *Br Heart J* 1982;48:555–562.

Froelicher VF, Wolthuis R, Fischer J, et al: Variations in normal ECG response to treadmill testing. *Am J Cardiol* 1981;47:1161–1167.

Froelicher VF, Wolthuis R, Keiser N, et al: A comparison of two bipolar electrocardiographic leads to lead V5. *Chest* 1976;70:611–616.

Goldberger AL, Bhargava V, Froelicher V, et al: Effect of myocardial infarction on high frequency QRS potentials. *Circulation* 1981;64:34–41.

Hollenberg M, Budge WR, Wisneski JA, et al: Treadmill score quantifies electrocardiographic response to exercise and improves test accuracy and reproducibility. *Circulation* 1980;61:276–285.

Hollenberg M, Wisneski JA, Gertz EW, et al: Computer-derived treadmill exercise score quantifies the degree of revascularization and improved exercise performance after coronary artery bypass surgery. *Am Heart J* 1983;106:1096–1104.

Hollenberg M, Zoltick JM, Go M, et al: Comparison of a quantitative treadmill exercise score with standard electrocardiographic criteria in screening asymptomatic young men for coronary artery disease. *N Engl J Med* 1985;313:600–606.

Hornsten TR, Bruce RA: Computer ST forces of Frank and bipolar exercise electrocardiograms. *Am Heart J* 1969;78:346–350.

Kardash MM, Boyle RM, Watson DA, et al: Assessment of aortocoronary bypass grafting using exercise ST segment/heart rate relation. *Br Heart J* 1984;51:386.

Kligfield P, Okin PM, Ameisen O, Borer J: Evaluation of CAD by improved method of exercise ECG: the exercise ST/HR slope. *Am Heart J* 1986;112:589–598.

Krishnan RK, Moghe CS: An approach to character generation using cubic splines. *Transactions on Consumer Electronics* 1983;29:25–32.

Lam JC, Chaitman BR, Hanson JS, et al: Comparative diagnostic value of exercise polarcardiography and 14-lead electrocardiography in the detection of coronary artery disease. *Am Heart J* 1985;110:1237–1241.

McHenry PL, Stowe DE, Lancaster MC: Computer quantitation of the ST-segment response during maximal treadmill exercise. *Circulation* 1968;38:691.

McManus CD, Teppner U, Neubert D: Estimation and removal of baseline drift in the electrocardiogram. *Comput Biomed Res* 1985;18:1–9.

Meyer CR, Keiser HN: Electrocardiogram baseline noise estimation and removal using cubic splines and state-space computation techniques. *Biomed Res* 1977;10:83–92.

Myers J, Ahnve S, Froelicher V, et al: A randomized trial of the effects of one year of exercise training on computer-measured ST-segment displacement in patients with coronary artery disease. *J Am Coll Cardiol* 1984;4:1094–1102.

Okin PM, Kligfield P, Ameisen O, et al: Improved accuracy of the exercise electrocardiogram: Identification of three-vessel coronary disease in stable angina pectoris by analysis of peak rate-related changes in ST segments. *Am J Cardiol* 1985;55:271–276.

Quyyumi AA, Raphael MJ, Wright C, et al: Inability of the ST segment/heart rate slope to predict accurately the severity of coronary artery disease. *Br Heart J* 1984;51:395.

Romano M, DiMaro T, Carella G, et al: Relation between heart rate and QT interval in exercise-induced myocardial ischemia. *Am J Cardiol* 1985;56:861–862.

Savvides M, Ahnve S, Bhargava V, et al: Computer analysis of exercise-induced changes in electrocardiographic variables. Comparison of methods and criteria. *Chest* 1983;84:699–706.

Savvides M, Froelicher V: Noninvasive non-nuclear exercise testing. *Cardiology* 1984;71:100–117.

Sheffield LT, Holt TH, Lester FM, et al: On-line analysis of the exercise electrocardiogram. *Circulation* 1969;40:935–944.

Silverton NP, Elamin MS, Smith DR, et al: Use of the exercise maximal ST segment/heart rate slope in assessing the results of coronary angioplasty. *Br Heart J* 1984;51:379.

Simoons ML: Optimal measurements for detection of coronary artery disease by exercise electrocardiography. *Comput Biomed Res* 1977;10:483–499.

Simoons ML, Boom HD, Smallenberg E: On-line processing of orthogonal exercise electrocardiograms. *Comput Biomed Res* 1975;8:105–117.

Simoons ML, Hugenholtz PG: Gradual changes of ECG waveform during and after exercise in normal subjects. *Circulation* 1975;52:570–577.

Simoons ML, Hugenholtz PG, Ascoop CA, et al: Quantitation of exercise electrocardiography. *Circulation* 1981;63:471–475.

Sketch MH, Mohiuddin MS, Nair-Mooss AN, et al: Automated and nomographic analysis of exercise tests. *JAMA* 1980;243:1053–1057.

Sullivan MA, Genter F, Savvides M, et al: The reproducibility of hemodynamic, electrocardiographic, and gas exchange data during treadmill exercise in patients with stable angina pectoris. *Chest* 1984;86:375–382.

Surawicz B, Knoebel SB: Long QT: Good, bad or indifferent? *J Am Coll Cardiol* 1984;4:398–413.

Taback L, Marden E, Mason HL, et al: Digital recording of electrocardiographic data for analysis by digital computer. *Med Electronics* 1959;6:167.

Thwaites BC, Quyyumi AA, Raphael MJ, et al: Comparison of the ST/heart rate slope with the modified Bruce exercise test in the detection of coronary artery disease. *Am J Cardiol* 1986;57:554–556.

Turner AS, Nathan MC, Watson OF, et al: The correlation of the computer quantitated treadmill exercise electrocardiogram with cinearteriographic assessment of coronary artery disease. *NZ Med J* 1979;89:115–118.

Van Tellingen C, Ascoop CA, Rijneke RD: On the clinical value of conventional and new exercise electrocardiographic criteria: A comparative study. *Int J Cardiol* 1984;5:689–695.

Watanabe K, Bhargava V, Froelicher V: Computer analysis of the exercise ECG: A review. *Prog Cardiovasc Dis* 1980;22:423–446.

Watanabe K, Bhargava V, Froelicher V: The relationship between exercise-induced R-wave amplitude changes and QRS vector loops. *J Electrocardiol* 1981;14:129–138.

Wolthuis RA, Froelicher VF, Hopkirk A, et al: Normal ECG waveform characteristics during treadmill exercise testing. *Circulation* 1979;60:1028–1035.

Wolthuis RA, Hopkirk A, Fischer JR, et al: Development of new criteria for computer interpretation of exercise electrocardiograms in a largely asymptomatic population. *Int J Cardiol* 1982;2:203–217.

Yanowitz F, Froelicher VF, Keiser N, et al: Quantitative exercise ECG in the evaluation of patients with early coronary artery disease. *Aerospace Med* 1974;45:443–448.

3 SPECIAL METHODS: VENTILATORY GAS EXCHANGE MEASUREMENTS

The guidelines for measurement of maximal oxygen uptake are (1) dynamic exercise of a large portion of the muscle mass, (2) progressive increases in work load to fatigue, (3) precise gas measurement techniques, and (4) minimal exercising time to lessen the effect of endurance. These guidelines have been followed using different exercise protocols and devices, and similar results have been obtained.

To measure oxygen uptake, the concentration of oxygen in expired air must be measured. Also, the volume of air expired is measured using a tissot, air bags, or flow meters, and then the amount of oxygen consumed by the body can be determined. Because the measurement of maximal oxygen uptake requires a nose clip, mouthpiece, breathing valves, weather balloons, and gas analysis equipment, it is not practical to perform in clinical practice. Though the automated systems have been validated, this has been in academic centers with skilled people using them. They are expensive and are limited by technical difficulties in both measuring airflow during exercise and by a lack of reliability of the gas analyzers.

Maximal oxygen uptake and treadmill work load are directly related. This relationship has correlation coefficients of $+.8$ to $.9$. There is, however, a wide scatter around the regression line that is due to wide variations in mechanical efficiency among individuals (Fig 3–1). Care should be taken so that patients do not support their weight or allow themselves to be dragged by the hand rails, since this reduces the amount of work performed.

Bruce has suggested a method of estimating functional aerobic impairment (FAI). Normally FAI should be zero because observed maximal oxygen uptake should be the same as that predicted. Bruce constructed a nomogram to determine FAI. On one side is treadmill time in his protocol, and on the other is age. Between these two lines are sloped lines with percent increments of FAI for sedentary and active individuals. By drawing a straight line through age (from which the maximal oxygen uptake can be predicted) and the treadmill time, an estimate of aerobic impairment can be read from the sloped lines. Previous studies demonstrated a poor correlation between age and VO_2 in healthy males even when activity levels were considered (Fig 3–2). This is due to the many factors that affect an individual's aerobic capacity in addition

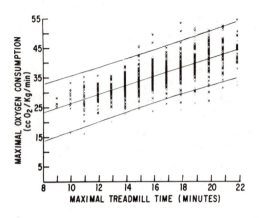

FIG 3–1.
Relationship of treadmill time to measured ventilatory oxygen consumption (VO_2) using a progressive treadmill protocol in healthy pilots.

to his current activity level, including past activity level, genetic endowments, mechanical efficiency, previous testing experience, and the specificity of training. Thus, this nomogram is based on two relatively poor relationships, which thereby limit its ability to predict functional capacity. It is preferable to estimate an individual's maximal oxygen uptake from the work load reached while performing a treadmill test. This estimation facilitates comparison between different treadmill protocols and avoids the problem arising from the fact that the same performance time in different protocols does not mean that the same work load was performed. Serial treadmill testing is complicated by the occurrence of adaptation, learning and habituation which increase treadmill time without an increase in maximal oxygen uptake.

The introduction of total treadmill time as a measure of a patient's aerobic capacity in medical practice has had advantages and disadvantages. The advantages are that an understanding of exercise physiology is not necessary for analyzing exercise test results and that, if the same protocol is used, test results can easily be compared. These advantages are outweighed by many disadvantages.

A true test of aerobic capacity is best limited to a total exercise time of 10 minutes, as endurance really becomes the key factor thereafter. Endurance is much more difficult to assess and is much more influenced by peripheral factors than by central factors. Comparison of total treadmill time locks one into a fixed treadmill protocol, and for the best physiologic testing, work loads should be adjusted for the individual patient, rather than the patient having to adapt to the protocol. Some patients can reach higher exercise levels if the grade is mainly increased rather than the speed. At high levels of performance, it is usually best to increase speed rather than grade because of the awkwardness of running on a treadmill at a steep incline.

Physicians will often ask "How long did the patient walk?" and not be concerned with what work load they reached. In performing serial treadmill tests, the improvement that a patient can achieve in total time because of learning makes it appear as if they improved their exercise capacity. Though it takes a greater understanding of exercise physiology and interaction with the patient, it would be much better to tailor each exercise test for the patient being tested. Rather than consider total time, which should be about 10 minutes, aerobic capacity should be estimated from the highest treadmill speed and grade at which the patient equilibrates. Though the gross relationships between total treadmill time in a fixed protocol or the work load achieved and total body oxygen consumption are adequate for clinical purposes, it is hoped that an inexpensive automated system for airflow and gas analysis will be developed that can accurately measure oxygen consumption. Such a system is needed for the evaluation of serial changes in the aerobic capacity after interventions.

This chapter describes gas analysis instrumentation, explains the gas exchange parameters that can be obtained during exercise testing and shows their reproducibility, demonstrates the inaccuracy of estimating maximal oxygen uptake, and explains why measuring gas exchange in patients with coronary heart disease can be helpful.

INSTRUMENTATION

Air Collection. The measurement of gas exchange variables during exercise requires that the patient have a mouthpiece in place that seals tightly, the nose closed with a clip, and no major eardrum leaks. Although face masks are available that cover the nose and mouth (making speaking possible), these usually leak during exercise at expiratory flows greater than 50 L/min.

Air Volume Measurement. Expired gas analysis requires that all expired gases be analyzed for total volume as well as oxygen and carbon dioxide content. Accurate measurement requires water content to be

FIG 3–2.
Relationship of age to measured VO_2 in the Bruce protocol in healthy subjects with activity status considered.

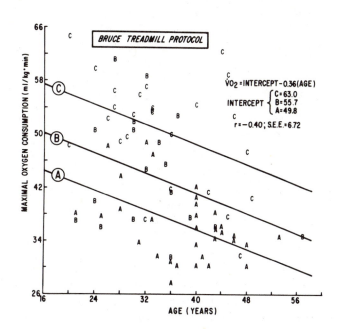

accounted for by adjusting for standard pressure and temperature. As originally performed, all expired gases were collected in a tissot. This device is an inverted open metal cylinder suspended in a larger open cylinder filled with water. Filling the inner cylinder with expired air causes it to raise in the water, and the displacement volume is known at each point along the height of the cylinder. Expired air is sampled for the content of CO_2 and O_2 and compared to the contents of room air or whatever gases are inspired. Other methods of measuring air volume require Douglas bags or weather balloons. The latter are more prone to leaks and tears but are more convenient. A turret that rotates from one bag to the next at each time interval is helpful. Each bag is sampled for the CO_2 and O_2 content.

In order to make measurements "on-line," various types of flow meters have been used including: mass transducers, Fleisch pneumotachometers, hot wire devices, small propellers or turbines, and dry gas meters. A Fleisch pneumotachometer measures the pressure drop due to the Venturi effect caused by airflow through a tube; the "hot wires" drop in temperature when cooled by air, and the propellers are spun by airflow. One problem with these devices is the difficulty of measuring ventilatory gas volume directly from a rapidly breathing individual. The phasic nature of breathing affects these devices. They are more effectively utilized if the air is stored in a bag or a weather balloon and drawn out at a steady flow rate through the flow meter. However, most commercial devices try to measure flow directly from the patient and are not as accurate as "off-line" methods. "On-line" analysis also requires a mixing chamber from which expired gases are sampled.

Gas Analyzers.   There are numerous types of gas analyzers. Though the mass spectrometer has the advantages of needing only a small sample size and making rapid accurate measurements, it is the most expensive and least reliable due to dependence on a vacuum. This device also has the advantage that it can analyze other gases such as acetylene. Infrared devices are used to measure CO_2 since CO_2 absorbs in the infrared spectra. Calcium zirconium high temperature fuel cells and biochemical membrane reactions (polargraphic) or paramagnetic devices are used to analyze oxygen content. The polargraphic technique is troublesome because of the short and uncertain life span of the sensor membrane.

Breath-by-Breath Analysis.   Recent devices perform breath-by-breath analyses. They make it possible to indirectly measure cardiac output (by CO_2 rebreathing) and study oxygen kinetics. Because this technique requires rapid response from the gas analyzers (since the gases are sampled at the mouthpiece and a mixing chamber is not used), it is best utilized in the research laboratory and does not offer advantages for clinical testing.

Gas Exchange Information From Exercise Testing.   The primary measurements of gas exchange during exercise testing are pulmonary airflow or ventilation (L/min) and the percentage of carbon dioxide ($FECO_2$) and oxygen (FEO_2) in expired air. The derived information from these basic measurements are presented below.

Maximal oxygen uptake (VO_2 max) is considered the best index of aerobic work capacity and maximal cardiorespiratory function. The collection and analysis of an expired gas sample taken during the last minute of an exercise test is used to directly determine VO_2 max. Maximal oxygen uptake is reached when there is no further increase in oxygen uptake despite further increases in workload.

Plateauing of Peak Oxygen Uptake.   Taylor et al. established the criteria of plateauing of peak oxygen uptake as a decrease in oxygen uptake or an increase of less than 150 ml/min or 2.1 ml/kg/min with an increase in work load. His original research was done using interrupted progressive treadmill protocols. With interrupted protocols, stages of exercise could be separated by rest periods ranging from minutes to days. Taylor found that 75% of his subjects fulfilled these criteria. Using continuous treadmill protocols, Pollock found that 69%, 69%, 59%, and 80% of subjects plateaued when tested using the Balke, Bruce, Ellestad, and Astrand protocols, respectively. Froelicher et al. found that only 33%, 17%, and 7% of his subjects met these criteria during testing with the Taylor, Balke, and Bruce protocols, respectively. This study also showed that there were no significant differences between these three types of protocols for maximal heart rate, VO_2 max, or blood pressure. Taylor later reported that plateauing does not occur in continuous treadmill protocols.

Plateaus most likely appear in progressive protocols because of hanging on or because of incomplete air sample collections. Whether plateauing occurs or not depends upon the subject's health, fitness, and motivation, but also on the criteria applied, equipment used, and methodology. Samples of small duration may better show plateauing while 30-second to one-minute samples may not unless the subject is allowed to hang on or lose the mouthpiece seal. Also, extrapolating from collections of irregular, short-time intervals may lead to an artificial plateau.

Gas Exchange Anaerobic Threshold (ATGE).   During progressive exercise, ventilation follows a linear relationship with oxygen uptake until 50% to 80% of maximal work capacity is exceeded. This point of relative hyperventilation is hypothesized to be related to tissue hypoxia and anaerobic metabolism. An increase in blood lactic acid has been reported to correlate with this breakpoint in ventilation. Wasserman et al. labeled this point of hyperventilation as the "anaerobic threshold." They theorized that ventilation was increased due to the increase in carbon dioxide production secondary to the buffering of lactic acid ($H_2CO_3 \leftrightharpoons H_2O + CO_2$).

However, studies with normal subjects and patients with McArdle's disease have shown that the relationship between the onset of blood lactic acid accumulation and the departure from linearity of ventilation can be altered. Hagberg et al. studied the ventilatory response of four patients who lacked muscle phosphorylase and therefore the ability to produce lactic acid during exercise. Although no change in blood lactic acid occurred during exercise, these patients exhibited an abrupt change in ventilation at approximately 77% of VO_2 max. Hughes et al. exercised normal subjects on a bicycle ergometer in a glycogen-depleted state and in a normal state of glycogen availability, at two pedal frequencies (60 and 90 rpm). When the subjects were glycogen depleted, the oxygen uptake prior to the increase of blood lactic acid was significantly higher than the oxygen uptake prior to the point of hyperventilation. When glycogen was available, with an increased pedal frequency, the oxygen uptake prior to lactate accumulation was lower than the oxygen uptake prior to the point of hyperventilation.

Although the mechanism for exercise hyperventilation is unclear, Hughes reported a very good test-retest correlation of .82 for determining the gas exchange anaerobic threshold (ATGE). In addition, Hughes and Davis and Gass were unable to alter the ATGE expressed as percentage of VO_2 max by any intervention. Table 3–1 summarizes the criteria used by various researchers for determining the ATGE. Figure 3–3 graphically displays these measurements. Davis et al. and Weber et al. have reported reproducibility of measuring ATGE during treadmill testing. When testing healthy subjects, Davis reported a test-retest correlation of .72. Weber tested patients with chronic heart failure and found a correlation of .87 for repeated determinations of the ATGE. Previously, investigators have shown habituation during treadmill walking to occur between subsequent tests. Davis did not refer to the previous treadmill experience of his subjects while Weber had all the subjects perform two treadmill tests prior to initiating the study. The reproducibility of the ATGE may be improved if the subject is given prior treadmill experience.

The gas exchange anaerobic threshold can be used as an important point of submaximal exercise for several reasons. First, previous research has shown variability in the rate at which oxygen uptake attains a steady state value above and below the gas exchange anaerobic threshold. Previous work by Davis and Weber as well as our laboratory, show the gas exchange anaerobic threshold to be a reproducible parameter. In addition, while the relative percentage of peak oxygen uptake at which the gas exchange anaerobic threshold occurs is significantly higher for angina patients (74%) when compared to either coronary artery disease patients limited by fatigue (57%) or normal subjects (61%), the absolute oxygen uptake value expressed in ml/kg/min is similar between the two subgroups of coronary artery disease patients. The higher percentage is due to the pathologically lowered VO_2 max in the angina patients. Thus, within a given population, the gas exchange anaerobic threshold

TABLE 3–1.
Criteria for Gas Exchange Anaerobic Threshold*

INVESTIGATOR	GAS EXCHANGE PARAMETERS
Davis et al.	Departure from linearity for VE, VCO_2, and an abrupt increase in R and the fraction of expired oxygen (FEO_2).
Withers et al.	An increase in the ventilatory equivalent for O_2 (VE/VO_2) without an increase in the ventilatory equivalent for CO_2 (VE/VCO_2) and an increase in FEO_2 without a decrease in $FECO_2$.
Reinhard et al.	The minimum VE/VO_2 value
Wasserman et al.	VE, VCO_2 increase rapidly while VO_2 continues linear

*Recommended and utilized by various researchers.

FIG 3–3.

Illustration of the gas exchange variables that can be measured during exercise to determine ATGE.

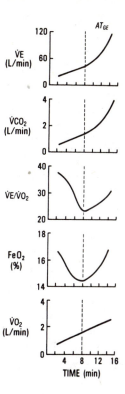

seems to be a relatively constant, reproducible, physiologic point during sub-maximal exercise.

Gas exchange anaerobic threshold has the potential of being a more important measurement than maximal oxygen consumption. For one thing, a patient need not be exercised to the maximum. For another, the level that the patient can perform during activities at a submaximal level without becoming anaerobic may have more relevance to tolerating and performing daily activities than maximal capacity. Also, in patients with limited cardiac output and limited maximal oxygen consumption, an improvement in anaerobic threshold could mean that they can better tolerate a higher level of submaximal exercise. This measurement may also better estimate fitness and predict performance than other measurements. However, more research is needed to demonstrate the clinical value of anaerobic threshold.

Oxygen Kinetics. Oxygen uptake kinetics describe the rate at which oxygen uptake reaches a steady state value (VO_2ss). Early investigations by Margaria et al. and DiPrampero et al. described the kinetics of oxygen uptake as a first-order function reaching a steady state within two minutes. Whipp et al. and Linnarsson et al. reported similar oxygen kinetics for levels of light or moderate work below the ATGE. However, at work loads above the ATGE, oxygen kinetics could be better described as a second-order function. Wasserman et al. found VO_2ss to occur after four minutes of exercise at work rates just below the ATGE. They also found that at work loads above the ATGE, VO_2ss occurred after approximately 10 minutes.

Linnarsson et al. proposed that the oxygen uptake kinetics above the ATGE were composed of a fast component similar to light or moderate work and a slow component continuing up to the sixth minute. The slow response component recognized in prolonged heavy work was assumed to result from raised body temperature, decreased carbohydrate oxidation, and fatigue. However, Wasserman et al. and Linnarsson et al. have proposed that the slow rate of adaptation above the ATGE is due to a lag in the circulatory response to the metabolic demand at the muscles. They believe that cardiac output rather than a redistribution of blood to the exercising muscle is the limiting factor for the delay in VO_2ss above the ATGE.

Sady reported slower oxygen uptake and heart rate kinetics in middle-aged men when compared to prepubescent boys. During this study, the subjects performed a single bout of maximal exercise for eight minutes. The slower rise to VO_2ss in the adults was attributed to a slower cardiovascular adjustment to exercise.

When the measured oxygen uptake is lower than the oxygen required for a work load, the energy difference is supplied by oxygen stores bound to myoglobin, high-energy phosphates and/or anaerobic glycolysis. Davis et al. have proposed that the amount of anaerobic work a person can do can be quantified from gas exchange information. The total oxygen deficit incurred during exercise, which can also be measured in recovery, equals the anaerobic capacity of a subject.

Respiratory Quotient. The respiratory exchange ratio or RQ equals the volume of carbon dioxide production divided by the oxygen uptake. RQ in conjunction with the determination of the oxygen deficit can provide a noninvasive index of carbohydrate metabolism relative to fat metabolism. Taylor used an RQ of 1.15 or greater as an index of attainment of maximal exercise, but this is not agreed upon.

Oxygen Pulse (O_2-Pulse). O_2-pulse is a noninvasive index of the physiologic efficiency of combined cardiopulmonary oxygen transport. It is calculated by dividing VO_2 by the heart rate. As work increases the O_2-pulse increases, and more importantly, at any given work load, the O_2-pulse is higher in the trained subject than in the untrained subject. Withers et al. expanded this concept to include the effect of training specificity on O_2-pulse. They reported a higher O_2-pulse for runners and cyclists when tested on their respective exercise mode. Karlsson et al. tested both trained and untrained subjects and reported a leveling off of the O_2-pulse at maximum levels of work. They felt this was the result of a decrease in stroke volume rather than a decrease in the arterial-venous O_2 difference. Heart disease patients tend to have a lower O_2-pulse when compared to normal adults. This appears to be the result of a decrease in the stroke volume secondary to the dysfunction of the left ventricle caused by infarction or ischemia.

Adequacy of Ventilation. The ventilatory response (VE) in L/min during exercise is controlled by two mechanisms, one for above and the other for below the ATGE. They are (1) the amount of ventilation required to eliminate carbon dioxide at work loads below the ATGE and (2) the amount of ventilation required to offset pH decreases secondary to lactic acidosis above the anaerobic or ATGE. Wasserman et al. state that the respiratory-limited patient may be unable to deplete oxygen in the muscle to a level that would stimulate glycolysis or be unable to increase ventilation sufficiently to compensate for the exercise-induced lactic acidosis. The hyperventilation required at heavy levels of work can aid in detecting the respiratory-limited patient. In contrast, patients with cardiovascular diseases tend to have the same ventilatory response to exercise as healthy individuals.

Mechanical Efficiency. Mechanical efficiency is the ratio of the absolute energy cost of a work load to the energy expenditure by the body to perform the work load. All "engines," even the human body, waste energy as heat in performing work and are not totally efficient. Since oxygen uptake is directly related to the total energy expenditure (1 L of oxygen yields 5 kcal of energy), the mechanical efficiency can be easily determined for a standard external work load. The total amount of energy released by the amount of oxygen consumed is divided into the actual work performed. Usually 80% of the energy is wasted as heat and the body is only about 20% efficient. Certain factors can increase oxygen uptake at standard work loads and decrease mechanical efficiency (Table 3–2). During treadmill testing, Withers et al. reported cyclists to be comparatively less efficient than runners. Studies at USAFSAM demonstrated a reduction in oxygen uptake and heart rate at similar work loads, consistent with an increase in mechanical efficiency during sequential exercise testing. Other investigators have demonstrated progressively more efficient motion using motion picture techniques in normals when treadmill tested up to 10 times. Studies involving serial treadmill testing should consider the changes in mechanical efficiency that can have an effect on results. Habituation increases total time on the treadmill by increasing submaximal efficiency rather than the time increase being due to an intervention (i.e., exercise training, drugs, surgery).

GAS EXCHANGE MEASUREMENTS IN PATIENTS WITH CORONARY HEART DISEASE

The safety of measuring gas exchange has been a concern when testing coronary patients. However, gas exchange can be measured safely during exercise

TABLE 3–2.
Factors Affecting Mechanical Efficiency

Weight (obesity) and stride length for weightbearing leg exercise.
Specific training for the device used for testing.
Experience with exercise on the device used (habituation, learning).
Body stability for isolated supine leg or arm exercise.
Motor coordination and neuromuscular system.

testing without complication or duress to the patient. Prior experience with the air collection system and proper instruction of hand signals for communication are necessary.

Testing the effects of medications or other interventions in patients with coronary artery disease should include the measurement of gas exchange. This is particularly the case since total treadmill time, which has been the major measurement for assessing drugs, can increase with serial treadmill testing without an increase in maximal oxygen consumption. In fact, this has occurred with the administration of placebo. Along with the accurate determination of VO_2 max, the continuous acquisition of gas exchange data can provide further information on the submaximal effectiveness of the intervention.

PREDICTING OXYGEN UPTAKE FROM TREADMILL TESTING IN HEART PATIENTS

The disadvantages of measuring oxygen uptake (i.e., cost of equipment, added personnel, time) can be avoided by predicting VO_2 max from performance characteristics during exercise tests. Early investigations correlating submaximal pulse rates with VO_2 max have been critically reviewed and are no longer recommended for the clinical setting. The most accepted methods today for estimating ventilatory oxygen uptake from the results of a progressive exercise test utilize maximal time and/or work load. Although shown to be reasonably accurate in normal populations, the application of these techniques to estimating oxygen uptake in coronary artery disease patients has been questioned. A particular problem in patients is the termination of a test due to angina, thus preventing the attainment of a true physiological maximal oxygen uptake. In this case, a measurement taken during the last minute of exercise is said to represent a symptom-limited peak oxygen uptake.

Roberts et al. investigated the relationship between oxygen uptake and both total treadmill time and work load in patients with coronary artery disease. The continuous acquisition of gas exchange throughout the exercise test was performed to investigate the possible physiological mechanism for the discrepancies in estimating oxygen uptake. Gas samples were collected through a Koegel low-resistance breathing valve into a series of evacuated weather balloons. Subjects had a nose clip in place throughout the gas collection period. The following parameters were derived from the gas exchange data: (1) ventilation (VE L/min; ATPS, STPD, BTPS); (2) oxygen uptake (VO_2; L/min, ml/kg/min); (3) carbon dioxide production (VCO_2; L/min) (4) respiratory exchange ratio ($R = VCO_2/VO_2$); (5) ventilatory equivalent for oxygen (VE/VO_2); and, (6) ventilatory equivalent for carbon dioxide (VE/VCO_2). The gas exchange anaerobic threshold was identified as the oxygen uptake prior to the systematic increase in VE/VO_2 without an increase in VE/VCO_2.

Peak oxygen uptake was determined as the highest value obtained during one-minute samples. The criteria outlined by Taylor of an increase in oxygen uptake of 150 ml/min or less with an increase in work load was used for determination of a plateau in oxygen uptake. The mean peak oxygen uptake for normals was significantly greater than for the coronary artery disease patients (41 versus 26 ml/kg/min). None of the normal subjects and only 9% of the patients fulfilled the criteria of Taylor for a plateau in oxygen uptake.

Correlation coefficients for peak oxygen uptake versus total time for normal subjects was .93 and .85 for the patients. Standard error of the estimate for normal subjects and patients was 2.56 ml/kg/min and 2.86 ml/kg/min, respectively.

Mean and standard deviation for oxygen uptake observed each 30 seconds in normal subjects and patients during the first five stages of the protocol are displayed in Figure 3–4. Statistically significant differences in oxygen uptake between normal subjects and coronary patients were observed from 30 seconds through one minute and 30 seconds, at two minutes and 30 seconds, and from five minutes through minute 10 of the protocol. The normal subjects attain a steady state for oxygen uptake during the first three stages while the coronary patients only do so at the first two stages. In addition, at each time period above the patient's mean gas exchange anaerobic threshold, there is a statistically significant difference in measured oxygen uptake between the two groups.

Table 3–3 presents the results from previously published data. Mean oxygen uptake values and correlation coefficients are comparable. Standard error of the estimate is in agreement with previous reports by Froelicher but somewhat lower than those reported by Bruce and higher than reported by Pollock. Mean oxygen uptake in our patients is similar to those presented by Bruce but somewhat lower than Haskell's patients tested 11 weeks post MI using a similar protocol. Correlation coefficients and standard error of the estimates are similar in the three studies.

FIG 3–4.
Plot of means for oxygen cost for treadmill work loads in normals and patients with coronary heart disease showing that above their anaerobic threshold, the patients are one MET lower than normals.

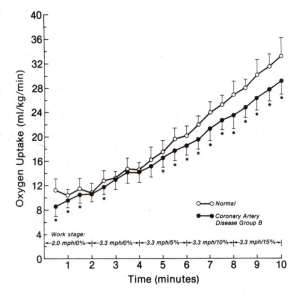

TABLE 3–3.

Studies Relating Oxygen Uptake to Treadmill Time in Normal Subjects and in Coronary Artery Disease Patients

AUTHOR	PROTOCOL	REGRESSION EQUATION X = TIME IN MIN	MEAN PEAK O_2 UPTAKE ± SD (ml/kg/min)	r	STANDARD ERROR OF THE ESTIMATE
Bruce et al.	Bruce	Y = 3.29x + 4.07	37.3 ± 8.2	0.93	4.9
Pollock et al.	Bruce	Y = 4.33x − 4.66	40.0 ± 7.2	0.88	0.096
	Balke	Y = 1.44x + 14.99	39.4 ± 5.9	0.92	0.25
Froelicher et al.	Bruce	Y = 3.18x + 0.59	44.5 ± 5.8	0.82	3.34
	Balke	Y = 1.25x + 9.42	41.6 ± 5.0	0.86	2.65
Roberts et al.	Modified Balke	Y = 3.91x − 8.88	36.8 ± 6.6	0.93	2.56
Bruce et al.	Bruce	Y = 2.3x + 9.48	25.5 ± 5.9	0.87	3.20
Haskell et al.	Naughton	N/A	27.7 ± 5.0	0.71	4.16
Roberts et al.	Modified Balke	Y = 2.57x + 2.13	26.4 ± 5.4	0.85	2.86

N/A = not available; r = correlation coefficient; SD = standard deviation.

Bruce was one of the first to present clinical data on the relationship between total treadmill time and oxygen uptake. However, he classified 53% of his subjects with only hypertension and no documented coronary disease as cardiac patients. Haskell presented favorable results for a protocol utilizing small increments in work (1 MET) and larger duration at each workload (three minutes) in coronary disease patients. This protocol resulted in a mean exercise time of 17 minutes with an upper limit of 28 minutes. But these patients were inadequately stressed since mean peak respiratory exchange ratio was 1.04.

In the Bruce, Pollock, and Froelicher studies, the subjects were similar in age and aerobic capacity and assumed to be free of coronary artery disease. Haskell's data is based on patients tested 11 weeks after an MI. Pollock's subjects were habituated to treadmill walking whereas Froelicher et al. randomized the order of treadmill tests and reported only small differences between testing periods. Bruce did not report on the previous treadmill experience of his subjects. Haskell's patients were tested three weeks after their heart attacks. The small standard error reported by Pollock may possibly be explained by the large proportion of subjects (69%) exhibiting a plateau in oxygen uptake compared to the subjects (17%) in the Froelicher and Bruce studies. Haskell did not report if a plateau in oxygen uptake had occurred. Pollock concluded that predictive equations appear to be specific to a certain population.

The low correlation between peak oxygen uptake and the gas exchange anaerobic threshold of r = .53 for the coronary patients suggests that the limiting factors associated with peak oxygen uptake, i.e., angina, in coronary artery disease patients occur above the gas exchange anaerobic threshold. The similar correlation coefficients between peak oxygen uptake and the gas exchange anaerobic threshold in normal subjects and the subgroup of patients limited by angina (r = .89 and .82, respectively) support this hypothesis. These correlation coefficients are similar to previously published values by Weltman (r = .85) but somewhat lower than the values reported by Matsumura (r = .95). However, in the Matsumura study, 34 were normal subjects and 47 were chronic heart disease patients, only two of which had ischemic heart disease. The Weltman data was obtained using normal subjects tested on a bicycle ergometer. The rather low correlation observed in the remaining patients limited by fatigue (r = .61) suggests that other medical factors such as claudication or lung disease affected their performance.

As shown in Figure 3–4, below the mean gas exchange anaerobic threshold, patients with coronary artery disease are able to reach a steady state within the two-minute duration of the workstage. Above the gas exchange anaerobic threshold, steady-state oxygen uptake is not observed within a work load for the coronary patients. This figure also shows that the oxygen uptake is similar for both groups below the mean gas exchange anaerobic threshold for the coronary patients. Above their gas exchange anaerobic threshold, the measured oxygen uptake of the coronary patients falls significantly below the normal group.

Even above the mean ATGE in normals, the measured oxygen uptake values are lower than the predicted oxygen uptake derived from equations utilizing the speed and grade of the treadmill. Early research reported oxygen uptake to attain a steady-state value within two minutes. However, investigations have observed slower oxygen uptake kinetics with a steady-state value attained within 4–6 minutes. These altered oxygen uptake kinetics have been attributed to age, previous training, and the relative work load. Auchincloss et al. found lower oxygen uptake values between coronary artery disease patients and normals at the onset of exercise and attributed this difference to a decreased cardiac output in the patients. Similarly, Coyle et al. reported that patients with asymptomatic ischemia were unable to increase oxygen uptake above their lactate threshold. They attributed this to decreased ventricular function and lower cardiac output when compared to normal subjects.

The slower rate of oxygen uptake could be due to a lag in the circulatory response to the metabolic demand at the peripheral muscles. Cardiac output rather than a redistribution of blood to the exercising muscle may be the limiting factor for the delay in steady-state oxygen uptake. To test this hypothesis, a subgroup of coronary artery disease patients with LV dysfunction were compared to the remainder of the patients. There was no statistical difference in age or peak oxygen uptake between these two groups that could account for differences in oxygen uptake kinetics. At all times above the gas exchange anaerobic threshold, the mean oxygen uptake was lower in the group with poor ventricular function. However, when compared to normals above their gas exchange anaerobic threshold, even the group with better ventricular function had lower oxygen uptake values.

REPRODUCIBILITY

Sullivan et al. studied 14 male patients with exercise test-induced angina and ST-segment depression with treadmill testing on three consecutive days to evaluate the reproducibility of expired gas analysis, including anaerobic threshold. The intraclass correlation coefficient (ICC) was used, which is a

TABLE 3–4.
Standard Deviation (SD) of Change of Two Measurements
and the Coefficient of Variation (CV) at Peak Exercise and
ATGE

	PEAK EXERCISE		ATGE	
VARIABLE	SD	CV %	SD	CV %
Time, sec	58	6	65	15
		±6		±9
VO_2, L/min	.150	6	.113	7
		±4		±4

generalization of the Pearson product-moment correlation coefficient for bivariate data. An estimate of the standard deviation of the change of two measurements (SD) and the coefficient of variation for peak exercise and the ATGE variables are provided in Table 3–4. The estimates of the standard deviation of the change of two measurements is important when performing power calculations for determination of sample size and/or the required change needed in a variable to detect significance. In addition, if SD is multipled by two, the change required in an individual to have a less than 5% chance of that change being due to measurement error is obtained. In order to compare to previous studies, the coefficient of variation was determined for the variables at each point of interest.

Peak exercise results for time and oxygen uptake by the ANOVA model to detect time trends revealed no significant change during the three days of testing in any of the measured variables. Oxygen uptake had a higher reliability coefficient ($r = .88$) and a smaller 90% confidence interval when compared to time ($r = .70$) consistent with a better correlation. Also, the mean changes in time (although not significant during the three days) were greater than the mean changes for VO_2 max.

VE/VO_2 was determined each minute by averaging the two 30-second samples. Two of the three independent observers agreed on the time of the ATGE in 100% of the exercise tests. All three observers agreed on 71% (30/42) of the tests. A second independent reading to determine the ATGE by the same three observers revealed similar results with agreement by two of the three observers on 100% (42/42) and total agreement on 69% (29/42) of the tests. When comparing the first reading to the second, there was agreement on 90% (38/42) of the exercise tests. An ICC of $r = .8$ and a 90% confidence interval of .63 to .91 was obtained for the oxygen uptake at ATGE.

SUMMARY

Because of time and cost advantages as well as the reported accuracy of estimating VO_2 max, the direct measurement of gas exchange has not been recommended for general clinical application. However, the continuous acquisition of gas exchange data throughout an exercise test can provide information regarding the physiological efficiency of the heart and lungs at submaximal as well as maximal work levels. Numerous investigators have been able to successfully use gas analysis techniques to test a variety of patients with cardiac disorders. As has been discussed, these measurements permit a better assessment of interventions. Measured VO_2 is a more reproducible and accurate measurement of cardiopulmonary performance than exercise work load or treadmill time.

The anaerobic threshold may have a more important impact on an individual's tolerance to everyday activities than VO_2 max. The ability to perform higher levels of submaximal exercise without becoming anaerobic or fatiguing would be more practical than performing maximal efforts. The collection of expired gases during exercise permits an estimate of the anaerobic threshold (ATGE).

Studies involving heart disease patients have reported lower measured VO_2 values when compared to estimated values obtained from treadmill work loads and/or performance time. These lower values, possibly influenced by underlying pathology, are due to the heart patient's lower aerobic capacity and higher relative work when compared to normal subjects. Above their anaerobic threshold, cardiac patients usually are consuming one MET less than normals would at the same work load. The slower oxygen kinetics as the relative work load increases can explain the large standard error for estimating oxygen uptake from treadmill time even in healthy populations.

BIBLIOGRAPHY

Allen CJ, Jones NL, Killian KJ: Alveolar gas exchange during exercise: A single-breath analysis. *J Appl Physiol: Resp Environ Exerc Physiol* 1984;57:1704–1709.

Asana K: Relationships of anaerobic threshold and onset of blood lactate accumulation with endurance performance. *Eur J Appl Physiol* 1983;52:51–56.

Astrand PO, Rodahl K: *Textbook of Work Physiology: Physiological Basis of Exercise*. New York, McGraw Hill Book Co, 1977, pp 333–342.

Banner AS, Green J, O'Connor M: Relation of respiratory water loss to coughing after exercise. *N Engl J Med* 1984;311:883–886.

Boucher CA, Anderson MD, Schneider MS, et al: Left ventricular function before and after reaching the anaerobic threshold. *Chest* 1985;87:145–150.

Brooks GA: Anaerobic threshold: Review of the concept and directions for future research. *Med Sci Sports Exerc* 1985;17:22–31.

Bruce R, Kusumi F, Niederberger M, et al: Cardiovascular mechanisms of functional aerobic impairment in patients with coronary heart disease. *Circulation* 1974;49:696–702.

Bruce RA, Hossack KF, Kusumi F, et al: Acute effects of oral propranolol on hemodynamic responses to upright exercise. *Am J Cardiol* 1979;44:132–140.

Bruce RA, Kusumi F, Hosmer D: Maximal oxygen uptake and nomographic assessment of functional aerobic impairment in cardiovascular disease. *Am Heart J* 1973;85:546–562.

Buchfuhrer MJ, Hansen JE, Robinson TE, et al: Optimizing the exercise protocol for cardiopulmonary assessment. *J Appl Physiol* 1983;55:1558–1564.

Caiozzo VJ, Davis JA, Ellis JF, et al: A comparison of gas exchange indices used to detect the anaerobic threshold. *J Appl Physiol* 1982;53:1184–1189.

Campbell E, Jones N: *Clinical Exercise Testing*. Philadelphia, WB Saunders Co, 1975, pp 1–268.

Convertino VA, Karst GM, Kirby CR, et al: Effect of simulated weightlessness on exercise-induced anaerobic threshold. *Aviat Space Environ Med* 1986;57:325–331.

Coyle EF, Martin WH, Ehsani AA, et al: Blood lactate threshold in some well-trained ischemic heart disease patients. *J Appl Physiol* 1983;54:18–23.

Davis JA: Anaerobic threshold: Review of the concept and directions for future research. *Med Sci Sports Exerc* 1985;17:6–18.

Dempsey JA: Is the lung built for exercise? *Med Sci Sports Exerc* 1986;18:143–55.

DiPrampero PE, Davies CTM, Cerretelli P, et al: An analysis of O_2 debt contracted in submaximal exercise. *J Appl Physiol* 1970;29:547–551.

Eldridge FL, Millhorn DE, Waldrop TG: Exercise hyperpnea and locomotion: parallel activation from the hypothalamus. *Science* 1981;211:844–846.

Eldridge JE, Giansiracusa RF, Jones RH, et al: Computerized detection of the lactate threshold in coronary artery disease. *Am J Cardiol* 1986;57:1088–1091.

Eldridge JE, Green-Ramsey CL, Hossack KF: Effects of the limiting symptom on the achievement of maximal oxygen consumption in patients with coronary artery disease. *Am J Cardiol* 1986;57:513–517.

Foster C, Jackson AS, Pollock ML, et al: Generalized equations for predicting functional capacity for treadmill performance. *Am Heart J* 1984;107:1229–1234.

Froelicher VF, Allen M, Lancaster MC: Maximal treadmill testing of normal USAF aircrewmen. *Aerospace Med* 1974;45:310–315.

Froelicher VF, Brammel H, Davis G, et al: A comparison of three maximal treadmill exercise protocols. *J Appl Physiol* 1974;36:720–725.

Froelicher VF, Brammell H, Davis G, et al: A comparison of the reproducibility and physiological response to three maximal treadmill protocols. *Chest* 1974;65:512–517.

Froelicher VF, Lancaster MC: The prediction of maximal oxygen consumption from a continuous exercise treadmill protocol. *Am Heart J* 1974;87:445–450.

Froelicher VF, Thompson AJ, Noquero I, et al: Prediction of maximal oxygen consumption: Comparison of the Bruce and Balke treadmill protocols. *Chest* 1975;68:331–336.

Froelicher VF, Yanowitz F, Thompson AJ, et al: Treadmill exercise testing at the USAF School of Aerospace Medicine: Physiological responses in aircrewmen and the detection of latent coronary artery disease. AGARDOGRAPH 1975;210:1–135.

Garrard C, Emmons C: The reproducibility of the respiratory responses to maximum exercise. *Respiration* 1986;49:94–100.

Hagberg JM, Coyle EF, Carroll JE, et al: Exercise hyperventilation in patients with McArdle's disease. *J Appl Physiol* 1982;52:991–994.

Hammond HK, Froelicher VF: Exercise testing for cardiorespiratory fitness. *Sports Med* 1984;1:234–239.

Haskell WL, Savin W, Oldridge N, et al: Factors influencing estimated oxygen uptake during exercise testing soon after MI. *Am J Cardiol* 1982;50:299–304.

Hickson RC, Bomze HA, Holloxzy JO: Faster adjustment of oxygen to the energy requirement of exercise in the trained state. *J Appl Physiol* 1978;44:877.

Hollmann W: Historical remarks on the development of the aerobic-anaerobic threshold up to 1966. *Int J Sports Med* 1985;6:109–116.

Hossack KF, Bruce RA, Kusumi F: Altered exercise ventilatory responses by apparent propranolol-diminished glucose metabolism: Implications concerning impaired physical training benefit in coronary patients. *Am Heart J* 1981;102:378–382.

Hughes EF, Turnier SC, Brook GA: Effects of glycogen depletion and pedaling speed on "anaerobic threshold." *J Appl Physiol* 1982;52:1598–1607.

Hughson RL, Green HL: Blood acid-base and lactate relationships studied by ramp work tests. *Med Sci Sports Exerc* 1982;14:297–302.

Hughson RL, MacFarlane BJ: Effect of oral propranolol on the anaerobic threshold and maximum exercise performance in normal man. *Can J Physiol Pharmacol* 1981;59:567–573.

Hughson RL, Smyth GA: Slower adaptation of VO_2 to steady state of submaximal exercise with beta blockade. *Eur J Appl Physiol* 1983;52:107–110.

Jones NL: Hydrogen ion balance during exercise. *Clin Sci* 1980;59:85–91.

Jones NL: Evaluation of a microprocessor-controlled exercise testing system. *J Appl Physiol* 1984;57:1312–1318.

Kirby TE: The CO_2 rebreathing technique for determination of cardiac output: Part II. *J Cardiac Rehabil* 1985;5:132–138.

Lewis SF, Haller RG, Cook JD, et al: Metabolic control of cardiac output response to exercise in McArdle's disease. *Respirat Environ Exerc Physiol* 1984;57:153–174.

Linnarsson D, Karlsson J, Fagraeis L, et al: Muscle metabolites and oxygen deficit with exercise in hypoxia and hyperoxia. *J Appl Physiol* 1974;36:399–402.

Margaria R, Mangili F, Luttica F, et al: The kinetics of oxygen consumption at the onset of muscular exercise in man. *Ergonomics* 1965;8:49–54.

Matsumura N, Nishijima H, Kojima S, et al: Determination of anaerobic threshold for assessment of functional state in patients with chronic heart failure. *Circulation* 1983;68:360–367.

Montoye HJ, Ayen T: Body size adjustment for oxygen requirement in treadmill walking. *Res Q* 1986;57:82–84.

Okada RD, Kanarck DJ: Left ventricular function before and after reaching the anaerobic threshold. *Chest* 1985;87:145–150.

Petersen ES, Whipp BJ, Davis JA, et al: Effects of beta-adrenergic blockade on ventilation and gas exchange during exercise in humans. *J Appl Physiol* 1983;54:1306–1313.

Powers SK, Beadle RE: Onset of hyperventilation during incremental exercise: a brief review. *Res Q* 1985;56:352–360.

Ready AE, Quinney HA: Alterations in anaerobic threshold as the result of endurance training and detraining. *Med Sci Sports Exerc* 1982;14:292–296.

Reinhard V, Muller PH, Schmulling RM: Determination of anaerobic threshold by ventilation equivalent in normal individuals. *Respiration* 1979;38:36–42.

Reybruck T, Ghesquiere J: Validation and determination of the "anaerobic threshold." Letter to the editor. *J Appl Physiol* 1984;57:610–613.

Roberts JM, Sullivan M, Froelicher VF, et al: Predicting oxygen uptake from treadmill testing in normal subjects and coronary artery disease patients. *Am Heart J* 1984;108:1454–1460.

Rowell CB, Taylor HL, Wang Y: Limitations to prediction of maximal oxygen intake. *J Appl Physiol* 1964;19:919–927.

Sullivan M, Ahnve S, Froelicher VF, et al: The influence of exercise training on the ventilatory threshold of patients with coronary heart disease. *Am Heart J* 1985;109:458–463.

Sullivan M, Froelicher V: Maximal oxygen uptake and gas exchange in coronary heart disease. *J Cardiac Rehabil* 1983;3:549–560.

Sullivan MA, Genter F, Savvides M, et al: The reproducibility of hemodynamic, electrocardiographic, and gas exchange data in patients with stable angina pectoris during treadmill exercise in patients with stable angina pectoris. *Chest* 1984;86:375–382.

Sullivan MA, Savvides M, Abouantoun S, et al: Failure of transdermal nitroglycerin to improve exercise capacity in patients with angina pectoris. *J Am Coll Cardiol* 1985;5:1220–1223.

Tanaka K, Matsuura Y, Matsuzaka A, et al: A longitudinal assessment of anaerobic threshold and distance-running performance. *Med Sci Sports Exerc* 1984:16:278–282.

Tesch PA, Kaiser P: Effects of beta-adrenergic blockade on O_2 uptake during submaximal and maximal exercise. *J Appl Physiol* 1983;54:901–905.

Thews G, Thews O: Nomograms for the pulmonary gas exchange at rest and during exercise. *Int J Sports Med* 1984;5:120–124.

Twentyman OP, Disley A, Gribbin HR, et al: Effect of beta-adrenergic blockade on respiratory and metabolic responses to exercise. *J Appl Physiol* 1981;51:788–793.

Wall JL, Charles J: The process of habituation to treadmill walking at different velocities. *Ergonomics* 1980;23:425.

Wasserman K: The anaerobic threshold measurement in exercise testing. *Chest* 1984; 5:77–87.

Wasserman K, Beaver WL, Davis JA, et al: Lactate, pyruvate, and lactate-to-pyruvate ratio during exercise and recovery. *J Appl Physiol* 1985;59:935–940.

Wasserman K, Whipp BJ: Exercise physiology in health and disease. *Am Rev Resp Dis* 1975;112:219–249.

Wasserman K, Whipp S, Koyal S, et al: Anaerobic threshold and respiratory gas exchange during exercise. *J Appl Physiol* 1973;35:236–243.

Weber KT, Janicki JS: Lactate production during maximal and submaximal exercise in patients with chronic heart failure. *J Am Coll Cardiol* 1985;6:717–724.

Weber KT, Janicki JS, Likoff MJ: Exercise testing in the evaluation of cardiopulmonary disease. *Chest* 1984;5:173–179.

Weber KT, Janicki JS, Maskin CS: Effects of new inotropic agents on exercise performance. *Circulation* 1986;73:III-196–III-204.

Whipp BJ: Exercise hyperventilation in patients with McArdle's disease. Letter to the editor. *J Appl Physiol* 1983;55:1638–1639.

Wilmore JH, Ewy GA, Morton AR, et al: The effect of beta-adrenergic blockade on submaximal and maximal exercise performance. *J Cardiac Rehabil* 1983;3:30–36.

Wilson JR, Ferraro N, Weber KT: Respiratory gas analysis during exercise as a noninvasive measure of lactate concentration in chronic congestive heart failure. *Am J Cardiol* 1983;51:1639–1643.

Withers RT, Sherman WM, Miller JM, et al: Specificity of the anaerobic threshold in endurance trained cyclists and runners. *Eur J Appl Physiol* 1981;47:93–104.

Wolthuis R, Froelicher VF, Fischer J, et al: New practical treadmill protocol for clinical use. *Am J Cardiol* 1977;39:697–700.

Wolthuis R, Froelicher VF, Fischer J, et al: The response of healthy men to maximal treadmill exercise. *Circulation* 1977;55:153–157.

Yeh M, Gardner R, Adams T, et al: "Anaerobic threshold": Problems of determination and validation. *J Appl Exerc Physiol* 1983;55:1178–1186.

4 INTERPRETATION OF SPECIFIC EXERCISE TEST RESPONSES

When interpreting the exercise test, it is important to consider each of its responses separately. Each type of response has a different impact on making a diagnostic or a clinical decision and must be considered along with the clinical information. A test should not be called abnormal (or positive) or normal (or negative); rather, the interpretation should specify which responses were abnormal or normal. Neither should the results be called subjectively or objectively positive or negative, but the particular responses should be recorded. The objective responses to exercise testing (exercise capacity, heart rate, blood pressure, electrocardiographic changes, and dysrhythmias) and subjective responses (patient appearance, the results of physical examination and symptoms, particularly angina) require interpretation and will be discussed below. As for the interpretation of all tests, the written summary should be directed to the physician who ordered the test and who will receive the report. It should contain information that helps in patient management and not vague "Med-speak." Interpretation depends on the application for which the test is used and on the population tested; this chapter is only a preparation for information available in later chapters.

EXERCISE CAPACITY OR FUNCTIONAL CAPACITY

Maximal oxygen uptake (VO_2 max) is the greatest amount of oxygen that a person can extract from inspired air while performing dynamic exercise requiring a large part of the total muscle mass. Since maximal oxygen uptake is equal to the product of cardiac output and arterial venous oxygen difference, it is a measure of the functional limits of the cardiovascular system. Maximal arterial venous oxygen difference is physiologically limited to 15 to 17 vol%. Thus, maximal AV O_2 difference behaves as a constant, making maximal oxygen uptake an indirect estimate of maximal cardiac output. Maximal oxygen uptake is dependent on many factors, including natural physical endowment, activity status, age, and sex, but it is the best index of exercise capacity and maximal cardiovascular function. The maximal oxygen uptake of the normal sedentary individual is approximately 30 ml O_2/kg/min and the minimal level for physical fitness is 40 ml O_2/kg/min. Aerobic training can increase maximal oxygen uptake by approximately 25%. This increase is dependent on the initial level of fitness and the age of the trainee, as well as the intensity, frequency, and length of training sessions. Individuals performing aerobic training such as distance running can have maximal oxygen uptakes as high as 60 to 90 ml O_2/kg/min. A mongrel dog easily exceeds these values, however. There is some convenience in measuring oxygen consumption in multiples of basal resting requirements. The MET is a unit of basal oxygen consumption or approximately 3.5 ml O_2/kg/min. This value is the oxygen requirement to maintain life in the resting state.

Figure 4–1 illustrates the relationship of maximal oxygen uptake to exercise habits and age. Though the three activity levels have regression lines that appropriately fit the data, there is much scatter around the lines and the correlation coefficients are poor. This finding demonstrates the inaccuracy involved with trying to predict maximal oxygen uptake from age and habitual physical activity. It is preferable to estimate an individual's maximal oxygen uptake from the work load reached while performing a treadmill test. This avoids the problem of comparing the same time performed on different treadmill protocols and of assuming that the same work load has been performed.

Patterson and colleagues studied 43 patients with cardiac disease and compared their functional classification by maximal oxygen uptake and by clinical assessment. When a discrepancy occurred, the hemodynamic data from cardiac catheterization usually indicated that maximal oxygen uptake more accurately reflected the degree of impairment. Patients began to experience limiting symptoms when maximal oxygen uptake was less than 22 ml O_2/kg/min (6 METs) and considered themselves severely limited when maximal oxygen uptake was 16 ml O_2/kg/min (4 METs) or less. When a patient's exercise

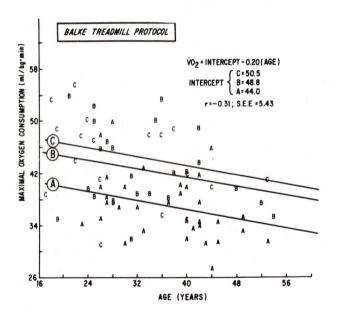

FIG 4–1.
Relationship of VO_2 max to current exercise status and age.

TABLE 4–1.
Activities That Correspond to Classes I to IV of the Specific Activity Scale (SAS)

Class I (≥ 7 METs)	A patient can perform any of the following activities: Carrying 24 pounds up eight steps Carrying an 80-pound object Shoveling snow Skiing Playing basketball, touch football, squash, or handball Jogging/walking 5 mph
Class II (≥ 5 METs)	A patient does not meet class I criteria but can perform any of the following activities to completion without stopping: Carrying anything up eight steps Having sexual intercourse Gardening, raking, weeding Walking 4 mph
Class III (≥ 2 METs)	A patient does not meet class I or class II criteria but can perform any of the following activities to completion without stopping: Walking down eight steps Taking a shower Changing bed sheets Mopping floors, cleaning windows Walking 2.5 mph Pushing a power mower Bowling Dressing without stopping
Class IV (≤ 2 METs)	None of the above

capacity is estimated from testing at less than 4 METs, prognosis is guarded. When technologic advances make the measurement of maximal oxygen uptake and even noninvasive measurement of cardiac output convenient and practical, it should be possible to determine limits, or discriminant values, for these measurements depending on age, activity status, and sex.

Functional classifications have been found to be too limited and poorly reproducible. One problem is that "usual activities" can decrease so that an individual can become greatly limited without having a change in functional class. A better approach is to use the specific activity scale (SAS) of Goldman shown in Table 4–1 or to question a patient regarding usual activities that have a known MET cost. Exercise testing to objectively determine exercise capacity is now usually used for determining disability rather than relying on functional classifications.

TREADMILL PERFORMANCE
AND CARDIAC FUNCTION

Exercise capacity determined by exercise testing has been proposed as a means to estimate ventricular function. A direct relationship appears to be supported by the fact that both resting ejection fraction and exercise capacity have prognostic value in patients with coronary heart disease. However, a marked discrepancy between resting ventricular function and exercise performance is frequently seen clinically. Additionally, exercise capacity is not determined by ventricular function in patients with cardiomyopathies. Exercise-induced ischemia could limit exercise in spite of normal resting ventricular function, and so patients with angina must be excluded and silent ischemia considered when evaluating an interaction.

We (McKirnan et al.) investigated the relationship between resting ventricular function and exercise performance in patients with a wide range of resting EF able to exercise to volitional fatigue. Radionuclide measurements of left ventricular perfusion and EF were compared with treadmill responses in 88 coronary heart disease patients free of angina pectoris. The exercise tests included supine bike radionuclide ventriculography, thallium scintigraphy, and treadmill testing with expired gas analysis. The number of abnormal Q-wave locations, EF, end-diastolic volume, cardiac output, exercise-induced ST-segment depression and thallium scar and ischemia scores were considered. Resting and exercise ejection fraction was highly correlated to thallium scar score but not to maximal oxygen consumption. Fifty-five percent of the variability in predicting treadmill time or estimated maximal oxygen consumption was explained by treadmill test-induced change in heart rate (39%), thallium ischemia score (12%), and resting cardiac output (4%). The change in heart rate induced by the treadmill test explained only 27% of the variability in measured maximal oxygen consumption. Myocardial damage predicted resting ejection fraction, and the ability to increase heart rate with treadmill exercise appeared as an essential component of exercise capacity. Exercise capacity and VO_2 max were only minimally affected by asymptomatic ischemia and were relatively independent of ventricular function.

Both estimated and measured VO_2 max correlated significantly with maximal heart rate, maximal rate pressure product, the change from rest to maximal for both heart rate and rate pressure product, resting ejection fraction, and maximal cardiac output ($P < .05$). A plot of resting ejection fraction versus measured maximal oxygen consumption is shown in Figure 4–2. This relationship was not improved by excluding patients with a respiratory quotient less than 1.1 or with a perceived exertion less than 17. Maximal ejection fraction, maximal end-diastolic volume, and thallium ischemia were significantly correlated with estimated VO_2 max alone ($p < .05$). In general, these correlations were somewhat higher for estimated than for measured VO_2 max. Resting ejection fraction correlated negatively with the sum of Q-wave areas on the resting electrocardiogram ($r = -.40$, $p < .01$) and thallium scar score ($r = -.72$, $p < .001$). Change in ejection fraction poorly correlated with the amount of ST-segment depression and thallium ischemia score.

A stepwise linear regression analysis was performed to predict (1) resting ejection fraction, (2) maximal treadmill time (estimated VO_2 max), and (3) measured VO_2 max. Parameters were divided into two categories: (1) central cardiac parameters that more specifically describe function, damage, and ischemia of the myocardium, and, (2) hemodynamic parameters routinely obtained during treadmill testing. For cardiac parameters, the thallium scar score explained most of the variability in resting ejection fraction (44%) with

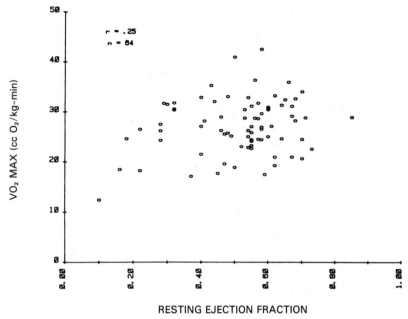

FIG 4–2.
Resting EF plotted against measured VO$_2$ max in a group of patients with coronary heart disease but not limited by angina.

ST depression laterally adding 6%. When treadmill parameters were added to the analysis, no real improvement in predictive power was obtained, but the same cardiac parameters explained slightly more of the variability in resting EF (56%). When treadmill parameters were considered alone, change in rate pressure product was selected first and could explain only 6% of the variability in resting ejection fraction.

When using cardiac parameters to predict treadmill time or VO$_2$ max, thallium ischemia, resting cardiac output, and maximal end-diastolic volume were chosen sequentially and combined to explain 19% of the variability. When these patients were separated into those with normal and those with abnormal resting ejection fraction (.50 being the discriminant value), predictive variables changed but no real improvement in explaining the variability in estimated VO$_2$ max was achieved. When treadmill parameters were added, the change in heart rate during treadmill exercise entered first, explaining 39% of the variability, followed by the thallium ischemia score (51%), and resting cardiac output (4%) to account for 55% of the variability in estimated VO$_2$ max or treadmill time. Separating patients by normal and abnormal resting ejection fraction did not improve the prediction. When treadmill parameters alone were considered, the change in heart rate with exercise alone explained 38% of the variability in the relationship with treadmill time or estimated VO$_2$ max. Change in heart rate explained 32% and 39% of the variability in estimated VO$_2$ max for patients with normal and abnormal resting ejection fraction, respectively.

The relationship between myocardial damage, ventricular function, and exercise capacity are poorly understood. Pfeffer and colleagues reported that ventricular performance was directly related to the amount of myocardium remaining after causing myocardial infarctions in rats. However, rats with smaller infarctions (4% to 30% of the left ventricle) had no discernable impairment in either baseline hemodynamics or peak indices of pumping and pressure generating ability when compared to sham-operated controls. This suggests that considerable damage to the left ventricle can occur before pump performance or oxygen transport are effected.

Carter and Amundsen reported a significant correlation ($r = .68$) between infarct size estimated from serum creatinine phosphokinase and exercise capacity at approximately three months post MI. This relationship improved ($r = .84$) after exercise training, implying that infarct size affects the response to training. In contrast, Grande and Pedersen reported an insignificant correlation between the enzyme estimate of infarct size and duration of work ($r = -.15$) performed in a progressive steady state protocol within two months post infarct. They observed significant correlations between infarct size and maximal heart rate ($r = .39$), maximal SBP ($r = -.32$), the increases in both SBP ($r = -.46$), and heart rate ($r = .39$) from rest to 100 watts. In our study, the thallium scar score, an estimate of myocardial damage, was not significantly correlated with VO_2 max or change in heart rate. However, there was a significant, negative correlation with maximal SBP, rate pressure product and change in rate pressure product from rest to maximal exercise.

DePace and colleagues studied resting left ventricular function, thallium-201 scintigraphy, and a QRS scoring scheme in myocardial infarction patients. For patients with prior MI, significant correlations between resting EF and QRS score ($r = -.51$) and between resting EF and thallium score ($r = .61$) were similar to the values for Q-wave areas ($r = -.40$) and thallium scar score ($r = -.72$) we obtained. Thallium score correlated poorly with QRS score in their study, but Q-wave sum was significantly correlated to thallium scar in our study ($r = .48$). A thallium defect has been correlated with pathological determination of infarct size and with the extent of asynergy obtained by contrast angiography. The thallium scar score was highly correlated to and predictive of resting ejection fraction. However, both parameters had poor correlations with exercise capacity. This implies that cardiac function only has a minor impact on determining VO_2 max.

Weber et al. classified 62 patients with chronic stable CHF into functional classes based on VO_2 max. Pulmonary capillary wedge pressure and direct Fick measurements of cardiac output were made at rest and during upright exercise. The most limited patients increased cardiac output by heart rate alone and had lower maximal heart rates, oxygen pulses, and changes in oxygen pulse from rest to maximal exercise. Patients were symptom-limited by exercise cardiac output rather than high filling pressures. These findings were supported by those of Litchfield and colleagues in six patients with severe ventricular dysfunction. A normal exercise capacity was achieved by increasing both heart rate and stroke volume and tolerating a high filling pressure during upright exercise. Other compensatory mechanisms included an increase in end-diastolic volume and elevated circulating catecholamines. Higginbotham et al. also examined determinants of upright exercise performance in 12 patients with severe left ventricular dysfunction using radionuclide angiography and invasive measurements. Multivariate analysis identified changes in heart rate, cardiac output, and AV O_2 difference with exercise as important predictors of VO_2 max. The resting ejection fraction did not correlate with VO_2 max nor did changes in ejection fraction, stroke counts or end-diastolic counts during exercise. These results are similar to our findings, but our study included coronary patients with a wide range of ejection fractions.

Increasing heart rate was the most important determinant to treadmill performance. Radionuclide techniques offered little to explain the variability in exercise capacity. This may be due to differences in posture for the two exercise studies. The change in ejection fraction from rest to maximal supine exercise had no predictive power, probably because of the complex nature of this response.

Adaptations in anaerobic metabolism may contribute to the poor ability of cardiac and treadmill parameters to predict measured and estimated VO_2 max. However, differences in AV O_2 difference may more simply explain our findings. The fact that patients with severely limited ventricular function can improve their exercise capacity without altering resting ventricular function provides further evidence for the poor relationship between resting ventricular function and exercise capacity. We can even hypothesize that exercise training could be used to increase exercise capacity and decrease the poor prognosis predicted by cardiac dysfunction.

In patients with a wide range of ejection fractions and without angina or pulmonary disease, ventricular function is only a weak determinant of exercise capacity. Patients were selected who were able to exercise to volitional fatigue since this relationship should be the strongest in them. Even in this select group, the relationship between ejection fraction and treadmill performance was poor. However, it would have been even poorer in an exercise laboratory when not as much concern would be given to seeing that volitional fatigue was the major endpoint or that the patients did not support themselves on the handrails. This concurs with the clinical impression that good ventricular function does not guarantee normal exercise capacity or vice versa. Even in patients free of angina, exercise limitations or expectations should not be determined by ejection fraction but rather by the patients' symptomatic response to exercise.

Ehsani et al. published a study similar to ours. Extensive measurements of systolic ventricular function were considered, but all of these were found not to predict maximal oxygen uptake. Resting ejection fraction did not correlate with maximal oxygen uptake, and there was weak correlation with peak exercise ejection fraction and maximal oxygen uptake. However, they did find that the change in ejection fraction from rest to maximal exercise correlated with maximal oxygen uptake ($r = .77$) and maximal heart rate ($r = .61$). Their patient population included only 27 asymptomatic patients with coronary artery disease able to perform maximal exercise. Their criteria and methodology are similar. Like Ehsani et al., we found that resting and exercise ejection fraction were not highly correlated with maximal oxygen consumption. In contrast, we also found that the change in ejection fraction did not correlate with estimated or measured oxygen consumption. We found maximal heart rate to correlate with maximal oxygen consumption. It is not clear why our groups have demonstrated different findings in regard to the change in ejection fraction. One difference between the studies is that none of our patients were taking beta blockers, while 18 of their patients were and the EF response to exercise can be normalized by beta blockers. The reproducibility of the exercise-induced change in EF over one year is very poor, and it does not correlate with other markers of ischemia. Both studies indicated that chronotropic incompetence is a significant factor in determining maximal oxygen uptake but considerable variability in maximal oxygen uptake remains unexplained. The importance of ventricular function in determining maximal oxygen uptake is far from resolved.

Maximal Cardiac Output.   There is a wide biologic scatter of maximal cardiac output and VO_2 max in healthy persons even when age, sex, and activity status are considered. Because both maximal cardiac output and maximal oxygen uptake decline with age, the effects of age and disease are usually difficult to separate. McDonough and colleagues measured maximal cardiac output in cardiac patients and found a decline in maximal cardiac output to be the major hemodynamic consequence of symptomatic coronary artery disease and one that resulted in functional impairment. Acute reduction in left ventricle performance, manifested by decreasing stroke volume and increasing pulmonary artery pressure, appeared to be the mechanism limiting cardiac output. As in other studies, maximal oxygen uptake was linearly related to maximal cardiac output. Hossack and colleagues measured cardiac output during treadmill exercise in 10 normal men and 77 patients with coronary heart disease using invasive techniques. These data were used to estimate limits of maximal cardiac output and stroke volume in normal subjects, and these normal standards were then used to evaluate the results in the patients. Patients with an ejection fraction of less than 50% had significantly impaired age-adjusted cardiac output and stroke volume.

MAXIMAL HEART RATE

Methods of Recording.   Although measuring a patient's maximal heart rate (HRmax) should be a simple matter, the different ways of recording rate and differences in the type of exercise used may affect its measurement. The best way is to use a standard ECG recorder and use the R-R intervals to calculate instantaneous heart rate. ECG paper speed must be calibrated regularly. Methods using the arterial pulse or capillary blush technique are much more affected by artifact than electrocardiographic techniques. Some investigators have used averaging over the last minute of exercise or in immediate recovery; both methods are inaccurate. Heart rate drops quickly in recovery and can be climbing steeply even in the last seconds of exercise. Premature beats can affect averaging and must be eliminated in order to obtain the actual heart rate. We prefer using the shortest three R-R intervals between the usual ECG complexes during the last 20 seconds of exercise for the maximal heart rate. In patients with atrial fibrillation, the QRS complexes occurring in 10 or 20 seconds are usually counted and multiplied by 6 or 3 to obtain the ventricular rate. Cardiotachometers are available but may fail to trigger or may trigger inappropriately on T-waves, artifact, or aberrant beats, thus yielding inaccurate results. Cardiotachometers have not been demonstrated to have the accuracy of the ECG paper technique.

Measures of Maximal Effort. Various objective measurements have been used to confirm that a maximal effort was performed. As maximal aerobic capacity is reached, the rate of oxygen consumption should plateau; increased work loads beyond this point should not result in further increases in oxygen consumed. Using gas analysis, Taylor has suggested that an RQ greater than 1.15 or a decrease in oxygen uptake or failure to increase oxygen uptake by 150 cc/min with increased work loads marks the "plateau" and should accurately reflect maximal oxygen uptake when using interrupted protocols. However, this plateau is infrequently seen in continuous treadmill protocols in our experience and may actually be due to holding on or incomplete expired air collection. This depends upon the sampling interval and the equipment utilized.

The Borg scale has been developed to subjectively grade levels of exertion. This method is best applied to match levels of perceived exertion during comparison studies. The linear scale ranges from 6 (very, very light) to 20 (very, very hard); the nonlinear scale ranges from 0 to 10, and both correlate with the percent of maximal HR being performed. Respiratory quotient, the ratio of carbon dioxide production to oxygen utilization, increases in proportion to exercise effort. Values of 1.15 are reached by most individuals at the point of maximal dynamic exercise. This requires gas exchange analysis during exercise. Lactic acid levels have been used but accurate measurements require mixed venous samples.

Type of Dynamic Exercise. Although steps, escalators, ladders and other devices are used, the three predominant types of exercise testing used clinically are treadmill and supine or upright bicycle ergometry. Position and type of exercise influences the heart rate responses.

Astrand and Saltin studied maximal oxygen uptake and heart rate in seven trained individuals using an upright bicycle ergometer and a treadmill. The bicycle was pedalled at a frequency of 50 rpm. Treadmill exercise yielded a mean maximal oxygen uptake 5% higher (p = .05) than that measured on the bicycle ergometer, but there was no difference in maximal heart rate. Hermansen and Saltin studied 55 trained men and demonstrated a 7% higher (p < .001) value on the treadmill running uphill than on the bicycle (50 rpm). However, the individual variation was large and the difference in oxygen consumption between treadmill and bike varied from +18.7% to −3.9%. There was no significant difference between the corresponding mean values for ex-

pired air volume, heart rate, and blood lactate level. Heart rate, minute ventilation, and blood lactate at submaximal levels were higher on the bike compared to the treadmill at the same oxygen consumption. There was an optimal
relationship between energy expenditure and the pedal or step frequency for
developing maximal oxygen consumption and, to ensure the highest possible
oxygen uptake, the treadmill inclination should be three degrees or more and
the pedalling frequency from 60 to 70 rpm.

Supine bicycle ergometry is used for radionuclide studies or for cardiac
catheterization studies. Due to changes in venous return and filling pressures,
the supine position results in lower resting heart rate and higher end-diastolic
volumes. As exercise begins, there is little change in stroke volume or end-
diastolic volume when compared to values obtained at rest. Because of the
unusual position and positional disadvantage, there usually is an element of
isometric exercise and a lower mechanical efficiency in the supine position.
In general, patients are not as able to give maximal efforts in the supine position; the HRmax is usually significantly lower while SBP is higher. Patients
with significant coronary heart disease may develop angina at a lower double
product in the supine than in the upright position which also contributes to
lower maximal heart rates.

Factors Limiting Maximal Heart Rate.   Several factors may
affect the HRmax during dynamic exercise (Table 4–2). Maximal heart rate
declines with advancing years, and possibly is affected by gender. Height,
weight, and even lean body weight apparently are not independent factors
affecting maximal heart rate. Sheffield and colleagues treadmill tested 100
asymptomatic females 19–69 years old, and concluded that the regression of
maximal heart rate on age in women was different than men, being about 5
beats/min lower. Some investigators report a substantial decrease in maximal
heart rates in well-trained athletes. Perhaps blood volume changes and cardiac hypertrophy can explain this. However, this has not been a consistent
finding. A group of elite marathon runners underwent maximal exercise testing and were found to have similar maximal heart rates to age-matched sedentary controls. While this point remains unsettled, it is possible that training
in early life may result in cardiac hypertrophy and/or dilation. Perhaps cardiac dimensions determine the maximal heart rate in individuals with a
healthy sinus node.

Altitude may affect the heart rate response to exercise. At sea level, atropine
administration does not impair maximal heart rate, implying the parasympathetic withdrawal is complete at maximal exercise. Astrand demonstrated,

TABLE 4–2.
Factors Influencing the Maximal Heart Rate

Age	Bed rest
Sex	Altitude
Level of fitness	Type of exercise
Cardiovascular	Method of recording
disease	True maximal exertion

however, that maximal heart rate decreases after prolonged exposure to hypoxia. Cunningham and colleagues have shown that catecholamine levels are elevated in plasma and urine at high altitudes. Hartly and coworkers examined maximal heart rate before and after the administration of atropine in five normal untrained men who lived at sea level all of their lives. The subjects were studied with bicycle ergometry at sea level and at 15,000-feet altitude. The maximal heart rates decreased a mean of 24 beats/min, and the maximal oxygen uptake decreased 26% at this altitude. Atropine administration did not affect HRmax at sea level but significantly increased HRmax at high altitude (165 to 176 beats/min). At high altitude, there is an increased parasympathetic tone at maximal exercise. This may be secondary to increased sympathetic tone and the baroreceptor reflex. Mean HRmax did not increase with the administration of supplemental oxygen so the impaired heart rate response was not due to hypoxia alone.

A major factor determining maximal exercise heart rate is motivation to exert oneself maximally. Older patients may be restrained by poor muscle tone, pulmonary disease, claudication, orthopedic problems, and other non-cardiac causes of limitation. The usual decline in HRmax with age is not as steep in people who are free from myocardial disease and stay active, but it still occurs.

Many studies have reported HRmax during treadmill testing in a variety of patients. Regressions with age have varied depending on the population studied and other factors. Table 4–3 and Figure 4–3 summarize these studies and are self-explanatory. Some of the major studies will be discussed.

Bruce and colleagues attempted to separate the effects of aging from the effects of cardiovascular disease on HRmax by analyzing their data on over 2,000 healthy middle-aged men and subgroups of over 2,000 ambulatory male patients with hypertension, coronary heart disease, or both. All men were given maximal treadmill tests, and the data from each subgroup was regressed on age and compared. Any substantial difference in slope would imply that disease, independently from age, influenced maximal heart rates. Bruce found an age-related decline in all groups with correlation coefficients ranging from −.3 to −.5. Applying the derived equations for a 50-year-old man would yield an estimated maximal heart rate of 177 for healthy men, 168 for hypertensives, and 151 beats/min for those with coronary heart disease.

Cooper and associates examined the maximal heart rate response to treadmill testing in over 2,500 men ranging in age from 10 to 80 years old with a mean of 43. Patients with abnormal resting electrocardiograms and those unable to give a maximal effort were eliminated from the study. Levels of cardiovascular fitness were determined by age-adjusted treadmill times using the Balke-Ware protocol; subjects were grouped into below average, above average, or average based on their results. Although their population as a whole showed a regression line with a slope similar to other studies, the data based on cardiovascular fitness showed significantly different slopes. These data suggest that those with less cardiovascular fitness achieve lower maximal heart rates and that these differences are more divergent at older ages. Those

TABLE 4–3.
Studies Evaluating the Relationship of Age to Maximal Exercise Heart Rate

STUDY	N	POPULATION STUDIED	MEAN AGE (SD OR RANGE)	MEAN HRMAX (SD)	REGRESSION LINE	CORRELATION COEFFICIENT	STANDARD ERROR OF THE ESTIMATE (BEATS/MIN)
Astrand*	100	Asymptomatic men	50 (20–69)	166 ± 20	Y = 211–.922(age)	NA	NA
Bruce	2,091	Asymptomatic men	44 ± 8	181 ± 12	Y = 210–.662(age)	–.44	14
Cooper	2,535	Asymptomatic men	43 (11–79)	181 ± 16	Y = 217–.845(age)	NA	NA
Ellestad†	2,583	Asymptomatic men	42 ± 7 (10–60)	173 ± 11	Y = 197–.556(age)	NA	NA
Froelicher	1,317	Asymptomatic men	38 ± 8 (28–54)	183	Y = 207–.64(age)	–.43	10
Lester	148	Asymptomatic men	43 (15–75)	187	Y = 205–.411(age)	–.58	NA
Robinson	92	Asymptomatic men	30 (6–76)	189	Y = 212–.775(age)	NA	NA
Sheffield	95	Men with coronary heart disease	39 (19–69)	176 ± 14	Y = 216–.88(age)	–.58	11‡
Bruce	1,295	Men with coronary heart disease	52 ± 8	148 ± 23	Y = 204–1.07(age)	–.36	25‡
Hammond	156	Men with coronary heart disease	53 ± 9	157 ± 20	Y = 209–1.0(age)	–.30	19

*Astrand used bicycle ergometry; all other studies performed on treadmill.
†Data compiled from graphs in reference cited.
‡Calculated from available data.
HRmax = maximal heart rate.
NA = not able to calculate from available data.

who are cardiovascularly fit tend to show less rapid declines in their maximal heart rates with age.

In an effort to clarify the relationship between maximal heart rate and age, Londeree and Moeschberger performed a comprehensive review of the literature compiling over 23,000 subjects aged 5 to 81 years. A stepwise multiple regression revealed that age alone accounted for 75% of the variability; other factors added only about 5% and included mode of exercise, level of fitness, and continent of origin but not sex. The 95% confidence interval, even when accounting for these factors, was 45 beats per minute (Fig 4–4). Heart rates at maximal exercise were lower on bicycle ergometry than treadmill and lower still with swimming. Their analysis revealed that trained individuals had a significant lowering of maximal heart rates.

Kostis and coworkers examined the relationships of maximal heart rates during exercise testing to the heart rate during the activities of daily living. Ninety-four men aged 16–65 who had been evaluated for chest pain with angiography and noninvasive testing and found to have no evidence of coronary or valvular heart disease were used in this study. All participants were studied by 24-hour ambulatory monitoring during normal daily activities and by a maximal treadmill test. A decline in maximal heart rate obtained during exercise with age was observed; the slope of this decline was similar to that observed in other studies. The slope of the decay of exercise maximal heart rate with age was similar to the slope of the decay of the intrinsic heart rate with age as reported by Jose and Taylor. A similar slope was also seen with the maximal heart rates observed during ambulatory monitoring. The minimal heart rates recorded by ambulatory monitoring were not age related and generally occurred at night when the subjects were sleeping.

At USAFSAM, we compared the cardiovascular responses to maximal treadmill testing using three different popular treadmill protocols to evaluate reproducibility among tests. The Bruce, Balke, and Taylor protocols were used in the evaluation of 15 healthy men. Each man performed one test per week for nine weeks, repeating each protocol three times in randomized order. The maximal heart rates achieved were reproducible within each protocol, and there were no significant differences in heart rate achieved among

FIG 4–3.

Plots of regression lines from the studies of maximal heart rate. See Table 4–3 for additional details.

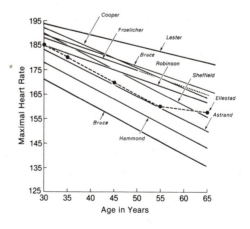

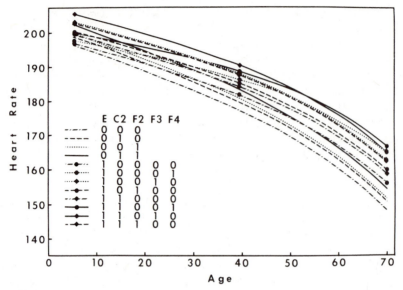

FIG 4–4.
Plots from literature review of studies involving multiple different types of dynamic exercise by Londeree and Moeschberger. Under E (ergometer), 0 = bicycle and 1 = treadmill; under C2 (European), F2 (sedentary), F3 (active), and F4 (endurance trained), 1 = class inclusion (i.e., a member of that category) and 0 = class exclusion.

the three protocols. Also, larger numbers of normals were studied as shown in Figure 4–5, which also shows the wide scatter.

Another factor that affects maximal heart rate and is important to clinical medicine is bed rest. Convertino and colleagues examined the cardiovascular responses to maximal exercise in normal man following 10 days of bed rest. A significant increase in HRmax was found following bed rest when compared to tests made before bed rest. It was suggested that lack of gravitational forces on baroreceptor mechanisms may have played a role in this accentuated heart rate response. Measurements of VO_2 max in both supine and upright positions revealed lower values with upright exercise. Oxygen consumption during maximal supine exercise was not impaired compared to measurements made before bed rest. Since maximal heart rates increased significantly but VO_2 max decreased, changes in heart volume are likely involved and may reflect changes in plasma volume during prolonged bed rest.

A consistent finding in population studies has been a relatively poor relationship of maximal heart rate to age. Correlation coefficients of $-.4$ are usually found with a standard error of the estimate of 10–25 beats/min. In general, this has not been "tightened" by considering activity status, weight, maximal respiratory quotient, or perceived exertion. An exercise program most likely has divergent effects on this relationship at the extremes of ages. Younger people may be able to achieve larger changes in cardiac dimensions than older people. This may affect maximal heart rate. Older individuals achieve a large learning effect whereby they are less afraid to give maximal effort and achieve higher HRmax on later testing when they are less apprehensive. Indiscriminant use of age-predicted maximal heart rate in making exercise prescriptions or in setting goals for treadmill performance should be avoided.

The physiological limits on maximal heart rate in normal people are determined by rapidity of sinus node recovery, cardiac dimensions, left ventricular filling, and contractile state. Systole has a relatively fixed time interval; when heart rate increases, relatively less time of the cardiac cycle is spent in diastole. It seems logical that a limit would be approached where an increase in heart rate would not effectively increase cardiac output due to decreased diastolic filling; not only would the heart receive less blood to pump thereby imposing mechanical limitations, but the degree of coronary artery perfusion would decrease, imposing metabolic constraints. Although this theoretical limitation is reasonable, there is little experimental work to support it. Astrand demonstrated no decrease in stroke volume in healthy exercising men as they approached maximal heart rates during treadmill exercise.

CHRONOTROPIC INCOMPETENCE (CI) OR HEART RATE IMPAIRMENT (HRI)

Ellestad and Wan analyzed the results from 2,700 patients tested in their treadmill laboratory, and defined a group below the 95% confidence limit for maximal heart rate regressed on age, as having "chronotropic incompetence."

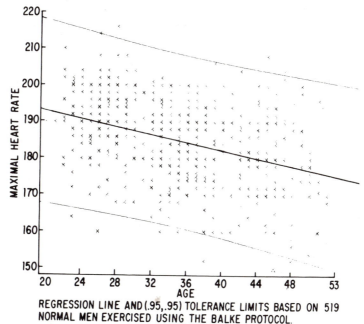

REGRESSION LINE AND (.95,.95) TOLERANCE LIMITS BASED ON 519 NORMAL MEN EXERCISED USING THE BALKE PROTOCOL.

FIG 4–5.
USAFSAM study of healthy pilots showing each individual's data point and illustrating the normal scatter.

Patients with no ST-segment depression who had CI had a four times greater incidence of coronary events than did those without CI in the four years after the test. The age-adjusted heart rate limits used for their study were published in Ellestad's text.

In a similar follow-up study of 1,500 patients who underwent angiography and treadmill testing, McNeer et al. found that those with a maximal exercise heart rate less than 120 beats/min had a 60% survival rate at four years versus a 90% survival in those who exceeded a maximal heart rate of 160 beats/min. Bruce et al. followed 2,000 clinically healthy men after screening them with treadmill testing and found that the inability to achieve a maximal heart rate 90% of that predicted for age had a four times increased risk for coronary events after five years. Chin et al. reported the only invasive hemodynamic study of patients with CI. They demonstrated a greater prevalence of three-vessel disease in patients with CI and ST-segment depression than in those with ST-depression and a normal heart rate response.

None of these studies considered the prevalence of exercise test-induced angina or evaluated other factors in their patients with CI. From previous studies of normal subjects and in evaluating patients with coronary heart disease, we have noted no distinguishing features in those with heart rate impairment. Therefore, Hammond et al. initiated a study to better characterize patients with CI.

Our patients represented a cross-section of persons with coronary heart disease, including those who had a myocardial infarction and coronary artery bypass surgery or angina pectoris, or both. Because our definition of CI required that patients have an impaired heart rate on two separate tests, our sample group was more rigidly defined than in previous studies. Patients who met the criteria for chronotropic incompetence had both a significantly lesser prevalence of bypass surgery and a greater prevalence of exercise-induced angina than did the other patients. It appears that the limited maximal heart rates were due to angina-limited effort; it also appeared that patients who had bypass surgery did not have as much heart rate impairment. Because of these differences, the 156 men were divided into subgroups based on whether or not they had angina and coronary bypass surgery. The mean heart rate of our patients with CI at a submaximal work load (5% grade) was significantly lower than that of the other patients except for those in the angina group (Table 4–4 and Fig 4–6).

This finding is in agreement with the data of Chin et al.; rate-pressure product, an estimate of myocardial oxygen consumption, was significantly lower in those patients with CI. There was a lower mean maximal oxygen consumption in all of the patients with CI except for the surgical bypass group. This demonstrates that patients with CI are functionally impaired. This difference retained significance in the group without angina and, therefore, symptom limitation is not the only explanation. Although peripheral adaptations are thought to be contributory to widening the arteriovenous oxygen difference in trained athletes, patients that are so quickly limited by their cardiovascular systems are not likely to benefit by this adaptation. Thus, the differences in maximal oxygen consumption must be due to the heart rate or the stroke vol-

TABLE 4–4.
Results of the Radionuclide Rest and Exercise Studies of the Five Study Groups Classified Into Those With Chronotropic Incompetence and Those With a Normal Heart Rate Response to Exercise

	ALL PATIENTS (n = 156)		NO ANGINA (n = 103)		ANGINA (n = 53)		BYPASS SURGERY (n = 58)		NO BYPASS (n = 98)	
	CI (n = 19)	NL (n = 137)	CI (n = 14)	NL (n = 89)	CI (n = 8)	NL (n = 45)	CI (n = 8)	NL (n = 50)	CI (n = 15)	NL (n = 83)
EDV (ml)	135 ± 80	132 ± 56	152 ± 66	130 ± 52	94 ± 35	136 ± 70	165 ± 84	112 ± 35	152 ± 86	137 ± 60
Rest Exer.	144 ± 66	154 ± 64	176 ± 52	151 ± 66	107 ± 43	160 ± 63	193 ± 84	125 ± 58†	157 ± 68	164 ± 60
EF at rest (%)	59 ± 14	52 ± 14	49 ± 18	52 ± 15	64 ± 8	53 ± 13*	49 ± 14	53 ± 14	57 ± 15	52 ± 15
EF at rest ≥ 50% (% patients)	83	66	57	66	100	68	63	67	79	66
ΔEF ≥ 10% with exer. (% patients)	17	33	36	36	14	24	13	39	21	30
Q max exer. (L/min)	8.5 ± 3.4	10.5 ± 4.0	9.7 ± 3.4	10.3 ± 3.6	6.7 ± 2.3	11.1 ± 4.6*	9.8 ± 4.6	9.0 ± 3.4	8.9 ± 3.4	11.2 ± 4.0
Thallium ischemia score	4.1 ± 4.2	3.4 ± 4.2	4.1 ± 5.5	2.6 ± 3.6	4.3 ± 5.6	5.1 ± 4.3	3.0 ± 4.2	2.1 ± 3.0	3.6 ± 4.3	4.4 ± 4.7
Thallium scar score	10.9 ± 5.6	12.4 ± 7.3	16.5 ± 9.1	11.3 ± 7.1*	9.9 ± 3.6	13.2 ± 6.4	14.5 ± 7.9	9.2 ± 5.6*	11.2 ± 6.0	13.9 ± 7.5

*p < 0.05.
†p = 0.01.
CI = chronotropic incompetence; ΔEF = maximal ejection fraction − ejection fraction at rest ÷ ejection fraction at rest × 100; EDV = end-diastolic volume; EF = ejection fraction; Exer. = exercise; NL = normal; Q max = maximal cardiac output.

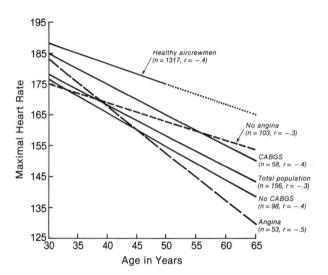

FIG 4–6.
Regression lines from the plots of maximal heart rate (HRmax) against age for the patient subgroups.

ume, or both. Because the degree of heart rate impairment is proportional to the degree of impairment in aerobic capacity, the most likely explanation is the limited heart rate. However, the mean level of aerobic impairment was above the 5-MET threshold that most studies have found to have a poor prognosis.

Exercise-Induced Angina Versus Myocardial Dysfunction. Much of what has been called "chronotropic incompetence" is related to early termination of exercise due to angina pectoris. Nevertheless, a significant number of patients are not limited by angina but have heart rate impairment. These patients also have significantly lower aerobic capacity than do age-matched patients with a normal heart rate response. Yet there were no significant differences in patients with and without CI regarding incidence of infarction, prevalence of congestive heart failure, exercise ejection fraction, or exercise-induced ST-segment depression. Two groups of patients with CI were characterized: those limited by angina and those limited by other factors. From the radionuclide testing, it appears that the patients with CI with angina have good mechanical myocardial reserve with less scar, higher ejection fraction, and lower end-diastolic volume. In contrast, the patients with CI without angina have more scarring, lower ejection fraction, and higher end-diastolic volume. This difference in the state of the myocardium was not apparent from clinical features, such as history of congestive heart failure, myocardial infarction, or pathologic Q-waves, but was only apparent from the results of radionuclide testing.

From previous studies, one would assume that patients defined as having CI during a treadmill test would have a poor prognosis. Therefore, we expected abnormal radionuclide studies and poor prognostic features to be concentrated in our patients with CI. However, we were surprised to find that most patients with CI stopped testing because of angina; in those without angina, the extent of myocardial damage was correlated to their impaired heart rate response. Previous studies overlooked the occurrence of angina and evidence for prior myocardial infarction in their examination of patients with so-called heart rate impairment. Patients with CI most likely represent a mixed group of patients with a variety of explanations for their impaired heart rate response including angina, myocardial dysfunction, sick sinus syndrome, and simply normal variation.

BLOOD PRESSURE RESPONSE

Systolic blood pressure should rise with increasing treadmill work load. Diastolic blood pressure usually remains about the same, but Korotkoff sounds can sometimes be heard all the way to zero in healthy young subjects. One group of investigators has suggested that a rising diastolic blood pressure is a sign of coronary heart disease. More likely, it is a marker for labile hypertension, which leads to coronary disease. The highest systolic blood pressure should be achieved at maximal work load. When exercise is stopped, approximately 10% of the people tested will drop their systolic blood pressure owing to peripheral pooling. To avoid fainting, patients should not be left standing for long. The systolic blood pressure that is elevated on resuming the supine position gradually returns to normal during recovery and then often drops below normal for several hours after the test. In spite of studies showing discrepancies between noninvasively and invasively measured blood pressure, the product of heart rate and systolic blood pressure, determined by cuff and auscultation, correlates excellently with measured myocardial oxygen consumption during exercise. Usually, an individual patient's angina pectoris will be precipitated at the same double product (systolic blood pressure times heart rate). This product is also an estimate of the maximal work load that the left ventricle can perform.

EXERTIONAL HYPOTENSION

Systolic blood pressure can rise above 280 mm Hg with no reported clinical implications or complications. An inadequate SBP rise can be due to aortic outflow obstruction or left ventricular dysfunction. Thomson and Kelemen reported that serious coronary artery disease was found in all their patients who developed hypotension along with angina during exercise testing. Six patients who had coronary artery bypass surgery had normal blood pressure responses to exercise testing without angina or ST-segment depression after their surgery. Studies by Morris and McHenry also support the diagnostic value of exercise-induced hypotension (EIH). However, they point out that it can be due to beta blockers, cardiomyopathies, and valvular heart disease as well as coronary artery disease. Hammermeister has reported data from the Seattle Heart Watch with EIH defined as a SBP drop below resting values.

This phenomenon also identifies patients at increased risk for the initiation of ventricular fibrillation in the exercise laboratory.

Weiner et al. investigated the reproducibility and prognostic significance of an exercise-induced decrease in SBP in 47 patients with such a reduction below the preexercise standing level in a consecutive series of 346 patients who underwent treadmill testing and cardiac catheterization during a three-year period. The prevalence of this abnormal finding was 11% in the total group but 21% in the 124 patients with three-vessel or left main coronary artery disease. Patients with an exercise-induced reduction in SBP were more likely to be male, have typical angina pectoris (class III or IV), and have had a prior MI than were patients without this finding. Although no complications occurred during the exercise tests of these 47 patients, the majority had severe ischemic responses, and 14 (30%) showed complex repetitive ventricular arrhythmias. Of the 47 patients, 24 received medical treatment and 23 underwent CABS. On repeat exercise testing in 42 patients, an abnormal SBP during exercise was consistently present in those medically managed (17 of 20) but entirely absent (0 of 22) in those who underwent CABS. The mean treadmill time, peak heart rate, and SBP were not significantly different in the initial and on repeat exercise tests in medical patients. However, in CABS patients, all of these variables were significantly higher in the repeat test. At a mean follow-up time of 37 months, the total cardiac mortality rate was 8% (2 of 24) in the medical group and 4% (1 of 23) in the CABS group.

Because of measurement difficulties, reproducibility limitations, and the different criteria used for defining EIH, its exact diagnostic or prognostic value is uncertain. Drops at high work loads or from high values are not as worrisome as other responses. When occurring with ST depression and/or angina, it must mean that much myocardium is in jeopardy. Table 4–5 lists the studies of EIH and the predictive values for left main and three-vessel coronary

TABLE 4–5.
Comparison of Reported Predictive Value of Exercise-Induced Hypotension for Left Main Coronary Stenosis and Three-Vessel Disease

FIRST AUTHOR	THREE-VESSEL DISEASE		LEFT MAIN STENOSIS	
	N/T	%	N/T	%
Thomson	11/15	73	5/15	33
Morris	15/22	68	3/22	14
Levites	4/25	16	1/25	4
Li	27/37	73	13/37	35
Weiner	19/47	40	7/47	15
Hammermeister	42/93	45	15/91	16
TOTAL	118/239	49	44/237	19

N = Number of patients with three-vessel disease or left main stenosis.

T = Total number of patients with exertional hypotension undergoing coronary arteriography.

disease. These studies are complicated by the inclusion of patients on beta blockers and those post MI. The exact sensitivity and specificity of this response for serious CAD or its impact on prognosis is uncertain.

EXERCISE/RECOVERY SBP RATIO

Amon and colleagues have reported that the normal decline in SBP during the recovery phase of treadmill exercise does not occur in some patients with CAD while in others the recovery values of SBP exceed the peak exercise values. To examine the diagnostic value of this observation, they studied 31 normal subjects and 56 patients undergoing treadmill exercise before coronary cineangiography. Because of large differences in peak exercise pressures between the two groups, recovery ratios were derived by dividing the SBP at one, two, and three minutes after exercise by the peak exercise SBP. The one-, two-, and three-minute ratios in the normal subjects declined steadily from 0.85 to 0.79 and to 0.73, respectively, while the ratios in the patients with CAD remained elevated at 0.97 to 0.93. With use of the upper limits defined by two SDs of the normal value, recovery ratios were compared with the occurrence of angina and with ST-segment depression on the exercise ECG in the patients with CAD. Abnormal ratios were more frequent in patients with CAD than in those with ST-segment depression and/or angina (42/56, 75%). Twenty of the patients with CAD who were on no medication underwent an additional treadmill test on a separate day and no significant differences were found in the ratios from the two tests. Ten additional patients with CAD underwent treadmill testing while on placebo and while on a beta blocker. There were no significant differences in the ratios from the two tests. Twenty-eight of the 31 (90%) normal subjects had normal recovery ratios. They concluded that the ratios of early recovery SBP to the peak exercise SBP are more sensitive than exercise electrocardiographic changes and angina for identifying patients with CAD.

NORMAL HR AND BP VALUES

The early emphasis placed on the exercise electrocardiogram tended to deemphasize other exercise responses. Measurements of these responses may improve the diagnostic value of exercise testing and may be useful for identifying the presence or the severity of coronary artery disease. The value of any measurement in providing diagnostic information from exercise testing depends on (1) the accuracy and completeness with which a measurement has been made in healthy individuals (reference values) and (2) the effectiveness with which certain limits of the measurement (discriminant values) separate healthy individuals from those subgroups with disease. The complete set of reference values presented in Figure 4–7 should help to determine discriminant values for separating patient groups. Using these discriminant values,

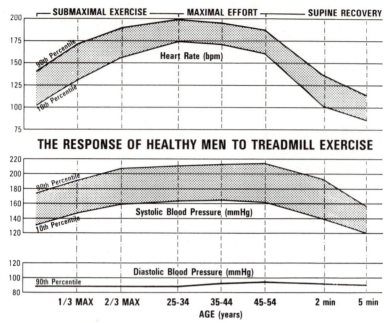

FIG 4–7.
The hemodynamic responses of over 700 healthy men to maximal treadmill exercise. The bands represent 80% of the population with 10% having values exceeding the upper limit and 10% with lower values.

sensitivity and specificity can be determined in a manner similar to that used for an abnormal ST-segment response. Many exercise test responses do not have a Gaussian distribution and require that nonparametric statistical tests be used. Therefore, discriminant values should be determined as percentiles rather than as standard deviations or confidence limits.

USING HEMODYNAMIC MEASUREMENTS TO ESTIMATE MYOCARDIAL OXYGEN CONSUMPTION

Though heart rate and stroke volume are important determinants of both maximal oxygen uptake and myocardial oxygen consumption, myocardial oxygen consumption has other independent determinants. It has been demonstrated that the relative metabolic loads of the entire body and those of the heart are determined separately and may not change in parallel with a given intervention. Although the heart receives only 4% of cardiac output at rest, it utilizes 10% of systemic oxygen uptake. The wide arteriovenous oxygen difference of 10 to 12 volumes percent at rest reflects the fact that oxygen in the blood passing through the coronary circulation is nearly maximally extracted. This value can be compared to the four volumes percent difference across the systemic circulation. When the myocardium requires a greater oxygen supply, coronary blood flow must be increased by coronary dilatation. During exercise, coronary blood flow can increase through normal coronary arteries up to five times the normal resting flow.

The increased demand for myocardial oxygen consumption required for dynamic exercise is the key to the use of exercise testing as a diagnostic tool for coronary artery disease. Myocardial oxygen consumption cannot be directly measured in a practical manner, but its relative demand can be estimated from its determinants, such as heart rate, wall tension (left ventricular pressure and diastolic volume), contractility, and cardiac work. Though all of these factors increase during exercise, increased heart rate is especially detrimental in patients who have obstructive coronary disease. Increased heart rate results in a shortening of the diastolic filling period, the time during which coronary blood flow is the greatest. In normal coronary arteries, dilation occurs. In obstructed vessels, however, dilation is limited and flow is decreased by the shortening of the diastolic filling period. This situation results in both inadequate blood flow and oxygen delivery.

Variable Threshold for Exercise-Induced Ischemia. It has been taught that exercise-induced ischemia occurs at the same rate-pressure product (heart rate times systolic blood pressure), unless an intervention has been effective or the coronary artery obstructions have worsened. However, changes in this threshold have been suggested to be due to coronary artery spasm. The effect of hyperventilation-induced alkalemia on angina was evaluated by Neill et al. in nine subjects with consistent exercise-induced chest pain and ST-segment depression. In five subjects who had arterial alkalemia while hyperventilating during exercise, the rate-pressure product during angina was 22×10^3 compared with 24×10^3 when they were breathing normally during exercise. The other four subjects appeared to hyperventilate, but were not alkalemic, and their rate-pressure product was not significantly different during repeat testing to angina. Thus, the threshold for angina during exercise was lowered in five patients in whom hyperventilation caused alkalemia. Was this effect due to coronary artery spasm or to changes in oxygen release from hemoglobin? A recent study by Waters et al. suggests that it is due to changes in coronary artery tone.

EXERCISE-INDUCED ARRHYTHMIAS (EIA)

Since exercise increases myocardial oxygen consumption, myocardial ischemia in the presence of coronary artery disease could predispose to ectopic activity during exercise. Exercise-induced supraventricular dysrhythmias are unusual and have not been related to coronary artery disease. Of major concern are exercise-induced premature ventricular contractions. Premature ventricular contractions occur in approximately one-third of asymptomatic men who perform a maximal treadmill test, and the prevalence is directly related to age. Premature ventricular contractions occur most frequently at maximal exercise and often are not reproducible on repeat testing. A subgroup of healthy men (approximately 2%) will have severe exercise-induced ventricular dysrhythmias. This group has three times the normal risk of developing coronary artery disease, but only about 10% of them will actually do so. Only 7% of those who develop coronary artery disease will have had so-called ominous ventricular dysrhythmias, and their premature ventricular contractions often occur at lower heart rates than they do in healthy subjects.

Dysrhythmias suppressed by acute exercise do not rule out the presence of coronary artery disease. Ambulatory monitoring and isometric exercise can identify premature ventricular contractions in more people than can dynamic exercise testing. The demonstration of the prognostic significance of exercise-induced ventricular dysrhythmias in coronary artery disease and the value of medical suppression will require careful follow-up studies. Studies have shown, however, that serious premature ventricular contractions detected by ambulatory monitoring performed three weeks after a myocardial infarction will identify patients at high risk. Ventricular dysrhythmias induced by exercise testing may be as predictive but more specific in these patients. In addition, the total information from an exercise test may be more helpful in patient management and more cost effective than ambulatory monitoring. In general, exercise-induced arrhythmias must be interpreted in relation to the medical condition of the individuals in whom they occur. This subject is discussed further in the chapter on applications.

THE ELECTROCARDIOGRAPHIC RESPONSE TO EXERCISE

The first attempt to evaluate the response of the electrocardiogram to exercise was performed by Einthoven. In 1908, he made several accurate observations in a postexercise electrocardiogram, including an increase in the amplitude of the P- and T-waves and depression of the J-junction. In 1953, Simonson studied the electrocardiographic response to treadmill testing of a wide age range of normal subjects, but did not have the benefit of computer analysis. In 1965, Blomqvist reported his classic description of the response of the Frank vectorcardiographic leads to bicycle exercise using computer techniques. Rautaharju and colleagues analyzed P-, ST-, and T-vector functions in the Frank leads at rest and during exercise. All P-wave vector functions increased during exercise and were compatible with right atrial overload whereas T-wave vectors decreased slightly. The ST-segment vector shifted clockwise, to the right, and upward.

Simoons and Hugenholtz reported Frank lead waveform changes during exercise in normal subjects. The direction and magnitudes of time-normalized P, QRS, and ST vectors and other QRS parameters were analyzed during and after exercise in 56 apparently healthy men between the ages of 23 to 62 years. The PR interval and the P-wave amplitude increased during exercise. Direction of the P vectors did not change consistent with right atrial overload. Surprisingly, no significant change in QRS magnitude was observed, and the magnitude in spatial orientation and the maximum QRS vectors remained constant. QRS onset to T-wave peak shortened. The terminal QRS vectors and the initial ST vectors gradually shortened and shifted to the right and superiorly. The T-wave amplitude lessened during exercise. In the first minute of recovery, the P and T magnitudes markedly increased, and then all measurements gradually returned to the resting level. There was an increase in S-wave duration in leads X and Y (14 to 24 msec). QRS right-axis shift was heart rate dependent. The ST-segment shifted toward the right superiorly and posteriorly, and T-wave magnitude increased markedly in the first minute of recovery. Shortening of the QRS complex (3 msec) was found in some young individuals during exercise.

Laciga and Koller made quantitative electrocardiographic measurements on 30 young healthy subjects at rest and during the stress of moderately acute stepwise exposure to a simulated altitude of 7,000 m. A complete 12-lead electrocardiogram was recorded during ascent and descent. With increasing altitude, P-wave amplitude became significantly increased in the inferior leads, the amplitude of the R-wave decreased progressively with altitude by about 10%, whereas the S-wave decreased and the R-wave in V5 increased by about 10%. A T-wave amplitude decrease was noted on occasion in both the limb and lateral precordial leads.

Riff and Carleton demonstrated in patients with atrioventricular (AV) dissociation that the duration of atrial repolarization (the atrial T-wave) can play a role in the normal rate-related depression of the J junction in inferior leads (AVF, II) and can increase S-wave amplitude. The effect of atrial repolarization on the ST-segments in the lateral leads is less important, but it affects a bipolar lead such as CM5, which contains anterior and inferior forces.

Using vectorcardiographic analysis after exercise testing, Kilpatrick found a higher sensitivity and specificity for coronary heart disease by using QRS criteria, including transient infarct patterns, rather than ST-segment changes. Such changes must be secondary to conduction abnormalities and not due to a loss of electrically active tissue. Other studies have found exercise-induced Q-waves to be of little diagnostic value.

Morales-Ballejo and colleagues analyzed the response of Q-waves in lead CM5 in 50 patients with coronary artery disease and in 50 normal subjects before and immediately after exercise. The septal Q-wave in lead CM5 was smaller in patients with coronary disease than it was in normal subjects at rest and immediately after exercise. Disappearance of the Q-wave in lead CM5 along with ST-segment depression after exercise was 100% specific for coronary artery disease. They felt that low Q-wave voltage and its failure to increase after exercise indicated abnormal septal activation and reflected loss of contraction due to ischemia. Loss of the septal Q could be due to septal fibrosis that could be due to coronary disease.

Nohara et al. assessed changes in exercise septal Q waves in lead V5 by single photon emission computed tomography in 107 patients. Of 18 patients who had regression of Q-wave amplitude during exercise, 17 had a septal perfusion defect and all had left anterior descending stenosis at angiography. Of 48 patients who had progression or no change of Q-wave or a new Q-wave during exercise in lead V5, 90% did not have a septal perfusion defect; 56% of the 41 patients who had no Q-waves at rest or during exercise had a left anterior descending coronary stenosis. This still needs further validation prior to universal utilization.

R-WAVE CHANGES

Exercise-induced R-wave amplitude changes were studied by Kentala and colleagues in healthy individuals and in patients with known coronary disease. Physically active normal subjects and patients with coronary disease who responded well to an exercise program demonstrated an increased R-wave amplitude in lead V5 relative to preexercise supine rest measurements both on assumption of an upright posture and in response to exercise. The R-wave amplitude then decreased in the supine position postexercise. Such changes were not found in patients who did not benefit from physical conditioning. The significance of an R-wave index is thus unclear.

Diagnostic Sensitivity. Studies have suggested R-wave changes to be sensitive independently and, in combination with ST-segment changes, to be superior in sensitivity to ST-segment changes alone. R-wave changes have been considered particularly useful in patients with nonspecific ST segments and in patients with left bundle branch block. Bonoris compared exercise-induced R-wave amplitude changes and ST-segment depression in 266 patients, many of whom were specifically chosen as false positive or false negative responders (48% sensitivity and 59% specificity using ST-segment criteria). Using R-wave criteria, the sensitivity was improved to 63% with a specificity of 79%. In a second study, 45 subjects with angiographically normal coronary arteries were evaluated; 41 (91%) demonstrated a decrease in R-wave amplitude with exercise. Among 44 patients with angiographic coronary disease, R-wave amplitude increased in 26 patients (59%) with severe coronary disease, and decreased in 18 patients (41%) with normal or minimally abnormal resting ventriculograms and less severe coronary artery disease.

Uhl and Hopkirk examined R-wave amplitude changes in 44 asymptomatic men with left bundle branch block. Among the seven men with angiographically significant coronary artery disease, all demonstrated an increase in the amplitude of the R-wave from rest to maximal exercise. In only 10 of the 37 men with normal angiograms did exercise induce an increase in R-wave amplitude, resulting in a sensitivity of 100% and a specificity of 73%.

Yiannikas and colleagues used the sum of the change in R-wave amplitudes in V4, 5, and 6 to investigate the response of 50 men with ST-T wave changes on their resting ECGs. Four of six subjects who increased R-wave amplitude during exercise had angiographically significant coronary artery disease, and the other two had cardiomyopathies. Greenberg et al. were able to improve the sensitivity of the exercise test from 50% to 76% by including R-wave criteria in 50 patients without compromising specificity or predictive value.

Baron et al., using the mean of the R-wave changes inferiorly and laterally, reported that of 62 patients with coronary artery disease, 61 (98%) increased the amplitude of the R-wave with exercise. The mean increase in R-wave amplitude was greatest among patients with multivessel disease and with either hypokinesia or akinesia.

Nearly as many studies have been unable to demonstrate that changes in the R-wave amplitude during exercise are useful clinically. Eenige van et al. were unable to improve sensitivity using R-wave amplitude changes as compared to ST-segment changes. This was despite the use of several lead systems, clinical subsets of patients, and different criteria for abnormal. Wagner et al. examined 73 patients with angiographic coronary artery disease, 28 patients with minimal disease, and 40 normals to compare the diagnostic value of R-wave changes with the ST-segment. R-wave criteria resulted in a sensitivity of 52% and a specificity of 63%, compared with 88% and 72%, respectively, using ST-segment criteria. No significant correlation was found between the extent of angiographically determined coronary artery disease and R-wave changes. Deanfield et al. demonstrated ST-segment depression to be associated with both a decrease and an increase in R-wave amplitude. There were no clinical or angiographic differences between patients who increased or those who decreased R-wave amplitude during exercise. Voyles and coworkers reported R-wave amplitude to have a variable directional response in 7 of 10 serially tested patients with exertional angina. All 10 patients had reproducible ST-segment responses in serial tests.

R-Wave Amplitude Changes and Left Ventricular Function. Gottwik et al. compared orthogonal Frank VCGs and angiographically determined left ventricular ejection fraction to study their relationship with R-wave amplitude. Summation of the R-waves in the orthogonal leads significantly correlated with ejection fraction at rest ($r = .78$). Amplitudes in these leads had a 92% accuracy rate in predicting whether an ejection fraction was greater or less than 50%. Askenazi and coworkers demonstrated a significant correlation ($r = .61$) between resting ejection fraction and sum of the orthogonal R-wave amplitudes in 73 patients. Greenberg and colleagues found that of 24 patients with an abnormal decrease in ejection fraction during exercise, 18 (75%) increased the amplitude of the R-wave. Seventeen of these 18 (94%) had multivessel coronary disease. All 18 normal subjects decreased their R-wave amplitudes from rest to maximal exercise and had normal ejection fraction, volume, and wall motion responses to exercise.

Battler et al. at UCSD found poor correlations between ejection fraction and R-wave amplitude at rest and during exercise in 60 patients ($r = .50$ and .51, respectively). Further, there was no significant relationship between changes in R-wave amplitude and changes in left ventricular ejection fraction during exercise in these patients or in 18 normals. Luwaert et al. studied 252 patients evaluated for chest pain, and demonstrated a significant although low correlation between the sum of the orthogonal R-waves and resting ejection fraction (r = .22). Eenige van and coworkers studied the value of R-wave amplitude changes during exercise in determining ejection fraction, end-diastolic pressures, and left ventricular wall motion. No useful diagnostic information was obtained using R-wave changes in this study.

Mechanism of R-Wave Amplitude Changes. Brody's demonstration of a relationship between left ventricular volume and R-wave amplitude has since gained support. More recently, however, several investigators have presented evidence against this concept. Battler and colleagues demonstrated a poor correlation between changes in R-wave amplitude and left ventricular volume. This has been corroborated by others. Talbot and colleagues have reported an inverse association between end-diastolic volume and R-wave voltage. Lerken et al. reported that the endocardial QRS amplitude decreased during volume increases in dogs. Deanfield and colleagues reported that R-wave amplitude was essentially unaffected by both increases or decreases in left ventricular volume.

That cardiac enlargement secondary to congestive heart failure may cause a decrease in R-wave amplitude also contradicts the Brody hypothesis. Further, if R-wave amplitude changes were strictly the result of changes in volume, one would expect R-wave amplitude to increase when changing from standing to supine, since diastolic volume would increase. However, this change in R-wave amplitude does not necessarily occur. Since the R-wave has been shown to correlate with systolic volume and ejection fraction, an association with contractility has been suggested. Axis shifts have been implicated as the cause of changes in R-wave amplitude. However, the shift of the QRS and ST-segment vector toward the right and posteriorly is a normal response to exercise. David et al. performed an experiment that was strongly against the concept that R-wave amplitude changes are due mainly to changes in ventricular volume. After inducing ischemia in dogs, R-wave amplitude continued to increase despite clamping of the vena cava, which reduced ventricular volume.

Ellestad has recently rejected the R-wave/volume relationship and suggested that the increase in R-wave amplitude that accompanies myocardial infarction, exercise, or coronary spasm is secondary to ischemia-induced changes in the electrical properties of the myocardium. This is supported by experimental data from David and coworkers. After inducing myocardial ischemia in dogs, they demonstrated that biphasic R-wave changes directly correlated with changes in intramyocardial conduction times, whereas intracardiac dimensional changes and R-wave changes were unrelated.

UCSD R-Wave Study. The acquisition of exercise ECGs by computer offered an opportunity to relate R-wave changes with ischemic ST-segment shifts. The ECG changes were analyzed spatially; that is, they were recorded in three dimensions, enabling optimal representation of global myocardial electrical forces. Patients were separated into groups achieving maximal heart rates higher and lower than the mean maximal heart rate achieved of 161 beats per minute. Data on asymptomatic normals has borne out that the R-wave amplitude typically increases from rest to submaximal exercise, perhaps to a heart rate of 140 beats/min, then decreases to the maximal exercise endpoint. Therefore, if a patient were limited by exercise intolerance, whether due to objective or subjective symptoms or signs, the R-wave amplitude would increase from rest to such an endpoint. Such patients may be demonstrating a normal R-wave response but be classified "abnormal," since the severity of disease causes a lower exercise tolerance and heart rate.

In Table 4–6, patients within each heart rate group (those achieving greater than, and those less than the median maximal heart rate attained of 161 beats/min) are listed, and comparisons are made between those increasing, and those decreasing spatial R-wave amplitude from standing rest to maximal exercise. The data indicate that there are no differences in ischemic variables, exercise capacity, or any of the indices of left ventricular function between patients increasing or decreasing spatial R-wave amplitude. The analysis was repeated after excluding patients with anterior Q-waves with no significant differences.

In order to study the value of exercise-induced R-wave amplitude changes as an index of left ventricular function and ischemia, computerized spatial R-wave amplitude measurements were obtained in 95 patients—30 who increased and 65 who decreased spatial R-wave amplitude during the exercise testing. Patients were classified into groups attaining a higher (N = 48) and lower (N = 47) than the median maximal heart rate. Within these two groups, patients with increasing or decreasing spatial R-wave amplitude were ana-

TABLE 4–6.
Differences in Ischemic and Functional Variables Between Patients With Increasing and Decreasing Spatial R-Wave Amplitude From Rest to Maximal Exercise

	MAXIMAL HEART RATE >161 BEATS/MIN SPATIAL R-WAVE AMPLITUDE		MAXIMAL HEART RATE <161 BEATS/MIN SPATIAL R-WAVE AMPLITUDE	
	INCREASE (n = 16)	DECREASE (n = 32)	INCREASE (n = 14)	DECREASE (n = 33)
Change during exercise of				
R-wave amplitude (%)	4.72 ± 6	−16.0 ± 9*	9.43 ± 10	−11.1 ± 5*
VO$_2$ max (L/min)	2.48 ± 6	2.47 ± 5	1.72 ± 13	2.0 ± 4
ST segment displacement, lead X (mV)	−0.09 ± 0.09	−0.05 ± 0.15	−0.07 ± 0.13	−0.06 ± 0.12
ST segment displacement, spatially (mV)	0.19 ± 0.08	0.24 ± 0.14	0.19 ± 0.10	0.16 ± 0.10
Angina during the test (%)	19	16	43	37
Thallium-201 ischemia score	2.3 ± 4.4	4.5 ± 3.7	3.9 ± 5.4	3.3 ± 4.3
Ejection fraction (%)	3.5 ± 17	2.7 ± 19	3.2 ± 18	1.4 ± 15
Resting ejection fraction	52 ± 13	54 ± 14	55 ± 14	56 ± 11

*p < 0.001. Values are mean ± SD.

lyzed for differences in maximal ventilatory oxygen consumption, ST-segment depression laterally and spatially, left ventricular ejection fraction at rest, change in ejection fraction during exercise, and thallium ischemia. We were unable to demonstrate any differences in ischemic variables or in left ventricular function between patients increasing or decreasing spatial R-wave amplitude.

S-Wave Changes.   During exercise there is an increase in the S-wave in the lateral precordial leads. Katzeff and Edwards hypothesized that this increase in the S-wave reflects the normal increase in cardiac contractility during exercise and that its absence is indicative of ventricular dysfunction. It is more likely, however, that the increase in S-wave is caused by exercise-induced axis shifts and conduction alterations.

U-Wave Changes.   In a study by Gerson and coworkers, 248 patients underwent exercise testing using leads CC5 and VL, 36 of whom had exercise-induced U-wave inversion. Of 71 patients with significant left anterior descending or left main disease and no prior MI, 35% had U-wave inversion compared to only 4% of 57 patients without left anterior descending or left main disease and only 1% of 82 patients who had no coronary artery disease. U-wave inversion was diagnosed if a discrete negative deflection within the TP segment relative to the PR segment occurred during or after exercise. Inverted U-waves were not diagnosed if the exercise heart rate increased to a level such that the QT interval could not be accurately measured. This has not been confirmed by other researchers, and McHenry now feels it is an artifact of his bipolar ECG lead system.

Junctional Depression.   Mirvis and colleagues studied junctional depression during exercise using left precordial isopotential mapping. During exercise, junctional depression was maximal along the left lower sternal border. In the early portion of the ST-segment, they found a minimum isopotential along the lower left sternal border that was continuous with terminal QRS forces in both intensity and location. The late portion of the ST-segment had a minimum isopotential located in the same areas as that observed at rest (i.e., the upper left sternal border). These observations suggested that junctional depression was the result of competition between normal repolarization and delayed terminal depolarization forces. Junctional depression was most marked along the left lower sternal border; most subjects did not exhibit these changes in only V5 and V6. Also, the slope of the ST segment varied from site to site and was directly correlated to magnitude and direction of the J-point deviation. Thus, junctional depression is the result of the presence of negative potentials over the left lower sternal border during early repolarization. These negative potentials responsible for physiologic junctional depression could be caused by delayed activation of basal areas of the left and right ventricles, which leads to accentuated depolarization-repolarization overlap.

Blood Composition Shifts.   During exercise, there are elevations in plasma osmolality, potassium, sodium, calcium, phosphate, lactate, and proteinase. There is a constant and gradual increase for both males and females in these measurements regardless of environmental conditions. Sodium and potassium rapidly return to normal after exercise. During respiratory acidosis, there is a loss of potassium from the musculoskeletal system that is increased by muscular activity. Potassium enters the myocardium during acidosis and exits after exercise. The mechanism for this variance between myocardial and skeletal muscle is not known. Serum potassium increases immediately postexercise, and this increase may be related to postexercise T-wave changes. The increase in potassium during exercise contrasts with the decrease in T-waves during exercise. There is no explanation as to why there should be a postexertional T-wave peak due to hyperkalemia when there is no T-wave peak during exercise.

Coester and colleagues drew arterial samples for blood gases and electrolytes at rest, during the last minute of maximal bicycle exercise, and at recovery. The amplitude of the T- and P-waves increased in bipolar lead CH5 reached a maximum in the first two minutes after exercise. All electrolytes measured were increased at the end of exercise, with potassium up 60% and phosphorus up 53%. Potassium dropped the most rapidly below resting values, along with plasma bicarbonate. ECG alterations were not closely related in time with any single factor such as potassium, but they appeared to reflect an interaction of the changes in mineral balance. The normal right-axis and posterior-axis deviation of the QRS complex and decreasing R-wave amplitude could be due to right ventricular overload, respiratory-induced descent of the diaphragm, changes in thoracic impedance, or changes in ventricular blood volume. A patient has been reported who developed left anterior hemiblock during exercise that responded in a normal rightward fashion after coronary artery bypass surgery. The decreased T-wave amplitude may be related to decreased end-systolic volume, changes in sympathetic tone, electrolyte concentration changes, or shifts in the T-wave vector. Other factors may also contribute to the changes in the exercise ECG, such as positional changes in the electrodes, changes in action potentials, electrolyte or hematocrit changes, changes in intracardiac blood volume, and augmentation of the atrial repolarization wave. The effect of age must be considered because there is extensive normal variation related to age. For example, greater ST-segment depression and greater right-axis deviation occur in older persons.

USAFSAM NORMAL EXERCISE ECG STUDY

Using computer techniques, we analyzed data from 40 low-risk normal subjects utilizing measurements of amplitude, intervals, and slope which were then processed and analyzed for treadmill times on the basis of electrocardiographic component and lead.

Figure 4–8 shows the waveforms measured using median values of the mea-

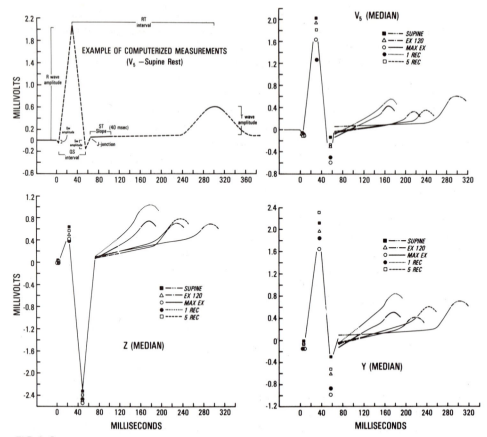

FIG 4–8.
Illustrations of the plots of the median ECG data from the 40 normals.

surements of all 40 subjects for leads V5, Y, and Z. These figures demonstrate the specific waveform alterations that occur in response to maximal treadmill exercise. Supine, exercise to HR 120, maximal exercise, one-minute recovery, and five-minute recovery were chosen as representative times for presentation of these median-based simulated waveforms.

There is depression of the J-junction and the tall peaked T-waves at maximal exercise and at one-minute recovery that can be an early sign of ischemia, but are seen here in normal subjects. Along with the J-junction depression, marked ST upsloping is seen. J-junction depression did not occur in Z lead (which is equivalent to and of the same polarity as V2). As the R-wave decreases in amplitude, the S-wave increases in depth. The QS duration shortens minimally, but the RT duration decreases in a larger amount.

Q-Wave, R-Wave, and S-Wave Amplitudes. In leads CM5, V5, CC5, and Y, the Q-wave shows very small changes from the resting values; however, it does become slightly more negative at maximal exercise.

Measurable Q-wave changes were not noted in the Z lead. Changes in median R-wave amplitude are not detected until near-maximal and maximal effort are approached. At maximal exercise and on into one-minute recovery, a sharp decrease in R-wave amplitude is observed in CM5, V5, and CC5. These changes are not seen in the Z lead. The lowest median R-wave value in Y occurred at maximal exercise, with R-wave amplitude increasing by one-minute recovery. In leads CM5, V5, and CC5, the lowest R-wave amplitude was seen at one-minute recovery. This different temporal response in R-waves in the lateral versus inferior leads is unexplained. There is little change in S-wave amplitude in Z. In the other leads, however, the S-wave became greater in depth or more negative, showing a greater deflection at maximal exercise, and then gradually returning to resting values in recovery. A decrease in the QS interval occurred, and it was shortest at maximal exercise. By three minutes of recovery, QS interval returned to normal. A steadily decreasing RT-interval duration was observed as exercise increased. The shortest interval was seen at maximal exercise and one-minute recovery. Changes in this interval followed changes in heart rate.

ST-Slope, J-Junction Depression, and T-Wave Amplitude. The amplitude of the J-junction in lead Z was very little changed through exercise, but elevated slightly in recovery. The location of the J-junction (QRS) end in Z was determined by using the Z-lead signal alone rather than by a three-dimensional method, so it is relatively inaccurate. It appears that the lead system affects the anterior-posterior presentation of the ST vector more than anticipated. Careful studies applying spatial determination of QRS end are needed to see whether the J-junction shifts anteriorly or posteriorly. The J-junction was depressed in all other leads to a maximum depression at maximal exercise; then it gradually returned toward but not to preexercise values slowly in recovery. There was very little difference between the three left precordial leads. A dramatic increase in ST-segment slope was observed in all leads and was greatest at one-minute recovery.

These changes returned toward pretest values during later recovery. The greatest or steepest slopes were seen in lead CM5, which did not show the greatest ST-segment depression. A gradual decrease in T-wave amplitude was observed in all leads during early exercise. At maximal exercise, the T-wave began to increase, and at one-minute recovery the amplitude was equivalent to resting values, except in leads Y and Z where they were greater than at rest. However, there was a great deal of overlap.

Percent R-Wave Changes. Figure 4–9 illustrates the percent change of R-wave amplitude for each individual compared with his R-wave at supine rest in V5 and Y. At lower exercise heart rates, the great variability of R-wave response was apparent, and many normal individuals had significant increases in R-wave amplitude. Though most showed a decline at maximum exercise, some normal subjects had an increase, whereas others showed very little decrease. At one-minute recovery, there was a greater ten-

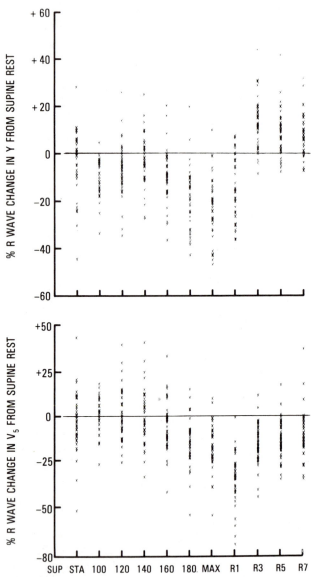

FIG 4–9.

Percent of R-wave amplitude change during treadmill exercise from supine rest in V5 and Y. SUP = supine; STA = standing; MAX = maximal exercise; RX = x minutes in recovery.

dency toward a decline in lead V5 but not in Y. Further into recovery, R-wave amplitude remained decreased in lead V5 but increased in Y.

We have safely exercised most of our patients with severe coronary heart disease to high exercise levels and have found declines in R-wave amplitude. If changes were due to left ventricular volume alterations, all normal individuals would respond in the same direction with standing.

ABNORMAL ST-SEGMENT CHANGES

Epicardial electrode mapping usually records ST-segment elevation over areas of severe ischemia and ST-segment depression over areas of lesser ischemia. ST-segment depression is the reciprocal of the injury effect occurring in the endocardium as viewed from an electrode overlying normal epicardium. ST-segment elevation seen from the same electrode reflects transmural injury or, less frequently, epicardial injury. On the surface electrocardiogram, exercise-induced myocardial ischemia can result in one of three ST-segment manifestations: elevation, normalization, or depression.

ST-SEGMENT ELEVATION

Fortuin and Friesinger reported the angiographic and clinical findings and two-year follow-up of 12 patients with 0.1 mV or more ST-segment elevation during or after exercise. These patients were selected from 400 patients who had coronary angiography and exercise testing. Seven of them had previous myocardial infarctions, and 9 of the 10 with angina developed it during the exercise test. One patient with atypical chest pain had normal coronary arteries and improved during the follow-up. Seven of eight with exercise-induced ST-segment elevation in lead V3 had left anterior descending coronary disease. All four with inferior elevation had right coronary disease. None had ST-segment elevation at rest, but many had Q-waves or T-wave inversion or both. Within two years, four of the patients died, one had a documented MI, and two became unstable.

Bobba and associates presented four similar patients with exercise-induced ST-segment elevation. They noted an increase in R-wave amplitude in the leads with ST-segment elevation and ST-segment depression in other leads.

Hegge and coworkers found 11% of the patients they studied with maximal treadmill testing and coronary angiography to have exercise-induced ST-segment elevation in the postexercise 12-lead electrocardiogram. This relatively high prevalence of ST-segment elevation is probably explained by inclusion of V1 and V2, leads not monitored in other studies. The ST-segment elevation was present in precordial leads only in 12 patients, in the inferior leads only in five patients, and in both in one patient. Seventeen patients had severe coronary artery disease in the arteries supplying the appropriate area and the remaining patient had a normal coronary angiogram.

Chahine and colleagues reported the prevalence of exercise-induced ST-segment elevation in 840 consecutive patients to be 3.5%. CM5 and CM6 were the only leads monitored, so lateral wall ST-segment elevation was all that could be detected. Only about 20% of those who had coronary artery disease showed ST-segment elevation. Sixty-four percent of the patients with left ventricle dyskinesia displayed ST-segment elevation. Manvi and Ellestad presented results in 29 patients with coronary artery disease who had abnormal left ventriculograms. ST-segment elevation occurred in 48%, 33% developed ST-segment depression, and the remaining 19% had no changes. ST-segment elevation occurred in 1.3% of 2,000 exercise tests.

Simoons and colleagues investigated the spatial orientation of exercise-induced ST-segment changes in relation to the presence of dyskinetic areas, as demonstrated by left ventriculography. In patients with an anterior infarct, the ST vectors were widely scattered, but were most often directed to the left, anterior, and superior. Patients with an inferior myocardial infarction had ST-segment vectors rightward and anterior, and also inferiorly if inferior dyskinesia was present. Anteriorly orientated ST-segment changes were associated with anterior or apical scars in patients with anterior infarcts. Thus, ST-segment vector shifts associated with dyskinesia resulted in ST-segment elevation over the dyskinetic area. In patients with dyskinetic areas, the direction of the ST-segment changes varied so widely that only the magnitude of the changes could be used as a criterion for exercise-induced ischemia.

Sriwattanakomen and colleagues reviewed 1,620 exercise tests and found 3.8% to have ST-segment elevation when all leads except aVR were evaluated. They then correlated exercise-induced ST-elevation with the coronary arteriography and left ventriculograms of 38 patients, 37 of which had significant coronary disease. In 27 patients with Q-waves, 25 had significant disease and ventricular aneurysms, whereas among 11 patients with no Q-waves and significant disease, only two had ventricular aneurysms. One patient had a ventricular aneurysm but no coronary disease. The sites of ST elevation correctly localized the area of ventricular aneurysm in 30 of 33 instances and determined the diseased vessels in 38 of 40 instances. They concluded that ST elevation during exercise in the absence of Q-waves indicates significant proximal disease without ventricular aneurysm, whereas with Q-waves, ST elevation is indicative of ventricular aneurysm in addition to significant proximal disease. Ischemia and abnormal wall motion may independently or additively underlie the mechanism for ST-segment elevation during exercise.

Longhurst and Kraus reviewed 6,040 consecutive exercise tests and found 106 patients (1.8%) without previous myocardial infarctions who had exercise-induced ST-segment elevation. Criterion was 0.5 mm elevation in a 15-electrode array. Forty-six of these patients with ST-segment elevation had ventriculography and coronary angiography. Coronary disease was detected in 40 of 46, with nearly equal numbers having one-, two-, and three-vessel disease. Ventriculograms were normal in 36 of 40 patients. Of 21 patients with anterior ST-segment elevation, 86% had left anterior descending obstruction. There was no anatomic correlation in those with lateral or inferior-posterior exercise-induced elevation.

Dunn and colleagues performed exercise thallium scans on 35 patients with exercise-induced ST-segment elevation and coronary artery obstruction. Ten patients developed exercise ST-segment elevation in leads that showed no Q-waves on the resting electrocardiogram. The site of elevation corresponded to a reversible perfusion defect and a severely obstructed coronary artery. Associated ST-segment depression in other leads occurred in seven patients, but only one had a second perfusion defect at the site of depression. Three of the 10 patients had a wall motion abnormality at the same site. Twenty-five patients developed exercise ST-segment elevation in leads with Q-waves. The site of the elevation corresponded to a severe stenosis and a thallium perfusion defect that persisted on the four-hour redistribution scan. Associated ST-segment depression in other leads occurred in 11 patients, and eight had a second perfusion defect at the site of the depression. In all 25 patients, there was a wall motion abnormality at the site of the Q-wave. Therefore, without a previous infarct, ST-segment elevation indicates the site of severe transient ischemia; associated ST-segment depression is usually reciprocal. In patients with Q waves, exercise-induced ST-segment elevation may be due to ischemia around the infarct, abnormal wall motion, or both. Association ST-segment depression may be due to a second area of ischemia rather than being reciprocal. Chaitman has shown that exercise-induced coronary artery spasm can cause ST elevation. Figures 4–10 and 4–11 show examples of ST-segment elevation in a normal resting electrocardiogram and over Q-waves, respectively.

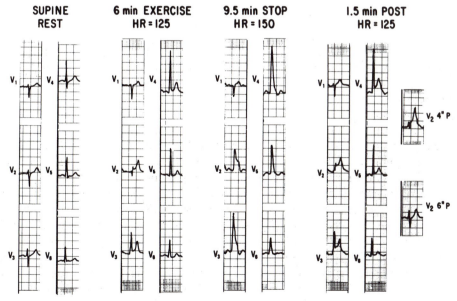

FIG 4–10.

Exercise-induced ST elevation in an ECG without diagnostic Q-waves. The patient has severe angina, septal ischemia on a thallium scan and a tight left anterior descending lesion on cardiac catheterization.

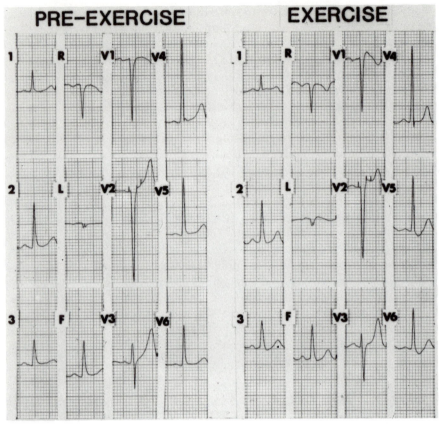

FIG 4–11.
Exercise-induced ST elevation in an ECG with anterior Q-waves secondary to an anterior MI. The patient did not have angina nor a postexercise thallium defect that "filled in." (Thirty-eight-year-old male. Status: post anterior wall myocardial infarction).

Bratt has assessed the value of lead V4R during exercise testing for predicting proximal stenosis of the right coronary artery. In 107 patients, a Bruce exercise test with the simultaneous recording of leads I, II, V4R, V1, V4, and V6 was followed by coronary angiography. ST-segment changes were recorded in the conventional leads and in lead V4R. Seventy-nine of the 107 patients were studied because of inadequate control of angina pectoris. In the 46 patients who had a previous MI, the infarct location was inferior in 28 and anterior in 18. Seven of the 14 patients without MI and significant proximal stenosis in the right coronary artery showed an ST-segment deviation of 1 mm or greater in lead V4R during exercise. This was also observed in 11 of 18 patients with an old inferior wall infarction and proximal occlusion of the right coronary artery. None of the 53 patients without significant proximal stenosis in the right coronary artery showed exercise-related ST-segment changes in lead V4R. Exercise-related ST-segment deviation in lead V4R (elevation in 17 and depression in four patients) had a sensitivity of 56%, a specificity of 96%, and a predictive accuracy of 84% in recognizing proximal stenosis in the right coronary artery.

ST elevation means something different when it occurs over pathological Q-waves (or an old transmural MI site) versus when it occurs in a normal ECG. Unfortunately, many of the studies have not made that distinction nor considered location.

ST-SEGMENT NORMALIZATION OR ABSENCE OF CHANGE

Another manifestation of ischemia can be no change or normalization of the ST-segment due to cancellation effects. Electrocardiographic abnormalities at rest, including T-wave inversion and ST-segment depression, have been reported to return to normal during attacks of angina and during exercise in some patients with ischemic heart disease. This cancellation effect is a rare occurrence, but it should be kept in mind. The ST segment and T-wave represent the uncancelled portion of ventricular repolarization. Since ventricular geometry can be roughly approximated by a hollow ellipsoid open at one end, the widespread cancellation of the relatively slowly dispersing electrical forces during repolarization is understandable. Patients with severe coronary artery disease would be most likely to have cancellation occur, yet they have the highest prevalence of abnormal tests. Manvi and Ellestad reported that 20% of the patients with dyskinesia and coronary artery disease had normal tests, and Chahine and coworkers reported that about 25% of their patients with dyskinesia and coronary artery disease normalized or minimally elevated their ST segments during exercise. Nobel and colleagues reported normalization of both inverted T-waves and depressed ST segments in 11 patients during exercise-induced angina. When exercise testing fails to produce ST-segment depression or elevation in a patient with known coronary artery disease, this could be due to two or more severely ischemic myocardial segments causing cancelling ST-segment vectors. Sweet and Sheffield reported a patient with minor ST-segment depression and T-wave inversion in lead V5 who normalized, or "improved" his electrocardiogram during treadmill testing only to have an acute infarction 10 minutes after the test. This normalization of ST-segment depression should thus be considered ST-segment elevation.

The prevalence of the cancelling of surface ST-segment changes by multiple ischemic ST vectors is not known. The inability of patients to give an adequate effort are more likely explanations for the majority of false negative exercise tests in patients with multivessel coronary artery disease. In those with single-vessel disease, the decreased sensitivity of exercise testing is most likely due to insufficient myocardial ischemia to cause surface ECG changes.

ST-SEGMENT DEPRESSION

The most common manifestation of exercise-induced myocardial ischemia is ST-segment depression. The standard criterion for this type of abnormal response is horizontal or downward sloping ST-segment depression of 0.1 mV or more for 80 msec. It appears to be due to generalized subendocardial ischemia. A "steal" phenomena is likely from ischemic areas because of the effect of extensive collateralization in the subendocardium. ST depression does not localize the area of ischemia as does ST elevation or help to indicate which coronary artery is occluded. The normal ST-segment vector response to tachycardia and to exercise is a shift rightward and upward. The degree of this shift appears to have a fair amount of biologic variation. Most normal individuals will have early repolarization at rest, which will shift to the isoelectric PR-segment line in the inferior, lateral, and anterior leads with exercise. This shift can be further influenced by ischemia and myocardial scars. When the later portions of the ST-segment are affected, flattening or downward depression can be recorded. Both local effects and the direction of the spatial changes during repolarization cause the ST-segment to have a different appearance at the many surface sites that can be monitored. Weiner demonstrated that the more leads with these apparent ischemic shifts, the greater the severity of disease. Figure 4–12 shows ST-segment depression in multiple leads in a patient with triple-vessel disease.

The probability and severity of coronary artery disease are directly related to the amount of J-junction depression and are inversely related to the slope of the ST segment. Because of these related factors, computer measurements such as the ST index and the ST integral which take into account both slope and depression should prove to be superior to classic criteria. Downsloping ST-segment depression is more serious than is horizontal depression, and both are more serious than upsloping depression. However, patients with upsloping ST-segment depression, especially when the slope is less than 1 mV/sec, probably are at increased risk. If a slowly ascending slope is utilized as a criterion for abnormal, the specificity of exercise testing will be decreased (more false positives) although the test may become more sensitive. One electrode can show upsloping ST depression while an adjacent electrode shows horizontal or downsloping depression. If an apparently borderline ST segment with an inadequate slope is recorded in a single precordial lead in a patient highly suspected of having coronary artery disease, multiple precordial leads should be scanned before the exercise test is called normal. An upsloping depressed ST segment may be the precursor to abnormal ST-segment depression in the recovery period or at higher heart rates during greater work loads. It is preferable to call tests with an inadequate ST-segment slope but with ST-segment depression borderline response, but added emphasis should be placed on other clinical and exercise parameters. Examples of the different criteria for ischemic ST depression are shown in Figure 4–13.

R-Wave Adjustment. The degree of exercise-induced ST depression can be influenced by R-wave amplitude, and perhaps should be

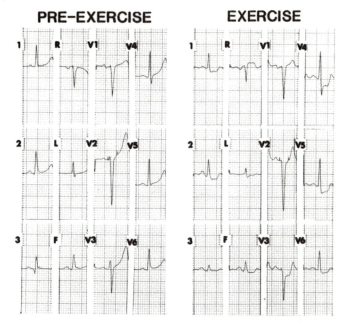

FIG 4–12.

Typical ST-segment depression in multiple leads in a patient with angina and three-vessel CAD. (Sixty-year-old male. Status: post inferior wall myocardial infarction).

normalized to a standard voltage. The average "gain factor" correction of R-wave amplitude should be approximately 25 mm (i.e., average R-wave voltage in V5). In the studies by Hollenberg et al., the magnitude of ST-segment depression was calibrated to a standard R-wave amplitude of 12 mm in lead V5 and 8 mm in lead aVF. Hakki et al. determined the influence of exercise R-wave amplitude on ST segment depression in 81 patients with coronary disease. Among the 26 patients who had an exercise R-wave amplitude in lead V5 < 11 mm, only 8% had an abnormal exercise ECG versus 49% of the 55 patients who had an exercise R-wave amplitude > 11 mm. The sensitivity of the exercise test was low in this study and 64% of the patients had inconclusive results. Exercise thallium scintigraphy increased the sensitivity of the test in patients with low R-wave amplitude.

EXERCISE-INDUCED ST-SEGMENT DEPRESSION NOT DUE TO CORONARY ARTERY DISEASE

Table 4–7 lists some of the conditions that can possibly result in false positive responses. Simonson has suggested that in a population with a high prevalence of heart disease other than coronary artery disease, an abnormal exercise

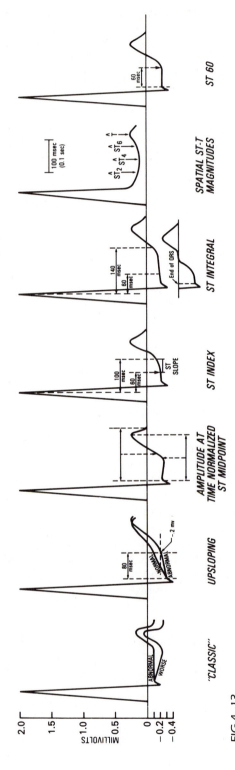

FIG 4–13.
Examples of the criteria for ST-segment depression.

test would be as diagnostic for that disease as it would be for coronary artery disease in populations with a high prevalence of coronary artery disease. Digitalis and other drugs can cause exercise-induced repolarization abnormalities in normal individuals. Patients who have had abnormal responses and who have anemia, electrolyte abnormalities, or are on medications should be retested when these conditions are altered. Meals and even glucose ingestion can alter the ST segment and T-wave in the resting ECG and can potentially cause a false positive response. To avoid this problem, all electrocardiographic studies should be performed after at least a four-hour fast. This requirement is also important because of the hemodynamic stress put on the cardiovascular system by eating. After eating, exercise capacity is decreased and angina occurs sooner.

Women. Sex has an effect on the exercise ECG that is not explained by hormones alone. Estrogen given to men does not increase the rate of false positive responses. Bruce has suggested that the lower specificity of exercise-induced ST-segment depression in women is due to hemodynamic or hemoglobin concentration differences. Table 4–8 summarizes the studies that have evaluated the exercise ECG in women.

Digoxin. Sundqvist et al. studied the effect of digoxin on the electrocardiogram at rest and during and after exercise in 11 healthy subjects. Exercise was performed on a heart rate-controlled bicycle ergometer with stepwise increased loads up to a heart rate of 170 beats/min. The subjects were studied after digoxin at two dose levels and after withdrawal of digoxin. Administration of digoxin induced significant ST-T depression at rest and during exercise even at the small dose. The ST-T changes were numerically small and dose-dependent. There was usually junctional depression and no downsloping, but six individuals had as much as a millimeter of ST depression. The most pronounced ST depression occurred at a heart rate of 110 to 130 beats/min. At higher heart rates, the ST depression was less pronounced

TABLE 4–7.

Conditions and Circumstances That Can Cause a False Positive Exercise Test

Valvular heart disease	Left ventricular hypertrophy
Congenital heart disease	Wolff-Parkinson-White syndrome
Cardiomyopathies	Preexcitation variants
Pericardial disorders	Mitral valve prolapse syndrome
Drug administration	Vasoregulatory abnormality
Electrolyte abnormalities	Hyperventilation repolarization
Nonfasting state	abnormalities
Anemia	Hypertension
Sudden excessive exercise	Excessive double product
Inadequate recording equipment	Improper lead systems
Bundle branch block	Incorrect criteria
Improper interpretation	

TABLE 4–8.
Studies Evaluating the Predictive Value of Exercise ECG
Abnormalities in Women

PRINCIPAL INVESTIGATOR	YEAR	NO.	SENSITIVITY (%)	SPECIFICITY (%)
Caru	1978	168	73	74
Cahen	1978	100	88	92
Sketch	1975	56	50	78
Detry	1977	45	89	63
Linhart	1974	98	71	78
Lesbre	1978	150	66	77
Broustet	1978	84	50	70
Barolsky	1979	92	60	68
Weiner	1979	580	76	64
Guiteras val	1982	112	79	66
Manca	1979	508	88	73
Bengtsson	1981	194	—	85

but still statistically significant. During the first minutes after exercise, no significant digitalis-induced ST-T depression was seen. This type of reaction is not usually seen in myocardial ischemia. Fourteen days after withdrawal of the drug, there were no significant digitalis-induced ST-T changes.

Left Bundle Branch Block.   Whinnery and associates reported 31 asymptomatic men who serially developed left bundle branch block and who were studied with both maximal treadmill testing and coronary angiography. They demonstrated that there can be a marked degree of exercise-induced ST-segment depression in addition to that found at rest in healthy men with left bundle branch block. No difference was found between the ST-segment response to exercise in those with or without significant coronary artery disease. Thus, the ST-segment response to exercise testing cannot be used to make diagnostic decisions on patients with left bundle branch block.

Right Bundle Branch Block.   Whinnery also reported the response to maximal treadmill testing 40 asymptomatic men with acquired right bundle branch block. There was no exercise-induced ST-segment depression in the inferior and lateral leads. Friedman and associates reported exercise-induced ST-segment depression in the anterior precordial leads in patients with right bundle branch block. This is most apparent in the right precordial leads with an rSR' or a notched R-wave; these leads often show a downsloping ST-segment at rest, and such a finding is thus not indicative of myocardial ischemia. Figure 4–14 shows ST depression in lateral leads in a patient with angina and Figure 4–15 shows no ST depression in lateral leads in a subject without coronary heart disease.

Vasey reviewed the records of 2,584 consecutive patients who underwent both treadmill testing and coronary angiography to determine the relation between exercise-induced acceleration-dependent LBBB and the presence of

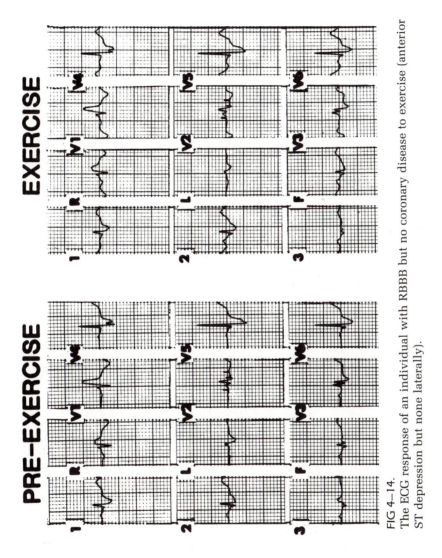

FIG 4–14.
The ECG response of an individual with RBBB but no coronary disease to exercise (anterior ST depression but none laterally).

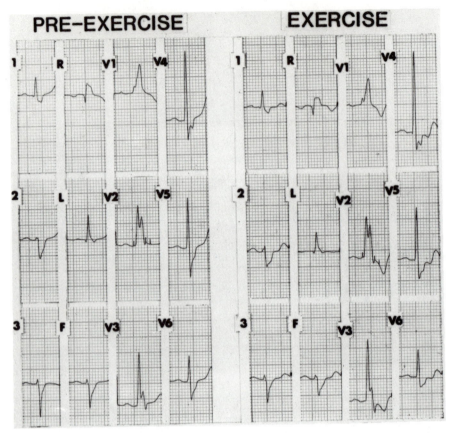

FIG 4–15.
The ECG response to exercise of an individual with RBBB and coronary disease
(ST depression laterally).

CAD. Rate-dependent LBBB during exercise was identified in 28 patients
(1.1%) who were categorized according to their presenting symptoms: classic
angina pectoris, atypical chest pain, symptomatic arrhythmias, and those who
were asymptomatic. Asymptomatic individuals were being screened for silent
CAD. CAD was present in 7 of 10 patients who presented with classic angina
pectoris, but 12 of 13 patients presenting with atypical chest pain had normal
coronary arteries. All 10 patients in whom LBBB developed at a heart rate of
125 beats/min or higher were free of CAD, whereas 9 of 18 patients in whom
LBBB developed at a heart rate of less than 125 beats/min had CAD. Normal
coronary arteries were present in three patients who presented with angina
and in whom both chest pain and LBBB developed during exercise. They
concluded that (1) patients who present with atypical chest pain and have
rate-dependent LBBB are significantly less likely to have CAD than patients
who present with classic angina; (2) the onset of LBBB at a heart rate of 125
beats/min or higher is highly correlated with the presence of normal coronary

arteries, regardless of patient presentation; and, (3) patients with angina in whom both chest pain and LBBB develop during exercise may have normal coronary arteries.

Other Causes.   Individuals with the left ventricular hypertrophy and strain pattern on their resting ECG are at high risk for coronary artery disease. Healthy individuals with the Wolff-Parkinson-White syndrome can have exercise-induced ST-segment depression. Some individuals with preexcitation, a short PR interval, and a normal QRS complex may have a false-positive exercise test. A group of patients with the prolapsing mitral valve syndrome were reported to have abnormal exercise tests but normal coronary angiograms. In individuals with this syndrome, false positive responses are apparently more common, occurring in approximately 25%.

Individuals with vasoregulatory asthenia and orthostatic or vasoregulatory abnormalities can have abnormal exercise-induced ST-segment changes without coronary artery disease. The same can be said for those with hyperventilation repolarization changes prior to treadmill testing, or these maneuvers can be reserved only for patients who have an abnormal response. Such changes are unusual and have rarely been responsible for false positive tests. Orthostatic and hyperventilation changes have been associated with the mitral valve prolapse syndrome. When they do occur with exercise-induced changes, the interpretation of ischemia should be avoided, and the clinician must rely on other parameters to make a diagnosis.

Persons with hypertension or an excessive SBP × HR product during exercise could hypothetically have a physiologic imbalance between myocardial oxygen supply and demand. An excessive number of false positives were not found, however, in one reported population of mild hypertensives. Barnard and coworkers demonstrated that a sudden high work load of treadmill exercise can yield ST-segment depression in healthy individuals on this basis. Foster and associates could not reproduce the ST-segment depression with sudden strenuous bicycle exercise even though ejection fraction dropped in their normal subjects. A recorder with an inadequate frequency response can either artifactually induce ST-segment depression in normal subjects or show upsloping depression when horizontal depression is actually present. Use of the proper equipment should avoid this type of distortion. In conclusion, the conditions discussed above can be avoided and should not be the major causes of false positive responses in a good exercise testing laboratory. The most common cause of a false positive test should be the normal variant in a patient who has a physiologic ST-segment vector that is similar to that produced by ischemia.

ST-segment depression occurring at low heart rates and other patterns may be highly predictive of coronary disease. McHenry has suggested that depression only occurring during recovery is indicative of a false positive. Careful analysis of the time-occurrence patterns in two studies has failed to confirm this or to identify any pattern indicative of a false positive response (Table 4–9).

TABLE 4–9.
Analysis of Time Occurrence Patterns of ST-Segment Depression in Two Studies Screening Asymptomatic Men (One Using Incidence Endpoints and the Other Angiography)*

OCCURRENCE TIME	140 MEN WITH ABNORMAL TREADMILL RESPONSE IN A FOLLOW-UP STUDY			111 MEN WITH ABNORMAL TREADMILL RESPONSE IN AN ANGIOGRAPHIC STUDY	
	OCCURRENCE RATE (%)	RISK RATIO†	PREDICTIVE VALUE (%)	OCCURRENCE RATE (%)	PREDICTIVE VALUE (%)
Exercise only	9	7.4	23	11	8
Recovery only	36	4	12	42	28
Exercise and recovery	55	12	25	47	39
All abnormal responders	100	14.3	20	100	30.6

*From Froelicher et al.
†Times that for normal subjects.

ST SHIFT LOCATION AND ISCHEMIA

Many clinicians use the ST-segment shifts observed in different leads to imply ischemia in underlying areas of myocardium. Validating the localization of ischemia with coronary angiography has several limitations. First, collaterals may adequately perfuse areas of the heart served by an obstructed artery. Second, coronary angiography cannot quantify the degree to which an infarcted area of the heart remains ischemic. Finally, the validity of relating anatomic lesions visualized at rest to exercise-induced changes in the electrocardiogram, both only inferring ischemia, is questionable. These limitations partially explain the difficulty correlating electrocardiographic alterations with the specific number or location of coronary angiographic obstructions. With the advent of coronary artery bypass surgery, precise localization of critical ischemia has assumed more than academic interest. Localization could help to direct surgical intervention to the site of jeopardized myocardium and/or the source of angina pectoris. We therefore utilized exercise thallium perfusion imaging as a measure of myocardial ischemia because of the demonstrated relationship between thallium uptake and myocardial blood flow. The purpose of this investigation was to define the relationship between localized areas of ischemia visualized by thallium imaging and changes observed in the electrocardiogram. Comparison to the results of others is also made.

UCSD Localization Study.   We (Abouantoun et al.) studied 54 patients with stable coronary heart disease, all with exercise-induced thallium scintigraphic defects. Their exercise ECG test results were compared to their thallium images and also to 14 low-risk normal subjects. Exercise data was analyzed for spatial ST vector shifts using a computer program in order to most accurately classify ST-segment depression and elevation. Thallium ischemic defects detected in our patients included areas in the septum and the inferior, lateral, and anterior walls. Twenty-six of these 54 patients also had coronary angiography for classification and comparison as having either localized or generalized disease. None of the scintigraphic ischemic sites or angiographic diseased areas could be specifically identified by exercise-induced ST vector shifts. Therefore, the surface exercise electrocardiogram cannot be used to localize ischemia to specific areas of myocardium.

The most accurate method of localizing exercise-induced ST-segment shifts is to use the time-coherent Frank X, Y, Z vector leads, since these leads best approximate particular cardiac areas, and yet correspond to changes in the standard ECG. Therefore, rather than listing complex combinations of ST shifts seen in the standard 12-leads, the direction and amplitude of ST-segment vector shifts was utilized. Measurements and plots of the spatial ST vector at a point 40 msec after QRS end were analyzed. This does not directly take slope into account, and so there can be normal and abnormal ST shifts for the same vector amplitude. Analysis was performed on data gathered at rest and at maximal or near maximal exercise. Spatial vector length was calculated as the square root of $(X^2 + Y^2 + Z^2)$ where X, Y, and Z are the vector lengths in these axes.

All the normal subjects had normal resting and exercise electrocardiograms except for one who had false positive ST depression in the inferior leads. Angina pectoris developed in 27 out of the 54 patients with thallium ischemia during treadmill testing. Abnormal ST-segment changes were seen in 48 (89%) of the patients, and in six patients the ST response was normal, even though they reached a mean maximal heart rate of 140.

Comparison with Other Localization Studies. Fuchs et al. evaluated the 12-lead ECG for localizing the site of coronary artery disease in 134 patients with angiographically documented single-vessel coronary disease. They reviewed 10 years of cardiac catheterization at John Hopkins Hospital to select these patients who had ECGs recorded during myocardial infarction, spontaneous rest angina, and/or treadmill exercise. Q-wave location correctly identified the location of the coronary lesion in 98% of the cases, ST elevation in 91%, T-wave inversion in 84%, and ST depression in only 60%. No response could separate right from left circumflex coronary artery disease. ST-segment elevation was recorded in 20 of the 56 patients who underwent exercise testing. All 56 had angina during the test. An association was found only between elevation in limb lead III and right coronary artery disease.

Simoons et al. studied the exercise-induced spatial ST vector shifts 30 and 80 msec after QRS end in 34 patients who had coronary angiography and thallium exercise scans because of clinically important chest pain. The electrocardiogram was normal at rest in 30. Twenty-two had significant coronary artery obstructions and 12 had normal angiograms. Four of these "normals" (33%) had abnormal exercise tests as well as chest pain. They found that in patients with exercise thallium ischemia defects, the ST vectors were posteriorly oriented in 15 of 22 and anteriorly oriented in 9 of 12 of those without ischemia defects. However, they could find no systematic difference in the ST vector direction of patients with anteroseptal compared to patients with posterolateral perfusion defects in accordance with our findings. In addition, the same investigators found a higher prevalence of posterior shifts in a better defined group of "normals" again in accordance with our findings. The results of Ascoop et al. using a similar vector approach for the ST vector 70 msec after QRS end differ from our findings. They found a vector shift out of the left inferior anterior octant to have predictive accuracy for angiographic coronary disease. But these findings are at variance with the work of other investigators including Niederberger et al. and Blomquist.

The false positive rate was as expected in such a population due to the less than perfect specificity of the exercise electrocardiogram. The direction of the exercise-induced ST-segment shifts in normals is mixed and is compatible with the normal variation possible during exercise as found by Simoons. Why this shift occurs is not known, but it may be due to relative ischemia in the subendocardium that is a normal exercise phenomenon.

During exercise, 70% of our patients had ST-segment vectors directed to the right superior-anterior octant and 17% to the right superior-posterior octant. This suggests that the right superior-anterior octant is the most common ischemic octant, though 21% (3 out of 14) of the normals had exercise-induced ST-segment vector shifts into the right superior-anterior octant as well.

Twenty-four percent of our patients had isolated septal ischemic defects. This corresponds to lesions of the left anterior descending coronary artery. This area has been the one identified with the greatest reproducibility by our scoring methods. Eighty-five percent of these patients had exercise ST-vectors going into the right superior-anterior octant. Since many normals and most of our other thallium ischemia patients have ST-vectors in the same octant, this direction of ST displacement does not necessarily characterize septal ischemia on the surface electrocardiogram. This is also the case in patients with combined anterior thallium ischemia defects, which also must be due to left anterior descending disease.

Lateral defects occurred in 17% of our patients; this area on thallium scans is second only to the inferior area for poorest reproducibility. Twenty-two percent of our patients had combined inferior defects. These two patterns seem to reflect occlusions in the left circumflex and right coronary artery. No direction of ST-vector shifts separated these from the others. This lack of distinguishing features for localization of ischemia is confirmed by the subgroup who had angiography.

The ST patterns seen in these patients are due to transmural ischemia. The ischemic vector "up the long axis" of the left ventricle is most likely due to global subendocardial ischemia; therefore, the transmural ischemic areas must "steal" from the subendocardium. This would explain why the majority of people have ST-vectors extending during exercise into the right superior quadrants—this is the direction of the open cone of the left ventricle. Localized transmural ischemia results in generalized subendocardial ischemia which slows electrical conduction, changing the action potentials, as is seen in myocardial infarction. The ST changes registered during exercise are partially dependent upon the location of scar tissue. ST-segment elevation or depression, or various combinations of ST-segment shifts, do not localize ischemia to myocardial areas or to the arteries that supply these areas. For instance, ST-segment shifts in II and AVF do not necessarily mean that there is inferior ischemia (or right coronary artery disease) nor do shifts in V5 mean that there is lateral ischemia (or left coronary artery disease).

SUBJECTIVE RESPONSES

Careful observation of the patient's appearance is necessary for the safe performance of an exercise test and is helpful in the clinical assessment of a patient. Patients who exaggerate their limitations or symptoms and those unwilling to cooperate are usually easy to identify. A drop in skin temperature during exercise can indicate an inadequate cardiac output with secondary vasoconstriction and can be an indication for not encouraging a patient to a higher work load. Neurologic manifestations such as lightheadedness or vertigo can also be indications of an inadequate cardiac output.

Findings on physical examination can be helpful, but their sensitivity and specificity have not been demonstrated. Gallop sounds, a mitral regurgitant murmur, or a precordial bulge could be due to left ventricular dysfunction. An S3 can sometimes be heard in normals after exercise, but a new S4 brought out by exercise has been said to be specific for coronary heart disease. The physical findings of congestive heart failure, including rales and neck vein distention, should be encountered rarely in patients referred for exercise testing. However, some exercise testing laboratories use the sitting position for the recovery period to avoid problems with the patient who develops orthopnea. It is preferable to have patients lie supine after exercise testing and allow those who develop orthopnea to sit up. Also, severe angina or ominous dysrhythmias following exercise can be lessened by allowing the patient to sit up. Attempts to make the findings of the physical examination less subjective include the use of phonocardiography, apexcardiography, and cardiokymography. Left ventricular ejection time can be determined by the ear densitigram and its first derivative more easily than by trying to obtain a carotid pulse tracing.

Chest Pain.   Weiner and coworkers reported 281 consecutive patients studied with treadmill testing and coronary angiography with the following responses: (1) 76 patients with ST-segment depression and treadmill test-induced chest pain; (2) 85 patients with ST-segment depression and no chest pain; (3) 40 patients with treadmill test induced-chest pain who had no ST-segment changes; and (4) 80 patients with neither chest pain nor ST-segment changes. They found that 91% of the first group, 65% of the second group, 72% of the third group, and only 35% of the fourth group had significant angiographically determined coronary artery disease. Cole and Ellestad followed 95 patients with abnormal treadmill tests. At five-year follow-up, the incidence of coronary artery disease was 73% in those with both chest pain and an abnormal ST-segment response compared with 43% in those who only had an abnormal ST-segment response. Mortality was also twice as high in those with both ST-segment changes and chest pain induced by the treadmill test. The results of these studies suggest that ischemic chest pain induced by the exercise test predicts the presence of coronary artery disease as well as ST-segment depression, and when they occur together, they are even more predictive of coronary artery disease than either is alone. It is important, however, that a careful description of the pain be obtained from the patient to ascertain that it is typical rather than atypical angina.

OBSERVER AGREEMENT IN INTERPRETATION

The complexity of not only the human body but also the human mind has created measurements, that when applied to medical diagnosis lead to observations with large variability, i.e., ST-segment displacement. The inherent subjective nature of these medical observations require questioning of the results of most diagnostic methods, not only in regard to accuracy or validity but also agreement (among different interpretors for a given test). Attempts at describing or assessing agreement have been complex and variable as evidenced in the literature by the numerous terms used: agreement, variability, consistency, within-observer correlation coefficients of disagreement, and many others. Agreement has two subgroupings: intraobserver, referring to agreement of the individual observer with himself on two separate occasions; and interobserver, referring to agreement among two or more individuals. Nearly all diagnostic areas of cardiology have been scrutinized for agreement, including the clinical examination, the rest-and-exercise ECG, echocardiography, and nuclear cardiology. Even the gold standard, coronary angiography, has been examined for observer variability. These studies will be briefly reviewed.

In one of the few studies of agreement concerning the cardiac physical examination, Raftery and Holland found that two cardiologists had excellent agreement on heart size and murmurs (greater than 94% agreement), but agreement on extra sounds was in a range of 72% to 92%. They found best agreement between cardiologists as opposed to three nonspecialists. In a study assessing agreement of three physicians as to the presence or absence of tibial or dorsalis pedis artery pulses, Meade and colleagues found an interobserver agreement in approximately 70% and 80%, respectively, and intraobserver agreement ranging from 73% to 87%, respectively.

The echocardiogram has been criticized not only for problems in technical reproducibility (the ability to give the same image on a second study) but also for its observer agreement in interpretation. Schieken and colleagues evaluated the echocardiogram as a possible tool for studying large groups in long-term studies and considered inter- and intraobserver agreements for measuring left heart dimensions using standard criteria. Using correlation coefficients, they found a within-observer intraclass correlation coefficient (another method of describing intraobserver agreement) range of .87 to .98 for various dimensions. They found an interobserver coefficient range of .86 to .98, except for the left ventricular posterior wall measurement, which had a coefficient of .57. They attributed their relatively high intra- and interobserver agreements to the use of standardized measurement criteria, which defined technically acceptable interfaces and standard measurement techniques. Crawford and colleagues compared their methods to the standards recommended by the American Society of Echocardiography, and found their own standards more accurate. Their study not only supports the use of standard reporting forms for increased precision but also stresses the importance of finding a standard that will give the greatest precision and agreement. Unfortunately, they did not address the problem of interinstitutional agreement.

Felner and associates evaluated experimental factors, both in interpretation and in testing protocol (subject gender, day and time of testing, and subject position) that might be involved in the variability of echocardiographic measurements. Using a variance component model, they determined the relative contribution of various factors to the total variability in measurement. As expected, the subject variance was a major component in all measurements, but technician, subject position, and day-to-day variance were minimal except for heart rate and right ventricular internal dimension. The interpreter variance component, however, was significant, particularly in measuring interventricular septal and posterior left ventricular wall thicknesses. Intrainterpreter variability in measurement was as large or larger than was interinterpreter variability. To ensure greater agreement, they stressed the necessity of reading echocardiograms either using one interpreter on two separate occasions or by using two interpreters.

The electrocardiogram and vectorcardiogram have been noted to have a low level of observer agreement (or high reader variability). Segall had a group of physicians interpret 100 electrocardiograms as normal, old myocardial infarction, or nonspecifically abnormal. Although only paired interobserver correlation was calculated, he did note that 70% or more of the 20 readers were only able to agree on 77 of the 100 ECGs. Using the same reporting categories, Davies and nine experienced electrocardiographers interpreted 100 ECGs on two separate occasions at two or more weeks apart. He found that at least two-thirds of his readers agreed on 78% of the ECGs and that complete agreement occurred in only 29% of the cases. Interobserver correlations of readings were not calculated, but intraobserver consistency or agreement was done on each of the experienced nine readers and showed an intraobserver agreement with a range of 81% to 93%. In another study, Acheson noted a 90% intraobserver agreement in one reader and an overall agreement of 60%.

Simonson evaluated 10 observers in their interpretation of 114 vectorcardiograms (VCG) and 105 electrocardiograms (ECG). In addition to an excellent review of the literature comparing the diagnostic value of the VCG and ECG, he and his colleagues looked at many areas of interpretation, such as diagnostic accuracy of various myocardial conditions and comparisons between the VCG and ECG. They also addressed inter- and intraobserver variation (another form of agreement, but more in terms of lack of agreement than agreement). Among the observers, he found a wide variation in making the correct interpretation for five conditions, as evidenced by wide standard deviations for the average correct or incorrect diagnoses.

Blackburn had 14 observers (from seven separate institutions) interpret 38 individual exercise electrocardiographic tests as to normal, abnormal, or borderline. Five readers repeated the readings. In only nine of the 38 (24%) exercise ECGs was there complete agreement among the 14 readers, and only 22 ECGs (58%) were read in agreement. This low value may be due to the fact that Blackburn's study did not allow a dichotomous decision because there was the third interpretation of borderline. In terms of intraobserver agreement, there was a wide range from 58% to 92% and an average still less than ours for a dichotomous decision. Blackburn attributed this wide variation in both inter- and intraobserver agreement to (1) the absence of defined criteria, (2) technical problems such as noise, and (3) differences in opinion as to ST-segment upsloping. Strict criteria such as the Minnesota code and computer analysis have been recommended as a means to increase agreement in electrocardiography.

Detre and colleagues studied observer agreement in detecting a lesion with 50% or more diameter occlusion in 13 coronary angiograms. These angiograms were reviewed by 22 readers on two separate occasions. Interobserver variability (observer disagreement) was measured in terms of both standard deviation, agreement index, and pairwise disagreement index. Detre found results midway between chance expectation and 100% agreement. This study demonstrated considerable inter- and intraobserver variability (low agreement) and found the lowest interobserver agreement among those who were least consistent, even with themselves (intraobserver agreement). There was also a strong correlation between observer experience and intraobserver consistency, that is, experienced observers usually agreed on two readings.

Zir and colleagues had four readers, two radiologists, and two cardiologists assess coronary artery stenoses and wall motion abnormalities in 20 patients. He found a striking degree of interobserver variability, particularly in the interpretation of arterial or ventricular wall segments with the highest percentage of positive findings. Galbraith and associates also correlated interobserver variability in the evaluation of coronary angiograms with postmortem pathologic findings. They found that in spite of the presence of coronary artery disease, angiographic interpretations of significant lesions (50% or more angiographic diameter occlusion) were noted in only approximately 80% of the arteries with such occlusions on pathologic examination. In addition, they found that when the majority opinion of angiographic interpretation was used, it added little to accuracy. This result was attributed to the large influence of a dominant, persistent, or senior reader on consensus interpretation and would suggest perhaps that first, individual reader assessment may give a less biased interpretation, and second, that accuracy may be more a function of the reader than of the angiogram.

Chaitman and colleagues looked at both subjective evaluations (estimations) and objective evaluations (measurements from frame tracings) of angiographic film for volume, ejection fraction, and wall motion. Less interobserver variability (greater agreement) was demonstrated between the objective observers than between the subjective observers, particularly with respect to volume measurements. There was even less agreement when comparing objective observer measurements to those of the subjective observers in all areas. Best inter- and intraobserver agreement occurred in ejection fraction measurements especially in the objective intraobserver measurement of ejection fraction, in which a .99 correlation was noted. Unfortunately, only one observer was tested for intraobserver agreement.

REPRODUCIBILITY OF TREADMILL TEST RESPONSES

We (Sullivan et al.) studied 14 male patients with exercise test-induced angina and ST-segment depression with treadmill testing on three consecutive days to evaluate the reproducibility of certain treadmill variables. Computerized ST-segment analysis and expired gas analysis, including anaerobic threshold, were evaluated for reproducibility using an intraclass correlation coefficient analysis (ICC). The ICC is a generalization of the Pearson product-moment correlation which is not affected by the addition or multiplication of a given number of observations and provides a better indication of reproducibility than does the coefficient of variation.

An estimate of the standard deviation of the change of two measurements (SD) and the coefficient of variation for peak exercise, the onset of angina, and the ATGE variables are provided in Table 4–10. The estimates of the standard deviation of the change of two measurements is important when performing power calculations for determination of sample size and/or the required change needed in a variable to detect significance. In addition, if SD is multiplied by 1.96, the change required in an individual to have a less than 5% chance of that change being due to measurement error is obtained. In order to compare our results with previous studies, the coefficient of variation was determined at each point of interest.

Oxygen uptake had a higher reliability coefficient (r = .88) and a smaller 90% confidence interval when compared to treadmill time (r = .70) consistent with a better correlation. The double product and heart rate were highly reproducible (r = .90 and r = .94, respectively). In addition, the 90% confi-

TABLE 4–10.
Standard Deviation of Change of Two Measurements (SD) and the Coefficient of Variation (CV) at Peak Exercise, the Onset of Angina, and the Gas Exchange Anaerobic Threshold (ATGE)

VARIABLE	PEAK EXERCISE		ONSET OF ANGINA		ATGE	
	SD	CV, %	SD	CV, %	SD	CV, %
Time (sec)	58	6 ± 6	65	11 ± 6	65	15 ± 9
Vo_2 (L/min)	.150	6 ± 4	.152	6 ± 4	.113	7 ± 4
Double product ($\times 10)^3$	2.6	9 ± 5	2.0	8 ± 5	2.2	8 ± 6
Heart rate (beats/min)	7	4 ± 2	6	4 ± 2	8	4 ± 4
ST60 X (mV)	.06	34 ± 25	.03	31 ± 25	.03	45 ± 29
ST60 GD (mV)	.05	23 ± 21	.04	25 ± 16	.05	53 ± 34

dence interval for both double product and heart rate was small. The ST60 displacement in lead X and the lead of greatest displacement were very reproducible (r = .83).

Onset of angina results for time, oxygen uptake, double product, ST60 lead X, and ST60 lead with the greatest ST-segment displacement (mV) were analyzed. As with peak exercise values, there was no significant time trend in any of the measured variables during the three days of testing. Reliability coefficients for time were as high as peak exercise values, but again, oxygen uptake had a higher reliability coefficient (r = .81) and a smaller 90% confidence interval when compared to time (r = .70). The double product was not nearly as reproducible, but heart rate was very reproducible (r = .89) and had a small 90% confidence interval. The ST60 displacement was similar to peak values.

Two of the three independent observers agreed on the time of the ATGE in 100% of the exercise tests. All three observers agreed on 71% (30/42) of the tests. A second independent reading to determine the ATGE by the same three observers revealed similar results with agreement by two of the three observers on 100% (42/42) and total agreement on 69% (29/42) of the tests. When comparing the first reading to the second, there was agreement on 90% (38/42) of the exercise tests. The ICC and the 90% confidence interval for oxygen uptake (r = .80) was similar to that obtained for the onset of angina (r = −.81). The ATGE double product was as reproducible (r = .74) as the double product obtained at the onset of angina (r = .75), and had a similar 90% confidence interval. The heart rate at the ATGE was reproducible (r = .83) and had a small 90% confidence interval.

In summary, measured oxygen uptake displayed better reproducibility than treadmill time at peak exercise, the onset of angina, and the gas exchange anaerobic threshold. The double product, heart rate, and ST-segment displacement in lead X were found to be reproducible at peak exercise, the onset of angina, and the ATGE. Gas exchange analysis provided accurate physiological determinants of exercise capacity in patients with angina pectoris. Noninvasive estimates of myocardial oxygen demand and ischemia were reproducibly determined.

CONCLUSIONS

The interpretation of the exercise test is not a simple skill, but requires the understanding of physiology and pathophysiology. Not all medical professionals can adequately interpret an exercise test. Training and experience are required as they are in other diagnostic procedures. All of the results of the test must be considered. Attempts shouid be made to make the interpretation reliable by using good methods and following the above suggestions. When properly interpreted, the exercise test is one of the most important diagnostic and clinically helpful tests in medicine.

Observer agreement is best when using dichotomous interpretations and the worst (most variability) when using more complex descriptions such as those involved in specifying location or overlapping areas. Several possible modes for improvement include (1) simple dichotomous decisions, (2) standardized report forms such as the one used in this study, (3) multiple observers or one very experienced reader, (4) multiple blinded or unbiased interpretations, and (5) computer analysis. Computer analysis of the exercise electrocardiogram and measurement of gas exchange variables can be highly reproducible. However, as long as human judgment with all its complexities remains the basis for the final interpretation, some variation will always have to be accepted. The human element is what keeps medical diagnosis an art.

ST-segment depression is a representation of global subendocardial ischemia, with a direction determined largely by the placement of the heart in the chest. ST depression does not localize coronary artery lesions. ST depression in the inferior leads (II, AVF) is most often due to the atrial repolarization wave that begins in the PR segment and can extend to the beginning of the ST segment. Severe transmural ischemia, resulting in wall motion abnormalities, causes a shift of the vector in the direction of the wall motion abnormality. However, preexisting areas of wall motion abnormality (i.e., scar) usually indicated by a Q-wave also cause such a shift resulting in ST elevation without ischemia being present. When the resting ECG shows Q-waves of a prior MI, ST elevation is due to ischemia or wall motion abnormalities or both, whereas accompanying ST depression can be due to a second area of ischemia or merely reciprocal changes. When the resting ECG is normal, however, ST elevation is due to severe ischemia (spasm or a critical lesion), and accompanying ST depression is reciprocal.

Cardiac radionuclide imaging has been used to demonstrate the relation of QRS amplitudes to left ventricular function and volume changes and ischemia during exercise. Exercise-induced R-wave and S-wave amplitude changes do not correlate with changes in left ventricular volume, ejection fraction, or ischemia. The concensus of many studies is that such changes do not have diagnostic value.

The nonelectrocardiographic responses should be appreciated for their information content which often exceeds or modifies the information from the ST segments. Exercise capacity and LV function are relatively independent and abnormalities of the hemodynamic responses (SBP, exercise capacity, HR) can be determined either by myocardial ischemia or damage. The same exercise test responses can have a different meaning from one population or clinical grouping to another, and so interpretation depends upon the application of the test.

BIBLIOGRAPHY

Abouantoun S, Ahnve S, Savvides M, et al: Can areas of myocardial ischemia be localized by the exercise electrocardiogram? A correlative study with thallium-201 scintigraphy. *Am Heart J* 1984;108:933–941.

Ahnve S, Sullivan M, Myers J, et al: Computer analysis of exercise-induced changes in QRS duration in patients with angina pectoris and in normal subjects. *Am Heart J* 1986;111:903.

Akiyama T, Richeson JF, Ingram JT, et al: Effects of varying the electrical conductivity of the medium between the heart and the body surface on the epicardial and precordial electrocardiogram in the pig. *Cardiovasc Res* 1978;12:697–702.

Amon KW, Richards KL, Crawford MH: Usefulness of the postexercise response of systolic blood pressure in the diagnosis of coronary artery disease. *Circulation* 1984;70:951–956.

Ask P, Oberg PA, Odman S, et al: ECG electrodes—A study of electrical and mechanical long-term properties. *Acta Anaesthesiol Scand* 1979;23:189–206.

Astrand I: Aerobic work capacity in men and women with special reference to age. *Acta Physiol Scand* 1960;49,169:1–82.

Barlow JB: The "false positive" exercise electrocardiogram: value of time course patterns in assessment of depressed ST segments and inverted T-waves. *Am Heart J* 1985;110:1328–1335.

Barnard R, MacAlpin R, Kattus A, et al: Ischemic response to sudden strenuous exercise in healthy men. *Circulation* 1973;48:936.

Baron DW, Lisley C, Sheiban I, et al: R-wave amplitude during exercise: relation to left ventricular function in coronary artery disease. *Br Heart J* 1980;44:512–517.

Battler A, Froelicher VF, Gallagher KP, et al: Effects of changes in ventricular size on regional surface QRS amplitudes in the conscious dog. *Circulation* 1980;62:174–180.

Battler A, Froelicher VF, Slutsky R, et al: Relationship of QRS amplitude changes during exercise to left ventricular function and volumes and the diagnosis of coronary artery disease. *Circulation* 1979;60:1004–1013.

Benge W, Litchfield RL, Marcus ML: Exercise capacity in patients with severe left ventricular dysfunction. *Circulation* 1980;61:955–959.

Bengtsson C, Grimby G, Lindquist O, et al: Prognosis of women with exercise-induced ECG changes: results from a longitudinal population study. *Cardiology* 1981;68:9–14.

Berkenboom GM, Abramowicz M, Vandermoten P, et al: Role of alpha-adrenergic coronary tone in exercise-induced angina pectoris. *Am J Cardiol* 1986;57:195–198.

Berman JL, Wynne J, Cohn PF: Multiple-lead QRS changes with exercise testing: diagnostic value and hemodynamic implications. *Circulation* 1980;61:53–61.

Blair SN, Lavey RS, Goodyear N, et al: Physiologic responses to maximal graded exercise testing in apparently healthy white women aged 18 to 75 years. *J Cardiac Rehabil* 1984; 4:459–468.

Blomqvist G: The Frank lead exercise electrocardiogram. *Acta Med Scand* 178:1–98, 1965.

Bonoris PE, Greenberg PS, Castellanet MJ, et al: Significance of changes in R-wave amplitude during treadmill stress testing: angiographic correlation. *Am J Cardiol* 1978;41:846–851.

Bonoris PE, Greenberg PS, Christison GW, et al: Evaluation of R-wave amplitude changes versus ST-segment depression in stress testing. *Circulation* 1978;57:904–910.

Borer JS, Rosing DR, Miller RH, et al: Natural history of LVEF during one year after acute MI: comparison with clinical, ECG, and biochemical determinations. *Am J Cardiol* 1980;46:1–12.

Braat SH, Kingma H, Brugada P, et al: Value of lead V4R in exercise testing to predict proximal stenosis of the right coronary artery. *J Am Coll Cardiol* 1985;5:1308–1311.

Bricker TJ, Porter CJ, Garson A, et al: Exercise testing in children with Wolff-Parkinson-White syndrome. *Am J Cardiol* 1985;55:1001–1004.

Brody DA: A theoretical analysis of intracavitary blood mass influence on the heart-lead relationship. *Circ Res* 1956;4:731–738.

Bruce RA, Fisher FD, Cooper MN, et al: Separation of effects of cardiovascular disease and age on ventricular function with maximal exercise. *Am J Cardiol* 1974;34:757–763.

Carter CL, Amundsen LR: Infarct size and exercise capacity after myocardial infarction. *J Appl Physiol: Respirat Environ Exerc Physiol* 1977;42:782–785.

Chadda KD, Cohen J, Werner BM, et al: Observations on serum and red blood cell magnesium changes in treadmill exercise-induced cardiac ischemia. *J Am Coll Nutr* 1985;4:157–163.

Chahine RA, Raizner AE, Ishimori T: The clinical significance of exercise-induced ST-segment elevation. *Circulation* 1976;54:209–213.

Chaitman BR, Bourassa MG, Wagniart P, et al: Improved efficiency of treadmill exercise testing using a multiple lead ECG system and basic hemodynamic exercise response. *Circulation* 1978;57:71–79.

Chin CF, Messenger JC, Greenberg PS, et al: Chronotropic incompetence in exercise testing. *Clin Cardiol* 1979;2:12–18.

Christison GW, Bonoris PE, Greenberg PE, et al: Predicting coronary artery disease with treadmill stress testing: changes in R-wave amplitude compared with ST-segment depression. *J Electrocardiol* 1979;12:179–185.

Coester N, Elliott JC, Luft UC: Plasma electrolytes, pH, and ECG during and after exhaustive exercise. *J Appl Physiol* 1973;34:677.

Cohen D, Kaufman LA: Magnetic determination of the relationship between the ST-segment shift and the injury current produced by coronary artery occlusion. *Circ Res* 1976;36:414.

Convertino V, Hung J, Goldwater D, et al: Cardiovascular responses to exercise in middle-aged man after 10 days of bedrest. *Circulation* 1982;65:134–140.

Cooper KH, Purdy JG, White SR, et al: Age-fitness adjusted maximal heart rates. *Med Sport* 1977;10:78–88.

Cunningham WL, Becker ES, Kreuzer F: Catecholamines in plasma and urine at high altitudes. *J Appl Physiol* 1965;20:607–610.

Daniels S, Iskandrian AS, Hakki AH, et al: Correlation between changes in R wave amplitude and left ventricular volume induced by rapid atrial pacing. *Am Heart J* 1984;April:711–717.

David D, Kitchen JG, Michelson EL, et al: R-wave amplitude responses to rapid atrial pacing: a marker for myocardial ischemia. *Am Heart J* 1984:53–61.

David D, Masahito N, Chen CC, et al: R-wave amplitude variations during acute experimental myocardial ischemia: An inadequate index for changes in intracardiac volume. *Circulation* 1981;63:1364–1371.

David D, Naito M, Michelson E, et al: Intramyocardial conduction: A major determinant of R-wave amplitude during acute myocardial ischemia. *Circulation* 1982;65:161–167.

Deanfield J, Davies G, Mongiadi F, et al: Factors influencing R-wave amplitude in patients with ischemic heart disease. *Br Heart J* 1983;49:8–14.

deCaprio L, Cuomo S, Vigorito C, et al: Influence of heart rate on exercise-induced R-wave amplitude changes in coronary patients and normal subjects. *Am Heart J* 1984;107:61–68.

DeLanne R, Barnes JR, Brouha L: Changes in osmotic pressure and ionic concentrations of plasma during muscular work and recovery. *J Appl Physiol* 1959;14:804.

DePace NL, Iskandrian AS, Hakki A, et al: Use of QRS scoring and thallium-201 scintigraphy to assess left ventricular function after myocardial infarction. *Am J Cardiol* 1982;50:1262–1268.

Dougherty JD: The relationship of QRS amplitude to the frontal QRS axis and the heart-electrode distance. *J Electrocardiol* 1971;4:249–260.

Dunn RF, Freedman B, Bailey IK, et al: Localization of coronary artery disease with exercise electrocardiography: Correlation with thallium-201 myocardial perfusion scanning. *Am J Cardiol* 1981;48:837–843.

Ehsani AA, Biello D, Seals DR, et al: The effects of left ventricular systolic function on maximal aerobic exercise capacity in asymptomatic patients with coronary artery disease. *Circulation* 1984;70:552–560.

Ekmekci A, Toyoshima H, Kwoczynski JK, et al: Angina versus giant R- and receding S-wave in myocardial ischemia and certain nonischemic conditions. *Am J Cardiol* 25:522–529.

Ellestad MH: Commentary: The mechanism of exercise-induced R-wave amplitude changes in coronary heart disease. *Arch Intern Med* 1982;142:963–965.

Ellestad MH, Wan MKC: Predictive implications of stress testing—Follow-up of 2,700 subjects after maximal treadmill stress testing. *Circulation* 1975;51:363–369.

Feldman T, Borow KM, Neumann A, et al: Relation of electrocardiographic R-wave amplitude to changes in left ventricular chamber size and position in normal subjects. *Am J Cardiol* 1985;55:1168–1174.

Feldman T, Childers RW, Borow KM, et al: Change in ventricular cavity size: Differential effects on QRS and T-wave amplitude. *Circulation* 1985;72:495–501.

Foster C, Dymond DS, Carpenter J, et al: Effect of warm-up on left ventricular response to sudden strenuous exercise. *J Appl Physiol* 1982;53:380–383.

Fox KM, England D, Honathan A, et al: Inability of exercise-induced R-wave changes to predict coronary artery disease. *Am J Cardiol* 1982;49:674.

Fox KM, Hakki AH, Iskandrian AS, et al: Relation between electrocardiographic and scintigraphic location of myocardial ischemia during exercise in one-vessel coronary artery disease. *Am J Cardiol* 1984;53:1529–1531.

Fox KM, Selwyn A, Oakley D, et al: Relation between the precordial projection of S-T segment changes after exercise and coronary angiographic findings. *Am J Cardiol* 1979;44:1068–1075.

Freeman G, Hwang MH, Danoviz J, et al: Exercise induced "Mobitz Type II" second degree AV block in a patient with chronic bifascicular block (right bundle branch block and left anterior hemiblock). *J Electrocardiol* 1984;17:409–412.

Fuchs RM, Achuff SC, Grunwald L, et al: Electrocardiographic localization of coronary artery narrowings: Studies during myocardial ischemia and infarction in patients with one-vessel disease. *Circulation* 1982;66:1168–1175.

Gavazzi A, DeServi S, Cornalba C, et al: Significance of the walk-through angina phenomenon during exercise testing. *Cardiology* 1986;73:47–53.

Gerson MC, Morris SN, McHenry PL: Relation of exercise-induced physiologic ST-segment depression to R-wave amplitude in normal subjects. *Am J Cardiol* 1980;46:778–782.

Gerson MC, Phillips JF, Morris SN, et al: Angina pectoris: Clinical and experimental difference between ischemia with ST elevation and ischemia with ST depression. *Am J Cardiol* 1961;7:412.

Gordon NF: Effect of selective and nonselective beta-adrenoceptor blockade on thermoregulation during prolonged exercise in heat. *Am J Cardiol* 1985;55:74D–78D.

Grande P, Pedersen A: Myocardial infarct size and cardiac performance at exercise soon after myocardial infarction. *Br Heart J* 1982;47:44–50.

Greenberg PS, Ellestad M: Ability of R-wave change during stress testing to accurately detect coronary disease in the presence of left bundle branch block at rest. *Angiology* 1980;31:230–237.

Greenberg PS, Ellestad M, Berge R, et al: Radionuclide angiographic correlation of the R-wave, ejection fraction, and volume responses to upright bicycle exercise. *Chest* 1981;80:459–464.

Greenberg PS, Ellestad MH, Berg R, et al: Correlation of R-wave and EF changes with upright bicycle stress testing. *Circulation* 1980;62:111–200.

Greenspan M, Anderson GJ: The significance of exercise-induced Q-waves. *Am J Med* 1979;67:454.

Gupta R, Gupta S: Comparison of QRS score and treadmill performance for assessing ventricular function after myocardial infarction. *Am Heart J* 1984;108:266–269.

Haiat R, Halphen C, Derrida JP, et al: Pseudonormalization of the repolarization during transient episodes of myocardial ischemia. *Am Heart J* 1977;94:390–391.

Hakki A, Iskandrian AS, Kutalek S, et al: R-wave amplitude: A new determinant of failure of patients with coronary heart disease to manifest ST segment depression during exercise. *J Am Coll Cardiol* 1984;3:1155–1160.

Hakki AH, DePace NL, Colby J, et al: Implication of normal exercise electrocardiographic results in patients with angiographically documented coronary artery disease. *Am J Med* 1983;75:439–444.

Hakki AH, Munley BM, Hadjimiltiades S, et al: Determinants of abnormal blood pressure response to exercise in coronary artery disease. *Am J Cardiol* 1986;57:71–75.

Hamer J, Boyle D, Sowton E: The transmission of electrical forces from the heart to the body surface. *Br Heart J* 1965;27:365–373.

Hammermeister KE, DeRouen TA, Dodge HT, et al: Prognostic and predictive value of exertional hypotension in suspected coronary heart disease. *Am J Cardiol* 1983;51:1261–1266.

Hammond HK, Kelly TL, Froelicher VF: Noninvasive testing in the evaluation of myocardial ischemia: Agreement among tests. *J Am Coll Cardiol* 1985;5:59–69.

Hartley LH, Vogel JA, Cruz JC: Reduction of maximal exercise heart rate at altitude and its reversal with atropine. *J Appl Physiol* 1974;36:362–365.

Higginbotham MB, Morris KG, Conn EH, et al: Determinants of variable exercise performance among patients with severe left ventricular dysfunction. *Am J Cardiol* 1983;51:52–60.

Hirzel HO, Leutwyler R, Krayenbuehl HP: Silent myocardial ischemia: Hemodynamic changes during dynamic exercise in patients with proven coronary artery disease despite absence of angina pectoris. *J Am Coll Cardiol* 1985;6:275–284.

Hirzel HO, Senn M, Nuesch K, et al: Thallium-201 scintigraphy in complete left bundle branch block. *Am J Cardiol* 1984;53:764–769.

Hlatky M, Botvinick E, Brundage B: Diagnostic accuracy of cardiologists compared with probability calculations using Bayes' rule. *Am J Cardiol* 1982;49:1927–1931.

Holland RP, Arnsdorf MF: Nonspatial determinants of electrograms in guinea pig ventricle. *Am Physiol Soc* 1981:148–160.

Holland RP, Brooks H: The QRS complex during myocardial ischemia: An experimental analysis in the porcine heart. *J Clin Invest* 1976;57:541–550.

Holland RP, Brooks H: TQ-ST segment mapping: Critical review and analysis of current concepts. *Prog Cardiovasc Dis* 1977;40:110–129.

Hollenberg M, Mateo GO, Massie BM, et al: Influence of R-wave amplitude on exercise-induced ST depression: Need for a "gain factor" correction when interpreting stress electrocardiograms. *Am J Cardiol* 1985;56:13–17.

Hollenberg M, Zoltick JM, Go M, et al: Comparison of a quantitative treadmill exercise score with standard electrocardiographic criteria in screening asymptomatic young men for coronary artery disease. *N Engl J Med* 1985;313:600–606.

Homans DC, Sublett E, Dai XZ, et al: Persistence of regional left ventricular dysfunction after exercise-induced myocardial ischemia. *J Clin Invest* 1986;77:66–73.

Horan LG, Andreae RL, Yoffee HF: The effect of intracavitary carbon dioxide on surface potentials in the intact canine chest. *Am Heart J* 1961;61:504–514.

Inoue H, Takenaka K, Murayama M, et al: Effects of acute changes in left ventricular size on surface potential in man. *Jpn Heart J* 1982;May:279–292.

Irving JB, Bruce RA: Exertional hypotension and postexertional ventricular fibrillation in stress testing. *Am J Cardiol* 1977;39:849–851.

Ishikawa K, Berson AS, Pipberger HV: Electrocardiographic changes due to cardiac enlargement. *Am Heart J* 1971;81:635–643.

Iskandrian AS, Hakki A, Mintz GS, et al: Changes in R-wave during exercise: A correlation with left ventricular function and volumes. *Cardiovasc Rev Rep* 1983;3:245–252.

Jose AD, Collison D: The normal range and determinants of the intrinsic heart rate in man. *Cardiovasc Res* 1970;4:160–167.

Jose AD, Taylor RR: Autonomic blockade by propranolol and atropine to study intrinsic myocardial function in man. *J Clin Invest* 1969;48:2019–2031.

Kansal S, Roitman D, Sheffield TL: Stress testing with ST-segment depression at rest. *Circulation* 1976;54:636–639.

Kaplan MA, Harris CN, Aronow WS, et al: Inability of the submaximal treadmill stress test to predict the location of coronary disease. *Circulation* 1973;62:250–256.

Kentala E, Luurela O: Response of R-wave amplitude to posterior changes and to exercise. *Ann Clin Res* 1975;7:258–263.

Kostis JB, Moreyra AE, Amendo MT, et al: The effect of age on heart rate in subjects free of heart disease: Studies by ambulatory electrocardiography and maximal exercise stress test. *Circulation* 1982;65:141–145.

Kovacs SJ: The duration of the QT interval as a function of heart rate: A derivation based on physical principles and a comparison to measured values. *Am Heart J* 1985;110:872–880.

Kveselis DA, Rocchini AP, Rosenthal A, et al: Hemodynamic determinants of exercise-induced ST-segment depression in children with valvular aortic stenosis. *Am J Cardiol* 1985;55:1133–1139.

Lair GT, Ribeiro MD, Louie EK, et al: Early augmentation of R-wave voltage after coronary artery occlusion: A useful index of myocardial injury. *J Electrocardiol* 1979;12:89–95.

LaMonte CS, Freiman AH: The electrocardiogram after mastectomy. *Circulation* 1965;32:746–754.

Lerman J, Mele E, Chiozza M, et al: Effects of nitrate on R-wave variations after exercise in coronary heart disease differences in patients with and without angina pectoris. *Chest* 1981;81:137–141.

Levites R, Baker T, Anderson GJ: The significance of hypotension developing during treadmill exercise testing. *Am Heart J* 1978;95:747–753.

Levken J, Chatterjee K, Tyberg JV, et al: Influence of left ventricular dimensions on endocardial and epicardial QRS amplitude and ST-segment elevations during acute myocardial ischemia. *Circulation* 1980;61:679–689.

Levkin J, Chatterjee K, Tyberg JV, et al: Pronounced dependence of ventricular endocardial QRS potentials on ventricular volume. *Br Heart J* 1978;40:891–901.

Lew AS, Prigent F, Maddahi J: Exercise-induced precordial ST-segment elevation due to right ventricular ischemia. *Am Heart J* 1986;111:172–174.

Lie H, Ihlen H, Rootwelt K: Significance of a positive exercise ECG in middle-aged and old athletes as judged by echocardiographic, radionuclide, and follow-up findings. *Eur Heart J* 1985;6:615–624.

Litchfield RL, Kerber RE, Benge JW, et al: Normal exercise capacity in patients with severe left ventricular dysfunction: Compensatory mechanisms. *Circulation* 1982;66:129–134.

Londeree BR, Moeschberger ML: Influence of age and other factors on maximal heart rate. *J Cardiac Rehabil* 1984;4:44–49.

Longhurst J, Kraus W: Exercise-induced ST elevation in patients without myocardial infarction. *Circulation* 1979;60:616.

Luwaert R, Cosyns J, Rousseau M, et al: Reassessment of the relation between QRS forces of the orthogonal electrocardiogram and left ventricular ejection fraction. *Eur Heart J* 1983;4:103–109.

Madias JE, Krikelis EN: Transient giant R-waves in the early phase of acute myocardial infarction: Association with ventricular fibrillation. *Clin Cardiol* 1981;4:339–349.

Manca C, Dei Cas L, Bernardini B, et al: Comparative evaluation of exercise ST response in healthy males and females. *Cardiology* 1984;71:341–347.

Manoach M, Gitter S, Grosman E, et al: Influence of hemorrhage on the QRS complex of the electrocardiogram. *Am Heart J* 1971;82:55–61.

Manoach M, Grossman E, Varnon D: Some considerations regarding the importance of blood, heart and tissue conductivity with regard to QRS amplitude changes after hemorrhage. *Am Heart J* 1971;71:726.

Mark AL: The Bezold-Jarisch reflex revisited: Clinical implications of inhibitory reflexes originating in the heart. *J Am Coll Cardiol* 1983;1:90–102.

Matsuda Y, Ogawa H, Moritani K, et al: Coronary angiography during exercise-induced angina with ECG changes. *Am Heart J* 1984;108:959–965.

McDonough JR, Danielson RA, Willis RE, et al: Maximal cardiac output during exercise in patients with coronary artery disease. *Am J Cardiol* 1974;33:23–29.

McKirnan MD, Sullivan M, Jensen D, Froelicher V: Treadmill performance and cardiac function in selected patients with coronary heart disease. *J Am Coll Cardiol* 1984;3(2):253–261.

McNeer JF, Margolis JR, Lee KL, et al: The role of the exercise test in the evaluation of patients for ischemic heart disease. *Circulation* 1978;57:64–70.

Mirvis DM: Ability of standard ECG parameters to detect the body surface isopotential abnormalities of pacing induced myocardial ischemia in the dog. *J Electrocardiol* 1985;18:77–86.

Mirvis DM, Ramanathan KB, Wilson JL: Regional blood flow correlates of ST-segment depression in tachycardia-induced myocardial ischemia. *Circulation* 1986;2:363–373.

Morales-Ballejo H, Greenberg P, Ellestad M, et al: Septal Q-wave in exercise testing: Angiographic correlation. *Am J Cardiol* 1981;48:247–253.

Morris DD, Rozanski A, Berman DS, et al: Noninvasive prediction of the angiographic extent of coronary artery disease after myocardial infarction: Comparison of clinical bicycle exercise, electrocardiographic and ventriculographic parameters. *Circulation* 1984;70:192–201.

Morris SN, Phillips JF, Jordan JW, et al: Incidence of significance of decreases in systolic blood pressure during graded treadmill exercise testing. *Am J Cardiol* 1978;41:221–226.

Mukharji J, Kremers M, Lipscomb K, et al: Early positive exercise test and extensive coronary disease: Effect of antianginal therapy. *Am J Cardiol* 1985;55:267–270.

Murayama M, Kawakubo K, Nakajima T, et al: Different recovery process of ST depression on postexercise electrocardiograms in women in standing and supine positions. *Am J Cardiol* 1985;55:1474–1477.

Myers J, Ahnve S, Froelicher VF, et al: Spatial R-wave amplitude changes during exercise: Relation with left ventricular ischemia and function. *J Am Coll Cardiol* 1985;6:603–608.

Neill WA, Pantley GA, Nakornchai V: Respiratory alkalemia during exercise reduces angina threshold. *Chest* 1981;80:149–153.

Niederberger M: Values and limitations of exercise testing after myocardial infarction (monograph). Wien: Verlag Bruder Hollinek, 1977, pp. 3–45.

Nobel RJ, Rothbaum DA, Knoebel SB, et al: Normalization of abnormal T-waves in ischemia. *Arch Intern Med* 1976;136:391.

Nohara R, Kambara H, Suzuki Y, et al: Septal Q-wave in exercise testing: Evaluation by single-photon emission computed tomography. *Am J Cardiol* 1985;55:905–909.

Noneman JW, Popio KA, Sheps DS: Exercise-induced ST-segment elevation in a patient with effort angina pectoris and normal coronary arteries. *J Am Coll Cardiol* 1983;2:1232–1235.

O'Hara MJ, Subramanian B, Davies AB, et al: Changes of Q-wave amplitude during exercise for the prediction of coronary artery disease. *Int J Cardiol* 1984;6:35–45.

Patterson J, Naughton J, Pietras R, et al: Treadmill exercise in assessment of the functional capacity of patients with cardiac disease. *Am J Cardiol* 1972;30:757.

Pfeffer MA, Pfeffer JM, Fishbein MC, et al: Myocardial infarction size and ventricular function in rats. *Circ Res* 1979;44:503–512.

Piters KM, Colombo A, Olson HG, et al: Effect of coffee on exercise-induced angina pectoris due to coronary artery disease in habitual coffee drinkers. *Am J Cardiol* 1985;55:277–280.

Podrid PJ, Graboys T, Lown B: Prognosis of medically treated patients with coronary artery disease with profound ST-segment depression during exercise testing. *N Engl J Med* 1981;305:1111.

Poyatos ME, Lerman J, Estrada A, et al: Predictive value of changes in R-wave amplitude after exercise in coronary heart disease. *Am J Cardiol* 1984;54:1212–1215.

Rakita L, Borduas JL, Rothman S, et al: Studies on the mechanism of ventricular activity. XII. Early changes in the RS-T segment and QRS complex following acute coronary artery occlusion: Experimental study and clinical applications. *Am Heart J* 1954;48:351–372.

Rebuzzi AG, Loperfido F, Biasucci LM: Transient Q-waves followed by left anterior fascicular block during exercise. *Br Heart J* 1985;54:107–109.

Riff DP, Carleton RA: Effect of exercise on the atrial recovery wave. *Am Heart J* 1971;82:759–763.

Robertson D, Kostuk WJ, Ahuja SP: The localization of coronary artery stenoses by 12-lead ECG response to graded exercise test: Support for intercoronary steal. *Am Heart J* 1976;91:437–444.

Rose KD, Dunn FL, Bargen D: Serum electrolyte relationship to electrocardiographic change in exercising athletes. *JAMA* 1966;195:155.

Rudy Y, Plonsey R, Liebman J: The effects of variations in conductivity and geometrical parameters on the electrocardiogram, using an eccentric spheres model. *Circ Res* 1979;44:104–111.

Sarma JSM, Sarma RJ, Bilitch M, et al: An exponential formula for heart rate dependence of QR interval during exercise and cardiac pacing in humans: Revaluation of Bazett's formula. *Am J Cardiol* 1984;54:103–108.

Sarma RJ, Sanmarco ME: Reversal of exercise-induced hemodynamic and electrocardiographic abnormalities after coronary artery bypass surgery. *Circulation* 1982;65:684–689.

Sato I, Tomobuchi Y, Funahashi T, et al: Poor responsiveness of heart rate to treadmill exercise in vasospastic angina. *Clin Cardiol* 1985;8:206–212.

Scardi S, Pivotti F, Pandullo C, et al: Exercise-induced intermittent angina and ST-segment depression. *Am J Cardiol* 1985;55:1427–1428.

Schiffer F, Hartley LH, Schulman CL, et al: Evidence for emotionally-induced coronary arterial spasm in patients with angina pectoris. *Br Heart J* 1980;44:62–66.

Sheffield LT, Malouf JA, Sawyer JA, et al: Maximal heart rate and treadmill performance of healthy women in relation to age. *Circulation* 1978;57:79–84.

Sheps DS, Ernst JC, Briese FW, et al: Exercise-induced increase in diastolic pressure: Indicator of severe coronary artery disease. *Am J Cardiol* 1979;43:708–712.

Simoons ML, Hugenholtz PG: Gradual changes of ECG waveform during and after exercise in normal subjects. *Circulation* 1975;52:570–577.

Specchia G, DeServi S, Falcone C, et al: Significance of exercise-induced ST-segment elevation in patients without myocardial infarction. *Circulation* 1981;63:46–53.

St John Sutton MG, Plappert T, Crosby L, et al: Effects of reduced left ventricular mass on chamber architecture, load, and function: A study of anorexia nervosa. *Circulation* 1985; 72:991–1000.

Starling MR, Moody M, Crawford MH, et al: Repeat treadmill exercise testing: Variability of results in patients with angina pectoris. *Am Heart J* 1984;107:298–303.

Stiles G, Rosati R, Wallace A: Clinical relevance of exercise-induced S-T segment elevation. *Am J Cardiol* 1980;46:931.

Stuart RJ, Ellestad MH: Upsloping S-T segments in exercise stress testing. *Am J Cardiol* 1976;37:19–22.

Sundqvist K, Atterhog JH, Jogestrand T: Effect of digoxin on the electrocardiogram at rest and during exercise in healthy subjects. *Am J Cardiol* 1986;57:661–665.

Suwa M, Hirota Y, Nagao H, et al: Incidence of the coexistence of left ventricular false tendons and premature ventricular contractions in apparently healthy subjects. *Circulation* 1984;70:793–798.

Sweet RL, Sheffield LT: Myocardial infarction after exercise-induced electrocardiographic changes in a patient with variant angina pectoris. *Am J Cardiol* 1974;33:813.

Talbot S, Kilpatrick D, Jonathan A, et al: QRS voltage of the electrocardiogram and Frank vectorcardiogram in relation to ventricular volume. *Br Heart J* 1977;39:635–643.

Thomson PD, Kelemen MH: Hypotension accompanying the onset of exertional angina. *Circulation* 1975;52:28–32.

Tubau JF, Chaitman BR, Bourassa MG, et al: Detection of multivessel coronary disease after myocardial infarction using exercise stress testing and multiple ECG lead systems. *Circulation* 1980;61:44–52.

Uhl GS, Hopkirk AC: Analysis of exercise-induced R-wave amplitude changes in detection of coronary artery disease in asymptomatic men with left bundle branch block. *Am J Cardiol* 1979;44:1247–1250.

Val PG, Chaitman BR, Waters DD, et al: Diagnostic accuracy of exercise ECG lead systems in clinical subsets of women. *Circulation* 1982;65:1465–1473.

Vasey C, O'Donnell J, Morris S, et al: Exercise-induced left bundle branch block and its relation to coronary artery disease. *Am J Cardiol* 1985;56:892–895.

Wagner S, Cohn K, Selzer A: Unreliability of exercise-induced R-wave changes as index of coronary artery disease. *Am J Cardiol* 1980;44:1241–1245.

Watanabe K, Bhargava V, Froelicher VF: The relationship between exercise-induced R-wave amplitude changes and QRS vector loops. *J Electrocardiol* 1981;14:129–138.

Weber KT, Kinasewitz GT, Janicki J, et al: Oxygen utilization and ventilation during exercise in patients with chronic cardiac failure. *Circulation* 1982;65:1213–1222.

Weiner DA, McCabe CH, Cutler SS, et al: Decrease in systolic blood pressure during exercise testing: Reproducibility, response to coronary bypass surgery and prognostic significance. *Am J Cardiol* 1982;49:1627–1631.

Wiens RD, Lafia P, Marder GM, et al: Chronotropic incompetence in clinical exercise testing. *Am J Cardiol* 1984;54:74–78.

Williams ME, Gervino EV, Rosa RM, et al: Catecholamine modulation of rapid potassium shifts during exercise. *N Engl J Med* 1985;312:823–827.

Woelfel AK, Simpson RJ, Gettes LS, et al: Exercise-induced distal atrioventricular block. *J Am Coll Cardiol* 1983;2:578–581.

Wolthius RA, Froelicher VF, Hopkirk A, et al: Normal electrocardiographic waveform characteristics during treadmill exercise testing. *Circulation* 1979;60:1028–1035.

Wright S, Rosenthal A, Bromberg J, et al: R-wave amplitude changes during exercise in adolescents with left ventricular pressure and volume overload. *Am J Cardiol* 1983;52:841–846.

Wroblewski EM, Pearl FJ, Hammer WJ, et al: False positive stress tests due to undetected left ventricular hypertrophy. *Am J Epidemiol* 1982;115:412–417.

Yiannikas J, Marcomichelakis J, Taggart P, et al: Analysis of exercise-induced changes in R-wave amplitude in asymptomatic men with electrocardiographic ST-T changes at rest. *Am J Cardiol* 1981;47:238–243.

Zalman F, Goldberger A, Shabetai R: Transient Q-waves during exercise in hypertrophic cardiomyopathy. *Am J Cardiol* 1985;56:491.

Zir LM, Miller SW, Dinsmore RE, et al: Interobserver variability in coronary angiography. *Circulation* 1976;53:627.

5

APPLICATIONS OF STANDARD EXERCISE TESTING

Exercise is the true test of the heart because it is the most common stress that humans undertake. The exercise test is the most practical and useful procedure in the clinical evaluation of cardiovascular status. The common clinical applications of exercise testing to be discussed in this book are listed in Table 5–1. Two applications that require extensive review, exercise testing of post MI patients (Chapter 6) and screening of apparently healthy individuals (Chapter 7), are covered in separate chapters. Less common uses, some of which are touched upon in this chapter, are listed in Table 5–2.

DIAGNOSIS OF CHEST PAIN AND OTHER CARDIAC FINDINGS

To evaluate a test for a disease, one must demonstrate how well the test distinguishes between those individuals with and those without the disease. Evaluation of exercise testing as a diagnostic test for coronary artery disease depends on the population tested, which must be divided into those with and those without coronary artery disease by independent techniques. Coronary angiography and clinical follow-up for coronary events are two methods of separating a population into those with and those without coronary disease.

Limitations of Coronary Angiography. It has been demonstrated in studies comparing angiographic and pathologic findings that coronary angiography usually underestimates the pathologic severity of coronary artery disease. Coronary angiography can be interpreted as normal when severe coronary artery disease is present. This can be due to total cutoff of an artery at its origin, by diffuse atherosclerotic narrowing of an artery, and by failure to use axial views to visualize proximal left coronary artery lesions. Another limitation of coronary angiography is that coronary artery spasm as a cause of ischemia may be missed because it is often transient. Also, coronary angiographic interpretation is subject to variability owing to observer error, as has been previously described. Recent studies using Doppler flow techniques and videodensitometric techniques have shown a wide discrepancy between angiographic lesions and coronary flow reserve.

146

TABLE 5–1.
Common Clinical Applications for Exercise Testing

Diagnosis of chest pain or other cardiovascular abnormalities or
    historical manifestations
Prognostication and estimation of disease severity (identification of
    those better treated with interventions)
Evaluation of post MI patients
Screening
Exercise prescription
Functional classification (disability evaluation)
Evaluation of therapies

TABLE 5–2.
Less Common Uses of Exercise Testing Specifically for
Evaluating Patients With Certain Conditions or Situations

Preoperatively
Intermittent claudication
Valvular heart disease
Dysrhythmias
Unstable angina
Hypertension

Limitations of Other Endpoints.   There are some important
limitations of using clinical events and pathologic endpoints to separate coronary artery disease patients and disease-free groups. Coronary disease events
and symptoms can be due to relatively minor lesions. Hemorrhage into nonobstructive plaques or thrombosis can cause symptoms or even death. Spasm
has been demonstrated to occur proximal to relatively minor lesions. Pathologic studies have shown that approximately 7% of people dying from a clinically diagnosed myocardial infarction have insignificant or no coronary atheroma. Coronary angiographic studies have shown that some patients with
classic angina pectoris and myocardial infarction can have normal coronary
angiograms. In spite of these limitations, coronary angiography and the observation of clinical symptoms or coronary events are the most practical endpoints that distinguish individuals with from those without coronary artery
disease.

Predictive Accuracy Definitions.   Sensitivity and specificity
are the terms used to define how reliably a test distinguishes diseased from
nondiseased individuals. Sensitivity is the percentage of total times that a test
gives an abnormal result when those with the disease are tested. Specificity
is the percentage of times that a test gives a normal result when those without
the disease are tested. This is different from the colloquial use of the word
specific. The method of calculating these terms is shown in Table 5–3.
   A basic step in applying any testing procedure for the separation of normals
from patients with disease is to determine a value measured by the test that
best separates the two groups. A problem is that there is usually a consider-

TABLE 5–3.
Definitions and Calculation of Terms Used to Demonstrate the
Diagnostic Value of a Test

$$\text{Sensitivity} = \frac{TP}{TP + FN} \times 100 \qquad\qquad \text{Relative risk} = \frac{\dfrac{TP}{TP + FP}}{\dfrac{FN}{TN + FN}}$$

$$\text{Specificity} = \frac{TN}{FP + TN} \times 100 \qquad \text{Predictive value of abnormal test} = \frac{TP}{TP + FP} \times 100$$

TP = true positives or those with abnormal test and disease; FN = false negatives or those with normal test and with disease; TN = true negatives or those with normal test and no disease; FP = false positives or those with abnormal test and no disease.

Predictive value of an abnormal response is the percentage of individuals with an abnormal test who have disease.

Relative risk, or risk ratio, is the relative rate of occurrence of a disease in the group with an abnormal test compared to those with a normal test.

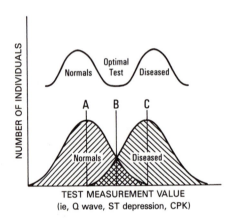

FIG 5–1.
Bell-shaped curves illustrating the distribution of the number of individuals with test results expressed as continuous variables.

able overlap of measurement values of a test in the groups with and without disease. Two bell-shaped normal distribution curves, one for the test variable in a population of normals and the other for this variable in a population with disease are illustrated in Figure 5–1. Along the vertical axis is the number of patients and along the horizontal axis could be the value for such measurements as Q-wave size, exercise-induced ST-segment depression, or CPK. Note that there is considerable overlap between the two curves. The optimal test would be able to achieve the most marked separation of these two bell-shaped curves minimizing the overlap. Unfortunately, most of the tests currently used for the diagnosis of coronary artery disease, including the exercise test, have a considerable overlap of the range of measurements for the normal population and for those with heart disease. Therefore, problems arise when a certain value is used to separate these two groups (i.e., 0.1 mV of ST-segment depression, a 10 mm Hg drop in systolic blood pressure, less than 5 METs exercise capacity, 3 consecutive premature ventricular contractions). If the value is set far to the right (i.e., 0.2 mV of ST-segment depression) in order to identify nearly all the normals as being free of disease, giving the test a high specificity, then a substantial number of those with the disease are called normal. If a value is chosen far to the left (i.e., 0.5 mm ST-segment depression) that identifies nearly all those with disease as being abnormal, giving the test a high sensitivity, then many normals are identified as abnormal. If a value is chosen that equally mislabels the normals and those with disease, the test will have its highest predictive accuracy. However, there may be reasons for wanting to adjust a test to have a relatively higher sensitivity or relatively higher specificity than possible when predictive accuracy is optimal. However, sensitivity and specificity are inversely related. That is, when sensitivity is the highest, specificity is the lowest and vice versa. Any test has a range of inversely related sensitivities and specificities that can be chosen by specifying a certain discriminant or diagnostic value.

Further complicating the choice of a discriminant value is that many diagnostic procedures do not have values established that best separate normals from those with disease. Even the Q-wave on the standard resting electrocardiogram or exercise-induced ST-segment depression have uncertainty regarding what is the best discriminant value (or cutpoint) and what the sensitivity and specificity of the currently used criteria are.

Once a discriminant value is chosen that determines a test's specificity and sensitivity, the population tested must be considered. If the population is skewed toward individuals with a greater severity of disease, the test will have a higher sensitivity. For instance, the exercise test has a higher sensitivity in individuals with triple-vessel disease than in those with single-vessel disease. Also, a test can have a lower specificity if it is used in individuals more likely to give false positive results. For instance, the exercise test has a lower specificity in individuals with mitral valve prolapse and in women.

The sensitivity and specificity of exercise-induced ST-segment depression can be demonstrated by analyzing the results obtained when exercise testing and coronary angiography have been used to evaluate patients. From these studies, the exercise test cutpoint of 0.1 mV horizontal or downsloping ST-segment depression has approximately 84% specificity for angiographically significant coronary artery disease; that is, 84% of those without significant angiographic disease had a normal exercise test.

These studies demonstrated a mean 66% sensitivity of exercise testing for angiographic coronary artery disease with a range of 40% for one-vessel disease to 90% for three-vessel disease. Most of these studies, however, used only the criterion of 0.1 mV horizontal or downsloping ST-segment depression to indicate an abnormal exercise test, and in many of them only a single lead was recorded. Sensitivity decreased for the milder degrees of coronary artery disease, but it is likely that some patients with single-vessel coronary disease do not have myocardial ischemia. If ST-segment elevation, heart rate and blood pressure response, exercise capacity, and symptomatology are considered, the sensitivity of the exercise test will be higher.

Two additional terms that help to define the diagnostic value of a test are its relative risk and predictive value. Table 5–3 also shows how these terms are calculated. The relative risk is the relative chance of having disease if the test is abnormal as compared with the chance of having disease if the test is normal. The predictive value of an abnormal test is the percentage of those persons with an abnormal test who have disease. Predictive value cannot be estimated directly from a test's demonstrated specificity or sensitivity. Predictive value is dependent upon the prevalence of disease in the population tested. Table 5–4 illustrates how a test with a 70% sensitivity and a 90% specificity performs in a population with a 5% prevalence of disease. Since 5% of 10,000 men have disease, 500 men have disease. In the middle column are the number of men with abnormal tests, and in the far right column are the number with normal tests. Since the test is 70% sensitive, 350 of those with disease will have abnormal tests and are true positives. The remaining 150 have normal tests and are false negatives. Since the test is 90% specific, 90% of the 9,500 without disease are true negatives, whereas the remainder are false positives. To calculate the predictive value, the number of true positives is divided by the number of those with an abnormal test. Table 5–4 also shows the performance of a test with the same 70% sensitivity and 90% specificity in a population with a 50% prevalence of disease. The predictive value of an abnormal response is directly related to the prevalence of the disease in the population tested. There are more false positive responses when exercise testing is used in a population with a low prevalence of disease than when it

TABLE 5–4.
Test Performance Versus Predictive Value and Risk Ratio: A Model in a Population of 10,000

DISEASE PREVALENCE	SUBJECTS	NUMBER WITH ABNORMAL TEST	TEST PERFORMANCE	NUMBER WITH NORMAL TEST
5%	500 diseased	450 (TP)	90% sensitivity	50 (FN)
		350 (TP)	70% sensitivity	150 (FN)
	9,500 nondiseased	2,850 (FP)	70% specificity	6,650 (TN)
		950 (FP)	90% specificity	8,550 (TN)
50%	5,000 diseased	4,500 (TP)	90% sensitivity	500 (FN)
		3,500 (TP)	70% sensitivity	1,500 (FN)
	5,000 nondiseased	1,500 (FP)	70% specificity	3,500 (TN)
		500 (FP)	90% specificity	4,500 (TN)

	PREDICTIVE VALUE OF ABNORMAL TEST		RISK RATIO*	
DISEASE PREVALENCE	5	50	5	50
Sensitivity/Specificity				
70%/90%	27%	88%	27	3
90%/70%	14%	75%	14	5
90%/90%	32%	90%	64	9
66%/84%	18%	80%	9	3

*Times that for normal subjects.
 TP = true-positive test result; FP = false-positive test result; FN = false-negative test result; TN = true-negative test result.

is used in a population with a high prevalence of disease. This fact explains the greater number of false positives found when using the test as a screening procedure in an asymptomatic group as opposed to when using it as a diagnostic procedure in patients with symptoms most likely due to coronary artery disease. Also, in Table 5–4 are the calculations for a test with a sensitivity and specificity of 90% and for a test with a sensitivity of 90% and a specificity of 70%.

Probability Analysis.   The information most important to a clinician attempting to make a diagnosis is the probability of the patient having the disease once the test result is known. Such a probability cannot be accurately estimated from the test result and the diagnostic characteristics of the test alone. It also requires knowledge of the probability of the patient having the disease before the test is administered. Bayes' Theorem states that the probability of a patient having the disease after a test is performed will be the product of the disease probability before the test and the probability that the test provided a true result.

The probability of a test result being true can be shown as the likelihood ratio, which is the ratio of true results to false results. In the case of an abnormal test result, the positive likelihood ratio equals

$$\frac{\text{Percent with disease with abnormal test}}{\text{Percent without disease with abnormal test}} \text{ or } \frac{\text{Sensitivity}}{1 \text{ minus specificity}}$$

In the case of a normal test result the negative likelihood ratio equals

$$\frac{\text{Percent without disease with normal test}}{\text{Percent with disease with normal test}} \text{ or } \frac{\text{Specificity}}{1 \text{ minus sensitivity}}$$

By analyzing the statements in the equations on the left side, it can be seen that they are equivalent to the numerators and denominators in the equations on the right.

The likelihood ratio is an indicator of the diagnosticity of a test; the higher it is, the greater the diagnostic impact of the test. Using conventional techniques of analyzing ST-segment depression with a cut point of 0.1 mV, the maximal or near-maximal exercise test has a sensitivity of approximately 66% and a specificity of 84%. Therefore, the likelihood ratio for an abnormal test result equals

$$\text{Positive likelihood ratio} = \frac{0.66}{1 \text{ minus } 0.84} = 4.0$$

and the likelihood ratio for a normal test result equals

$$\text{Negative likelihood ratio} = \frac{0.84}{1 \text{ minus } 0.66} = 2.5$$

Bayes' Theorem may be expressed in the following fashion:

$$\frac{\text{Posttest odds}}{\text{of disease}} = \frac{\text{Pretest odds}}{\text{of disease}} \times \frac{\text{Likelihood ratio}}{\text{of the test results}}$$

The clinician often makes this calculation intuitively when he suspects as a false result the abnormal exercise test of a 30-year-old woman with chest pain (low prior odds or probability). The same abnormal response would be accepted as a true result in a 60-year-old man with typical angina (high prior odds or probability).

Angiographic studies have been used to investigate the prevalence of significant coronary artery disease in patients with different chest pain syndromes. Because chest pain is the presenting complaint in the majority of patients referred for a diagnostic exercise test, the nature of the pain would seem a practical basis for estimating the prior probability of coronary artery disease. Approximately 90% of the patients with true angina pectoris have been found to have significant angiographic coronary disease. In patients presenting with atypical angina pectoris, approximately 50% have been found to have significant angiographic coronary disease. Atypical angina refers to pain that has an unusual location, prolonged duration, or inconsistent precipitating factors or that is unresponsive to nitroglycerin. Figure 5–2 demonstrates the calculation of the probability of coronary artery disease in such patients.

The 50-year-old male patient with typical angina pectoris has a 90% probability or 9:1 chance of having significant coronary artery disease. An abnormal exercise test increases these odds from 9:1 to 36:1. Such an impressive change in odds represents a relatively small increase in the probability of disease from 90% to 98%. Because such a patient still has a 75% probability of disease after a negative test, coronary angiography may yet be required to definitely rule out coronary disease. The greatest diagnostic impact of such a

	PRE-TEST ODDS	LIKELIHOOD RATIO	POST-TEST ODDS	POST-TEST PROBABILITY
ANGINAL	9 : 1	ABNORMAL TEST (x4)	36:1	(36/37) =98%
		NORMAL TEST (x2.5)	9:2.5	(9/12)=75%
ATYPICAL ANGINA	1 : 1	ABNORMAL TEST (x4)	4:1	(4/5)=80%
		NORMAL TEST (x2.5)	1:2.5	(1/4)=25%
NON-ANGINAL	1 : 9	ABNORMAL TEST (x4)	4:9	(4/13)=31%
		NORMAL TEST (x2.5)	1:23	(1/24)=4%
ASYMPTOMATIC	1 : 19	ABNORMAL TEST (x4)	4:19	(4/23)=17%
		NORMAL TEST (x2.5)	1:48	(1/49)=2%

FIG 5–2.
The impact of clinical presentation and exercise test results on the probability of disease.

circumstance would be in patients with atypical angina. An abnormal test result would increase the odds from 1:1 to 4:1, the probability of disease to 80% and, for practical purposes, establish the diagnosis. With a normal test, the probability of coronary disease would be reduced to 27%.

An important but often neglected assumption in using Bayes' Theorem is that the sensitivity and specificity do not depend on the variables that determine the pretest probability. For example, if the pretest probability is determined using knowledge of the patient's sex, then the theorem will not be completely valid since the specificity of the test depends on sex (i.e., specificity is lower in women). Likewise, if the pretest probability is based on the character of the chest pain reported, any dependence of specificity on this symptom will invalidate the application of the theorem. Since there is evidence that exercise test results (ST depression) are more sensitive in patients with typical angina pectoris because they have more severe disease, this would appear to invalidate the theorem's application. Actually, this problem is not as serious as one might imagine as long as the number of variables determining the pretest probability is relatively small. Perhaps more caution is needed in applying the theorem to the results of tests and populations of patients different from those used to determine sensitivity and specificity. Detrano et al. have produced results that suggest that such an erroneous application can produce relatively large errors in posttest probabilities.

An example will help illustrate these principles. If a 50-year-old woman without prior MI and atypical angina and 0.15 mV ST-segment depression has a pretest probability of 0.40, the posttest probability can be calculated from Bayes' Theorem.

$$\text{posttest probability} = \frac{.40Se}{.40Se + .60\ (1 - Sp).}$$

If one uses a sensitivity of 0.90 and a specificity of 0.90 from a study done on men with severe typical angina, the result would be:

$$\text{posttest probability} = \frac{.40 \times .90}{.40 \times .90 + .60 \times .20} = .75$$

However, if a more appropriate study done on women with atypical chest pain produced a sensitivity of 0.70 and a specificity of 0.65, then using these appropriate values:

$$\text{posttest probability} = \frac{.40 \times .70}{.40 \times .70 + .60 \times .35} = .57$$

A clinician who refers patients with greater than 70% disease probability by coronary angiography would mistakenly refer this patient if he had used the inappropriate sensitivity and specificity. The clinician who does not calculate disease probabilities but instead uses intuition might also err if he assumed the test to be as accurate for his 50-year-old female patient as it is for men with severe angina.

Even though a test may not have an important impact on disease probability in a patient, the test can be used for other purposes, such as demonstrating the severity or prognosis of a disease or the result of a therapeutic intervention. In addition, any test only gives a probability statement; how this impacts an individual patient depends on the Art of Medicine.

Methodological Problems With Studies Evaluating the Diagnostic Value of Exercise Testing.   In order to determine why exercise testing remains controversial as a diagnostic test for coronary artery disease, Philbrick et al. undertook a methodological review of 33 studies comprising 7,501 patients who had undergone both exercise tests and coronary angiography. These studies were published between 1976 and 1979 and had to include at least 50 patients (Table 5–5). Seven methodologic standards were declared necessary: (1) adequate identification of the groups selected for study, (2) adequate variety of anatomic lesions, (3) adequate analysis for relevant chest pain syndromes, (4) avoidance of a limited challenge group (in order to prevent excessively limiting the study group by excluding patients with clinical conditions that might cause false negative or false positive results), (5) avoidance of workup bias (occurring when the results of the exercise test influences patient selection), (6) avoidance of diagnostic review bias (i.e., bias that can occur when the result of the exercise test is allowed to influence the interpretation of the coronary angiogram), and (7) avoidance of test review bias (occurring when the result of the coronary angiogram is allowed to influence the interpretation of the exercise test). Of these seven methodologic standards for research design, only the requirement for an adequate variety of anatomic lesions received general compliance. Less than half of the studies complied with any of the remaining six standards: adequate identification of the groups selected for study; adequate analysis for relevant chest pain syndromes; avoidance of a limited challenge group; and avoidance of workup bias, diagnostic review bias, and test review bias. Only one study met as many as five standards.

These methodologic problems help explain the wide range of sensitivity (35% to 88%) and specificity (41% to 100%) found for exercise testing. The variations could not be attributed to the usual explanations: definition of anatomic abnormality, exercise test technique, or definition of an abnormal test. Determining the true value of exercise testing requires methodologic improvements in patient selection, data collection, and data analysis. Another important consideration is the exclusion of patients post MI. These patients most often have obstructive coronary artery disease and have altered exercise test responses.

Detry et al. evaluated modern approaches to exercise testing including computer averaging of the ECG, multivariate analysis of results, compartmental diagnostic approach and probabilistic interpretation of the results. These methods were tested in a group of 387 patients who had computer-assisted maximal exercise tests. Because of the problems of including patients with prior MI in such studies, they were carefully excluded. In 284 symptomatic patients, the diagnosis was made by arteriography and 103 healthy men were included. The computer averaged ECG signals of X, Y, and Z recorded at maximal exercise, maximal heart rate, blood pressure and work load, and the onset of angina pectoris during exercise were entered into a multivariate step-

TABLE 5–5.
Angiographic Studies Evaluating the Diagnostic Value of Exercise Testing

INVESTIGATOR	YEAR	CASES (n)	SENSITIVITY (%)	SPECIFICITY (%)
Hultgren	1967	55	66	100
Eliasch	1967	65	84	81
Demany	1967	75	64	49
Mason	1967	84	78	89
Kassenbaum	1968	68	47	97
Roitman	1970	100	73	82
Newton	1970	52	57	81
Fitzgibbon	1971	160	48	80
Cohn	1971	110	86	73
McConahay	1971	100	35	100
Ascoop	1971	96	59	94
Martin	1972	100	62	89
McHenry	1972	166	81	95
Kellerman	1973	74	54	96
Bartel	1974	465	65	92
Piessens	1974	70	65	83
Rios	1974	50	83	89
Sketch	1975	251	53	88
Borer	1975	89	49	41
Jelinek	1976	153	45	89
Goldschlager	1976	153	45	89
Santinga	1976	283	73	78
Detry	1977	98	55	85
Chaitman	1978	100	88	82
McNeer	1978	1222	53	91
Balnave	1978	70	81	100
Berman	1978	164	84	67
Weiner	1978	302	76	76
Chaitman	1979	200	84	72
Weiner	1979	2045	79	69
Aldrich	1979	181	40	92
Raffo	1979	100	91	96
Borer	1979	75	63	95
	Averages		66	84

(Modified from Philbrick et al.)

wise discriminant analysis. The pretest likelihood for coronary artery disease was calculated from age and history; the posttest likelihood was calculated from Bayes' Theorem, and the average information content of several diagnostic methods was assessed in categorical and compartmental models.

By multivariate analysis, five variables collected at maximal exercise were selected, including the heart rate, the ST-segment level, the onset of angina during the test, the work load, and slope of the ST-segment in lead X. The average information content of the analysis using five variables was 44% in a categorical model versus 55% in a compartmental model. For comparison, the information content of the analysis using the ST-segment alone was only 16% and 27%, respectively. The classification provided by the analysis of the ST-segment changes was barely better than one provided by the simple history. The probabilistic use of a multivariate and compartmental analysis of the data leads to a significantly better and more accurate classification of the patients (83% correct classification). Since the history of MI is almost always associated with significant coronary artery narrowings and those with anterior Q-waves or LVH have ST shifts not due to ischemia, it is important to exclude such patients in studies dealing with the diagnostic value of exercise testing.

Another problem with determining specificity is including enough normals and the problem of the definition of normals. Should they be low-risk individuals or individuals with clean coronary arteries? Rosanski has pointed out that the decline of specificity in other forms of exercise testing may well be due to pretest and posttest reference bias. Analysis of the ST-segments in Detry's study achieved results similar to that in the literature. The best cut-point was .095 mV, a value very close to the commonly used diagnostic criteria of .10 mV. Computer analysis was not an improvement over visual reading. Detry concluded that the value of exercise testing for the diagnosis of CAD is limited if one persists in using the classic univariate and categorical interpretation of ST-segment changes only. To be clinically relevant, diagnostic exercise testing requires first the consideration of other exercise test responses, and second, the analysis of these parameters in a compartmental and probabilistic way. This approach is facilitated by computer quantification and processing of the data.

Other investigators have attempted to combine exercise ECG variables in a nonlinear fashion. Usually this involves an intuitively derived or empirical scale requiring greater ST depression when ST segments are upsloping or calculating the rate of change of ST-segment shifts with heart rate. Detrano et al. have compared some of these rules for modifying the ST-segment response in a group of 303 consecutive subjects without prior MI who were referred for angiography to Cleveland Clinic. They calculated sensitivities and specificities of the ST-segment changes adjusted for ST slope, R-wave amplitude, and heart rate change. They found that only by adjusting for heart rate change could accuracy be significantly improved.

Microprocessor analysis of digitized ST segments during exercise has permitted the application of various algorithms. Though cardiologists agree that computerized analysis simplifies the evaluation of exercise ECG, there has been less agreement as to whether accuracy is enhanced (see Chapter 2). Detrano et al. have produced evidence to refute the results of Sketch and Hollenberg in a large group of patients without prior MI who were referred for angiography to Cleveland Clinic. In their study, neither the algorithm developed by Hollenberg nor the ST index proposed by McHenry were superior to careful visual analysis of ST-segment shifts induced by exercise. This issue has not been resolved and clinicians should be cautious when trusting commercial microprocessors to analyze exercise tracings.

Detrano et al. reported 154 patients referred to Cleveland Clinic for coronary arteriography who were prospectively studied with exercise electrocardiography, exercise thallium scintigraphy, cinefluoroscopy for coronary calcifications, and coronary angiography. Pretest probabilities of coronary disease were determined based on age, sex, and chest pain type. These and pooled literature values for the conditional probabilities of test results based on disease state were used in Bayes' Theorem to calculate posttest probabilities. The results of the three noninvasive tests were compared for statistical independence, a necessary condition for their valid use in the Bayesian model. The test results were found to be independent from one another in the diseased and nondiseased patients. Some dependencies that did occur between the test results and the clinical variables of age and sex were not sufficient to invalidate the model. Sixty-eight patients had at least one major coronary artery obstruction greater than 50%. When these patients were divided into low, intermediate, and high probability subgroups according to their pretest probabilities, noninvasive test results analyzed by Bayesian probability analysis appropriately advanced 17 of them by at least one probability subgroup while only seven were moved backward. Of the 76 nondiseased patients, 34 appropriately retreated into a lower probability subgroup while 10 incorrectly moved up. Detrano concluded that posttest probabilities calculated from Bayes' Theorem more accurately classified diseased and nondiseased patients than did pretest probabilities, thus demonstrating the theorem's utility.

SUMMARY OF THE DIAGNOSTIC UTILIZATION OF EXERCISE TESTING

In studies that took into account the number of coronary arteries involved, all found increasing sensitivity of the test as more vessels were involved. The most false negatives were found among patients with single-vessel disease, particularly if the diseased vessel was not the left anterior descending artery.

No matter what techniques are used, there is a reciprocal relationship between sensitivity and specificity. The more specific a test is (i.e., the more able it is to determine who is disease free), the less sensitive it is. The values for sensitivity and specificity can be altered by adjusting the criterion used for abnormal. For instance, when the criterion for an abnormal exercise-induced ST-segment response is altered to 0.2 mV depression, making it more specific for coronary artery disease, the sensitivity of the test can be reduced by half. For unknown reasons, the specificity of the ST-segment response is decreased when the test is used in women and in patients who have ST-segment depression at rest, left ventricular hypertrophy, vasoregulatory abnormality, or mitral valve prolapse.

DETERMINATION OF PROGNOSIS

Exercise testing can be used to determine the prognosis for patients with coronary artery disease. The results of an exercise test can help to estimate the risk of mortality and morbidity. Studies have demonstrated that the severity of angiographic coronary artery disease is directly related to the work load that can be performed. Exercise-induced hypotension, extremely limited exercise capacity, chronotropic incompetence, marked ST-segment depression, downsloping ST-segment depression, five or more leads with ischemic depression, ST-segment depression beginning at a low heart rate, systolic blood pressure drop, and inverted U-waves are more predictive of severe coronary artery disease and left ventricular dysfunction than is 0.1 mV of horizontal ST-segment depression only at maximal exercise. Patients who can achieve a normal work load, a normal maximal heart rate, and a normal maximal systolic blood pressure during treadmill testing appear to have a better prognosis than do those unable to do the same. Patients without chest pain during exercise testing also appear to do better.

Identifying which patients could increase longevity from coronary artery bypass surgery is helpful in clinical decision making. From current information, it appears that patients with left main or three-vessel disease will have improved survival if treated surgically. However, this expectation is most realizable in those patients with moderately reduced resting left ventricular ejection fractions (less than 50% to greater than 30%).

McNeer and colleagues demonstrated that a combination of exercise test parameters were both diagnostically and prognostically important. Their study involved 1,472 patients who underwent exercise testing and coronary angiography and were then followed for at least one year. Ninety-seven percent of the patients who had abnormal ST-segment depression in the first or second stage of the Bruce protocol had significant coronary artery disease. More than 60% had three-vessel disease, and more than 25% had significant narrowing of the left main coronary artery. Those who achieved the fourth stage and did not have abnormal ST-segment responses had less than 15% prevalence of three-vessel disease and less than 1% prevalence of left main coronary disease. Patients able to exercise to or beyond stage 4 and who were able to achieve a maximal heart rate of 160 or greater beats/min or with a normal ST-segment response or both had a one-year survival of almost 100%. Patients forced to stop exercising in stages 1 or 2 with a low heart rate response and with abnormal ST-segment depression had a one-year survival of 85%.

Weiner and colleagues reported a study of 436 consecutive patients referred for suspected or known coronary artery disease who were able to undergo both exercise testing and coronary angiography. All patients underwent treadmill testing using the Bruce protocol, and 12-lead electrocardiograms were obtained during exercise. A lesion of the left main coronary artery was considered significant if it had greater than 50% diameter narrowing, and this criterion was 70% in other vessels. Fifty-five patients were excluded because of left ventricular hypertrophy, digoxin therapy, left bundle branch block, and for the attainment of less than 85% maximal predictive heart rate (of these 55, two had left main coronary artery disease, and four had three-vessel disease; thus, the predictive value of being excluded was about 10%). Four patient groups were defined by angiographic findings: (1) 35 with left main disease, (2) 89 with three-vessel disease without left main disease, (3) 188 patients with either one- or two-vessel disease, and (4) 124 patients with no significant coronary disease. Of the 35 patients with left main disease, most had disease of other coronary arteries, and nearly half had three-vessel disease. Exercise test responses that were considered included the amount of ST-segment depression, configuration, onset, and duration and the number of leads in which it occurred. Hemodynamic responses included treadmill time, systolic blood pressure, and maximal heart rate. Other measurements included angina, premature ventricular contractions, and abnormal R-wave response in lead V5.

Ninety-seven percent of patients with left main disease had at least 0.1 mV of ST depression, and 91% had 0.2 mV or more of ST-segment depression. Patients with left main disease as a group were distinguished from patients with three-vessel disease by an early onset and longer persistence of ST-segment depression, as well as by a greater number of leads in which the depression occurred. A fall in systolic blood pressure occurred in 23% of the patients with left main disease versus 17% of those with triple-vessel disease and 6% of those with single- or double-vessel disease. As an indicator of either left main or three-vessel disease, a fall in SBP had a predictive value of 66% and a sensitivity of 19%. The criterion of 0.3 mV or more of ST-segment depression occurred in 44% of such patients and had only a slightly lower predictive value (64%). Combined analysis of test variables disclosed that the development of 0.2 mV or more of downsloping ST-segment depression beginning in stage 1, persisting for at least six minutes into recovery, and involving at least five ECG leads had the greatest sensitivity (74%) and predictive value (32%) for left main coronary disease. This abnormal pattern identified either left main or three-vessel disease with a sensitivity of 49% and a predictive value of 74%.

Bruce and colleagues demonstrated noninvasive screening criteria for patients who had improved four-year survival after coronary artery bypass surgery. Their data have come from 2,000 men with coronary heart disease enrolled in the Seattle Heart Watch who had a symptom-limited maximal treadmill test. These subjects received usual community care, which resulted in 16% of them having coronary artery bypass surgery in nonrandomized fashion. The diagnosis of coronary heart disease was based on a history of angina, myocardial infarction, or cardiac arrest. Cardiomegaly was determined by physical and chest x-ray examinations. The patients were divided into three groups. One group had only myocardial ischemia manifested by exercise test-induced normal ST-segment elevation or depression and/or angina. The second group could have myocardial ischemia, but had to have "left ventricular dysfunction" manifested by at least two of the following: cardiomegaly, less than 4 METs exercise capacity, and less than 130 mm Hg maximal systolic blood pressure. A third group had none of the above. Comparisons were then made within each group between the operated and unoperated patients, and surprisingly little difference was found. However, life table analysis showed a significantly higher survival rate of 94% at four years among the operated patients, as compared with the 68% survival of the unoperated patients in the group with left ventricular dysfunction. If the 4.6% death rate due to surgery in those with "ischemia" only was reduced, perhaps the patients who were operated on in that group would have had a significantly improved survival as well. The European randomized trial of coronary artery bypass surgery demonstrated that patients with 0.2 mV of exercise-induced ST-segment depression had improved mortality if in the surgical cohort, but CASS and the VA CABS Cooperative Trial failed to demonstrate that. Thus, it remains controversial whether patients with exercise-induced ST depression can expect improved survival if they undergo CABS.

Bruce et al. added to their analysis of the Seattle Heart Watch by applying noninvasive criteria in a learning set for exercise enhanced risk assessment for events due to coronary heart disease, to a test series in a later population sample. In this series, subsequent follow-up in 5,308 men enrolled in the learning series of the Seattle Heart Watch during 1971 to 1974 were compared with findings in 3,065 men enrolled from 1975 to 1981. Of the 8,373 men, 4,105 or almost half were classified before exercise testing as asymptomatic healthy individuals. Another 1,374 men had hypertension, and 2,894 had prior clinical manifestations of coronary heart disease including angina, MI, cardiac arrest, or cardiac death. Men in the same age and risk groups for each pretest clinical classification showed similar gradients of risk. Age-standardized event rate showed a reduction longitudinally in healthy men and in patients who underwent coronary bypass surgery. The majority of events occurred in men with only increased risk rather than high risk.

The study by Podrid and colleagues has placed some doubt on the use of exercise testing to identify high-risk patients. They were reacting to the current practice of often referring patients with severe ST-segment depression to coronary angiography. They contend that the prevailing view is that such patients have far advanced multivessel disease and that coronary artery bypass surgery is the only way to improve their outlook. In their select group of patients referred because of profound ST-segment depression, they did not find a bad prognosis. In 142 patients with coronary artery disease and severe ST-segment depression with a mean follow-up of 59 months, mortality was only 1.4%, and only 1.3% had coronary artery bypass surgery per year. Sixty-six percent of these patients had a prior myocardial infarction and 70% had angina. This low mortality suggests an unusual selection process resulting from the referral patterns to this group of physicians. This study points out that it is necessary to consider multiple variables when predicting the risk of ischemic heart disease. A relatively low-risk group can be found in any population identified using one risk predictor, such as the ECG response to an exercise test, by excluding other risk predictors.

Weiner et al. analyzed the CASS data to attempt to identify predictors of mortality in medically treated patients with coronary artery disease. This study was based on analysis of 16% of the registry of patients with no previous coronary artery bypass surgery who were able to undergo a standard or modified Bruce protocol within one month of their catheterization. During the mean follow-up of four years, 212 or 5% died. This represents a low annual mortality, and approximately 40% of the patients had a prior MI and 36% underwent coronary artery bypass surgery during a three-year minimal follow-up. Standard clinical variables including chest pain, congestive heart failure, physical exam, family history, risk factor index, drugs, and cardiac catheterization findings were included. Exercise test variables included limiting symptoms, PVCs, peak heart rate, peak systolic blood pressure, ST-segment response, and final exercise stage. Thirty variables were analyzed in 4,000 patients. Regression analysis demonstrated that seven variables were independent predictors of survival. A high-risk subgroup (annual mortality about 5%) was identified consisting of patients with either congestive heart failure or ST-segment depression and a final exercise stage in the Bruce protocol of one or less (5 METs or less). When all 30 variables were analyzed jointly, the left ventricular contraction pattern and the number of diseased vessels were the best predictors of survival. In a subgroup of 572 patients with three-vessel disease and good LV function, the probability of survival at four years ranged from 53% for patients only able to achieve stage 1/2 to 100% for patients able to exercise into stage 5 (MET level of 10). Thus, in patients with defined coronary pathoanatomy, clinical and exercise variables primarily relating to left ventricle function are helpful in assessing prognosis. The following are some of the univariate risk ratios generated by some of the variables: age greater than 60—2.5x, prior MI—2.4x, CHF—5x, cardiac enlargement—9x, digoxin—4x, less than stage 1—2x, more than 0.1 mV ST-segment depression—1.4x.

The presence of congestive heart failure was the most potent clinical predictor of survival when the clinical and exercise test variables were analyzed. Two other significant clinical variables, prior MI and cardiac enlargement, were also related to ventricular dysfunction. These results confirmed two other large studies involving multivariate analysis of clinical data. Hammermeister et al. identified the clinical variables of cardiac enlargement, use of diuretics, S3 gallop, and CHF as predictive of survival among 47 variables analyzed from the Seattle Heart Watch study. Harris et al. in Sydney found that class IV heart failure, cardiac enlargement, and a history of MI were 3 of the 12 clinical variables independently predictive of survival. The two exercise predictors of survival were duration of exercise and the ST-segment response. Hammermeister et al. also identified the exercise duration and the blood pressure and heart rate response as the most important exercise predictors of survival. They failed to demonstrate that the ST-segment response was an independent predictor. Podrid and coworkers analyzed the prognostic significance of 0.2 mV of ST-segment depression during exercise testing in 142 selected patients and found that the annual mortality was only 1.4%. Survival of patients varied from 0.5% to 2% per year depending on exercise capacity. In Weiner's study, the annual mortality in 730 patients with 0.2 mV was 3.6% and ranged from 5.6% for those with a low exercise capacity to 2% for those achieving stage 3.

Wyns et al. evaluated the independent prognostic information provided by exercise testing in a population with a high prevalence (82%) of stable coronary artery disease. Survival rates were calculated with the life table method in 372 men, mean age 48 years, referred for coronary arteriography. A previous MI was noted in 146, and 248 had typical angina (80 had both). During a mean follow-up of 29 months (1 to 8 years), 32 patients died and 27 patients had nonfatal events (MI or hospitalization for disabling angina). Both a coronary heart disease history (typical angina pectoris and/or an old MI) and the exercise test results (abnormal if angina and/or ST segment shifts of 0.1 mV or more) had a significant prognostic value for the five-year survival rate (P < 0.001). In patients with an MI and/or angina, the five-year cummulative survival rate was 76% if the exercise test was abnormal versus 94% if it was normal (P < 0.001). The following eight noninvasive and two invasive variables were submitted to Cox regression analysis: age, typical angina pectoris, previous MI, maximal heart rate and work load, maximal ST segment shift; angina pectoris during exercise testing, number of diseased vessels, and wall motion score. By univariate analysis, the age and the maximal work load were the only noninvasive predictive variables for survival or cardiac events (P < 0.05). By multivariate analysis, and combining all noninvasive and invasive variables, survival was predicted by the wall motion score, the presence or absence of three-vessel disease, and age. Considering all events, besides the three variables listed above, the maximal work load during exercise testing contributed significantly (P < 0.001) and independently to the model. Thus, even in populations with a high prevalence of coronary artery disease, exercise capacity provides prognostic information that is not available either from the history or from cardiac catheterization. Unfortunately, the ST-segment response was confused by combining both elevation and depression with angina and by not excluding elevation over Q waves. In contrast, analysis of the Duke University data base has found ST-segment depression to have prognostic value.

Dagenais et al. analyzed the factors influencing the five-year survival rate in 220 patients with at least 0.2 mV of horizontal or downsloping ST-segment depression during exercise testing. They confirmed previous observations that survival was inversely proportional to the duration of exercise. All patients who achieved stage IV of the Bruce protocol survived, whereas the survival rates for patients who terminated exercise during stages III, II, and I were 86, 73 and 52%, respectively.

Blumenthal et al. validated the ability of a strongly positive exercise test to predict left main coronary disease even in patients with minimal or no angina. The criteria for a markedly positive test included (1) early ST-segment depression, (2) 0.2 mV or more of depression, (3) downsloping ST depression, (4) exercise-induced hypotension, (5) prolonged ST changes after the test, and (6) multiple areas of ST depression. Table 5–6 summarizes nine studies that evaluated the predictive value of an exercise test for identifying patients with left main coronary disease as cited and discussed by Blumenthal et al.

The Montreal Heart Institute has applied multivariate techniques to compare the diagnostic yield of multiple noninvasive tests including exercise testing for diagnosis and for determining the severity of coronary disease. The data provide models whereby the posttest risk of disease can be estimated. In a study of 92 symptomatic women without previous MI, Hung et al. used a stepwise linear discriminate analysis of 41 clinical, exercise ECG, fluoroscopic and thallium scintigraphic variables to determine which data were

TABLE 5–6.

Left Main Disease and Exercise Testing: Studies Evaluating the Predictive Value and Sensitivity of the Exercise Test for Identifying Patients With Left Main Coronary Artery Disease (see Appendix B for two additional studies)

PRINCIPAL INVESTIGATOR	YEAR	NO. WITH LEFT MAIN DISEASE (TOTAL)	CRITERION	PREDICTIVE VALUE (%)	SENSITIVITY (%)
Cheitlin	1975	11 (106)	0.2 mV depression	24	100
Goldschlager	1976	15 (410)	0.1 mV downsloping	8	67
McNeer	1978	108 (1,472)	0.1 mV in stage I or II	23	47
Nixon	1979	26 (115)	Angina or 0.1 mV depression at low work load	19 26	96 54
Levites, Anderson	1978	11 (75)	0.2 mV depression abnormal in stage I	50 24	82 63
Morris	1978	18 (460)	Exertional hypotension	14	17
Weiner	1981	35 (436)	"Markedly positive" Exertional hypotension	32 23	74 23
Blumenthal	1981	14 (40)	0.2 mV depression Anterior and inferior depression Exertional hypotension	38 57 75	100 93 21
Sanmarco	1980	29 (378)	0.3 mV only Exertional hypotension Both	15 15 27	24 28 35

Predictive value = % of those with abnormal response who have left main disease as defined by criteria; sensitivity = % of those with left main disease who have an abnormal response as defined by the investigators.

most predictive of coronary disease and/or multivessel disease. The analyses selected a reversible thallium defect, coronary calcification, and character of chest pain as the variables most predictive of coronary disease. Cardiac fluoroscopy score, thallium score, and extent of ST-segment depression were the variables most predictive of multivessel disease. The same investigators used multiple logistic regression analysis to assess the incremental diagnostic yield of exercise ECG and thallium scintigraphy, and cardiac fluoroscopy to clinical data in predicting the likelihood of coronary disease and/or multivessel disease in 171 symptomatic men. The most significant predictive variable for coronary disease was thallium and, for multivessel disease, the amount of exercise performed. Each noninvasive test incrementally improved predictive accuracy over clinical variables alone. However, the addition of cardiac fluoroscopy to the exercise ECG and thallium scan did not improve specificity. When the analyses were confined to multivessel disease as the endpoint, the addition of thallium scintigraphy to the exercise ECG only marginally improved specificity. The risk estimates determined by these and other multivariate models require prospective evaluation.

It appears that individual clinical or exercise test variables are unable to detect left main coronary disease because of their low sensitivity or predictive value. However, a combination of the amount, pattern, and duration of ST-segment response and exercise capacity is highly predictive and reasonably sensitive for left main or three-vessel coronary disease. The question remains of how to identify those with abnormal resting ejection fractions, who will benefit with prolonged survival after coronary artery bypass surgery. Perhaps those with a normal resting ECG will not need surgery for increased longevity because of the associated high probability of normal ventricular function.

EVALUATION OF EXERCISE CAPACITY

The exercise test can be used to evaluate the exercise capacity of asymptomatic individuals or of patients with various forms of heart disease. Patients who exaggerate their symptoms or who mainly have a psychologic impairment often can be identified. Exercise testing can more accurately measure the degree of cardiac impairment than a physician's assessment of exercise capacity. Rightly so, it is now used more than functional classifications based on "usual activity" to determine disability. As previously described, maximal oxygen uptake, either directly measured or estimated, is the best noninvasive measurement of the functional capacity of the cardiovascular system. Being unable to exercise at a maximal oxygen consumption of 18 ml O_2/kg/min or 5 METs (equivalent to finishing the first stage of the Bruce protocol) has been found to have a poor prognosis in numerous studies in spite of either medical or surgical treatment. The determination of a patient's exercise capacity affords an objective measurement of the degree of cardiac impairment and can be useful in patient management. Exercise testing can also be used to evaluate the effects of training, whether it be part of an athletic program, a fitness program, or a rehabilitation program. A maximal oxygen uptake of 40 ml O_2/kg/min is the lowest level of fitness, and measurements of up to 80 ml O_2/kg/min can be obtained in Olympic-class long distance runners. Following a trainee's progress in an exercise program with serial exercise testing can optimize the training program and is often a good way to encourage adherence.

EVALUATION OF DYSRHYTHMIAS

An exercise test can be used to evaluate patients with dysrhythmias or to induce dysrhythmias in patients with the appropriate symptoms. The dysrhythmias that can be evaluated include premature ventricular contractions (PVCs), sick sinus syndrome, and various degrees of heart block. Ambulatory monitoring or isometric exercise often detects a higher prevalence of dysrhythmias, including more serious dysrhythmias than does dynamic exercise testing. The findings in each of these tests, however, may have different significances.

Lown believes that maximal exercise testing is useful for detection of arrhythmias and assessment of antiarrhythmic drug efficacy. Because few reports document the safety in patients with malignant ventricular arrhythmias, Lown and colleagues reviewed the complications of symptom-limited exercise in 263 patients with such arrhythmias who underwent a total of 1,377 maximal treadmill tests. Seventy-four percent of the population studied had a history of ventricular fibrillation or hemodynamically compromising ventricular tachycardia, and the remainder had experienced ventricular tachycardia in the setting of either recent MI or poor left ventricular function. A complication was defined as the occurrence of arrhythmia during exercise testing—ventricular fibrillation, ventricular tachycardia, or bradycardia—that mandated immediate medical treatment. Complications were noted in 24 patients (9.1%) during 32 tests (2.3%), whereas 239 patients (90.9%) were free of complications during 1,345 tests (97.7%). There were no deaths, MIs, or lasting morbid events. Clinical descriptors associated with complications included male sex, presence of coronary artery disease, and a history of exertional arrhythmia. Clinical variables previously considered to confer increased risk during exercise, such as poor left ventricular function, high-grade ventricular arrhythmias before or during exercise, exertional hypotension, and ST depression, were not predictive of complications. Occurrence of a complication was also unaffected by the use of antiarrhythmic drugs at the time of exercise. Complication frequency in their study group was compared with that in a reference population of 3,444 cardiac patients without histories of symptomatic arrhythmia who underwent 8,221 exercise tests. Of these, four subjects (0.12%) developed ventricular fibrillation (0.05% of tests) without fatality or lasting morbidity. They concluded that maximal exercise testing can be conducted safely in patients with malignant arrhythmias and that clinical variables previously thought to confer risk during exercise are not predictive of complications.

Lown and colleagues also compared the provocation of PVCs in a standard exercise test with provocation of PVCs in an abbreviated form of testing (Mini) that seemed to approximate more closely the demands of daily activities. The Mini protocol was as follows: the treadmill was kept at 12% elevation; speed began at 1.7 mph and was increased every 15 seconds to the following levels—2.5, 3.4, 4.2, 5.5, 6.0 mph. It was then kept at 6.5 mph until the test was completed. The study involved 52 patients with known or suspected history of ventricular arrhythmia—42 men and 10 women, average age 49 years. Hemodynamic and ST-segment changes were similar during both forms of testing. Thirty-seven patients (71%) undergoing a standard exercise test exhibited PVCs, whereas 32 (62%) did so during Mini testing. Of 13 patients with repetitive PVCs, standard exercise testing as well as Mini provoked the same degree of PVCs in 10. In two patients, the yield of these complex forms of PVCs was higher with Mini and in one patient with standard exercise testing. This abbreviated protocol may be useful for patients undergoing serial exercise studies to assess drug efficacy for the suppression of PVCs.

Woelfel et al. studied 14 patients with exercise-induced ventricular tachycardia (VT) with serial treadmill testing. Those with reproducible VT were treated with a beta-blocking agent and later with verapamil. In 11 patients (79%), VT of similar rate, morphologic characteristics, and duration was reproduced on two consecutive treadmill tests performed 1 to 14 days apart. Beta blockade prevented recurrent VT during acute testing in 10 of 11 patients and during chronic therapy in 9. Eight patients had a consistent relation between a critical sinus rate and the onset of VT. In these patients, successful therapy correlated with preventing achievement of the critical sinus rate during maximal exercise. They also found verapamil to be effective in this group.

Sami et al. performed a retrospective study to examine the prognostic significance of exercise-induced ventricular arrhythmia in patients with stable CAD who were included in the multicenter patient registry of the Coronary Artery Surgery Study. The population included 1,486 patients selected from 1975 to 1979, and followed an average of 4.3 years. All underwent a standard Bruce exercise test and had CAD by cardiac catheterization at entry. Patients were classified depending on whether they had minimal or significant CAD. They were further subclassified depending on whether they had exercise-induced ventricular arrhythmia (EIA). Patients with minimal CAD and EIA (16 patients) and 229 patients without had similar clinical and angiographic characteristics except for the average (EF), which was 50% for those with and 64% for those without PVCs. One hundred and thirty patients with significant CAD and EIAs had a higher prevalence of previous MI, a lower mean EF and a higher proportion with at least two vessel disease than those without EIAs and significant CAD (1,111 patients). The five-year event-free survival was not influenced by the presence of EIA; it was 76% and 88% in those with minimal CAD or with EIAs, respectively, and 71% and 76% in both groups with significant CAD, respectively. Using a stepwise Cox regression analysis of selected clinical and angiographic risk factors, the only independent significant risk factors that were found for cardiac events were the number of coronary arteries diseased and the EF.

Califf et al. at Duke studied the prognostic information provided by ventricular arrhythmias associated with treadmill testing in 1,293 consecutive non-surgically treated patients undergoing an exercise test within six weeks of cardiac catheterization. The 236 patients with simple ventricular arrhythmias (at least one PVC, but without paired complexes or ventricular tachycardia) had a higher prevalence of significant CAD (57% versus 44%), three-vessel disease (31% versus 17%), and abnormal left ventricular function (43% versus 24%) than did patients without ventricular arrhythmias. Patients with paired complexes or ventricular tachycardia had an even higher prevalence of significant coronary artery disease (75%), three-vessel disease (39%), and abnormal left ventricular function (54%).

In the 620 patients with significant CAD, patients with paired complexes or ventricular tachycardia had a lower three-year survival rate (75%) than patients with simple ventricular arrhythmias (83%) and patients with no ventricular arrhythmias (90%). Ventricular arrhythmias were found to add independent prognostic information to the noninvasive evaluation, including history, physical examination, chest x-ray, ECG, and other exercise test variables (p = 0.03). Ventricular arrhythmias made no independent contribution once the cardiac catheterization data were known. In patients without significant coronary artery disease, no relation between ventricular arrhythmias and survival was found.

Weiner et al. investigated the determinants and prognostic significance of ventricular arrhythmias during exercise testing. Eighty-six patients with such arrhythmias were identified from a consecutive series of 446 patients who underwent treadmill testing and cardiac catheterization. The prevalence of these arrhythmias was 19% in the total group but increased to 30% in the 120 patients with three-vessel or left main CAD. Patients with exercise-induced arrhythmias were more likely to have three-vessel or left main CAD, a lower resting EF, 0.2 mV of ST depression, and more severe segmental wall motion abnormalities than patients without this finding. Repeat exercise testing in 22 patients with exercise-induced arrhythmias after CABS revealed that persistence of these arrhythmias was associated with either severe wall motion abnormalities preoperatively or residual ST depression during the postoperative exercise testing. At a mean follow-up period of 5.3 years, the presence of exercise-induced ventricular arrhythmias was not associated with increased cardiac mortality in the medically treated patients.

Although exercise-induced VT, whether sustained or nonsustained, is usually associated with significant organic heart disease, its prevalence, associated characteristics, and prognostic significance in a population are unknown. Fleg and Lakatta studied the prevalence of VT associated with maximal treadmill exercise in 597 male and 325 female volunteers, aged 21 to 96 years, from the Baltimore Longitudinal Study on Aging who were without apparent heart disease. Ten subjects, 7 men and 3 women, with exercise-induced VT were identified, representing 1.1% of those tested; only one was younger than 65 years. All episodes of VT were asymptomatic and nonsustained. In 9 of 10 subjects, VT developed at or near peak exercise. The longest run of VT was 56 beats; multiple runs of VT were present in four subjects. Two subjects had exercise-induced ST segment depression, but subsequent exercise thallium results were negative in each. Compared with a group of age- and sex-matched control subjects, those with asymptomatic, nonsustained VT displayed no difference in exercise duration, maximal heart rate, or the prevalence of coronary risk factors of exercise-induced ischemia as measured by the ECG and thallium scintigraphy. Over a mean follow-up period of two years, no subject developed symptoms of heart disease or experienced syncope or sudden death. Exercise-induced VT in apparently healthy subjects occurred mainly in the elderly, was limited to short, asymptomatic runs of three to six beats usually near peak exercise, and did not predict increased cardiovascular morbidity or mortality rates over a two-year follow-up.

The diagnostic and prognostic utility of exercise-induced ventricular arrhythmias is obviously limited. The above cited studies found a sensitivity of only 30% for the most severe form of coronary disease. In many cases exercise-induced arrhythmias are probably causally related to myocardial scar and/or dysfunction and only indirectly to ischemia. For this reason, the arrhythmias themselves have not been consistently shown to add independent information.

EVALUATION OF PATIENTS
WITH ATRIAL FIBRILLATION

The reported prevalence of atrial fibrillation (AF) has varied widely, but it is directly related to age. Kannel et al., in a 22-year analysis from the Framingham Study, described the onset of chronic AF in 49 of 2,325 males and 49 of 2,866 females. This represents an overall 2% chance of developing AF in 20 years. They noted a direct relationship between the incidence of AF and age ranging from approximately 0.2% cases at 25–34 to greater than 3% at 55–64 years of age. Only 30 men and 18 women had no history of concomitant cardiovascular disease, and the other 50 cases were preceded more frequently than controls by congestive heart failure and rheumatic heart disease while males had in addition stroke and hypertension as precursors. Stroke was an antecedent predictor of AF, suggesting transient or intermittent AF as a possible cause of cerebral emboli. There was an increased mortality associated with the onset of AF: within six years, 60% of males and 45% of females died. In a 30-year follow-up of 43 individuals with AF but without cardiovascular disease, Framingham researchers found them to have an increased risk for strokes. In a similar population study from Mayo Clinic, individuals with "lone AF" were found to have a good prognosis. Rose et al. screened 18,403 male civil servants and found the prevalence of AF to be 0.2% in those 40 to 49, 0.4% in those 50 to 59, and 1% in those 60 to 64. Those with AF had a mortality more than three times that of age-matched peers. Campbell et al. studied 2,254 subjects over the age of 65 and found the prevalence of AF to be 2%. They also noted a higher prevalence (5%) in subjects over the age of 75 years. Thus, studies document that AF is an important clinical problem that will increase in prevalence as the population grows older. One problem managing patients with chronic AF has been how to obtain the optimal medical control of their cardiovascular response to exercise.

RESPONSE TO EXERCISE IN PATIENTS
WITH ATRIAL FIBRILLATION (AF)

Submaximal Exercise Testing.   Several authors have noted that patients in AF have an inordinately fast ventricular response during the first stage of an exercise test. Aberg et al. noted that the largest increment in ventricular rate occurred during the first stage of exercise and was greater than 45% of the total increase in heart rate. Likewise, Hornsten and Bruce have noted an increase in ventricular response from 83 to 152 bpm during stage I and a maximal response of 176 at least two stages later. In fact, most studies evaluating pharmacologic efficacy in HR control have used only a submaximal exercise level to evaluate HR decrease. Most studies used only a submaximal level to evaluate and have focused on HR control rather than exercise capacity.

In calculating percent change in HR at the submaximal stages (i.e., 3.0 mph/ 0% grade and anaerobic threshold) in a study we did at the Long Beach VA, we took the HR at that level, subtracted resting HR, and divided by the difference between maximal HR and resting HR. Our findings are consistent with a rapid increase in HR during the lowest work loads with smaller incremental changes approaching maximal. This contrasts with the linear relationship between HR and work load in subjects in normal sinus rhythm.

Brown and Goble evaluated the effect of propranolol in six patients with chronic AF. Three had rheumatic valvular disease, and the others had treated thyrotoxicosis. Each subject was tested at three similar levels of exercise determined on the first test. In spite of marked reductions in heart rate and blood pressure at all levels of exercise, the study was abbreviated because three patients had dramatic deterioration. David et al. used timolol to control resting and submaximal exercise heart rate (bicycle exercise at 300 kiloponds for one minute followed by two minutes at 450 kiloponds). They found digoxin to be ineffective both at regular and high doses and that timolol alone reduced heart rate more effectively than digoxin at high or low dose. A study by Yehalom compared practolol to placebo in 28 patients. Each patient underwent submaximal bicycle exercise at 200 to 300 kiloponds. They noted a significant decrease in resting and exercise HR in the slow and fast HR groups with the addition of practolol. Klein et al. described the use of verapamil in 23 patients treated with digoxin for chronic AF and noted a decrease in heart rate at rest and during submaximal bike exercise. The "slow" heart rate group demonstrated little response to verapamil. Redfors studied 11 subjects in AF who were placed on increasing amounts of digoxin. A nonlinear increase in heart rate occurred at low dose but became more linear at higher doses of digoxin. Digoxin had the least effect on heart rate at maximum work loads.

Maximal Exercise Testing.   Hornsten and Bruce compared 25 males and 40 females in chronic AF to a similar population matched by age, sex, and cardiac functional status but in sinus rhythm. Maximal treadmill tests were performed using the Bruce protocol. They noted significantly decreased heart rates at rest (83 vs. 76), at submaximal (152 vs. 124), and maximal work loads (176 vs. 150), and in recovery for the patients in AF compared to those in sinus rhythm. The mean exercise time for males in AF was 371 seconds (predicted VO_2 of 18 ml/kg/min) as compared to 377 seconds for males in sinus rhythm; for females in AF, 283 seconds (predicted VO_2 of 25/ml/kg/min) versus 272 seconds for those in sinus rhythm. All of the patients had rheumatic heart disease which explains the mean functional aerobic impairment (FAI) of 35%.

Aberg et al. performed two bicycle tests on 24 patients in chronic AF, all of whom had valvular heart disease. The first test was performed with the patient on a "maintenance" lower dose and the second on a high dose of digoxin. During exercise, heart rate was lower on higher doses of digoxin ranging from 5 to 25 bpm. There was a higher work load at a heart rate of 110 in subjects on the higher dose, but there was no significant change in maximum work; mean maximum heart rate was 157 with an estimated VO_2 of 12 ml/kg/min from a bicycle mean work load of 283 kiloponds. The functional aerobic impairment of 60% was secondary to the intrinsic heart disease. Aberg et al.

also studied 195 patients with a mean age of 47 years in chronic AF who had advanced valvular heart disease, all of whom were on digitalis. Each test involved "steady-state" bicycle ergometry with progressively increasing work loads at 100 kiloponds. The work load at a heart rate of 110 was reduced as was the mean maximum work load when comparing them to normals and the FAI was 60%. Mean maximum work load was 275 kpm/min which is equivalent to an estimated VO_2 of 12 ml/kgm/min. The largest percentage increase in heart rate occurred from rest to load I (approximately 45%) with less of an increase in the other two loads. Aberg et al. performed a third study involving 15 patients with advanced valvular heart disease to look at reproducibility of heart rates on two consecutive bicycle tests. The initial mean maximum heart rate was 138 bpm at a work load of 337 kiloponds (estimated VO_2 of 13 ml/kg/min) and an FAI of 55%. They noted that patients with a high work capacity had less of a heart rate change between tests than those with a low work capacity.

Davidson and Hagan studied seven men and four women with a mean age of 55 years who were in chronic AF; 10 had rheumatic valvular disease. Maximal treadmill tests were performed before and after each digoxin dosage change. Two patients were on propranolol. Heart rate response at stage I fell from a mean of 163 bpm to 146 bpm at optimal digoxin dose. There was no significant change in heart rate response at maximal exertion—176 bpm to 166 bpm—but two minutes into recovery, a mean heart rate of 98 fell to 86 bpm at optimal dosaging. Duration of exercise increased from 3.6 minutes to 5.2 minutes. Khalsa et al. studied 11 patients with maximal bicycle exercise prior to DC cardioversion. Nine were NYHA class II or worse and most had enlarged hearts on chest x-ray. They reached a mean maximal HR of 142 and a mean work load of 98 W.

Lang et al. studied 20 patients in chronic AF on digoxin therapy with an optimal verapamil dose followed by a double-blind crossover. Bicycle testing was performed with three-minute stages up to maximal effort. Heart rate was significantly lowered at rest and during all work loads, but SBP was only lowered at maximum effort. Maximum exercise duration was increased from 219 seconds to 292 seconds. Again FAI was high since they included patients with NYHA class II or III.

Molajo et al. described the use of Corwin, a new beta (partial) agonist in 10 patients in chronic AF taking digoxin. Two were NYHA class III and the rest were I and II. Eight of 10 subjects had rheumatic mitral valve disease and one had ischemic heart disease. The study was a two-week/phase, double-blind, crossover study with a one-week washout interim period. A maximum symptom-limited Bruce protocol was used. Heart rate (HR) response was significantly reduced while on Corwin: resting HR fell from 80 to 73, three-minute exercise HR from 132 to 105, and peak exercise from 162 to 120. Mean maximum exercise time increased from 215 seconds to 257 seconds while on Corwin. Functional aerobic impairment was 55% and is consistent with the intrinsic heart disease and the NYHA class II or worse in seven of their patients.

In a multicenter study, DiBianco et al. evaluated the effects of Nadolol on the HR response to maximal treadmill exercise in 20 patients with AF of greater than 2.5 months duration. The study involved a randomized, double-blind, crossover comparison of nadolol and placebo. The treadmill protocol used was a modified maximal Bruce protocol that began with a three-minute stage at 1.7 mph and 0% grade. Digoxin was continued at a stable dose in 17 of 20 patients. The heart rate reduction was significant at rest (92 to 73), at three minutes submaximal exertion.(153 to 111), and maximum effort (175 to 126). There was a decrease in exercise time from 466 seconds on placebo (estimated Vo_2 of 25 ml/kg/min) to 380 seconds (estimated VO_2 of 21 ml/kg/min) while on nadolol. The authors focused mainly on heart rate control rather than on the exercise capacity. The FAI of 40% is consistent with intrinsic heart disease, no doubt present in their patients with cardiomyopathy or rheumatic heart disease.

We (Atwood et al.) studied 34 consecutive male volunteers ranging in age from 49 to 87 years with chronic AF (greater than six months duration). Acutely ill patients, those with angina, on beta blockers and/or calcium antagonists and those with severe lung disease or thyroid dysfunction were excluded. All but one patient was taking digoxin. None of the patients was in congestive heart failure at the time of the study and all were functional class I or II. All patients had normal left ventricular function by echocardiography except for those with the diagnosis of cardiomyopathy. Patients were exercised on a treadmill using individualized protocols designed such that the maximal exercise test lasted between 10 to 12 minutes. Respiratory gas exchange variables were determined continuously throughout the exercise test. The number of QRS complexes multiplied by 10 in a six-second rhythm strip at the end of each minute was used to determine heart rate. Analysis of hemodynamic and pulmonary gas exchange variables was performed at a submaximal work load reached by all tested (3.0 mph/0% grade), the gas exchange anaerobic threshold (ATGE), and maximal exertion. These results are listed in Table 5–7. Our patients in chronic atrial fibrillation had decreased values of absolute ml O_2 at ATGE but had a mean percent of maximal oxygen uptake at ATGE comparable to a population in normal sinus rhythm. VO_2 and heart rate at maximal effort demonstrated a wide scatter in relationship to age due to the small number of patients and the diversity of heart diseases included.

Table 5–8 summarizes the results of the nine studies of maximal testing for comparison with our findings. Our study was the first to provide measured oxygen uptake. FAI is calculated by the formula: estimated VO_2 (from work load performed, i.e., treadmill time) minus predicted VO_2 (from age) divided by predicted VO_2 max. We obtained a higher aerobic capacity probably by excluding patients in congestive heart failure and including more patients with "lone" AF, fewer patients with valvular heart disease, and a majority of patients with normal LV function by echocardiogram. Using the equation of max HR equals 206 minus .6 times age (206 − [.6 × 60]), the mean maximal HR of 171 for our population is exactly as expected for this age group in normals. Consistent with other studies, the mean submaximal heart rate in our study was inordinately high and exhibited the greatest percent increment at that time.

TABLE 5–7.
Results of Exercise Testing in 34 Patients With Chronic Atrial Fibrillation

VARIABLE	TOTAL POPULATION (N = 34)	AGE 49–<60 (N = 8)	60–<70 (N = 15)	70–87 (N = 11)	<65 (N = 16)	>65 (N = 18)
Age	66 ± 8.9	55.8 ± 3.2	64.5 ± 2.8	75.6 ± 6	59.1 ± 4.2	72.3 ± 6.4
Weight	79 ± 13.2	80.4 ± 9.8	82.8 ± 14.7	73 ± 11	82.1 ± 12.6	76.4 ± 13.2
Rest SBP (standing)	138 ± 23	136 ± 20	134 ± 24	145 ± 20	135 ± 22	141 ± 21
HR	92 ± 21	97 ± 23	91 ± 18	90 ± 24	97 ± 21	87 ± 19
Measurements at 3 mph/0% grade						
VO$_2$	14.9 ± 2	14.6 ± 2	14.9 ± 2.2	15 ± 1.5	14.2 ± 1.8	15.7 ± 1.9
HR	141 ± 20	149 ± 19	139 ± 20.4	139 ± 21	147 ± 20	136 ± 20
SBP	163 ± 19	157 ± 18	165 ± 17	165 ± 23	157 ± 16	170 ± 19
PE	12.1 ± 2.9	12.8 ± 2.1	11.6 ± 3.6	12.3 ± 2.3	12 ± 3	12 ± 3
RER	0.88 ± 0.08	0.88 ± 0.1	0.88 ± 0.07	0.88 ± 0.08	0.87 ± 0.08	0.9 ± 0.08
%dHR*	62	62	59	68	57	67
Measurements at Anaerobic Threshold						
% Max VO$_2$	70 ± 9	68 ± 10	72 ± 9	65 ± 7	70 ± 10	68 ± 8
VO$_2$	15.4 ± 3.2	15 ± 2.6	15.7 ± 3.3	15.4 ± 4.4	15.2 ± 2.6	15.8 ± 4.1
HR	143 ± 25	139 ± 31	145 ± 25	142 ± 23	146 ± 27	139 ± 23
SBP	167 ± 19	164 ± 20	168 ± 21	168 ± 17	162 ± 20	173 ± 17
PE	13 ± 2.3	12.7 ± 1.3	12.9 ± 3	13.2 ± 1.3	13 ± 2	13 ± 3
RER	0.85 ± 0.06	0.82 ± 0.07	0.87 ± 0.05	0.84 ± 0.04	0.86 ± 0.06	0.84 ± 0.04
%dHR†	58	50	67	72	56	71
Measurements at Maximum Exertion						
VO$_2$	21.3 ± 4.1	22.1 ± 3.8	21.8 ± 4	19.9 ± 4.5	21.8 ± 3.6	20.8 ± 4.6
HR	171 ± 30	181 ± 37	172 ± 32	162 ± 21	184 ± 36	160 ± 19
Age-predicted MaxHR‡	165	171	162	159	169	161
SBP	176 ± 23	166 ± 15	180 ± 20	179 ± 23	169 ± 14	183 ± 23
PE	17.6 ± 3.5	18.1 ± 1.2	18.4 ± 1.4	15.9 ± 2.2	18 ± 1	17 ± 5
RER	1.05 ± 0.09	1.07 ± 0.06	1.08 ± 0.08	1.01 ± 0.12	1.08 ± 0.08	1.02 ± 0.1
VE	67.1 ± 15.4	71.1 ± 14	69.8 ± 13.6	57.8 ± 19.8	72.7 ± 13.2	60.7 ± 17.6

*%dHR = [subHR − restHR/MaxHR − restHR] × 100.
†%dHR = [ATGE HR − restHR/MaxHR − restHR] × 100.
‡Age-predicted MaxHR = 206 − .62 × age.
Key: VO$_2$ = ventilatory oxygen uptake; SBP = systolic blood pressure; HR = heart rate in beats per minute; PE = perceived exertion; RER = respiratory exchange ratio or respiratory quotient (RQ); VE = expired gas volume.
Values shown are mean ± SD.

TABLE 5–8.
The Results of Maximal Exercise Testing In Patients With Atrial Fibrillation

INVESTIGATOR	HORNSTEN	ABERG	ABERG	ABERG	KHALSA	DAVIDSON	LANG	MOLAJO	DIBIANCO	ATWOOD
Year	1968	1972	1972	1977	1979	1979	1983	1984	1984	1986
No. Patients	65	179	24	15	11	11	20	10	20	34
Mean age	50	47	45	45	56	55	59	52	60	66
Exercise protocol	Bruce	Bike	Bike	Bike	Bike	Bruce	Bike	Bruce	Modified Bruce	Modified B-W
Mean Max HR	176	134	157	138	142	176	169	162	175	171
est METs	5	3.5	3.5	4	5.7	6.5	4.5	5	7	8
est VO$_2$	18	12	12	13	20	23	15	18	25	27
FAI	35%	60%	60%	55%	30%	50%	50%	55%	40%	14%
Measured VO$_2$	—	—	—	—	—	—	—	—	—	21

Max = maximal; HR = heart rate; est = estimated; MET = 3.5 ml O$_2$/kg/min; VO$_2$ = ventilatory oxygen consumption in ml O$_2$/kg/min; FAI = functional aerobic impairment; B-W = Balke-Ware protocol.

THE EFFECT OF DRUGS ON EXERCISE PERFORMANCE IN PATIENTS WITH CHRONIC AF

In patients with chronic AF, the primary goal of therapy is to control the rapid heart rate response at rest and during exercise. Digoxin has been the drug of choice to control resting heart rate. However, digoxin has limited effectiveness in controlling heart rates during exercise or other stresses. The concomitant use of beta-adrenergic or calcium channel-blocking agents with digoxin has been recommended as a better means of controlling heart rate.

A concern with beta-adrenergic blockade therapy is the possible reduction in cardiac output resulting not only from reduction in maximal heart rate but also from the depression of myocardial function. If a significant reduction in cardiac output occurs, maximal oxygen uptake would be decreased, causing a reduction in exercise capacity. Studies in normal subjects have provided conflicting results as to the effect of beta-adrenergic blocking agents on maximal oxygen uptake and other ventilatory variables associated with aerobic capacity. Similarly, in studies of patients with AF, the effects of beta-adrenergic blockade on maximal exercise capacity have been inconclusive, and none of the studies have included measurements of ventilatory parameters. To investigate the effect of maximum dose (600 mg) Celiprolol, a beta-1 selective adrenergic blocker, on hemodynamic and respiratory gas exchange variables in patients with chronic AF during maximal exercise testing, Atwood performed the following study.

Nine male patients (mean age of 65 years) with chronic AF, eight treated with digoxin, underwent a randomized, double blind maximal dose Celiprolol/placebo study using exercise testing with measured ventilatory parameters to assess the effect of beta-adrenergic blockade on exercise capacity. We observed a significant decrease in heart rate and SBP at the submaximal workload of 3 mph/0% grade during Celiprolol administration which is similar to previous data obtained in normal subjects and patients in AF. Celiprolol did not alter gas exchange variables such as minute ventilation, oxygen uptake, and respiratory exchange ratio is consistent with studies in normal subjects.

A significant decrease in heart rate and systolic blood pressure occurred at the ATGE during Celiprolol therapy which is similar to data acquired in normal subjects and patients with coronary artery disease patients taking beta-adrenergic blockers. The observed reduction in oxygen uptake at the ATGE during Celiprolol is consistent with Peterson et al. but not with studies by Sklar and Hughson and MacFarlane. The discrepancies with these studies appear attributable to: (1) medication and dosage level used—Celiprolol at maximum dose versus propranolol at moderate dose, (2) chronicity of administration—for one week versus one oral dose, (3) population differences—young normal subjects versus older heart disease patients, (4) pharmacokinetics and testing times—two hours after Celiprolol which reaches its peak level two to four hours later versus in the Sklar study four hours after propranolol which peaks at one to two hours, and (5) differences in testing protocols.

In subjects in normal sinus rhythm, the effect of beta-adrenergic blockade on maximal oxygen uptake has been controversial. Authors have noted either a decrease in oxygen uptake with beta-adrenergic blockade or no change at all. Wilmore et al. list several possible causes for such variable findings, some of which include type of beta-adrenergic blocker (selective or nonselective with or without intrinsic sympathomimetic activity), method of medication administration (intravenous or oral), timing of test with respect to peak medication effect, length of time on medication (hours, days, weeks), dosage level (high versus low), exercise protocol (using treadmill or cycle ergometry), subject motivation and age, and even the statistical analysis used.

Few studies in patients with AF have addressed the effect of beta-adrenergic blockade on maximal exertion. DiBianco et al., in a multicenter trial involving 20 subjects in AF, looked at the exercise heart rate response to AF while on placebo and digoxin versus nadolol and digoxin. They noted not only a reduction in heart rate and systolic pressure but also a significant reduction in exercise time from placebo of 466 seconds to 380 seconds while on nadolol. This implied a reduced exercise capacity, but the authors focused on the reduced heart rate response and the safety of nadolol. In another study with 10 patients, Molajo et al. noted a reduction of maximal heart rate but also noted a significant increase in exercise time from 215 seconds during the placebo and digoxin phase to 257 seconds while on digoxin and Corwin, a beta-adrenergic antagonist with partial beta-agonist activity and some positive inotropic properties. However, the improved exercise time was 40 seconds in the same stage II of the Bruce protocol. In addition, the population tested had mild to moderate congestive heart failure and the Bruce protocol with its rigorous first stages explains why this population had such a low total treadmill time.

From a clinical standpoint, the addition of a beta blocker for heart rate control in patients with chronic AF makes sense when the only goal is to reduce myocardial oxygen demand through reduction of heart rate such as in patients with angina pectoris. However, in adding beta-blocker therapy, there is the risk of compromising VO_2 because of the negative chronotropic and inotropic effects associated with these agents. Maximum dose of beta blockade exerted negative chronotropic and inotropic effects, consequently leading to decreased exercise capacity, but perhaps a lower dose would have normalized heart rate without a change in VO_2 oxygen uptake.

Treatment with Diltiazem.   Since a calcium antagonist may offer chronotropic control but less negative inotropic effect, it could be more advantageous in the treatment of atrial fibrillation. Therefore, Atwood tested these patients after stabilizing them on diltiazem. They exhibited an improvement in treadmill time and no decrease in VO_2 max with good heart rate control. This leads us to believe that diltiazem is the agent of choice for these patients.

Clinically, the decrease in the ATGE and reduction in oxygen uptake at higher work loads becomes important in patients who desire an active lifestyle. Since the patient perceives an equivalent amount of work as being harder during beta-adrenergic blockade, his or her motivation to engage in previous activities may be affected. Results from the present study suggest that the use of beta-adrenergic blockers in patients with AF is a double-edged sword. The effective control of submaximal exercise heart rates must be weighed against the impairment in oxygen delivery at moderate to heavy work loads. The key to therapy in AF patients would appear to be normalizing the heart rate response to exercise without affecting the ATGE or maximal oxygen uptake, and this can be done with a calcium antagonist.

EVALUATION FOR AN INDIVIDUALIZED EXERCISE PROGRAM

The exercise test can be used to evaluate the safety of participating in an exercise program and can help formulate an exercise prescription. Because of the wide scatter of maximal heart rate when plotted against age, it is much better to determine an individual's maximal rate, in order to assign a target for training, rather than give a predicted value. In certain individuals, it would be advantageous to objectively evaluate their response to exercise in a monitored situation prior to embarking on an exercise program. In adult fitness or cardiac rehabilitation programs, an exercise test can be used to safely progress an individual to a higher level of performance. Also, the improvement in exercise performance secondary to training demonstrated by an exercise test can be an effective incentive and encouragement to people in such programs.

EVALUATION OF TREATMENTS

The exercise test can be used to evaluate the effects of both medical and surgical treatment. The effects of various medications, including nitrates, digitalis, and antihypertensive agents, have been evaluated by exercise testing. Though exercise testing has been used to evaluate patients before and after coronary artery bypass surgery, the reported studies have not given a definitive answer, mainly because of alterations in medications after surgery. One problem with using treadmill time or work load rather than measuring maximal oxygen uptake in serial studies is that people learn to perform treadmill walking more efficiently. Treadmill time or work load can increase during serial studies without any improvement in cardiovascular function. Thus, it is important to include the measurement of maximal oxygen uptake when the effects of medical or surgical treatment are being evaluated by treadmill testing.

EVALUATION OF ANTIANGINAL AGENTS

Reproducibility. Since studies using standard exercise testing are required by the FDA prior to approval of antianginal agents, it is important to know the reproducibility of exercise variables in angina patients.

The NIH group studied the reproducibility of selected variables during an upright bicycle test in patients with angina pectoris. However, there is little information on the reproducibility of hemodynamic and ECG data in angina patients during treadmill testing. Weber and Sklar have used the gas exchange anaerobic threshold (ATGE) as a relative exercise point in the evaluation of different pharmacological interventions. Angina patients have exceeded the ATGE during exercise testing, and so this variable should be helpful in evaluating various interventions.

To evaluate reproducibility, we (Sullivan et al.) studied 14 angina patients with three consecutive days of treadmill testing. A random effects analysis of variance (ANOVA) model was used to measure reliability and to determine any trends in the test results. The intraclass correlation coefficient (ICC), a generalization of the Pearson product-moment correlation coefficient for bivariate data, served as the measure of reliability.

Prior studies evaluating the changes of work performance in patients with angina pectoris have concentrated on improvements in total exercise time. Smokler and Lasvik, using moderately severe angina as an endpoint, have observed coefficients of variation (standard deviation divided by the mean × 100) of approximately 5% for total treadmill time. Similar results were obtained: coefficient of variation of 6% for peak time. However, when the interclass coefficient (ICC) was determined to test for reproducibility, a rather low value of r = .70 was obtained. The addition of a given amount to each observation of a parameter would increase the mean without affecting the standard deviation and thus lower the coefficient of variation. The ICC, like the Pearson product-moment correlation coefficient, is not affected by the addition or multiplication of a given number to the observations. An example of this is observed at peak exercise where there is a lower coefficient of variation (6%) than at the onset of angina (11%); but reproducibility, as defined by the ICC, is the same (r = .70).

During sequential exercise testing, McGraw reported an increase in total treadmill time in angina patients. In a previous serial study of normal subjects, increases in total treadmill time were reported without changes in maximal oxygen uptake. In this study, we observed better reproducibility for oxygen uptake when compared to time at each analysis point.

The ability to reproducibly determine anginal pain during exercise testing is critical to the evaluation of therapeutic interventions. Previous investigations have included a baseline exercise test in which the patient becomes familiar with the exercise testing equipment and staff. Studies by Redwood and Astrom have stressed the importance of a properly designed exercise test protocol when evaluating patients with stable angina pectoris. In our study, the baseline test familiarized the patient with the equipment and staff and evaluated their exercise capacity. From this, an individualized protocol was designed to allow the patient sufficient time on the treadmill before stopping due to anginal pain. Redwood has suggested that exercise capacity at the onset of angina can be optimally evaluated using a progressive exercise test that elicits anginal pain within three to six minutes.

Also, increments in work should not exceed 20 W or approximately 2 METs for a 75-kg man. In our study, the onset of anginal pain occurred at a mean of approximately six minutes. In the individualized protocols, the increments in work did not exceed 2 METs and in most cases were approximately 1 MET. The advantage of the individualized protocol over one protocol for all patients is that it provides a gradual increase in work and is specific for each patient's exercise capacity.

The criteria for stopping the exercise test was the patient's subjective anginal pain corresponding to that level of pain at which they would normally stop to take a sublingual nitroglycerin. The use of the Borg pain scale produced a wide range of numerical endpoints. It would appear that there is individual variation in the amount of tolerable anginal pain prior to stopping an activity.

As summarized in Table 4–10 in Chapter 4, the reproducibility of the double product, a noninvasive estimate of myocardial oxygen demand, was excellent at peak exercise ($r = .90$), but somewhat low at the onset of angina and the ATGE ($r = .75$ for both). The poorer reproducibility at the onset of angina and the ATGE may be explained by the fact that blood pressure was measured every two minutes. The observed improvement in the ICC for the heart rate when compared to double product at the onset of angina ($r = .89$) and the ATGE ($r = .83$) and a slight increase at peak exercise ($r = .94$) supports this contention. Thus, when systolic blood pressure is difficult to obtain, heart rate may be used as a reproducible noninvasive estimate of myocardial oxygen demand.

Studies involving angina patients by Linden and Lasivik have reported high coefficients of variation for the amount of ST-segment displacement. However, here again, the failure of the coefficient of variation to depict a reproducible variable is evident. When considering the ICC for lead X, the reproducibility is good, ($r = .80$) at peak exercise, the onset of angina, and ATGE, although the coefficients of variation range from 31% to 45%. Although not nearly as reproducible at the onset of angina or ATGE ($r = .65$), the lead with the greatest ST-segment displacement is reproducible at peak exercise ($r = .83$).

Conclusions from our study of modern exercise testing techniques in patients with stable angina pectoris include the following: (1) measured oxygen uptake should be used instead of total exercise time because it is a more reproducible measure of aerobic exercise capacity; (2) the gas exchange anaerobic threshold is a reproducible submaximal exercise variable at which to evaluate myocardial ischemia and myocardial oxygen demand; (3) a pretrial exercise test allows the patient to become familiar with the exercise testing staff, the equipment, and the nature of his/her anginal endpoints; (4) the treadmill protocol should be designed for the patient's exercise capacity with 2 METs or less increments per stage; (5) computerized techniques for ECG analysis provide reproducible measurement of ST-segment displacement; and (6) statistical methods based on the estimate of the measurement error associated with a particular variable can be used by the clinician and/or investigator to better plan and evaluate an intervention.

Waters et al. investigated the frequency and mechanism of variable threshold angina by performing seven treadmill tests in each of 28 patients with stable effort angina and exercise-induced ST segment depression. Each patient had tests at 8 a.m. on four days within a two-week period and on one of these days had three additional tests at 9 a.m., 11 a.m., and 4 p.m. Time to 0.1 mV ST depression increased from 277 ± 172 seconds on day 1 to 319 ± 186 seconds on day 2, 352 ± 213 seconds on day 3, and 356 ± 207 seconds on day 4 ($p < 0.05$). Rate-pressure product at 0.1 mV ST depression remained constant. Similarly, time to 0.1 mV ST depression increased from 333 ± 197 seconds at 8 a.m. to 371 ± 201 seconds at 9 a.m. and 401 ± 207 seconds at 11 a.m. and decreased to 371 ± 189 seconds at 4 p.m. ($p < 0.01$). Again, rate-pressure product at 0.1 mV ST depression remained constant. The standard deviation for time to 0.1 mV ST depression was 22 ± 11%. The standard deviation for rate-pressure product at 0.1 mV ST depression was significantly less at 8.4 ± 2.8%. In 78 (40%) of the 196 tests, time to 0.1 mV ST depression was less than 80% or greater than 120% of the patient's mean; in contrast, rate-pressure product at 0.1 mV ST depression was less than 80% or greater than 120% of the patient's mean in only three tests (1.5%). They found considerable variability in exercise tolerance in patients with effort angina, even when rate-pressure product at the onset of ischemia remained fixed. They concluded that a history of variable threshold angina does not necessarily imply variations in coronary tone.

EVALUATION OF LONG-ACTING NITRATES

It has been difficult to demonstrate the efficacy of long-acting nitrate preparations in the treatment of angina pectoris. More objective measurements during exercise testing are available that could make this possible, but they rarely have been applied. A key question we have tried to answer whether gas exchange variables and computerized ST-segment analysis accurately and reproducibly detect beneficial changes during exercise in angina patients treated acutely with sublingual nitrates or after treatment with long-acting nitrate preparations. Do these beneficial changes persist after chronic administration of the long-acting agents for two weeks?

The use of organic nitrates in the treatment of angina dates back to the 19th century when the English physician Brunton discovered the vasodilator activity of amyl nitrate by inhalation, and noted the immediate but transient relief of anginal pain. Subsequent findings by Murrell in 1879 established the use of sublingual nitroglycerin for the treatment of anginal pain as well as its use as a prophylactic agent prior to exertion.

Symptoms of effort angina are produced by a transient imbalance between the supply and demand of myocardial oxygen. The deficiency in myocardial oxygen is a result of increased myocardial demand in the face of restricted myocardial blood flow. Effort angina pectoris must be distinguished from spontaneous angina pectoris, in which coronary spasm plays an important role. Typical effort angina is highly predictive of obstructive coronary artery disease. However, only one-third of all patients examined at necropsy with significant coronary atherosclerosis have a history of angina pectoris. It is not clear why some patients with obstructive coronary artery disease have pain while others having the same degree of obstruction do not manifest this symptom. The chest pain associated with angina is usually relieved promptly by sublingual nitroglycerin.

The initial reports of the pharmacologic activity of a long-acting nitrate were by Krantz and coworkers in 1939. A group of nitrates of the anhydrides of certain sugar alcohols were examined for the effect of each agent (given intravenously) on blood pressure in the dog. The investigators were able to show that no significant amount of nitrate ion appeared in the blood, and thus the vasodilator effect was probably due to the organic nitrate compounds. Isosorbide dinitrate was one of the most active agents.

Some of the discrepancies in results in earlier animal studies related to the rapidly fluctuating hemodynamic state after intravenous administration. The time interval after drug injection and whether measurements are continuous or intermittent must be considered. During the first few minutes, cardiac output may rise, fall, or remain unchanged; hence, the decrease in pressure seen at this time was thought to be largely due to a fall in peripheral resistance. After 15 minutes, a fall in cardiac output was more consistent, and was believed to be more important in the persistence of the lowered blood pressure. A fall in left ventricular filling pressure observed early might be due to an increase in cardiac contractile force or decreased filling time (due to reflex tachycardia), but at later times, the fall was probably due to direct venous vasodilation, with a decrease in venous return.

Why are there controversy and disparate results with clinical studies of the use of the long-acting nitrates? Some explanations for this include the following: (1) acute (single-dose) effects can be demonstrated for the long-acting preparations, but when the agents are given chronically, tolerance can develop; (2) there is a definite placebo effect involved in the treatment of angina; (3) nitrate blood levels are difficult to measure, but some modes of delivery clearly do not result in effective blood levels; (4) acute peaks of nitrates in the blood may be more effective than a chronic level; and, (5) treadmill time or work load is not a reproducible measurement, and more objective measurements using expired gases and computerized ST-segment analysis rarely have been used.

Most studies evaluating antianginal agents have relied on changes in treadmill time to assess drug efficacy. VO$_2$ max has been rarely performed in patients with angina. Endpoints in anginal patients are often subjective, and the grading of angina to arrive at a consistent endpoint has not resolved this problem. Therefore, researchers have looked at submaximal endpoints as measures of change. These have included ST-segment depression, anginal threshold, the heart rate and blood pressure response to exercise, and more recently, anaerobic threshold. Angina patients should be able to walk longer on the treadmill because they become anaerobic later because of improved cardiac performance during exercise due to an antianginal medication. This has not been demonstrated yet but offers the opportunity to more objectively and safely evaluate antianginal agents. An additional methodology is to assess ST-segment changes using computer methodology and see if this objective estimate of myocardial ischemia is altered by antianginal agents.

Measurements should be made at the following points:

1. Supine and sitting HR and BP. Rationale: the action of nitrates may be through dropping BP. Previous studies have found a relationship between a change in VO_2 and a drop in BP. If this is demonstrated, a nitrate effect could be documented or titrated in the office by changes in resting BP.
2. Standard work load. We have used 3.0 mph/5% grade as a "standard" submaximal work load that most angina patients can achieve.
3. Submax HR and double product. These are chosen specifically for each individual using his baseline testing. The HR and the double product where definite abnormal ST depression is first seen is the value used for subsequent comparisons.
4. Ventilatory anaerobic threshold. Point chosen by gas analysis techniques where VE and VO_2 separate.
5. Onset of angina. Patients' first appreciation of usual angina.
6. Maximal exercise. Last 30 seconds of treadmill exercise.

With these considerations, we designed several studies to evaluate the effects of long-acting nitrates on treadmill test variables. Figure 5–3 illustrates the design of such a study. The following methods were used for the studies herein described.

INDIVIDUALIZED MAXIMAL TREADMILL PROTOCOL

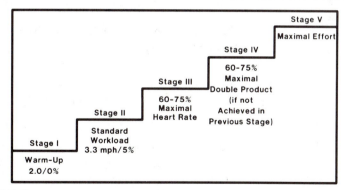

FIG 5–3.
Design of a study to evaluate antianginal agents with serial treadmill testing. Each stage is two minutes in duration. Stages III, IV, and V are determined from a submaximal modified Balke-Ware treadmill test done the day before. The 60%–75% levels are specific for each patient depending on his test responses to the treadmill test off the drug.

Testing Procedures.   The patients were exercised on a calibrated motor driven treadmill. Following the baseline test, the patients underwent exercise testing at the same time of day one week later. The baseline test was given to evaluate their current clinical condition and allow them to become familiar with the procedure. All testing was done in the fasting state, with no food eaten for at least three hours. Individualized protocols were designed to provide small increments in work to allow the patients sufficient time on the treadmill before reaching a symptom-limited endpoint. These protocols conformed to guidelines for testing patients with stable angina pectoris outlined by Redwood et al. The patients' subjective perception of anginal pain was evaluated using the Borg scale. The patients were taught the proper hand signals to indicate the severity of anginal pain. The points of analysis were the onset of anginal pain and peak angina, corresponding to that level of pain at which the patient would normally stop exercise to take a sublingual nitroglycerin.

Oxygen Uptake.   Patients breathed through a Koegel valve; expired gas was collected continuously in meteorological balloons each minute during the exercise test. Mixed expired oxygen and carbon dioxide were measured with an Applied Electrochemistry S-3A O_2 analyzer and a Gould Godart Mark IV capnograph. Expired volumes were determined by evacuating the balloons through a dry gas meter calibrated with a tissot at a fixed flow rate. The peak oxygen uptake was the last $\geq$ 30-second sample obtained prior to the symptom-limited endpoint.

The following measurements were derived from the gas exchange data: minute ventilation (VE, L/min-BTPS); oxygen uptake (VO_2, ml/kg/min, L/min); carbon dioxide production (VCO_2, L/min); respiratory exchange ratio (RER, VCO_2/VO_2); and the ventilatory equivalent for oxygen (VE/VO_2).

EVALUATION OF PENTAERYTHRITOL TETRANITRATE

We evaluated the efficacy of oral sustained release pentaerythritol tetranitrate (PETN) in 11 stable angina pectoris patients using a double blind, randomized study design.

Results.   Treadmill exercise testing with the direct measurement of expired gas exchange variables was determined at 1, 6, and 10 hours after administration of PETN or matching placebo. Changes in resting, standing and supine heart rates (mean increases four and five beats/min, respectively; p<.025), and supine systolic blood pressure, (mean decrease 9 mm Hg; p<.025), were observed one hour post PETN. There were no significant changes in any of the resting hemodynamic variables measured at 6 and 10 hours. One and six hours after PETN, ventilation and the ventilatory equivalent for oxygen were increased at peak exercise (p<.025). Furthermore, at one hour, trends toward increased peak oxygen uptake and carbon dioxide production were observed ($.05 < p < .10$). Total treadmill time did not differ between PETN and placebo at any time period investigated. The small sample size and possible nitrate tolerance are suggested as possible explanations for the lack of significant changes in other hemodynamic and gas exchange variables.

Parker has demonstrated partial tolerance to the hemodynamic effects of isosorbide dinitrate within 48 hours of initiating therapy. Thadani et al. demonstrated that acute resting hemodynamic and exercise variables in angina patients are attenuated during chronic therapy. Resting hemodynamic changes that persisted for eight hours during acute therapy were demonstrable for only four hours during chronic therapy. Similarly, significant increases in exercise capacity were observed for eight hours after acute and only two hours during chronic therapy.

EVALUATION OF TRANSDERMAL NITROGLYCERIN (TDN)

Transdermal nitroglycerin systems are advertised to offer 24-hour relief from angina pectoris. The basis for this extended therapeutic effect was inferred from studies documenting constant plasma nitroglycerin levels 24 hours after transdermal application and from preliminary studies in patients with angina pectoris. However, recent controlled studies have produced conflicting results as to the efficacy of TDN systems in patients with angina. Thompson observed significant increases in treadmill time at 2 and 26 hours after application of individually titrated TDN patches. In contrast, other investigators have been unable to document significant changes in exercise capacity 24 hours after application of TDN, although increases in exercise time were observed at intervals up to eight hours.

We studied 16 patients with stable angina pectoris in a double blind crossover manner utilizing treadmill exercise testing with the direct measurement of total body oxygen uptake, 1 and 24 hours after application of a 20 cm^2 TDN system and identical placebo. Testing was performed after a three-day lead-in period on either an active patch or placebo. Points of analysis were peak angina and the submaximal work load occurring at four minutes of exercise. No statistically significant differences were observed between TDN and placebo in any of the resting hemodynamic or peak angina variables at 1 or 24 hours. A significant increase in the double product at the submaximal work load was observed one hour after TDN relative to placebo. However, no significant differences were observed in any of the other measured variables at the submaximal work load, 1 or 24 hours post TDN.

A chronically administered, once-daily application of 20 cm^2 TDN was ineffective in altering the exercise capacity in our patients with angina pectoris. A combination of factors appear responsible for this. In investigations demonstrating an increase in exercise capacity with TDN, a titration period was initiated prior to the study to determine the maximally tolerated dosage. This was not done in the present study. In addition, the timing of the initial test, one hour after application of the transdermal system, may have been too early to detect significant changes in exercise capacity because of inadequate blood nitroglycerin levels.

The development of tolerance is another explanation. Twenty-four hours after transdermal application, blood nitroglycerin concentrations have been observed to be similar to concentrations obtained at two and eight hours. However, changes in exercise capacity recorded at two and eight hours after transdermal application did not persist up to 24 hours. Although blood nitroglycerin levels at any time period after transdermal application are lower than those observed during oral nitrate therapy, the lack of effect observed at 24 hours in the present study may in part be due to a nitrate tolerance acquired during the three-day lead-in period. Tolerance to organic nitrates when given chronically occurs within 48 hours after initiating therapy.

There were no positive effects of TDN at a submaximal work load where reductions in myocardial oxygen supply and demand were hypothesized to occur. Future studies should consider interrupted administration to lessen tolerance and titration of the dose until a drop in resting blood pressure occurs.

CORRELATION OF CHANGES IN RESTING SYSTOLIC BLOOD PRESSURE (SBP) WITH EXERCISE CAPACITY

Although the effectiveness of nitrates for the long-term prophylaxis of exertional angina is controversial, investigations utilizing large doses have demonstrated persistent physiological effects. During a titration period, the observation of a 10 mm Hg decrease in resting SBP and/or a 10 beat/min increase in resting heart rate has been utilized in studies attempting to demonstrate an increase in exercise capacity following nitrate administration. These criteria have served a dual purpose of documenting physiological changes in variables known to affect myocardial oxygen demand and to identify subjects nonresponsive to nitrates prior to inclusion in a study. If after nitrate administration changes in blood pressure and/or heart rate are correlated with changes in exercise capacity, the utilization of these variables by the clinician could identify patients expected to improve exercise tolerance during nitrate therapy.

In order to determine if these practical criteria could predict improved exercise capacity in angina pectoris patients treated with nitrates, we (Sullivan et al.) included both nitrate responsive and nonresponsive subjects. Nineteen patients with stable angina pectoris were studied in a double-blind placebo controlled manner. Significant increases in resting heart rate and peak oxygen uptake and decreases in resting SBP were observed one hour postnitrate relative to placebo (p<.05). Changes in peak oxygen uptake and total treadmill time during nitrate administration relative to placebo correlated to changes in resting supine systolic and diastolic blood pressure (r = − .54 to − .62; p<.05) but not to changes in resting heart rate. The multiple regression correlation coefficient utilizing the changes in supine systolic and diastolic blood pressure during nitrate administration relative to placebo as independent variables was r = .66 when compared to changes in peak oxygen uptake. These results suggest that during administration of nitrates, a decrease in resting systolic and diastolic blood pressure is essential to insure increases in exercise capacity. Conversely, a lack of blood pressure response to nitrates is indicative of no improvement in exercise tolerance. Thus, in the clinical setting, these parameters should be utilized as the basis for nitrate titration.

Improvement in oxygen uptake and treadmill time was noted in 10 of 11 patients with a greater than 5 mm Hg drop in supine SBP. In five of the remaining seven patients without a greater than 5 mm Hg drop in supine SBP, there was no improvement in exercise capacity. Multiple regression analysis utilizing changes in resting supine systolic and diastolic blood pressure during nitrate administration relative to placebo as independent variables resulted in significant correlations with changes in oxygen uptake and total treadmill time.

This is the first statistical proof for the previously intuitive concept of equating changes in resting SBP with improvement in exercise capacity in angina pectoris patients receiving nitrates. Patients who had the greatest drop in systolic and diastolic blood pressure had the greatest increase in peak oxygen uptake and total treadmill time. Conversely, those patients in whom administration of nitrates did not affect resting blood pressure did not improve their exercise capacity.

Previous investigators have observed similar relationships between mean changes in resting blood pressure and mean changes in exercise capacity. Awar et al. investigated the cardiocirculatory effect of topical nitroglycerin using right heart catheterization and forearm plethysmography in nine angina patients. Although they did not directly address the issue of resting blood pressure changes, utilizing data from their study, it is possible to calculate a negative correlation (r = − .86; p<.01) between changes in resting mean arterial pressure and changes in exercise time. This calculation suggests that the greater the decrease in mean arterial pressure, the greater the increase in exercise capacity.

Studies demonstrating the positive effects of nitrates on exercise capacity have utilized a titration criteria of a 10 mm Hg fall in resting SBP or a 10 beat/min increase in heart rate. The increased heart rate criteria is based on the baroreceptor mediated rise in heart rate due to decreased arterial pressure. Reichek has emphasized the importance of individual nitrate titration to achieve an optimal physiologic response. Standard doses of nitrates produced variability in the hemodynamic and exercise response. These results suggest that clinicians should document changes in resting systolic and diastolic blood pressure in angina patients receiving nitrate therapy. It appears that the greater the drop in systolic and diastolic blood pressure, the greater the benefit. The magnitude of this change in blood pressure may be limited by symptoms such as headaches, hypotension, or possible nitrate tolerance during chronic administration. On the other hand, a lack of blood pressure response after nitrate administration suggests little or no therapeutic effect and warrants a reevaluation of therapy.

EVALUATION OF PERCUTANEOUS TRANSLUMINAL CORONARY ANGIOPLASTY

Wijns and colleagues at the Thoraxcenter evaluated exercise testing and thallium scintigraphy in predicting recurrence of angina pectoris and restenosis after a primary successful PTCA. In 89 patients, a symptom-limited exercise ECG and thallium scintigraphy were performed four weeks after they had undergone successful PTCA. No information is given on pre-PTCA testing. Patients were followed for 6 months or until recurrence of angina. They all underwent a repeat coronary angiography at six months or earlier if symptoms recurred. PTCA was considered successful if the patients had no symptoms and if the stenosis was reduced to less than 50% of the luminal diameter. Restenosis was defined as an increase of the stenosis or more than 50% luminal diameter. The ability of the thallium scintigram (presence of a reversible defect) to predict recurrence of angina was 66% vs. 38% for the exercise ECG (ST-segment depression or angina at peak work load). Restenosis was predicted in 74% of patients by thallium but only in 50% of patients by the exercise ECG. Thallium was highly predictive but the ECG was not. Restenosis had occurred to some extent already at four weeks after the PTCA in most patients in whom it was going to occur.

Bergan et al. reported follow-up data in 183 patients who had undergone PTCA at least one year earlier. The duration of follow-up ranged from one to five years. Subjective clinical information was obtained in all patients and exercise testing in 91. PTCA was initially successful in 141 patients (79%). Of the 42 patients in whom PTCA was unsuccessful, 26 underwent CABG while 16 were maintained on medical therapy. When compared to the medical patients at time of follow-up, successful PTCA patients experienced less angina (13% vs. 47%), used less nitroglycerin (25% vs. 73%), were hospitalized less often for chest pain (8% vs. 31%), and subjectively believed their condition had improved (96% vs. 20%). During exercise testing, the prevalence of angina was less (9% vs. 43%), and exercise duration was greater (8.2 minutes vs. 5.8 minutes) among PTCA patients. However, there were no significant differences in ST depression (26% PTCA patients vs. 55% medical patients). No pre-PTCA exercise testing is reported. There were no significant differences in the incidence of subsequent MI, mortality, or need for CABS. For these variables, no differences were seen between the CABG and PTCA groups.

Vandormael and colleagues reported the safety and short-term benefit of multilesion PTCA in 135 patients, 66 of whom had a minimum of six months follow-up. Primary success, defined as successful dilation of the most critical lesion or all lesions, occurred in 87% of the 135 patients. Complete revascularization was achieved in 46% of the 117 patients with a primary success. Of the 66 patients eligible for six-month follow-up, 80% had an uncomplicated course and required no further procedures. Clinical improvement by at least one angina functional class was observed in 90% of the patients. Cardiac events including a second revascularization procedure were significantly more common in patients who had incomplete versus complete revascularization. All patients who had a primary success demonstrated clinical improvement with a reduction in symptoms or improved exercise tolerance. Exercise-induced angina occurred in 11 (12%) and an abnormal exercise ECG in 30 (32%) of the 95 patients with post-PTCA exercise test data. Exercise-induced angina occurred in 1 (2%) of 46 patients with complete revascularization versus 10 (20%) of 49 patients with incomplete revascularization; an abnormal exercise electrocardiogram occurred in 9 versus 21 patients, respectively.

Of 57 patients who had paired exercise test data before and after angioplasty, exercise-induced angina occurred in 56% of patients before the procedure, compared with only 11% of patients after angioplasty. Exercise-induced ST segment depression of more than 0.1 mV occurred in 75% of patients before PTCA versus 32% of patients after the procedure. After patients were stratified according to completeness of revascularization, the number of patients with exercise-induced angina was reduced to zero when complete revascularization was obtained; the difference was less marked in the patients who had incomplete revascularization. The incidence of exercise-induced ST-segment depression of more than 0.1 mV was significantly reduced in patients who had complete and incomplete revascularization compared with preangioplasty.

Rosing et al. reported that exercise testing after successful PTCA exhibited improved ECG and symptomatic responses, as well as improved myocardial perfusion and global and regional left ventricular function (RNV). Sixty-six patients were studied before and after successful PTCA. Surprisingly, only 33% had abnormal ST-segment depression while 68% had angina during initial TM testing. Follow-up studies an average of eight months after the successful procedure showed 7% to have ST-segment depression or angina during treadmill studies, and there were no abnormal studies with thallium scintigraphy. RNV demonstrated similar EFs at rest before and after PTCA, but an improvement of 9 ± 10% (p < 0.001) in the exercise EF at follow-up. However, 52% of patients with paired data still had an abnormal RNV study after successful PTCA most likely due to a false positive result.

Ernst et al. in the Netherlands described the results of functional and anatomic follow-up of 25 patients who underwent PTCA. All patients had subjective and objective evidence of coronary artery disease mainly due to proximal discrete one-vessel disease. Patients were studied prior to, within 14 days after, and at four to eight months later. History, exercise ECG, thallium scintigraphy, and RNV were performed at rest in maximal exercise. The mean stenosis of a dilated vessel decreased significantly from 83% to 38%. The functional status of the patients improved as reflected by a decrease in anginal complaints, increase in negative ECGs, exercise level, and ejection fraction response. The ejection fraction response to exercise was the most reliable way to discover a possible restenosis in the late follow-up period.

EVALUATION OF CABS PATIENTS

Hultgren et al. analyzed the five-year effect of medical versus surgical treatment on symptoms and exercise performance in patients with stable angina who entered the Veterans Administration Cooperative Study from 1972 to 1974. Exercise testing revealed comparable changes to symptoms and physical performance. At one year, surgical patients had fewer tests stopped by angina compared with medical patients (28% versus 64%), a higher estimated oxygen consumption (26 versus 21 ml/kg/min), and treadmill duration (7.3 versus 4.9 min). Other measures of exercise performance were comparably improved. At five years, exercise performance of surgical patients remained superior to that of medical patients, but the treatment difference was smaller. The beneficial effect of surgical treatment in patients with stable angina was maintained, with only a modest increase in symptoms and a slight decrease in exercise performance at five years compared with one year. Benefits of surgery were still substantially superior to medical treatment at five years.

Ryan and the CASS group reported the results of exercise testing performed in 81% of the 780 patients randomized at entry. The cumulative survival at the end of seven-year follow-up was 90% for those assigned to surgical treatment and 88% for those assigned to medical therapy. The survival rates did not differ significantly from either those of the entire randomized cohort or those of the 149 patients who did not have a qualifying exercise test at baseline. No differences in important baseline characteristics existed between those who were or were not exercise tested at entry. Stratification of patients according to the degree of ST-segment depression and final exercise stage achieved during a Bruce treadmill test (final stage) failed to show any significant differences in seven-year survival rates between medically and surgically assigned patients. Additionally, no differences in survival were noted within either the medical or surgical groups regardless of the degree of ST-segment depression or the final stage achieved. The presence of exercise-induced angina, however, identified patients who had a survival advantage if assigned to surgical therapy, with a seven-year survival rate of 94% compared with 87% of medically assigned patients (p = .007). This advantage was observed primarily in the subset of patients with three-vessel coronary artery disease and impaired left ventricular function. Mortality is incredibly low and suggests that the population is highly selected toward a low-risk group.

Gohlke et al. evaluated exercise responses in patients with different angiographically defined degrees of revascularization with serial exercise tests in 435 patients one to six years after CABS. All patients had undergone postoperative angiography 2 to 12 months after CABS to determine the degree of revascularization achieved. Revascularization was complete in 182, sufficient in 176, and incomplete in 57 patients. Twenty patients had all grafts occluded. Exercise capacity, angina threshold, maximal double product, prevalence of $\geq$ 0.1 mV exercise-induced ST-segment depression, and the prevalence of the combination of ST-segment depression plus angina pectoris were determined in serial supine bicycle tests. Patients with complete, sufficient, and incomplete revascularization showed improvement of all exercise parameters for six, four, and one year after CABS, respectively. In those with the best result, the prevalence of ST-depression preoperative was 76% and was 20%, 22%, 20%, 27%, 34%, and 33% in successive years. The prevalence also decreased in patients whose grafts occluded. Patients with all grafts occluded had improvement of only some exercise parameters. Exercise capacity was improved by 50% in patients with complete and sufficient revascularization, at one year and still by 30% at five years. Surprisingly, it was also improved in patients with incomplete revascularization or with all grafts occluded.

To determine whether preoperative exercise testing adds important independent prognostic information in patients undergoing CABS, Weiner and the CASS group analyzed 35 variables in 1,241 enrolled patients. All patients underwent a treadmill test before CABS and were followed for seven years. Survival in this surgical cohort was 90.6%. Multivariate stepwise discriminant analysis identified the left ventricular score and the final exercise stage achieved as the two most important (p < .001) independent predictors of postoperative survival. In a subgroup of 416 patients with three-vessel coronary disease and preserved left ventricular function, the probability of postoperative survival at seven years ranged from 95% for those patients able to exercise to stage 4 to 83% for those whose ability was limited to stage 1 of exercise. Exercise capacity was found to be an important independent predictor of postoperative survival.

EVALUATION OF PATIENTS FOR SURGERY

Carliner et al. performed a prospective study of preoperative exercise testing in 200 patients older than 40 years scheduled for elective major noncardiac surgery under general anesthesia. The exercise test showed ST-segment depression in 32 patients (16%). The patients were followed with serial pre- and postoperative ECGs and determinations of CK and CK-MB. Six patients (3%) had primary postoperative endpoints: three (1.5%) died and three (1.5%) had MIs. Secondary endpoints of suspected postoperative myocardial ischemia/injury diagnosed by ECG or elevation in CK-MB levels occurred in 27 patients (14%). Endpoint events were more common in patients aged 70 years or older. Endpoint events were also more common in patients with an abnormal (positive or equivocal) exercise test response than in those with a negative response (27% vs. 14%); however, preoperative exercise results were not statistically significant independent predictors of cardiac risk. Using multivariate analysis, the only statistically significant independent predictor of risk was the preoperative ECG. Endpoint events were more common in patients with an abnormal than in those with a normal ECG (23% vs. 7%, p<0.002).

Because the results of exercise testing do not appear to add substantially to the risk separation provided by the ECG at rest, exercise testing is not recommended as a routine preoperative method for assessing perioperative risk in older patients who are being evaluated before major elective noncardiac surgery under general anesthesia.

EVALUATION OF PATIENTS WITH HBP

Franz has investigated the blood pressure response during and after exercise in 552 males in order to determine if an exercise test is suitable for differentiating normotensive subjects and hypertensive subjects. Patients suffering from mild hypertension showed significantly higher blood pressures at 100 W and after exercise than age-matched normotensives and significantly lower values than stable hypertensives. In addition, the systolic pressure response to bicycle exercise was significantly influenced by age. Using the upper limits of blood pressure during and after exercise, 50% of the patients with borderline hypertension could be classified as hypertensives. Their blood pressure response at 100 W did not significantly differ from the patients with mild hypertension. In contrast, in the 50% who reacted negatively to exercise testing, the systolic blood pressure response at 100 W was significantly lower than that of those demonstrating a positive reaction. They had exactly the same diastolic pressure value as the normotensives. This study suggests that the assessment of blood pressure during exercise is useful in distinguishing between normotensive and hypertensive patients and in making estimates of blood pressure response to daily stress more accurate.

SUMMARY

Despite over 30 studies involving more than 7,000 patients, some controversy exists regarding the diagnostic power of the exercise test. A clinically practical approach to "multivariate analysis" using all of the test responses appears to result in a 60% sensitivity and 80% specificity for "significant" coronary artery disease. The test is less sensitive for mild degrees of disease and less specific in certain subgroups of patients. The amount, pattern, and duration of ST-segment depression along with exercise capacity, HR, and SBP response are highly predictive and reasonably sensitive for left main and triple-vessel disease. Also, such combinations result in the best means of prognostication.

Exercise testing is replacing functional classifications as a means of determining the degree of disability. The results from studies determining the risk of exercise-induced PVCs and more serious ventricular dysrhythmias are mixed, but prognosis appears to relate more to the "company they keep." The studies evaluating antianginal agents have been greatly hampered by the increase in treadmill time that occurs merely by performing serial tests. The studies of CABS and PTCA are confounded by differences in medication states before and after intervention and by the low rate of abnormal preintervention studies in the patients undergoing PTCA who mostly have single-vessel disease. From one study, we must conclude that exercise testing has little value in evaluating patients prior to noncardiac surgery. There have been reports, some of which are cited, of other applications of exercise testing such as its use for evaluating patients with unstable angina, valvular heart disease, and intermittent claudication. These have not been discussed but are left for a future edition when more results are available.

BIBLIOGRAPHY

Aberg H, Strom G, Werner I: On the reproducibility of exercise tests in patients with atrial fibrillation. *Ups J Med Sci* 1977;82:27–30.

Abrams J: The brief saga of transdermal nitroglycerin discs: Paradise lost? *Am J Cardiol* 1984; 54:220–224.

Ades PA, Brammell HL, Greenberg JH, et al: Effect of beta blockade and intrinsic sympatho-mimetic activity on exercise performance. *Am J Cardiol* 1984;54:1337–1341.

Areskog NH: Exercise testing in the evaluation of patients with valvular aortic stenosis. *Clin Physiol* 1984;4:201–208.

Baker BJ, Wilen MM, Boyd CM, et al: Relation of right ventricular ejection fraction to exercise capacity in chronic left ventricular failure. *Am J Cardiol* 1984;54:596–599.

Berger E, Williams DO, Reinert S, et al: Sustained efficacy of percutaneous transluminal coronary angioplasty. *Am Heart J* 1986;111:233–236.

Blumenthal DS, Weiss JL, Mellits ED, et al: The predictive value of a strongly positive stress test in patients with minimal symptoms. *Am J Med* 1981;70:1005–1010.

Boden WE, Bough EW, Reichman MJ, et al: Beneficial effects of high-dose diltiazem in patients with persistent effort angina on B-blockers and nitrates: A randomized, double-blind, placebo-controlled crossover study. *Circulation* 1985;71:1197–1205.

Bove EL, Marvasti MA, Potts JL, et al: Rest and exercise hemodynamics following aortic valve replacement. *J Thorac Cardiovasc Surg* 1985;90:750–755.

Brown RW, Goble AJ: Effect of propranolol on exercise tolerance in patients with atrial fibrillation. *Br Med J* 1969;2:279–280.

Brown SE, Prager RS, Shinto RA, et al: Cardiopulmonary responses to exercise in chronic airflow obstruction. *Chest* 1986;89:7–11.

Bruce RA, Hossack KF, Kusumi F, et al: Acute effects of oral propranolol on hemodynamic responses to upright exercise. *Am J Cardiol* 1979;44:132–140.

Bruce RA, Hossack KF, Kusumi F, et al: Excessive reduction in peripheral resistance during exercise and risk of orthostatic symptoms with sustained-release nitroglycerin and diltiazem treatment of angina. *Am Heart J* 1985;109:1020–1026.

Brugada P, Facchini M, Wellens HJJ: Effects of isoproterenol and amiodarone and the role of exercise in initiation of circus movement tachycardia in the accessory atrioventricular pathway. *Am J Cardiol* 1986;57:146–149.

Butman SM, Olson HG, Butman LK: Early exercise testing after stabilization of unstable angina: Correlation with coronary angiographic findings and subsequent cardiac events. *Am Heart J* 1986;111:11.

Butman SM, Olson HG, Gardin JM, et al: Submaximal exercise testing after stabilization of unstable angina pectoris. *J Am Coll Cardiol* 1984;4:667–673.

Califf RM, McKinnis RA, McNeer M, et al: Prognostic value of ventricular arrhythmias associated with treadmill exercise testing in patients studied with cardiac catheterization for suspected ischemic heart disease. *J Am Coll Cardiol* 1983;2:1060–1067.

Carliner NH, Fisher ML, Plotnick GD, et al: Routine preoperative exercise testing in patients undergoing major noncardiac surgery. *Am J Cardiol* 1985;56:51–58.

Cerri B, Grasso F, Cefis M, et al: Comparative evaluation of the effect of two doses of Nitroderm TTS on exercise-related parameters in patients with angina pectoris. *Eur Heart J* 1984; 5:710–715.

Chaitman BR, Brevers G, Dupras G, et al: Diagnostic impact of thallium scintigraphy and cardiac fluoroscopy when the exercise ECG is strongly positive. *Am Heart J* 1984;108:260–265.

Chiang BY, Olsen DB, Gaykowski R, et al: Evaluation of treadmill exercise on total artificial heart recipients. *Trans Am Soc Artif Intern Organs* 1984;30:514–519.

Dagenais GR, Rouleau JR, Christen A, et al: Survival of patients with a strongly positive exercise electrocardiogram. *Circulation* 1982;65:452–456.

David D, Di Segni E, Klein HO, et al: Inefficacy of digitalis in the control of heart rate in patients with chronic atrial fibrillation: beneficial effect of an added beta adrenergic blocking agent. *Am J Cardiol* 1979;44:1378–1382.

Davidson D, Hagan A: Role of exercise stress testing in assessing digoxin dosage in chronic atrial fibrillation. *Cardiovasc Med* 1979;4:671–678.

Deering TF, Weiner DA: Prognosis of patients with coronary artery disease. *J Cardiopulmonary Rehabil* 1985;5:325–331.

Detrano R, Yiannikas J, Salcedo EE, et al: Bayesian probability analysis: A prospective demonstration of its clinical utility in diagnosing coronary disease. *Circulation* 1984;69:541–550.

Detry JMR, Luwaert RJ, Rousseau MF, et al: Diagnostic value of computerized exercise testing in men without previous myocardial infarction: A multivariate, compartmental and probabilistic approach. *Eur Heart J* 1985;6:227–238.

Diamond GA: An alternative factor affecting sensitivity and specificity of exercise electrocardiography. *Am J Cardiol* 1986;57:1175–1179.

DiBianco R, Morganroth J, Frietag JA, et al: Effects of nadolol on the spontaneous and exercise-provoked heart rate of patients with chronic atrial fibrillation receiving stable dosages of digoxin. *Am Heart J* 1984;108:1121–1127.

Ellestad MH, Wan MKC: Predictive implications of stress testing. *Circulation* 1975; 51:339–363.

Engler R, Ray R, Higgins CB, et al: Clinical assessment and follow-up of functional capacity in patients with chronic congestive cardiomyopathy. *Am J Cardiol* 1982;49:1832–1837.

Epstein SE, Robinson BF, Kahler RL, et al: Effects of beta-adrenergic blockade on the cardiac response to maximal and submaximal exercise in man. *J Clin Invest* 1965;44:1745–1752.

Ernst S, Hillebrand FA, Klein B, et al: The value of exercise tests in the follow-up of patients who underwent transluminal coronary angioplasty. *Int J Cardiol* 1985;7:267–279.

European Cooperative Group: Long-term results of prospective randomized study of coronary artery bypass surgery in stable angina pectoris. *Lancet* 1982;:1173–1180.

Fleg JL, Lakatta EG: Prevalence and prognosis of exercise-induced nonsustained ventricular tachycardia in apparently healthy volunteers. *Am J Cardiol* 1984;54:762.

Foster ED, Davis KB, Carpenter JA, et al: Risk of noncardiac operation in patients with defined coronary disease: The coronary artery surgery study (CASS) registry experience. *Ann Thorac Surg* 1986;41:42–50.

Franciosa JA: Exercise testing in chronic congestive heart failure. *Am J Cardiol* 1984;53:1447–1450.

Franz IW: Ergometry in the assessment of arterial hypertension. *Cardiology* 1985;72:147–159.

Froelicher VF, Atwood JE: *Cardiac Disease: A Logical Approach Considering DRGs.* Chicago, Year Book Medical Publishers, 1986.

Gohlke H, Gohlke-Barwolf C, Samek L, et al: Serial exercise testing up to six years after coronary bypass surgery: Behavior of exercise parameters in groups with different degrees of revascularization determined by postoperative angiography. *Am J Cardiol* 1983;51:1301–1306.

Goldman L: Classification systems for the serial assessment of cardiac functional status. *Prac Cardiol* 1983;9:40–57.

Goldman S, Probst P, Selzer A, et al: Inefficacy of "therapeutic" serum levels of digoxin in controlling the ventricular rate in atrial fibrillation. *Am J Cardiol* 1975;35:651–655.

Gooch AS, Natarajan G, Goldberg H: Influence of exercise on arrhythmias induced by digitalis-diuretic therapy in patients with atrial fibrillation. *Am J Cardiol* 1974;33:230–237.

Gorforth D, James FW, Kaplan S, et al: Maximal exercise in children with aortic regurgitation: An adjunct to noninvasive assessment of disease severity. *Am Heart J* 1984;108:1306–1311.

Graybiel A: Auricular fibrillation in an asymptomatic young man. Effects of exercise, digitalization, atropinization and the restoration of normal rhythm. *Am J Cardiol* 1964;14:828–836.

Greenberg PS, Ellestad MH, Clover RC: Comparison of the multivariate analysis and CAD-ENZA systems for determination of the probability of coronary artery disease. *Am J Cardiol* 1984;53:493–496.

Hanson P, Stevens R, Berkoff H, et al: Exercise capacity and cardiovascular responses to serial exercise testing in men and women after coronary artery bypass graft surgery. *J Cardiopulmonary Rehabil* 1985;5:389–397.

Hitzhusen JC, Hickler RB, Alpert JS, et al: Exercise testing and hemodynamic performance in healthy elderly persons. *Am J Cardiol* 1984;54:1082–1086.

Ho SWC, McComish MJ, Taylor RR: Effect of beta-adrenergic blockade on the results of exercise testing related to the extent of coronary artery disease. *Am J Cardiol* 1985;55:258–262.

Hollenberg M, Go M: Efficacy of transdermal nitroglycerin patches in patients with angina pectoris. *Cardiovas Rev Rep* 1984;5:328–340.

Hornsten TR, Bruce RA: Effects of atrial fibrillation on exercise performance in patients with cardiac disease. *Circulation* 1968;37:543–548.

Hossack KF, Bruce RA, Ivey TD, et al: Changes in cardiac functional capacity after coronary bypass surgery in relation to adequacy of revascularization. *J Am Coll Cardiol* 1984;3:47–54.

Hossack KF, Bruce RA, Ivey TD, et al: Improvement in aerobic and hemodynamic responses to exercise following aorta-coronary bypass grafting. *J Thorac Cardiovasc Surg* 1984;87:901–907.

Hossack KF, Kannagi T, Day B, et al: Long-term study of high-dose diltiazem in chronic stable exertional angina. *Am Heart J* 1984;107:1215–1220.

Hossack KF, Pool PE, Seagren SC, et al: Long-term monotherapy of angina with nitrates. *Aust NZ J Med* 1985;15:221–225.

Hughson RL, MacFarlane BJ: Effect of oral propranolol on the anaerobic threshold and maximum exercise performance in normal man. *Can J Physiol Pharmacol* 1981;59:567–573.

Huikuri HV, Korhonen UR, Linnaluoto MK, et al: Effect of coronary artery bypass grafting on left ventricular response to isometric exercise. *Am J Cardiol* 1984;54:514–518.

Hultgren HN, Peduzzik P, Ketre K, et al: The five-year effect of bypass surgery on relief of angina and exercise performance. *Circulation* 1985;72:V79–V83.

Hung J, Chaitman BR, Lam J, et al: Noninvasive diagnostic test choices for the evaluation of coronary artery disease in women: A multivariate comparison of cardiac fluoroscopy, exercise electrocardiography and exercise thallium myocardial perfusion scintigraphy. *J Am Coll Cardiol* 1984;4:8–16.

Hung J, Chaitman BR, Lam J, et al: A logistic regression analysis of multiple noninvasive tests for the prediction of the presence and extent of coronary artery disease in men. *Am Heart J* 1985;110:460–469.

Hung J, Lamb IH, Connolly SJ, et al: The effect of diltiazem and propranolol, alone and in combination, on exercise performance and left ventricular function in patients with stable effort angina: a double-blind, randomized, and placebo-controlled study. *Circulation* 1983;68:560–567.

James MA, Walker PR, Papouchado M, et al: Efficacy of transdermal glyceryl trinitrate in the treatment of chronic stable angina pectoris. *Br Heart J* 1985;53:631–635.

Kannel W, Abbott R, Savage D, et al: Epidemiologic features of chronic atrial fibrillation. *N Engl J Med* 1982;306:1018–1022.

Kansal S, Roitman D, Bradley EL, et al: Enhanced evaluation of treadmill tests by means of scoring based on multivariate analysis and its clinical application: a study of 608 patients. *Am J Cardiol* 1983;52:1155–1160.

Khalsa A, Olson S: Verapamil-induced ventricular regularity in atrial fibrillation. *Acta Med Scand* 1979;205:509–515.

Klein H, Pauzner H, Di Segni E, et al: The beneficial effects of verapamil in chronic atrial fibrillation. *Arch Intern Med* 1979;139:747–749.

Klein HO, Sareli P, Schamroth CL, et al: Effects of atenolol on exercise capacity in patients with mitral stenosis with sinus rhythm. *Am J Cardiol* 1985;56:598–601.

Lang R, Klein H, Segni E, et al: Verapamil improves exercise capacity in chronic atrial fibrillation: Double-blind crossover study. *Am Heart J* 1983;105:820–824.

Losse B, Kuhn H, Loogen F, et al: Exercise performance in hypertrophic cardiomyopathies. *Eur Heart J* 1983;4:197–208.

McConahay DR, Valdes M, McCallister BD, et al: Accuracy of treadmill testing in assessment of direct myocardial revascularization. *Circulation* 1977;56:548–552.

Melin JA, Piret LJ, Vanbutsele RJM, et al: Diagnostic value of exercise electrocardiography and thallium myocardial scintigraphy in patients without previous myocardial infarction: A bayesian approach. *Circulation* 1981;63:1019–1024.

Melin JA, Wuns W, Vanbutsele RJ, et al: Alternative diagnostic strategies for coronary artery disease in women: Demonstration of the usefulness and efficiency of probability analysis. *Circulation* 1985;71:535–542.

Molajo AO, Coupe MO, Bennett DH: Effect of corwin on resting and exercise heart rate and exercise tolerance in digitalized patients with chronic atrial fibrillation. *Br Heart J* 1984;52:392–395.

Murayama M, Kawakubo K, Nakajima T, et al: Different recovery process of ST depression on postexercise electrocardiograms in women in standing and supine positions. *Am J Cardiol* 1985;55:1474–1477.

NcNeer JF, Margolis JR, Lee KL, et al: The role of the exercise test in the evaluation of patients for ischemic heart disease. *Circulation* 1978;57:64–70.

Niemela K, Ikaheimo M, Takkunen J: Functional evaluation after aortic valve replacement. *Scand J Thor Cardiovasc Surg* 1983;17:221–225.

Nyberg G: The time of onset of action of sublingual nitroglycerin in exercise-induced angina pectoris. A methodological study. *Eur Heart J* 1985;6:625–630.

Okada RD, Kanarck DJ: Left ventricular function before and after reaching the anaerobic threshold. *Chest* 1985;87:145–150.

Olivari MT, Carlyle PF, Levine B, et al: Hemodynamic and hormonal response to transdermal nitroglycerin in normal subjects and in patients with congestive heart failure. *J Am Coll Cardiol* 1983;2:872–878.

Pandis J, Morganroth J, Baessler C: Effectiveness and safety of oral Verapamil in control exercise-induced tachycardia in patients with atrial fibrillation receiving digitalis. *Am J Cardiol* 1983;52:1197–1201.

Parker JO, Van Koughnett KA, Farrell B: Nitroglycerin lingual spray: Clinical efficacy and dose-response relation. *Am J Cardiol* 1986;57:1–5.

Parker JO, Van Koughnett KA, Fung HL: Transdermal isosorbide dinitrate in angina pectoris: Effect of acute and sustained therapy. *Am J Cardiol* 1984;54:8–13.

Patterson RE, Eng C, Horowitz SF, et al: Bayesian comparison of cost-effectiveness of different clinical approaches to diagnose coronary artery disease. *J Am Coll Cardiol* 1984;4:278–289.

Pearson SB, Banks DC, Patrick JM: The effect of beta-adrenoceptor blockade on factors affecting exercise tolerance in normal man. *Br J Clin Pharmacol* 1979;8:143–148.

Petersen ES, Whipp BJ, Davis JA, et al: Effects of beta-adrenergic blockade on ventilation and gas exchange during exercise in humans. *J Appl Physiol* 1983;54:1306–1313.

Petru MA, Crawford MH, Kennedy GT, et al: Long-term efficacy of high-dose diltiazem for chronic stable angina pectoris: 16-month serial studies with placebo controls. *Am Heart J* 1985;109:99–103.

Philbrick JT, Horwitz RI, Feinstein AR: Methodologic problems of exercise testing for coronary artery disease: Groups, analysis, and bias. *Am J Cardiol* 1980;46:807.

Pittner H: Pharmacodynamics and cardioselectivity of Celiprolol—a new beta-adrenoreceptor antagonist with intrinsic sympathomimetic activity. *Clin Res* 1982;30:635A.

Podrid PJ, Graboys T, Lown B: Prognosis of medically treated patients with coronary artery disease with profound ST segment depression during exercise testing. *N Engl J Med* 1981;305:1111.

Pryor DB, Harrell FE, Lee KL, et al: Estimating the likelihood of significant coronary artery disease. *Am J Med* 1983;75:771–780.

Pucci P, Zambaldi G, Cerisano G, et al: Evaluation of a new preparation of transdermal nitroglycerin for patients with angina of effort. *Giornale Italiano Cardiologia* 1983;13:167–171.

Raffestin B, Denjean A, Legrand A, et al: Effects of nifedipine on responses to exercise in normal subjects. *J Appl Physiol* 1985;58:702–709.

Redfors A: Plasma digoxin concentration—its relation to digoxin dosage and clinical effects in patients with atrial fibrillation. *Br Heart J* 1972;34:383–391.

Redwood DR, Rosing DR, Goldstein RE, et al: Importance of the design of an exercise protocol in the evaluation of patients with angina pectoris. *Circulation* 1971;43:618–628.

Reichek N, Priest C, Zimrin D, et al: Antianginal effects of nitroglycerin patches. *Am J Cardiol* 1984;54:1–7.

Reybruck T, Ghesquiere J: Validation and determination of the "anaerobic threshold." Letter to the editor. *J Appl Physiol* 1984;57:610–613.

Roberts JM, Sullivan M, Froelicher VF, et al: Predicting oxygen uptake from treadmill testing in normal subjects and coronary artery disease patients. *Am Heart J* 1984;108:1454–1460.

Rod JL: Predischarge symptom-limited exercise testing after cardiac valvular surgery. *J Cardiopulmonary Rehabil* 1985;5:561–566.

Rod JL, Foster C, Schmidt DH: Evaluation of percutaneous transluminal coronary angioplasty by symptom-limited graded exercise testing. *J Cardiac Rehabil* 1984;4:70–73.

Rod JL, Squires RW, Pollock ML, et al: Symptom-limited graded exercise testing soon after myocardial revascularization surgery. *J Cardiac Rehabil* 1982;2:199–205.

Rosing DR, Van Raden MJ, Mincemoyer RM, et al: Exercise, electrocardiographic and functional responses after percutaneous transluminal coronary angioplasty. *Am J Cardiol* 1984;53:36C–41C.

Rozanski A, Diamond GA, Forrester JS, et al: Should the intent of testing influence its interpretation? *J Am Coll Cardiol* 1986;7:17–24.

Ryan TJ, Weiner DA, McCabe CH, et al: Exercise testing in the coronary artery surgery study randomized population. *Circulation* 1985;72:V31.

Sady SP: Transient oxygen uptake and heart rate responses at the onset of relative endurance exercise in prepubertal boys and adult men. *Int J Sports Med* 1980;2:240.

Sami M, Chaitman B, Fisher L, et al: Significance of exercise-induced ventricular arrhythmia in stable coronary artery disease: A CASS project. *Am J Cardiol* 1984;54:1182.

Scardi S, Pivotti F, Fonda F, et al: Effect of a new transdermal therapeutic system containing nitroglycerin on exercise capacity in patients with angina pectoris. *Am Heart J* 1985;110:546.

Scardi S, Pivotti F, Pandullo C, et al: Exercise-induced intermittent angina and ST-segment depression. *Am J Cardiol* 1985;55:1427–1428.

Schneider MS, Kanarek DJ, Nelson KM: Positive training effects on anaerobic threshold during beta-adrenergic blockade in cardiac rehabilitation. *Circulation* 1982;66:186.

Scholl JM, Chairman BR, David PR, et al: Exercise electrocardiography and myocardial scintigraphy in the serial evaluation of the results of percutaneous transluminal coronary angioplasty. *Circulation* 1982;66:380.

Schwartz JB, Keefe D, Kates RE, et al: Acute and chronic pharmacodynamic interaction of verapamil and digoxin in atrial fibrillation. *Circulation* 1982;65:1163–1170.

Sklar J, Johnston GD, Overlie P, et al: The effects of a cardioselective (metroprolol) and a nonselective (propranolol) beta-adrenergic blocker on the response to dynamic exercise in normal men. *Circulation* 1982;65:894–899.

Sokoloff NM, Spielman SR, Greenspan AM, et al: Plasma norepinephrine in exercise-induced ventricular tachycardia. *J Am Coll Cardiol* 1986;8:11–17.

Sox HC: Exercise testing in suspected coronary artery disease. *Disease of the Month* 1985;31:7–66.

Sullivan M, Genter F, Savvides M, et al: The reproducibility of hemodynamic, electrocardiographic, and gas exchange data during treadmill exercise in patients with stable angina pectoris. *Chest* 1984;86:375–382.

Superko HR, Adams WC, Daly PW: Effects of ozone inhalation during exercise in selected patients with heart disease. *Am J Med* 1984;77:463–469.

Szlachcic J, Massie BM, Kramer BL, et al: Correlates and prognostic implication of exercise capacity in chronic congestive heart failure. *Am J Cardiol* 1985;55:1037–1042.

Tesch PA, Kaiser P: Effects of beta-adrenergic blockade on O_2 uptake during submaximal and maximal exercise. *J Appl Physiol* 1983;54:901–905.

Thadani U, Manyari D, Parker JO, et al: Tolerance to the circulatory effects of isosorbide dinitrate: rate of development and cross tolerance to glyceral trinitrate. *Circulation* 1980;61:526–535.

Thompson RH: The clinical use of transdermal delivery devices with nitroglycerin. *Angiology* 1983;34:23–31.

Vandormael MG, Chaitman BR, Ischinger T, et al: Immediate and short-term benefit of multilesion coronary angioplasty: Influence of degree of revascularization. *J Am Coll Cardiol* 1985;6:983–991.

Varnauskas E: The European trial of coronary artery bypass surgery. *Lancet* 1982;2:1173–1177.

Vasilomanolakis EC: Geriatric cardiology: When exercise stress testing is justified. *Geriatrics* 1985;40:47–57.

Violante B, Buccheri G, Brusasco V: Effects of beta-adrenoceptor blockade on exercise performance and respiratory response in healthy, physically untrained humans. *Br J Clin Pharmacol* 1984;18:811–815.

Wall JL, Charles J: The process of habituation to treadmill walking at different velocities. *Ergonomics* 1980;23:425.

Wasson JH, Sox HC, Neff RK, et al: Clinical prediction rules. Applications and methodological standards. *N Engl J Med* 1985;313:793–799.

Weber KT, Janicki JS, McElroy PA: Cardiopulmonary exercise testing in the evaluation of mitral and aortic valve incompetence. *Herz* 1986;2:88–96.

Weiner DA, Levine SR, Klein MD, et al: Ventricular arrhythmias during exercise testing: Mechanism, response to coronary bypass surgery, and prognostic significance. *Am J Cardiol* 1984;53:1553.

Weiner DA, McCabe CH, Cutler SS, et al: The efficacy and safety of high-dose verapamil and diltiazem in the long-term treatment of stable exertional angina. *Clin Cardiol* 1985;7:648–653.

Weiner DA, McCabe CH, Ryan TJ, et al: Assessment of the negative exercise test in 4,373 patients from the coronary artery surgery study (CASS). *J Cardiac Rehabil* 1982;2:562–568.

Weiner DA, Ryan TJ, McCabe CH, et al: The value of preoperative exercise testing in predicting long-term survival in patients undergoing aortocoronary bypass surgery. *J Cardiovasc Surg* 1983;70:I226–231.

Weiner DA, Ryan TJ, McCabe CH, et al: Prognostic importance of a clinical profile and exercise test in medically treated patients with coronary artery disease. *J Am Coll Cardiol* 1984;3:772–779.

Weintraub WS, Barr-Alderfer VA, Seelaus PA, et al: A sequential approach to the diagnosis of coronary artery disease using multivariate analysis. *Am Heart J* 1985;109:999–1005.

Whipp BJ: Exercise hyperventilation in patients with McArdle's disease. Letter to the editor. *J Appl Physiol* 1983;55:1638–1639.

Wijns W, Serruys PW, Reiber JHC, et al: Early detection of restenosis after successful percutaneous transluminal coronary angioplasty by exercise-redistribution thallium scintigraphy. *Am J Cardiol* 1985;55:357–361.

Wijns W, Serruys PW, Simoons ML, et al: Predictive value of early maximal exercise test and thallium scintigraphy after successful percutaneous transluminal coronary angioplasty. *Br Heart J* 1985;53:194–200.

Wilmore JH, Freund BJ, Joyner MJ, et al: Acute response to submaximal and maximal exercise consequent to beta-adrenergic blockade: Implications for the prescription of exercise. *Am J Cardiol* 1985;55:135D–141D.

Wilson JR, Martin JL, Schwartz D, et al: Exercise intolerance in patients with chronic heart failure: Role of impaired nutritive flow to skeletal muscle. *Circulation* 1984;69:1079–1087.

Winnford MD, Fulton DC, Crobett JR, et al: Propranolol-verapamil versus propranolol-nifedipine in severe angina pectoris of effort: A randomized, double-blind, crossover study. *Am J Cardiol* 1985;55:281–285.

Woelfel A, Foster JR, McAllister RG, et al: Efficacy of verapamil in exercise-induced ventricular tachycardia. *Am J Cardiol* 1985;56:292–297.

Wu SC, Mancarella SS, Fossa L, et al: Usefulness of stress testing for the evaluation of hypertensive heart disease in young hypertensive subjects. *Cardiology* 1984;71:277–283.

Wyns W, Musschaert-Beauthier E, Van Domburg R, et al: Progostic value of symptom limited exercise testing in men with a high prevalence of coronary artery disease. *Eur Heart J* 1985;6:939–945.

Yahalom J, Klein HO, Kaplinsky E: Beta-adrenergic blockade as adjunctive oral therapy in patients with chronic atrial fibrillation. *Chest* 1977;71:592–596.

Young DZ, Lampert S, Graboys TB, et al: Safety of maximal exercise testing in patients at high risk for ventricular arrhythmia. *Circulation* 1984;70:184–191.

SPECIAL APPLICATION: EXERCISE TESTING OF PATIENTS RECOVERING FROM MYOCARDIAL INFARCTION

Though the death rate for coronary heart disease (CHD) has been decreasing steadily since the middle 1960s, it still remains the leading cause of death in the United States. Four deaths in every 10 are due to cardiac disorders; of these, 90% can be attributed to coronary heart disease. The three distinct clinical manifestations of CHD are primary cardiac arrest, angina pectoris, and acute myocardial infarction (MI). MI has been carefully studied because most patients with this manifestation are admitted to coronary care units. Also, MI has a definable onset and can be diagnosed by objective means with established criteria (i.e., pain syndrome, ECG changes, enzyme patterns). The case fatality rate in MI patients is temporally related to onset. The risk of death is highest within the first 24 hours of onset of signs and/or symptoms and declines throughout the following year. Following the onset of a first MI in middle-aged males, 30% to 50% are dead within 30 days, and 85% of these deaths occur within the first 24 hours.

Those patients with a first MI who arrive at a hospital alive have a 10% to 18% risk of dying before discharge. The mortality thereafter falls from an annualized rate of 9% over months 2 through 6, to 4% for months 7 through 30, to 3% over the next three years. Other studies have suggested a mortality rate of 11% in the first three months after hospital discharge, and lower rates thereafter. Thus, after a short critical period, survivors of MI stabilize at a risk of dying that has been estimated as two to five times that of a comparable healthy peer group. Most return to work, particularly since physician and public attitudes have become more encouraging.

The pathophysiological determinants of prognosis are (1) the amount of viable myocardium and (2) the amount of myocardium in jeopardy. Inferences

198

can be made regarding these two determinants clinically if a patient has had congestive heart failure (CHF) or cardiogenic shock and continued chest pain or ischemia. Utilizing cardiac catheterization, they can be assessed by ejection fraction and the number of vessels occluded. The clinical findings manifested by abnormalities of these two determinants are the basis for several indices that have been used to predict risk. Clinical data have also been useful in triaging patients in regard to the necessary length of stay in the hospital. The criteria for a complicated MI are listed in Table 6–1. Patients without these criteria, i.e., those with uncomplicated MIs, can be discharged within five to seven days, while those with these criteria require longer hospitalization and closer observation.

Health care professionals must be able to advise post-MI patients as to what they should or should not do to improve their prognosis. One strategy has been to identify high-risk patients by using various clinical markers and test results. Clinical markers that have indicated high risk include prior MI, congestive heart failure, cardiogenic shock, tachycardia, continued chest pain, older age, and complicating illnesses. Procedures used to determine risk with some success have included the chest x-ray, routine ECG, ambulatory monitoring, radionuclide cardiac tests, high frequency averaged ECGs, electrophysiological studies, and exercise testing. The assumption has been that patients at high risk should be considered for intervention; the interventions are coronary artery bypass surgery (CABS) and percutaneous transluminal coronary angioplasty (PTCA).

May et al. from the NIH have reviewed the clinical trials performed to see if mortality can be altered in patients long-term post-MI. They report that there have been no randomized trials demonstrating CABS to be effective in the post-MI population for preventing recurrent MI or death. Despite the lack of proof that CABS alters prognosis after MI, strategies have been proposed based on exercise test results delineating which patients should have coronary angiography and be considered for CABS or PTCA. This appears reasonable since there are many more studies using exercise testing after MI to evaluate risk than studies performed with other techniques. However, careful review of the available studies indicates that there is little agreement on which exercise test responses indicate high risk.

Basic clinical questions remain unanswered. What exercise test responses indicate an increased risk for subsequent cardiac events? Do the clinical pa-

TABLE 6–1.

Characteristics That Lead to the Classification of Complicated MI

CHF
Cardiogenic shock
Large MI as determined by CPK and/or ECG
Pericarditis
Dangerous arrhythmias including conduction problems
Concurrent illnesses
Pulmonary embolus
Continued ischemia

rameters associated with MI (i.e., CHF, prior MI, MI location and type, shock, continued ischemia) have adequate predictive power, making the exercise test unnecessary? By summarizing the results of the studies using exercise testing in patients post MI, this chapter provides assistance to those who must decide the best long-term management of this population and to those designing studies to answer these questions.

This chapter begins with a summary of early studies and methodological studies that have provided useful information regarding the use of exercise testing in the MI population. The studies that have compared exercise test results with coronary angiography are also presented. The main part is devoted to a critique of the follow-up studies. Studies dealing with radionuclide exercise testing post-MI are reviewed in Chapter 8.

RISK VERSUS SAFETY OF EXERCISE TESTING EARLY POST-MI

The risk of death and major arrhythmias by performing an exercise test early after MI is small. However, the major experience is based on clinically selected MI patients; those without major complications such as heart failure, severe arrhythmias or ischemia, left ventricular dysfunction, or other severe diseases. Often only 50% or less of the post-MI patients have been exercise tested because of the concern their physicians have for the dangers of the test. However, researchers have safely used the test in high-risk patients.

The exercise test can determine the possible risk the patient may incur with exercise. It is certainly safer that adverse reactions be observed in controlled circumstances. The risk-benefit ratio of this procedure can be improved by a number of considerations. Although maximal exercise testing soon after MI has been reported, until approximately one month after MI, a submaximal limited test is more clinically appropriate. Arbitrarily, a heart rate limit of 140 beats/min and a MET level of 7 is used for patients under 40, and 130 beats/min and a MET level of 5 for patients over 40. Particularly for patients on beta blockers, a Borg-perceived exertion level in the range of 13 to 15 is used to end the test. In addition, conservative clinical indications for stopping the test should be applied. The physician providing medical care for the patient can gain valuable information about the patient by being there during the test and interacting with the patient.

EARLY AND METHODOLOGICAL STUDIES OF EXERCISE TESTING POST-MI

In one of the first studies establishing the safety of early exercise, Cain and colleagues reported their use of a graded activity program in 335 patients who were at least 15 days post an uncomplicated MI. The patients had been restricted to bed, chair, and commode. The ECG was monitored after the patient performed activities such as climbing stairs and walking up a grade. They concluded that ECG monitoring of early activity was a more reliable means of ascertaining the presence of coronary insufficiency than were physical signs or symptoms. Torkelson reported results in 10 patients post an uncomplicated MI. During the sixth week of an in-hospital rehabilitation program, a low-level treadmill test was performed using 1.7 mph at a 10% grade. He concluded that the treadmill test was valuable for discerning the exercise responses of MI patients.

Ibsen and colleagues reported the results of a maximal bicycle test in the third week after MI in 209 patients. They concluded that an exercise test was safe in such patients, it was an objective measure of physical work capacity, and it described the reaction to physical activity. They believed that because it was a maximal test, it gave a better basis for advising return to a normal life and was of great psychologic importance to the patient. No follow-up data was presented.

Niederberger presented the values and limitations of exercise testing after MI in a monograph published in Vienna in 1977. From his review and experience, he recommended a bicycle test beginning with a workload of 25 W increasing 25 W every two minutes. He found computerized ST-segment measurements to be reproducible, but a follow-up had not been completed.

Markiewicz and colleagues studied 46 men under the age of 70 using treadmill testing at 3, 5, 7, 9, and 11 weeks after their MI. The test at 3 to 5 weeks and the test at 7 to 11 weeks appeared to provide most of the information obtained in all five tests performed. In selected low-risk patients, they performed maximal treadmill testing at three weeks after MI and found that a low heart rate response suggested a poor prognosis.

Sivarajan and colleagues evaluated 41 post MI patients. They assessed symptoms, signs, and hemodynamic and ECG responses during and after three activities: sitting upright, walking to an adjacent toilet, and walking on a treadmill. These activities were studied at 3, 6, and 10 days, respectively, after infarction. They concluded that successful performance of these three activities provided useful criteria for discharge of a patient with MI.

EFFECT OF EXERCISE TESTING ON PATIENT AND SPOUSE CONFIDENCE

Taylor et al. evaluated the effects of the involvement of the wife in her husband's performance on a treadmill test three weeks after an uncomplicated acute MI. They compared 10 wives who did not observe the test, 10 who observed the test, and 10 who observed and performed the test themselves. In a counseling session after the treadmill test, wives were fully informed about the patient's capacity to perform activities. Perceived confidence in their husband's physical and cardiac capabilities were significantly greater among those wives who also performed the test than in the other two groups. In a similar study, Ewart demonstrated that the patient's confidence was enhanced by the test also.

PROTOCOL COMPARISONS

Handler and Sowton compared the Naughton and modified Bruce treadmill protocols in 20 patients six weeks after an MI. Estimated exercise capacity and ischemic responses were similar using both protocols. The only significant difference was the relatively long mean maximal exercise duration in the Naughton protocol. Starling et al. evaluated 29 uncomplicated post-MI patients with a heart-rate-limited and symptom-limited modified Naughton treadmill test and 31 similar patients with a symptom-limited modified Naughton and standard Bruce test at six weeks following MI. Predischarge, the symptom-limited Naughton test identified a greater number of patients with ST-segment depression or angina than did the heart-rate-limited test (21 vs. 13 patients). At six weeks following MI, the standard Bruce test identified significantly more ischemic abnormalities than did the symptom-limited modified Naughton test (20 vs. 13 patients). During the Bruce test, a higher double product was reached in a shorter time. However, rather than using the Bruce protocol, it is more logical that the post-MI test protocol be individualized to the patient and that the initial level should begin at 2 METs followed by 1 or 2 MET incremental stages.

REPRODUCIBILITY

Starling et al. evaluated the comparative predictive value of ST-segment depression or angina in 93 post-MI patients tested predischarge and 36 tested again at six weeks. They concluded that angina alone, regardless of the presence of ST-segment depression, was a better predictor of multivessel disease than ST-segment depression alone. Repeat testing was helpful for confirming this likelihood. Handler and Sowton evaluated the diurnal variation and reproducibility of abnormalities occurring during predischarge treadmill testing in 41 patients. Each patient was exercised using a symptom-limited Naughton protocol in the morning and the afternoon on two consecutive days. Ischemic abnormalities were poorly reproducible in any patient, but no significant diurnal variation occurred. The reproducibility of an ischemic result in all four tests was 66%. They could find no reason for the poor reproducibility of ST-segment depression or elevation and angina (i.e., hemodynamic or clinical). Starling et al. evaluated 89 patients with predischarge and six-week treadmill tests to determine the importance of doing repeat tests to identify abnormalities of known prognostic value. Nineteen patients completed only a predischarge exercise test, nine of whom experienced an early cardiac event precluding repeat testing. All nine had prognostically important treadmill abnormalities during the predischarge test. ST-segment depression was highly reproducible between the early and six-week test. Angina, inadequate blood pressure response, and ventricular arrhythmias showed limited reproducibility and substantial individual variability.

Experience from testing hundreds of post-MI patients has been that even the most carefully taken BP measurements are poorly reproducible, that treadmill time is influenced by many technical factors, that angina is highly subjective, but that ST-segment and oxygen-consumption measurements, though dependent upon instrumentation, can be very reproducible. The spontaneous hemodynamic improvements post MI and the effect of serial testing must be considered.

THE PROGNOSTIC VALUE OF PACING VERSUS EXERCISE TESTING

Tzivoni et al. compared right atrial pacing and treadmill testing in 111 patients recovering from acute MI prior to hospital discharge. Patients with predischarge congestive heart failure, chest pain, physical disability, or an age older than 70 were excluded. Ischemic responses were more frequent during pacing than during treadmill testing (41% vs. 34%). The results of the two tests were concordant in 102 patients. During a mean follow-up period of 16 months, 10 patients had recurrent MI and six died. These investigators found atrial pacing to be more sensitive for predicting both situations. Currently, they only use atrial pacing in patients unable to perform exercise tests.

THE PROGNOSTIC VALUE OF PROGRAMMED STIMULATION VERSUS EXERCISE TESTING

Denniss et al. did a one-year follow up study of 228 clinically well survivors of MI. Patients with inducible ventricular tachycardia or fibrillation had a higher mortality than those without inducible arrhythmias in the electrophysiological laboratory (26% vs. 6%). Exercise-induced ST-segment change of 0.2 mV or more was associated with a higher mortality than those with less than a 0.2 mV shift (11% vs. 4%). The electrophysiological (EP) study was performed one to four weeks post MI and the exercise test was maximal at two to eight weeks. ST depression and elevation were combined. Univariate analysis was performed and other exercise test variables were not considered. There was a 6% mortality in the 191 who underwent exercise testing and a 27% in those who did not. These results with EP studies in the post-MI population have not been confirmed.

PREDICTING MAXIMAL OXYGEN CONSUMPTION

Haskell et al. measured VO_2 during symptom-limited treadmill testing 3 and 11 weeks after an acute infarct. Twenty-two men underwent a standard modified Naughton protocol with 2.5% grade increments while the others underwent an accelerated protocol with 5% grade increments every three minutes.

Estimated VO_2 values were significantly higher than measured values in patients completing the accelerated protocol at 11 weeks, and holding on to the treadmill handrails significantly increased estimated VO_2 but did not affect measured VO_2. Roberts and colleagues, in a group of patients four months or more post MI, also found estimated VO_2 to exceed measured VO_2 when patients exceeded their anaerobic threshold. This usually amounts to approximately a one-MET difference when using tables based on normals for estimating oxygen consumption in post-MI patients.

SPONTANEOUS IMPROVEMENT POST-MI

Wohl and colleagues studied 50 patients after an acute MI. They found that in stable patients, there was an improvement at three weeks of the relationship between myocardial oxygen supply and demand as detected by ST-segment changes. There was a delayed improvement between three and six months in functional capacity associated with increased stroke volume and cardiac output. Haskell and DeBusk reported the cardiovascular responses to repeated treadmill testing at 3, 7, and 11 weeks after acute MI. Two symptom-limited tests were performed on 24 males (mean age 54 years) several days apart. All test variables measured at maximum effort increased significantly between 3 and 11 weeks. Thus, exercise capacity increased spontaneously after an MI, even in patients not in a formal exercise program.

EFFECT OF Q-WAVE LOCATION ON ST-SEGMENT SHIFTS

Castellanet et al. studied 97 patients with a prior transmural MI who underwent coronary angiography and treadmill testing. In patients with a previous inferior wall infarction, the ST-segment response had a high degree of sensitivity and specificity (approximately 90%) in detecting additional coronary disease. However, in patients with a previous anteroseptal MI, the ST response had much less sensitivity. In this group, a positive test suggested the presence of ischemia in the lateral or inferior posterior region. It was thought that the aneurysm generated an ischemic vector cancelling ST-segment changes and producing a false negative treadmill test. If the anterior infarction extended beyond V4, the sensitivity rate of treadmill testing dropped even further. Ahnve et al. used thallium scintigraphy and computerized ST vector shifts to evaluate the effect of Q-wave location on the relationship of ST shifts to ischemia. Anterolateral MIs had large ST-segment spatial shifts that did not indicate ischemia, while when shifts occurred in patients with inferior or subendocardial MIs ischemia was detected by thallium defects. It appears that large anterior MIs behave as if left bundle branch block were present and the ST shifts have a very low specificity for ischemia.

Atterhog and colleagues reported the electrocardiographic response to exercise at varying time points in 12 patients after an anterior MI. In their hospital, a submaximal bicycle test was performed three weeks after an acute MI as a routine procedure since 1968. Three weeks after MI, 10 of their 12 patients exhibited an exercise-induced rise in ST segments in anterior precordial leads over the infarcted area. This response decreased over the follow-up months, and some subjects had exercise-induced ST-segment depression. The ST-segment elevation was interpreted as a sign of ischemia in the infarcted zone and the rate at which this resolved was thought to have prognostic significance.

THE RESULTS OF EXERCISE TESTING AND CORONARY ANGIOGRAPHY

Exercise testing results would be clinically most helpful in deciding about CABS if the exercise test could predict which patients have anatomic findings associated with improved survival if CABS was performed, i.e., left main or triple-vessel disease along with an EF of 30% to 50%. However, the endpoint usually predicted has been multivessel disease (MVD). Angiographic studies are thought of as "instant epidemiology" since the investigator does not need to wait upon endpoints. However, those who undergo this invasive procedure are highly selected. The following angiographic studies are summarized in Table 6–2.

Weiner et al. reported 154 patients with a single MI who had exercise testing and coronary angiography. The patients averaged were one year post-MI. Eighty-three patients developed ST depression only, 22 had elevation with depression in other leads, 19 had elevation only, and 30 had no changes. Respectively, multivessel disease was present in 76%, 91%, 21%, and 13% of the above groups. Left ventricular aneurysms were present, respectively. in 31%, 68%, 79%, and 40%. ST depression (with or without ST elevation) predicted multivessel disease, ST elevation alone or no ST shift suggested single-vessel involvement, and elevation predicted LV aneurysm.

Paine et al. studied 100 consecutive patients with exercise testing and cardiac catheterization at a median of four months after MI. Of 31 patients with 0.1 mV of ST depression, 87% had two- or three-vessel disease while of 21 patients with no depression, 38% had two- or three-vessel disease. Fourteen patients had ST elevation and they had more LV damage.

Dillahunt and Miller exercise tested 28 patients from 10 to 18 days after MI and catheterized the same patients 4–20 weeks later. Among 11 patients with no symptoms, ST-segment changes, or arrhythmias during the treadmill test, eight had single-vessel disease (73%) and three had two-vessel disease. In contrast, among the 17 patients with any abnormality, 14 (82%) had three- or four-vessel disease. The EF was significantly lower in the 17 patients with an abnormal test.

Sammel et al. reported the results of exercise testing and coronary arteriography in 77 men under 60 years of age studied one month after MI. The 22

TABLE 6–2.
Studies Applying Exercise Testing in Post-MI Populations With Coronary Angiographic Correlation

				EXERCISE TEST CHARACTERISTICS			ANGIO	
INVESTIGATOR	YEAR	#EX TESTED	END POINTS	LEADS	PROTOCOL	TIME POST-MI	TIME POST-MI	AGE/% WOMEN
Weiner	78	154	ss, BPd, >4 mm, RVA	12LD	Bruce	2–36 mo	2–36 mo	25–65/12%
Paine	78	100	90% MHR,ss,IVCD,1 mm	V4–6	Bruce	4 mo	4 mo	48/7%
Dillahunt	79	28	ss, 1mm, >3PVC/min, 5 min	CM5,V2	Naughton	10–18 days	4–20 wk	42–69/21%
Sammel	80	77	ss, 6 METs	12LD	Green Ln	1 mo	1 mo	<60/0%
Fuller	81	40	HR 120,ss, 1mm, >5 PVCs	12LD	low Bruce	.9–18 days	5–12 wk	54/0%
Starling	81	57	ss, VT, BPd, HBP	12LD	Naughton	9–21 days	3–12 wk	56/7%
Boschat	81	65	85% MHR,1 mm	12LD	Bruce	2–12 mo	2–12 mo	50/2.5%
Schwartz	81	48	ss, BPd, VT, 2 mm, 75% MHR	12LD	low Bruce	18–22 days	3 wk	50/10%
DeFeyter	82	179	ss, VT	12LD	Bruce	6–8 wk	6–8 wk	28–65/10%
Akhras	84	119	ss	12LD	Bruce	2 wk	6 wk	50/6%
Morris	84	110	ss	12LD	UPR Bike	>6 wk	< 3 mo	56/12%
van der Wall	85	176	ss	12LD	Bruce/TH	6–8 wk	6–8wk	54/11%

Key: Investigator—the first author; year—year of publication; #EX TESTED—the number of patients exercise tested.
Exercise Test Characteristic Columns. End Points—endpoints for exercise testing; SS—signs and/or symptoms; HR, with a heart rate value—heart rate limit; Max—maximal effort; percent heart rate—percent of age predicted maximal heart rate chosen as a limit; MET—a maximal exercise level allowed to be reached as estimated from work load; Symptoms—symptoms alone were the endpoint; VT—ventricular tachycardia as an endpoint; mm—amount of ST shift taken as an endpoint; BPd—SBP drop; IVCD—intraventricular conduction defect. Leads—the ECG leads analyzed; 12 LD—the full 12 lead; CM5—a bipolar lead; V5—fifth precordial lead. Protocol—type of exercise study done; TM—treadmill; Green Ln—Green Lane hospital TM protocol; low Bruce—Bruce protocol with 0 and ½ stages which are 0% and 5% grade at 1.7 mph prior to stage 1 (10% grade at 1.7 mph). UPR—upright bike combined with radionuclide testing; Bruce/TH—Bruce protocol with Thallium imaging; time post-MI—mean time post-MI that the exercise test or angiography was done.

patients with exercise-induced angina had a greater proportion of myocardium supplied by significant lesions compared to the 55 patients free of angina. The combination of ST segment changes (0.1 mV or more depression or 0.2 mV or more elevation) and angina was 91% predictive of triple-vessel disease. All four patients with significant left main disease (≥75% stenosis) had both angina and ST-segment changes. It is difficult to compare their results to the other studies since the number of vessels diseased was not given. Instead, a scoring system was used that estimated muscle in jeopardy.

Fuller et al. performed submaximal exercise tests on 40 MI patients prior to discharge and performed catheterization 5–12 weeks after MI. Among the 15 patients with an abnormal treadmill test (angina and/or ST segment depression of 0.1 mV or more), 13 (87%) had significant multivessel disease versus 7 of 25 patients (28%) with a negative test. In a subgroup of 30 patients with a first MI, 89% with an abnormal test had MVD while 19% of those with a negative test had MVD. Among 18 patients with a first inferior MI, the test was even more predictive. The abnormal treadmill response before discharge was predictive for later angina both within the first month and later during a seven-month follow-up. Among the 15 patients with an abnormal test, 73% later had angina compared to 16% among the 25 patients with a negative test.

Boschat et al. from France have reported their results in 65 patients who sustained their first transmural MI and within four months had undergone

	POPULATION CHARACTERISTICS							ST DEPRESSION		ANGINA	
	MI %										
			TM		% WITH		%				
EXCLUSIONS	PR	SE	A	IP	ANGINA	MEDS	MVD	SENS	SPEC	SENS	SPEC
<85% MHR,BBB	0	27	33	41	45	No Dig	59	91	65		
USA,CHF	22	4	48	48	59	18% BB,23% Dig	66	41	88		
>Killip 2, HTN	?	21	50	29		7% Dig	61	23	100	29	100
>60,prMI,LBB	0	27	33	43	30	25%, BB,12% Dig	33	48	89		
>65,CHF	25	23	25	53	25	22% BB,10% Dig	50	65	ST &/or Ang		90
USA,CHF,HTN	19	25	37	39		25% Dig,33% BB	72	54	75	68	81
CHF,ANYM,USA	0	0	24	41	50	Stopped	65	60	?		
CHF,USA	25	31	54	35	15		71	56	ST &/or Ang		86
>65,BBB	8	12	35	45	29	Stopped	54	67	ST &/or Ang		67
Complic,BBB	?	?	?	?		Stopped	73	94	94		
Complic	0	0	53	47	31	Stopped	88	30	84	44	95
>70, BBB	0	0	43	57	30	Stopped	44	64	70	20	63
						Averages	59	58	82	40	83

Population Characteristics Including Age, Sex, Exclusions, MI Mix, and Medications. age/sex—mean age of patients and the percentage of women (w) included in the study. Exclusion—the "greater than" symbol excludes patients above a certain age. Other exclusion factors include congestive heart failure (CHF), unstable angina pectoris (USAP), cardiac drugs (drgs), subendocardial MI (se), women (w), complications (complic), and aneurysm (ANYM); MI %—the percentage of the types of MIs included in the study: PR—prior MI; A—transmural (Q-wave) anterior wall MI; I—transmural inferior and/or posterior MIs; SE—subendocardial or non-Q-wave MIs. % with Angina—percent of population with classical angina; Meds—the percentage of patients on digoxin (Dig) or a betablocker (BB) at the time of treadmill testing and often through the follow-up period. %MVD—percent of population with multivessel disease; STD—abnormal ST-segment depression; CP—chest pain induced by the exercise test; sens—sensitivity; spec—specificity. ST&/or Ang—abnormal ST depression and/or angina induced by the exercise test as the criteria for an abnormal response.

coronary angiography and treadmill testing. These 65 who had a treadmill test were out of a group of 80 patients (81%) who had coronary angiography. Approximately one-third of the 65 had post MI angina. No patients were receiving drugs that would interfere with heart rate or ST-segment analysis. Care was taken to see which patients had ST-segment elevation over Q-waves associated with depression in the opposite direction. Only half of the vessels supplying the infarcted areas remained occluded, meaning that half had undergone spontaneous recanalization. Multiple-vessel and diffuse disease was more common in inferior than anterior wall MIs. Only 28 (43%) had an abnormal test by ST-segment depression criteria, and abnormals were more common in the inferior MIs (54%). The clinical severity of the angina was directly related to abnormal tests while functional aerobic impairment closely correlated with the number of diseased vessels. ST segment elevation was noted in patients with wall motion abnormalities in the leads facing the areas of infarction and was associated with a lower ejection fraction, but was a poor indicator of MVD. ST-segment depression was only about 60% sensitive for MVD. The occurrence of ST-segment elevation in the leads facing the infarcted zone along with significant depression in the opposed leads always indicated that another major vessel was involved, but this occurred in only 25% of the cases presented. Patients who had both angina and exercise-induced ST segment depression usually had MVD.

Schwartz et al. reported 48 patients studied with an exercise test and coronary angiography three weeks after their MI. Among the 21 patients with an abnormal response (>0.1 mV ST-segment depression and/or angina), 90% had MVD versus 55% among the 27 patients with a normal test. Exercise-induced ST-segment elevation in 24 patients predicted a significantly lower EF and more abnormally contracting segments.

Starling et al. evaluated 57 uncomplicated patients with a symptom-limited Naughton treadmill test 9–21 days after MI and with coronary arteriography within 12 weeks. They found that ST-segment depression (0.1 mV or more) and/or angina during the exercise test had a superior sensitivity (88%) for detecting MVD compared to ST-segment depression alone (54%). Patients with an inadequate blood pressure response had MVD, and a significantly reduced EF (mean EF of 39%).

DeFeyter et al. found the prevalence of MVD was 63% in inferior and 42% in anterior MIs. Left ventricle impairment was more severe in anterior and prior MIs than in inferior or nontransmural MIs. When they considered an abnormal exercise response to be ST-segment depression and/or angina for diagnosing MVD, the sensitivity and specificity for MVD was low for anterior and inferior MIs, but an 80% sensitivity and a 91% specificity was obtained in 21 patients with non-Q-wave MIs. With the definition of an abnormal test as depression and/or angina and elevation, they analyzed the diagnostic value for combined MVD and advanced left ventricular wall motion abnormalities. A sensitivity of 41% and a specificity of 87% was obtained. In the whole group, the posttest risk for MVD with an abnormal exercise test (angina and/or ST depression) was 71% and for those with a negative test, it was 37%. They were the only investigators to analyze the non-Q-wave subset and found the highest predictive accuracy for ST depression in them.

Akhras reported results that are different from the other studies. Of their 119 patients with an uncomplicated MI, it is not clear what percentage had prior MI nor did they specify non-Q-wave and Q-wave MIs. Data on ventricular function is not given, but apparently patients with poor ventricular function were excluded. Ischemic area criteria (ST depression) were applied in the leads not affected by the MI. Incomplete information makes it impossible to compare their results to other studies.

Morris et al. compared the results from ECG and radionuclide ventriculography during upright bicycle testing in 110 patients undergoing coronary angiography after a single transmural MI. Patients with ECG evidence of combined anterior and inferior/posterior MIs were excluded as well as patients with normal coronary angiograms, valvular disease, or CABG. Testing took place between six weeks and three months after MI. Combining exercise test-induced chest pain, ST-segment depression, and hypotension yielded a sensitivity of 44% and a specificity of 80% for MVD. An abnormal EF response (less than a 5% rise) had a sensitivity of 76% and a specificity of 65%, or if a fall in EF equal to or greater than 5% was considered abnormal, the sensitivity was 43% and the specificity 95%. Wall motion abnormalities had a specificity of 75% or less for MVD. The authors pooled the medical literature for prediction of MVD in 963 patients from a total of 21 studies of post MI patients and found that during exercise testing, chest pain had a sensitivity of 57% and a specificity of 86% and that ST-segment depression had a sensitivity of 59% and a specificity of 74%. They found that exercise-induced chest pain and ST-segment depression occurred almost twice as frequently with treadmill as with bicycle exercise. They concluded that electrocardiographic and scintigraphic results do not identify patients with MVD after MI with high enough accuracy, and that ventriculography parameters (a fall in EF and wall motion worsening) have a similar specificity but a higher sensitivity.

Van der Wall et al. from Amsterdam reported their findings in 202 patients aged 70 years or less admitted to their CCU with a definite first transmural MI. Fifteen patients died and 11 refused to undergo angiography. The remaining 176 patients underwent a Bruce treadmill combined with thallium scintigraphy one to three days before coronary angiography. Patients with valvular heart disease, cardiomyopathy, and bundle branch block were excluded. All medications were withheld at least three days before the test. They concluded that thallium scintigraphy alone or combined with electrocardiography should not be used to predict the absence or presence of MVD in patients after a previous MI because of its inadequate sensitivity and specificity.

Veenbrink and colleagues from Utrecht have attempted to answer an important question: Is there an indication for coronary angiography in patients under 60 years of age with no or minimal angina pectoris after a first MI? They defined high-risk coronary artery disease as three-vessel disease, proximal stenosis to the left anterior descending, or stenosis of the left main. Criteria for a significant lesion was 70% or more, except in the left main where a 50% lesion was required. In addition to horizontal or downsloping ST depression, criteria for an abnormal exercise ECG response included U-wave inversion and upsloping ST-segment depression. ST depression was not considered abnormal if it accompanied ST-segment elevation over the infarcted area. Only patients with transmural MIs were included and were pretty much equally divided between anterior and inferior MIs. Cardiac catheterization was done approximately two months after the event. Ten percent of their patients had "high-risk" lesions; 11 patients had an abnormal exercise test including eight of the nine with high-risk disease. They concluded that coronary angiography in patients under 60 with no or minimal angina can be restricted to patients with an abnormal exercise test by their criteria, thus obviating the need for about 80% of coronary angiograms performed in this age group. Though this study had an admirable purpose, it is difficult to compare it to the other angiographic studies or to generalize their results because of the unusual exercise test criteria they used. No numerical data regarding patients with ST-segment depression alone or with other exercise findings were given.

Sia et al. in Australia evaluated the use of an early symptom-limited maximal exercise test in predicting coronary anatomy, left ventricular ejection fraction, and hemodynamics in 64 patients after an acute non-Q-wave MI. Ten of the patients were women, 28% had prior MIs, 11% were on beta blockers, and 83% were on calcium antagonists. Exercise tests and cardiac catheterization were performed at a median of six and seven days, respectively, after the

MI. Forty-one percent of the patients had a negative exercise test response (no angina, less than 1 mm of ST depression, and normal blood pressure responses). Twenty-five percent had a positive response (1 to 1.9 mm of ST depression or angina); 34% had a "strongly positive" exercise test response (at least 2 mm of ST depression or a 10 mm Hg drop in SBP). A negative response predicted the absence of three-vessel disease (at least 70% stenosis) or critical stenoses (at least 90% stenosis) involving major coronary arteries (negative predictive accuracy 92%), whereas a strongly positive response predicted their presence (positive predictive value 77%, specificity 88%).

SUMMARY OF THE ANGIOGRAPHIC STUDIES

For clinical purposes, it would be ideal if exercise testing identified patients with the angiographic lesions associated with improved survival after coronary artery bypass surgery (CABS). Given the current state of knowledge, such lesions would be triple-vessel or left main disease accompanied by an ejection fraction from 30%–50%. The angiographic studies have mainly been aimed at recognizing patients with any vessels occluded in addition to the vessel supplying the infarct site. These studies have had limited sensitivity and specificity for recognizing MVD which includes patients with two-vessel disease and patients with normal LV function. The high-risk subset is approximately only 20% to 30% of those with MVD.

What can be our expectations for identifying these patients? The exercise test can be expected to identify patients with much muscle in jeopardy due to lesions causing ischemia. However, it cannot be expected to recognize individuals with decreased ventricular function. Such patients are best recognized by a combination of prior history of MI or congestive heart failure, an abnormal ECG, and physical exam and chest x-ray findings. Many of the angiographic studies have attempted to use ST segment elevation to identify patients with left ventricular aneurysm. One could infer that those with left ventricular aneurysms have decreased ventricular function, but it would be better if the studies correlated the results with ejection fraction.

Other candidates for CABS are those in whom medical management cannot adequately control their angina. Exercise test-induced angina is of uncertain significance because it predicts neither the severity of underlying lesions nor relative risk. Patients with single-vessel disease who have angina can have peri-infarctional ischemia either due to the vessel associated with infarction not having recanalized or due to inadequate collaterals. Approximately 50% of the arteries responsible for an MI recanalize within six months. The effect of recanalization versus failure to recanalize has not been related to any MI subset.

These studies involve populations that are very select, often containing a higher prevalence of patients with angina than the usual post-MI population since they are more likely to undergo angiography. In some studies, an abnormal test result is considered angina and/or ST depression, and the results for each response cannot be separated. Few of these studies consider the other exercise test responses that have been associated with a poor prognosis; i.e., a low exercise capacity, PVCs, or an abnormal systolic BP. However, review of the studies demonstrates a limited sensitivity and specificity for MVD. Certainly the sensitivity for detecting those with left main and triple-vessel disease is higher but not 100%. On the other hand, the poor specificity could lead to more angiography than is necessary. This leads to unnecessary CABS since there is always the tendency to "do something," albeit the absence of data that survival is improved.

PROGNOSTIC STUDIES

This portion is based upon the analysis of published reports of longitudinal studies utilizing exercise testing in the early post-MI period with a follow-up for cardiac events. We have chosen the most commonly cited studies and those of particular instructive value. These studies have been carefully analyzed for their (1) methodology, (2) selection of sample, (3) detailed description of sample, and (4) description of statistical methods. The cardiac event endpoints chosen are reinfarction and death. Some studies combine these two endpoints to predict outcome. Some investigators combine reinfarction and death with soft endpoints such as angina, worsening of symptoms, or CABS. The latter is especially worrisome since the results of the test can influence who will have CABS and since CABS may affect mortality. These studies are summarized in Table 6–3. The studies are grouped and combined for meta-analysis by the institution at which they were performed. Each column is explained in the legend.

In the first study reviewed, Ericsson and colleagues reported their results of treadmill testing three weeks after an acute MI in 100 of 228 MI patients. Ventricular dysrhythmias were classified as occurring during monitoring, during rest before the test, and during and after the treadmill test. They considered PVCs if equal to or greater than 5 per minute and specifically as unifocal, multifocal, couplets, triplets, ventricular tachycardia, and ventricular fibrillation. During rest before the treadmill test, two had unifocal and multifocal PVCs. During and after the treadmill test, six had unifocal, eight had multifocal, seven had two or three in a row, and one had four or more PVCs in a row. The exercise ECG or other exercise responses were not considered. It was concluded that the treadmill test proved to be a sensitive method for demonstrating dysrhythmias in patients with recent MIs and that after a three-month follow-up, there was a higher mortality in those with PVCs (2 out of 19 with versus 2 out of 81 without PVCs). No formal statistical analysis was reported.

Kentala and associates have reported their findings in consecutive male patients discharged after acute MI in 1969 from the University of Helsinki Hospital. During this period, 298 males less than 65 years old were treated. Forty-five died in-hospital and the patients were selected for follow-up because of their availability and willingness to participate in a randomized trial of cardiac rehabilitation. Clinical parameters assessed included a careful history of prior activity level. Exercise testing was done at four to six weeks after infarction using a bicycle ergometer. Bipolar chest leads with the negative lead fastened to the forehead were recorded. An individualized work load with steps of 150 or 300 kiloponds was chosen with intervals of four minutes. The test was continued to maximum unless arrhythmias occurred or if the heart rate exceeded 150.

The prognostic power of clinical and ECG variables recorded soon after MI and in connection with the exercise test were analyzed by stepwise multiple discriminant analysis. In this analysis, eighteen clinical and electrocardiographic variables were chosen. They included the following: maximal exercise SBP, paradoxical apical pulsation, PVCs during hospital admission, forced vital capacity, T-wave negativity after exercise, age, terminal forces of the P-wave at rest, relative weight, resuscitated or not, physical work capacity, social classification, clinical cardiac failure, chest x-ray, PVCs during exercise, relative heart volume, ST-segment depression after exercise, initial and terminal notching of the QRS complex, and number of previous MIs. PVCs were classified according to the Scandinavian Committee.

The prognosis was correctly predicted in 86%, 80%, and 74% of cases at two-, four-, and six-year follow-up points. There were statistically significant differences between the important variables using stepwise multiple discriminant analysis made at the two-, four-, and six-year points. Based on the changes in discriminatory power of the variables during the two-, four-, and six-year follow-up periods, they proposed a natural history for their patients. Patients dying within two years had a low exercise systolic blood pressure. With longer follow-up, the exercise blood pressure had a weaker impact. At the four- and six-year points, an abnormal resting terminal P-wave was the best predictor of poor prognosis. This probably identified a group with mild heart failure. Sudden death was defined as when a patient expired within one hour of symptoms, and they were more common late in the follow-up period. For patients who suddenly died later, the T-wave changes after exercise, which possibly indicated subendocardial injury, were common. Patients with a high level of physical activity before infarction were less prone to die suddenly. Exercise-induced ST-segment depression did not identify a high-risk group at any point during follow-up, and had very little power in the discriminant function. Of the many factors considered, an abnormal apical impulse, T-wave inversion after exercise, prior resuscitation, sedentary life-style before infarction, and occurrence of PVCs during exercise were of discriminatory value in relation to sudden death. Frequency differences were tested with chi-square tests and differences between correlation coefficients by the Fisher Z-transformation. Analysis of variance was used to test for differences of group means.

Granath and colleagues performed exercise tests at three and nine weeks after an acute MI in 205 patients and followed them for two to five years. There was a relatively high mortality of 25%, but that rate was unadjusted for varying lengths of follow-up. The treadmill test was interrupted with angina

TABLE 6–3.
Studies Using Exercise Testing in Postmyocardial Infarction Populations With Follow-up to Determine Prognosis

| | | | EXERCISE TESTED | | EXERCISE TEST CHARACTERISTICS | | | | POPULATION CHARACTERISTICS | | | | | | |
| | | | | | | | | | | | MI % | | TM | | |
INVESTIGATOR	YEAR	POP. SIZE	#	%	END POINTS	LEADS	PROTOCOL	# WEEKS POST-MI	AGE/ %WOMEN	EXCLUSIONS	PR	SE	A	IP	DIG OR BB
1 Ericsson	73	184	100	54	HR140,ss	PC	TM	3	59/7	>65	25		51	43	35%D,1%BB
2 Kentala	75	298	158	53	Max	CH1-6	Bike	6-8	53/0	>65,Rehab	28	13	42	58	66%D
3 Granath	77	430	205	48	HR140,ss	12LD	TM/Bike	3&9	59/11	>65	18	?	48	33	10%BB
4 Smith	79	109	62	57	60%HR	12LD	GXT	3	60/7	?	?	?	?	?	?
5 Hunt	79	633	56	9	70%HR,ss	7LD	Bike	6	57/11	No complic	?	5	47	53	?
Srinivasan	81		154			7LD					?	?	?	?	?
6 Sami	79		200		ss	12LD	Naughton	3–52	57/10	CHF,USAP	8	9	29	62	8%D
Davidson	80	461	195	42	HR/ss	12LD	Stanford	3	53/0	>70,drgs,CHF	8	10	29	61	None
DeBusk	83	702	338	48	ss	12LD	Naughton	3	54/0	>70,CHF,USAP	?	?	?	?	3%D
7 Theroux	79	326	210	64	5 METs,70%HR	CM5	Naughton	1.6	52/0	>70CHF,USAP	34	18	31	50	40%BB,1%D
Waters	85	330	225	68					53/16		25	21	43	55	6%D,32%BB
8 Koppes	80	410	108	26	Submax/Max	12LD	Bruce	3&8	52/13	CHF,drgs,ANG	25	24	28	48	None
9 Starling	80	190	130	68	HR130/ss	V156	Naughton	2	53/14	USA,CHF	24	29	34	37	26%D,16%BB
10 Weld	81	325	236	73	4 METs,ss	V5	low Bruce	2	54/12	>70	21	?	?	?	12%BB,41%D
11 Saunamaki	81	404	317	78	ss	PC	Bike	3	57/20	AGE,CHF,ANG	10	?	32	?	20%D,2%BB
12 Velasco	81	958	200	21	30w,ss	PC	SupBike	2.5	60/22	>66,se,w	3	0	46	55	11%D,9%BB
13 DeFeyter	82	222	179	81	ss	12LD	Bruce	6-8	52/0	>65,referrals	8	12	35	45	Stopped
14 Jelinek	82		188		Symptoms	V456	Bike	1.5	52/10	ANG,CHF	18	28	29	42	?
15 Madsen	83	886	456	52	ss	9LD	Bike	2.6	51/7	>75,CHF,USAP	31	6	35	53	12%D,2%BB
16 Gibson	83	229	140	61	HR120,ss	3LD	Naughton	1.6	63/13	>65,CHF	19	26	35	53	2%D,61%BB
17 Norris	84	395	315	80	ss	?	2.5 mph	4	51/13	>60	0	27	29	42	30%BB
18 Williams	84	226	205	91	6 METs	3LD	Bruce	1.7	50/0	>70	23	22	33	45	16%D,19%BB
19 Jennings	84	503	103	20	5 METs,ss	V5	2 mph	1.7	56/18		?	?	51	49	4%D,10%BB
20 Fioretti	84	293	214	72	Symptoms	XYZ	Bike	2	54/13	>66,CHF,ANG	?	?			40%BB
	84	405	300	74					54/16	CHF,ANG	27		36	?	18%D,52%BB
21 Krone	85	1417	667	47	5 METs	3LD	low Bruce	2	?/20	>70	22	22	31	42	28%D,31%BB
Dwyer	85								60%<60						
22 Handler	85	296	222	75	5 METs,70%HR	3LD	Naughton	1.4	54/16	>65,CABS,BBB	?	21	42	37	1%D,17%BB
23 SCOR	85	1469	295	20	75%HR,ss	12LD	Mixed TM	1.7	58/18	MD judgment	21	18	38	44	26%D,53%BB
24 Jespersen	85		126		Max,ss	II,V46	Bike	3.4	57/14	>71,CHF,USA	0	36	31	33	13%D,20%BB
TOTAL			6178												

TABLE 6–3. (continued)

INVESTIGATOR	MEAN FU	RANGE FU	% CABS IN FU	MORTALITY IF ET YES/NO	RE MI IF ET YES/NO	EXERCISE TEST RISK MARKERS					STATISTICAL METHOD
						BP	PVC	EXCAP	ANGINA	ST	
Ericsson	3mo	3mo–?	?	5%/		NR	4×	?	?	NR	Descriptive
Kentala	6yr	?	0%	32%/	?	+	+	NR	NR	+*	UV; some DF
Granath	2–5yr	2–5yr	?	25%/		NR	2×*	2×	2×	6×*	UV
Smith	1.5yr	?	?	10%/17%	?	NR	—	NR	4×*	3×*	UV
Hunt	1yr	?	?	14%/18%	?	NR	?	NR	3×*	7×*	Descriptive, UV
Srinivasan	1.25yr	1–2yr	?	8%	?	NR	—	NR	NR	3×*	Not cited (UV)
Sami	19mo	2–51mo	10%	2%/	5%/	NR	—	+*	1	+*	UV
Davidson	26mo	1–60mo	10%	1.5%/	6%/	?	?	+*	1		MV-LR; LT, K-M &
DeBusk	34mo	?	6%	2.1%/5.5%	2%/	NR	NR	NR	NR	8×*	UV; Cox to select some variables
Theroux	1yr	1yr	5.7%	9.5%/	6%/	NR	2×	NR	—	13×*	UV
Waters	2yr	5–7yr	16%	11%–3%		+*	+	+	NR	8×*	UV (Cox), MV-Cox/ conditional wrt time
Koppes	2yr	?	?	2%/		?	?	?	?	?	UV
Starling	11mo	6–20mo	?	8%/	9%/	5×*	2×	NR	4×	4×	UV
Weld	1yr	?	?	9%/		5×*	2×*	19×*	2×	2×	MV-LR; UV est
Saunamaki	5.7yr	5–6yr	?	35.6%/	?	3×*	2×*	NR	NR	1	LT w/in clinical subsets
Velasco	3yr	3mo–6yr	?	11%/	3%/	3×	2×	NR	3×*	4×*	UV
DeFeyter	28mo	13–40mo	13%	6%/	7%/	NR	3×	+	2×	1	UV
Jelinek	2.3yr	10d–62mo	?	7%/	19%/	—	NR	+*	2×*	1	UV
Madsen	1yr	?	0%	6.6%/28%	4%/12%	+*	+*	+*	?	1	MV-DF, Cox; algorithm
Gibson	1.3yr	1–3yr	14%	5%/	6%/	NR	NR	NR	+	+	UV
Norris	3.5yr	1–6yr	24%	13%/33%	12%/	NR	NR	?	?	1	UV-LT; Cox cited
Williams	1yr	1yr	12%	6%/31%	6.8%/	2×	—	2×*	2×*	1	MV-DF; UV est
Jennings	1.2yr	?	5%	9%/21%	3%/	8×*	1	8×*	?	2×	UV
Fioretti	1yr	1yr	8%	9%/23%	4%/	+*	2×	+*	1		UV
		1yr		7%/28%		+*	+*	+*	3×*		MV-DF;algorithm
Krone	1yr	1yr	8%	5%/14%	5%/10%	8×*	2×	3×*	?	?	UV; MV-LR
Dwyer	1.2yr	?	12%	7%/	4%/	NR	?	?	1	2×	UV; MV-LR
Handler	1yr	6–36mo	9%	7%/15%		5×*	1	8×*	2×	3×	UV
SCOR	1yr	?	?	7%		1	2×	9×*	1	3×*	UV; MV-DF
Jespersen	1yr	1yr	<1%		2%	1	1	1	?		UV; K-M
						BP	PVCs	ExCap	Angina	ST	
No. of studies demonstrating											
Significant risk predictor						8	4	8	4	7	
No. with + effect						12	13	12	11	12	
No. with reported effect						15	20	14	16	19	

in 42 patients, dyspnea in 10 patients, and alarming ECG abnormalities that consisted of PVCs in 29 patients. Seven patients were stopped because of fatigue and 16 because their heart rate reached 140 beats per minute. In 101 patients, caution was the main reason for ending the exercise test with particular regard to earlier arrhythmias or the general condition. The first exercise test three weeks after the MI was performed on a treadmill, and the second test at nine weeks was performed with a bicycle. The endpoints of exercise testing were angina pectoris, dyspnea, and tachycardia. They defined tachycardia as a heart rate equal to or greater than 130 bpm at 33 W at the first week test or a heart rate equal to or greater than 130 bpm at 65 W during the bicycle test at the third week. The criteria for ventricular dysrhythmias was

---

PROSPECTIVE STUDIES

Investigator—first author; Year—year of publication; MI Pop. size—number of patients admitted to the hospital with MI over period of study; Exercise—the number of patients out of this MI population who underwent exercise testing; Tested %—the percentage of patients out of this MI population who underwent exercise testing.

Exercise Test Characteristic Columns. Endpoints–endpoints for exercise testing; SS—signs and/or symptoms; HR with a heart rate value—heart rate limit; Max—maximal effort; Percent heart rate—percent of age predicted maximal heart rate chosen as a limit; MET—maximal exercise level allowed to be reached as estimated from workload; symptoms—symptoms alone were the endpoint. Leads—lists the ECG leads analyzed; PC—precordial leads; 12 LD—the full 12 lead; CM5—a bipolar lead; V5—fifth precordial lead; XYZ—Frank vector leads. Protocol—type of exercise study done: TM—treadmill; GXT—Bruce protocol stopped at 85% of the age-predicted maximal heart rate; Stanford—Stanford version of the Naughton test; low Bruce—Bruce protocol with 0 and ½ stages which are 0% and 5% grade at 1.7 miles per hour prior to stage 1 (10% grade at 1.7 miles per hour). The Norris study at Greenlake used a 2.5-mph treadmill protocol with increasing grade. Time post MI—mean time post MI that the exercise test(s) were done.

Population Characteristics Including Age, Sex, Exclusions, MI Mix, and Medications. Age/sex—mean age of patients and percentage of women (w) included in the study; Exclusion—the "greater than" symbol excludes patients above a certain age. Other exclusion factors were congestive heart failure (CHF), unstable angina pectoris (USAP), cardiac drugs (drgs), subendocardial MI (se), women (w), complications (complic), and not in a rehabilitation program (Rehab). MI %—percentage of types of infarctions included in the study; PR—prior MI; A—transmural (Q-wave) anterior wall MI; I—transmural inferior and/or posterior MI; SE—subendocardial or non-Q-wave MIs. (Because some investigators did not distinguish the location of Q-waves only, the totals of SE, A, and IP can exceed 100%; 100—SE always equals the % of Q-wave MIs.) Meds—the percentage of patients on digoxin (Dig) or a beta blocker (BB) at time of treadmill testing and often through follow-up period. Mean FU—mean or median months or years of follow-up time; Range FU, % CABS in FU—percentage of patients included in the study who underwent CABS during follow-up period. Mortality—in those patients included in the study who underwent exercise testing (yes) and in those excluded from exercise testing for clinical reasons (no). Recurrent MI—percentage who had a repeat MI if exercise tested (yes) or if not exercise tested (no).

The next series of columns describes the exercise test risk markers. BP—abnormal SBP response; PVCs—abnormal PVCs seen; ExCap—abnormally low exercise capacity tolerance; Angina—induced by test; ST—abnormal ST-segment response (usually only depression). These are the responses to exercise testing that have been most commonly reported as having prognostic value. Risk ratio—univariate (UV) or multivariate (MV) analysis risk ratio. If significant statistically, the risk ratios are indicated by an asterisk. Nonsignificant risk ratios permit trends across studies to be detected. The risk ratio means that if the cutpoint value for this abnormality was reached, those with that abnormality have a certain times (×) risk of death as opposed to those without the abnormality. Only the hard endpoints of death (and in some studies, reinfarction) are considered. NR—results of prediction with the exercise test marker were not reported; LT—clinical life table, usually stratified; LR—logistic regression; K-M—Kaplan Meier; est—estimates; wrt—with regard to time; DF—discriminant function analysis; ?—insufficient data to test significance; 1—null effect; +—a positive nonsignificant association of usual high risk with death; —a negative nonsignificant association of usual high risk level with death; nX—n times increased risk of death with usual high risk level; Cox—proportion hazard regression model for survival analysis; algorithm—detailed specific algorithm displayed for clinical use.

not given. The investigators chose not to evaluate the ST segments because of the accepted difficulties of evaluating ST shifts after MI and because of medications.

The appearance of tachycardia at low work loads, major ventricular dysrhythmias, or anginal complaints during these early exercise tests was associated with a significantly increased mortality during the observation period. Exercise-induced PVCs proved to be of greater prognostic significance than those recorded at rest. They found the test valuable for evaluating the response to antidysrhythmic agents. Analysis of clinical data in the CCU failed to produce any differences between the survivors and those who died. However, there were more deaths among those patients who had a previous infarction (17/37) as compared to those with a first infarction (40/168). During exercise testing, nine weeks after infarct, PVCs were seen in 23% of the patients. During follow-up, 16 of these died compared to 25 of 134 without arrhythmias. Tachycardia during a submaximal workload (greater than 130 beats per minute) which was 33 W at three weeks and 65 W at nine weeks identified a high-risk group at both time periods. Angina pectoris at the time of the three-week test was not associated with an increased mortality but there was a twofold risk for those who reported it at the nine-week test. Granath et al. apparently utilized 2×2 chi-square tests to evaluate associations of each factor with survival, but they do not specify analysis techniques.

Smith and colleagues from Arizona did treadmill tests on 62 patients 18 days after admission for acute MI. They considered the standard exercise predictors including ST-segment elevation and ST-segment depression but not their location. Death and MI were similarly high both in the group with elevation and in the group with depression. There was no difference in the mean Norris Index for those exercise tested and those not tested. Thirty percent (6 of 20) of the patients who developed ST-segment depression either died or had another MI after discharge from the hospital versus only two (5%) of the 42 patients who did not have ST-segment depression during exercise. Chi-square tests and t-tests were used for statistical analysis. The extent of variation in follow-up time is not clear, but failure to adjust for the indicated unequal times could create serious bias.

THE ROYAL MELBOURNE HOSPITAL STUDIES

Hunt et al. reported their findings in 75 patients under 70 years of age. They selected their patients on the basis of having survived an MI complicated by arrhythmias and/or mechanical abnormalities. Only 56 were exercised to 70% age-predicted heart rate on a bike six weeks post MI. Significant cardiac arrhythmias to gain entry into the study were ventricular, atrial, or junctional arrhythmias occurring at a rate of more than 1 per 10 beats; transient second or third degree AV block; or LBBB. Mechanical abnormalities included rales, shock, enlarged heart, or x-ray signs of CHF. They were selected from 633 patients with MIs who met age and logistic criteria and were followed for one year. Of 11 patients with ST depression of 1 mm or more, 36% died while 4 of the 45 (11%) without depression died. Three of seven patients with angina died (43%) while 5 of 49 (10%) of those without angina during the exercise test died. Frequency counts in various categories, and chi-square significance tests were presented for comparisons among these patients. Selection restrictions to "intelligent, cooperative" patients as well as other criteria make it difficult to apply their findings to other populations.

Srinivasan, Hunt, and colleagues reported a second study of exercise testing in patients with electrical and/or mechanical complications during their acute MI. Criteria to gain entry into the study were the same as the previous study. They prospectively selected 154 patients who underwent an exercise test four to six weeks after discharge. The patients exercised on a bicycle until they were unable to continue or had reached 70% of age-predicted maximal heart rate. Patients were excluded if CHF, hypertension, chest pain, or unstable ECG changes persisted, or if they were more than 70 years of age. There was no modification of their medication treatment because of the test, but specifics were not given. Neither was a description of their MI mix or other clinical features provided. Seven-lead ECGs were recorded, and it is assumed that this included the lateral precordial leads since V4 was monitored throughout exercise. Exercise began at a work load of 75 W and was increased every minute by 25 W. Patients were followed from 12 to 24 months with a median of 15 months with reference to survival, recurrence of reinfarction, and angina pectoris; however, the analysis was based on deaths only.

The exercise test variables considered were ST-segment depression, PVCs as present or absent, and angina. Eighteen patients had abnormal ST-segment depression (0.1 mV), and nine of these developed chest pain during the test. A total of 13 patients died during follow-up (8%). Six of these deaths occurred among the 18 patients with ST-segment depression (33% mortality) while seven deaths occurred in the 136 patients with no ST-segment depression (5% mortality). Of the nine patients who had ST-segment depression and chest pain, four died whereas two of the nine patients with ST-segment depression and no pain died. Seven of the 136 patients without ST-segment depression had exercise test-induced chest pain and only one of these died. All of the patients in this study were selected because their hospital course was complicated either by heart failure and/or significant cardiac arrhythmias. No statistical analyses were cited, but apparently chi-square and t-tests were performed.

THE STANFORD STUDIES

Sami and colleagues studied the prognostic value of treadmill testing in 200 males who were tested serially approximately five times each from 3 to 52 weeks after MI. None of these patients had congestive heart failure or unstable angina, and they were a relatively low-risk group since only 2% died over the two years of follow-up. At three weeks, 100% of those who subsequently had an episode of cardiopulmonary resuscitation and 60% of those who required CABS had 0.2 mV of ST-segment depression during treadmill testing. Only 35% of those without an event had a similar amount of ST-segment depression. At five weeks and beyond, recurrent PVCs during serial treadmill testing occurred in 90% of those who had a recurrent MI and in only 47% of those without an event. Exercise-induced PVCs or ischemic ST-segment depression 11 weeks after infarction identified patients with an increased risk of subsequent coronary events, while the absence of either identified a group of patients who were free of problems. The major emphasis concerned events two years post MI, although only half had been followed for that time. Differences were compared by chi-square and t tests.

Davidson and DeBusk reported results of treadmill testing in 195 men tested three weeks after acute MI. Stepwise logistic analysis on a subset of 92 with at least two-year follow-up showed ST-segment depression equal to or greater than 0.2 mV, angina, and a work capacity of less than 4 METs to be risk markers. These results were confirmed in the 195 men using stratified life table analysis with log rank tests. The patients were followed for 1–64 months, and the 150 followed for at least one year had a 19% event rate; however, more than half of these endpoint events were coronary artery bypass surgery. The exercise test clearly could have biased this group of patients toward angiography and subsequent surgery. PVCs on a single treadmill test three weeks after MI had no independent prognostic value.

DeBusk et al. applied a stepwise risk stratification procedure sequentially combining historical, then clinical characteristics, and finally treadmill test results in a study population of 702 consecutive men less than 70 years of age and alive 21 days after an acute MI. Prior MI or angina, or recurrence of pain in the CCU identified 10% of the patients with the highest rate of reinfarction and death within six months (18%). Clinical contraindications to exercise testing identified another 40% with an intermediate risk (6.4%). Exercise test results included ST-segment shifts, the MET level, angina pectoris, peak heart rate, peak SBP, exertional hypotension, and PVCs. In the patients who underwent treadmill testing, an abnormal test ($\geq$ 0.2 mV depression and a heart rate less than 136) identified a high-risk group (9.7%) while those with a negative test had a 3.9% incidence of hard medical events. No other treadmill responses were predictive. A proportional hazards regression model was used to identify characteristics that significantly discriminated risk.

THE MONTREAL HEART INSTITUTE STUDIES

Theroux and colleagues studied the prognostic value of a limited treadmill test performed one day before hospital discharge after MI in 210 consecutive patients. These patients were followed for endpoints of heart disease for one year. Exercise capacity and the BP response were not considered. Sixty-five percent (28 of 43) who had angina during treadmill testing reported the onset of angina subsequently, according to the authors. This was statistically different from the 36% occurrence rate in those without chest pain during exercise testing. In those with a normal ECG response to exercise testing, there was a 2% mortality and a 0.7% sudden death rate; in those with ST-segment depression, there was a 27% mortality (17 of 64) and a sudden death rate of 16%. Statistical tests were performed using chi-square analysis.

Waters et al. reported an expansion of the initial study from the same institution. During 1976 and 1977, 12% of all patients admitted died in the hospital, 28% were excluded from the study, and 60% were included and underwent exercise testing. Mortality data was not reported on the 28% excluded from the study. Over the five- to seven-year follow-up of the 225 patients tested, 16% had CABS. They considered clinical and exercise test variables. ST elevation and depression were similar risk predictors, and so they were combined. PVCs were classified by any appearance during or immediately after exercise, the BP response was considered abnormal if SBP failed to increase by 10 mm Hg or more, and functional capacity was considered abnormal if the patient failed to achieve the target heart rate or work load. Target heart rate was considered to be 70% of predicted maximal heart rate and the maximal workload was 5 METs. Clinical variables included age, sex, previous MI, type, and ECG location of the MI, recurrence of pain in the hospital, treatment with beta-blocking drugs or digitalis at discharge, and a QRS score. In the first year, overall mortality was 11% and it was 3% per year afterwards. Exercise-induced ST-segment depression was present in 31% and generated a risk ratio of 7.8 for one-year mortality; 12% had ST elevation in CM5 and the risk ratio was slightly less than with ST-segment depression; 28% had PVCs, and 9% had a flat blood pressure response. Predictors by the Cox regression model differed from the first year to the second year of follow-up. During the first year, ST-segment shift in either direction, a flat blood pressure response or angina within the 48 hours after admission were predictors. During the second year, a history of prior MI, the QRS score, or PVCs were independent risk predictors.

Mortality curves were constructed using the product-limit method and compared univariately by log-rank test for discrete variables and by the Cox models with a single beta parameter for continuous variables. Variables significant by the univariate analysis were then analyzed with proportional hazard regression models; the variables retained in the model were selected in a stepwise manner. Possible time-dependent effects of predictors led to analysis by models fit to two separate time periods. Mortality to one year was analyzed by eliminating all follow-up data after one year; mortality after one year was analyzed separately removing the patients who died before one year.

Koppes et al. presented their results in a highly selected group of 108 patients with MI out of a group of 410 admitted to Wilford Hall Air Force Medical Center from 1975 to 1978 with a transmural or subendocardial acute MI. The 108 selected did not have congestive heart failure or angina pectoris after their infarct nor were they taking any cardiac drugs (i.e., digoxin, beta blocker, or antiarrhythmic). The major purpose of the study was to establish the normal hemodynamic responses during exercise testing in a group of uncomplicated infarct patients. A submaximal test was done at three weeks, and then a maximal test at eight weeks. Eighteen patients were not included in analysis because they were unable to do the 0, ½, and first stage of the Bruce protocol at three weeks or to exercise maximally at eight weeks because of angina or ST-segment depression. ST-segment depression, angina, and PVCs (classified as more than three, multifocal, couplets, and ventricular tachycardia) were considered. No other treadmill variables were considered and only unpaired t-testing was used. Death occurred in only two patients, one with ST-segment depression only and one with neither angina nor ST-segment depression. The rates of reinfarction, bypass surgery, or progression to functional class 3 or 4 are not presented. However, complications were said to be less in those with a nonischemic response. Among the 18 patients limited at the eighth week exercise test by cardiovascular signs or symptoms, there was a 56% complication rate. Unfortunately, the low mortality rate and the failure of the investigators to provide specific endpoints is difficult to make conclusions from the study. At the third stage of the Bruce protocol, there was no change in heart rate or rate pressure product between the third and the eighth week. This is in contrast with Sivarajan et al., who showed an increase in both and diastolic systolic blood pressure at a matched work load between the in-hospital and three-month test but no difference between a three-month test and a six-month test. Koppes et al. cite t-tests as their analysis technique to compare proportions of deaths in some of the patient subgroups. Such comparisons should be made using chi-square or Fisher's exact test for small sample size.

Starling et al. reported their results using treadmill testing in 130 patients after an uncomplicated MI. Approximately 30% of the patients considered were excluded because of angina at rest or during ambulation while still in the hospital, CHF, dangerous dysrhythmias, or hypertension. There was a relatively high rate of prior (24%) and subendocardial MIs (29%). Treadmill tests were done before hospital discharge from 7 to 24 days after MI (mean 15 days). Endpoints for the exercise test were a heart rate of 130, fatigue, angina, ventricular tachycardia, a decrease from peak systolic blood pressure of 20 or greater with continued exercise or a hypertensive blood pressure response (systolic of 200 mm Hg or greater and a diastolic blood pressure of 110 mm Hg or greater. ST-segment depression alone was not an endpoint. Abnormal findings were considered to be horizontal or downsloping ST-segment depression of 0.1 mV or more, angina pectoris, an abnormal blood pressure response defined as SBP increase of 10 mm Hg or less with a peak SBP of 140 or less or a decrease of 20 mm Hg or greater SBP from peak with continued exercise, and PVCs at a rate of five or more per minute or ventricular tachycardia.

Of the 130 patients, 123 had regular follow-up visits for at least six months; seven patients were lost to follow-up. Follow-up of the 123 ranged from 6–20 months; adjustment was apparently not done for varying length of follow-up. Events considered were unstable angina, recurrent MI, and cardiac death. Sixty percent of the patients had one or more treadmill exercise-induced abnormality: 32% had ST-segment depression, 28% had angina, and 14% had an inadequate blood pressure response. Of the 39% of patients with no abnormality, three had recurrent MI but there were no deaths. In those with ST-segment depression, four died and six had a recurrent MI. In those with angina, five died and four had a recurrent MI. In those with inadequate blood pressure response, three died and two had a recurrent MI. In the 15% who had PVCs, two died and one had recurrent MI. Twenty-three percent had two or more exercise-induced abnormalities and 6% had three simultaneous abnormalities. Since recurrent MI and cardiac death were infrequent, there was no significant difference between those with a specific abnormality and those with no abnormality although cardiac deaths occurred only in patients with an abnormality. When patients with ST-segment depression and angina were combined into one group and compared to those with no abnormality, they had a statistically greater incidence of cardiac death. When patients with either or both of these two manifestations and an inadequate blood pressure response were grouped together, they had an even higher incidence of death. Patients with exercise-induced abnormalities had a significantly reduced exercise tolerance compared to patients with no abnormality. The statistical techniques used were Student's t-test, chi-square, or Fisher's exact test.

Saunamaki and Andersen in Copenhagen reported the prognostic value of the exercise test three weeks post MI. Clinical predictors were not considered, and a maximal bike test was used. They considered the general prognostic importance of ventricular arrhythmias associated with the exercise test, left ventricular function, and ST-segment changes. Major ventricular arrhythmias were defined as 10 or more PVCs a minute, PVCs in pairs, three or more in a row, or ventricular fibrillation. Multiformed and R on T were rarely seen. The prognostic value of left ventricular function was investigated using the change in rate pressure product from supine rest to maximal exercise. The discriminating level of change in rate pressure product was found empirically, taking into consideration an age-dependent variation found in the male who stopped due to fatigue. There was no significant difference in survival between patients with an ST-segment deviation of at least 0.1 mV and those without ST-segment deviation. The change of rate-pressure product (HR $\times$ SBP) from rest to maximal exercise adjusted for age was empirically found to be discriminating. Mortality increased among patients with major PVCs. Those with a small increase in rate pressure product and/or arrhythmias had a five-year survival of 55% versus 80% in the others. In their 1982 study, they considered clinical parameters as well. Clinical subgroups were defined as (1) patients with clinical heart failure during hospitalization and/or previous MI, and (2) patients with anterior MI versus inferior or indefinite MI. Within each clinical group, exercise tests still determined a high-risk and low-risk group. The probability of survival in different risk strata was calculated according to Peto, death rate according to Nelson, and log rank testing was used to compare survival curves. Follow-up was complete as maintained for a mean of 5.7 years.

Velasco et al. from Spain reported their findings using exercise testing after an uncomplicated transmural MI. From 1973 to 1978, 958 patients with a preliminary diagnosis of MI were admitted to their CCU. Men less than 66 years old with a transmural MI who survived were considered for the study. Women and patients with subendocardial MIs were excluded. A total of 462 patients were selected and performed the exercise test before discharge. The investigators then selected the 200 patients who regularly attended the hospital for a checkup at the end of the third, sixth, and twelfth month as well as those who attended at least the first checkup and died before the second and those who died after the second visit. There were 260 patients lost to follow-up. The test was performed on the day before discharge ranging from 14 to 27 days with an average of 18 days. A bike test in the recumbent position with a constant load of 30 W for six minutes was performed. The exercise test was stopped for angina or dangerous dysrhythmias. They considered the following endpoints during exercise testing: (1) angina, (2) ST-segment depression, (3) increase in heart rate of 35 beats per minute or more, (4) poor SBP during exercise (equal to or less than 5 mm Hg), and (5) malignant PVCs defined as multifocal, paired early in more than 10% of the beats in at least one minute of exercise. Ventricular tachycardia (three or more consecutive beats) was also included.

Angina pectoris occurred in 9%, ischemic ST depression in 14%, abnormal increase in heart rate in 17%, poor systolic blood pressure rise in 9%, and malignant PVCs in 3% of the patients. During the period of observation, patients with an abnormal test response had a 21.5% death rate compared with 4% in those with a negative response. The mortality rate was 7.5% in patients without ST-segment changes and 32% in those with ST-segment changes. In patients with angina, the mortality rate was 29% versus 9% in those without angina. In patients with an excessive increase in heart rate during exercise (35 beats or more above the resting heart rate), mortality was 24% versus 8% in those without this response. Patients with a poor SBP response (equal to or less than 5 mm Hg) had a mortality rate of 27% versus 10% in those with a normal SBP rise. There was no significant difference in those with malignant PVCs. This study is flawed by the large dropout rate (over 50% of those tested chose not to be followed) and by the use of only univariate analysis. Chi-square testing was the only statistical method used. Possible biases due to selective loss to follow-up were not considered.

Weld and colleagues reported the results of low level exercise testing on 236 of 250 patients who had diagnosed acute MIs. Only 14 patients were excluded from this study because of contraindications. A progressive protocol of three stages, each lasting three minutes, with a maximal work load of 4 METs, was performed just prior to hospital discharge (mean hospital stay was 16 days). Forty-three percent had ventricular dysrhythmias and 51% had less than a 4-MET exercise capacity. Twenty-two percent had exercise-induced ST-segment depression in V5. This finding must be viewed with caution since half of the total population were taking digoxin. In a one-year follow-up performed for recurrent infarction and death, there was a 12% cardiac death rate.

They considered duration of exercise, ST-segment depression, and exertional PVCs. PVCs were classified by frequency and characteristics: pairs (two consecutive), ventricular tachycardia (three or more), multiformed (those that changed shape and timing). Exertional hypotension was considered a drop of 10 or 20 mm Hg during exercise. Multiple logistic regression was used to rank exercise duration, number of PVCs, and ST-segment depression in strength of association with cardiac death one year after MI. A stepwise analysis was used to test the independence of each, to determine their combined ability, and to determine if they added significantly to the predictive ability of routine clinical variables. Angina was not useful in predicting outcome. The investigators stated their belief that reduced exercise duration is an indicator of LV failure and owes its predictive value to this association.

The exercise test variables of duration, PVCs, and ST-segment depression ranked ahead of the clinical variables of vascular congestion, cardiomegaly, and prior MI in predictive value. This is the first study that considered standard clinical risk predictors along with the exercise test; the exercise test proved superior to the clinical variables. The exercise test variables ranked in the following order: (1) exercise duration, (2) PVCs, and (3) ST-segment depression. Patients unable to reach an exercise capacity of 4 METs had a relative risk of 15. Exertional hypotension (a maximal SBP of less than 130) generated an odds ratio of five, but a drop in SBP was not predictive. Standardized regression coefficients showed that all three exercise variables had a stronger association with one-year cardiac mortality than any of the clinical variables that constitute the Norris index. However, by this multivariate analysis, ST-segment depression was not statistically associated with one-year mortality. The predictive ability of the multiple logistic regression model was tested using a jackknife procedure. Contingency table analysis was used to relate individual exercise variables to other data and to outcome for comparisons to other studies.

De Feyter et al. from the Free University Hospital in Amsterdam have reported the prognostic value of exercise testing and cardiac catheterization six to eight weeks after MI. Their study provides data on a consecutive series of 179 survivors of acute MI who had a symptom-limited Bruce test. Out of a group of 222 patients treated, 22 refused, 7 had bundle branch block, 5 had technical difficulties, 3 died, 6 were lost to follow-up, and 43 were not evaluated. They considered the following exercise test variables: ST-segment depression, angina, ST-segment elevation, ventricular arrhythmias (classified as simple or unifocal [less than 10 beats per minute] and complex [greater than 10/min, multifocal, pairs, runs or ventricular tachycardia]), exercise time, blood pressure response, maximal heart rate, and magnitude of ST-segment shift. An inadequate blood pressure response was considered an increase of 10 mm Hg or less in SBP or peak SBP of 140 mm Hg or less. In this study, the following cardiac catheterization variables were also considered: number of vessels, ejection fraction, LVEDP, wall motion abnormalities, and LAD involvement.

The mean follow-up period was 28 months (ranging from 13 to 40), there were 11 cardiac deaths and 12 reinfarctions. Strata were compared at one, two, and three years. Fifty-eight patients with an exercise time of 10 minutes or more had a very low risk for cardiac death or reinfarction. No treadmill markers resulted in a higher risk group while three-vessel disease or a left ventricular EF of 30% or less did predict high risk. The mortality rate was 22% in patients with an EF less than 30% or with triple-vessel disease; 1% in patients with an EF greater than 30% or with one- or two-vessel disease. Clinical variables were not considered. Each variable was considered univariately with discrete variables considered as present or absent and continuous variables optimally dichotomized. The cumulative incidence in each subgroup was then calculated. Significant differences in performance in intergroup differences were calculated with a chi-square test.

Jelinek et al. from Melbourne have presented their findings in 188 patients with an uncomplicated MI who underwent bicycle testing on the day of discharge (about day 10) and returned to work at a median of six weeks post MI. Exclusion criteria were given but not the number in the total population nor the sex mix or medication status. They were followed for 10 days to 64 months with a median of 26 months. The bike test was symptom limited. They considered the total duration of exercise, maximal heart rate, maximal blood pressure, and ST-segment shifts. Secondary risk factors for recurrence of heart attack were found to be angina before the MI, angina on the exercise test, and radiological heart failure. There was no difference between the two groups for maximal work load, maximal heart rate, maximal systolic blood pressure, or maximal double product. There were 28 recurrent MIs including six sudden deaths, five fatal acute MIs, two late deaths post MI, and 15 nonfatal infarcts. The risk factors for total events were angina prior to MI, angina during exercise testing, and x-ray findings of CHF. No other variables were predictive including ST depression, but only chi-square analysis was performed.

Madsen has reported findings from symptom-limited bike testing at Grostrup Hospital in Denmark. The study population included 886 patients discharged between 1977 and 1980 after MI. Nearly 50% of the patients were excluded from testing because of age, CHF, or other clinical reasons. A bike protocol that started at 50 W increased 50 W each six minutes until maximal effort was used. During the one-year follow-up, few patients were on beta blockers and no one underwent CABS. Madsen considered angina, ST-segment depression, PVCs, duration of exercise, maximal heart rate, and maximal rate pressure product as possible risk markers. A variety of clinical markers were also considered. The most important exercise test variables were duration of exercise and PVCs. Prediction of death was not different with clinical or exercise test variables or their combination. For reinfarction, the predictive value was significantly higher for the exercise test variables than the combined set. Madsen found that clinical criteria from the hospitalization identified a high-risk group not eligible for exercise testing. According to the author, the prediction of death could not be improved by adding exercise data. Exercise test variables alone or added to clinical variables improved prediction of reinfarction compared to clinical variables alone, and clinical variables alone provide a better prediction of patients without reinfarction. Stepwise linear discrimant function analysis provided in the BMDP package was utilized. A prognostic score calculated from the patients' variables was compared to a breakpoint value to determine group membership (death or surviving). This was done with and without exercise test variables. The classification results reported were based on a jackknife procedure. Tests of differences in predictive values between analyses were based on McNemar's test. Madsen's results are similar to those of Weld who used multiple regression and the jackknife technique. Weld found exercise duration, PVCs during exercise, and x-ray pulmonary vascular congestion that were nearly the same variables as selected by Madsen.

Gibson et al. applied predischarge quantitative exercise thallium scintigraphy in 140 consecutive patients with an uncomplicated MI. The results were compared with submaximal treadmill testing and coronary angiography. During follow-up, seven patients died and nine suffered recurrent myocardial infarction. Included in their coronary events were clinical progression of angina pectoris. This confuses analysis since the test responses are compared between those with and without combined events. There was no difference in clinical characteristics between those with and those without events including EF. The only variables that were different during treadmill testing were achievement of target heart rate and the occurrence of angina. The presentation of data did not permit determination of the test modalities that were able to be compared to predict death or nonfatal recurrent MI. For the cutpoint values chosen, it appeared that no testing modality was significantly different for sensitivity of detecting those who were going to die. They ranged from the treadmill with the lowest sensitivity, to coronary angiography, to thallium scintigraphy, which had the greatest sensitivity for predicting a nonfatal MI. They mentioned that mortality was four times higher in those with ST depression and angina with borderline significance, that PVCs were not predictive, and that those with hypotension and ischemia had more complications. However, this univariate analysis is in question because sufficient data are not presented. This is a disappointing report since this study is one of the most complete but suffers from a lack of proper statistical analysis. The low mortality (5%) also seriously reduced the statistical power of the tests to detect differences between groups.

Norris et al. from Greenlane Hospital in New Zealand reported the determinants of reinfarction and sudden death in male survivors of a first MI aged younger than 60 years (mean 50) who underwent exercise testing and coronary angiography four weeks after MI. Between January, 1977, and June, 1982, 425 men suitable were admitted to the hospital. Of these, 7% died in the hospital, leaving 395 survivors. Of these, 315 (80%) underwent exercise testing and 325 (82%) underwent coronary angiography. Exercise testing was performed at 2.5 miles per hour starting at 0% grade and gradually increasing to 15%. Exercise was stopped at 15 minutes in the absence of symptoms or earlier if there was angina, breathlessness, fatigue. An abnormal response was considered to be ST depression, angina, or the inability to complete the 15 minutes. "Modern therapy" also included an impact on cigarette smoking: the 62% smoking rate at the time of infarction was reduced to 17%. Total cardiac mortality was best predicted by EF and by a coronary prognostic index dependent on age, history of infarct, and chest x-ray. Neither the severity of coronary artery lesions nor the results of exercise testing predicted mortality. Reinfarction could not be predicted by any clinical or angiographic variable. Statistical methods included univariate t-tests and log-rank tests of stratified life tables. Although use of the multivariate Cox proportional hazards regression model was mentioned in one sentence, no details were presented that would allow evaluation of its use.

Williams et al. from Ottawa Civic Hospital compared clinical and treadmill variables for the prediction of outcome after MI. They considered the relative prognostic merits of 15 clinical and 10 predischarge exercise test (including all 5 variables in Table 6–3) variables in 226 patients. A submaximal treadmill test was performed on 205 patients (88%) to a mean work load of 6 METs an average of 12 days after MI. The standard Bruce protocol was used, and leads V1, V5, and AVF were monitored. Of the population, 22% had non-Q-wave subendocardial infarctions and 34% had anterior transmural MIs. Sixteen percent were taking digitalis, 36% had exercise-induced ST-segment depression, and 23% had angina. During the first year of observation, 3.4% of the patients developed unstable angina, 6.8% had a recurrent infarction, and 6% died. Twelve percent underwent coronary bypass surgery. Among those who did not have a treadmill test, there was a 31% death rate. The predictors of death were found to be resting ST-segment depression, a high CPK, a poor exercise tolerance, and a history of prior MI. The authors concluded that the limited prognostic value of predischarge treadmill test does not justify its routine use for this purpose. Both univariate and multivariate techniques were used in this study. A stepwise linear discriminant analysis was performed to derive a discriminant function for prediction. Individual variables as predictors were univariately evaluated.

Jenning et al. at Newcastle on Tyne considered 1,253 patients admitted over one year to their CCU; 503 sustained an MI, but only 289 were less than 66 years of age. Of these 289, 18% died in the hospital and 36% were excluded from study because of LBBB, ischemic pain, or other complications; 49 could not be tested prior to discharge for logistic reasons. Transmural and subendocardial MIs were not specified. Six patients underwent CABS and were not included in follow-up. The treadmill test had one-MET increments for each of its four stages. Patients with an HR response greater than 130 were considered to have an excessive response. Exertional hypotension was considered as a fall in SBP of 10 mm Hg from the resting value or a drop of 20 from a previous exercise value. Ten percent were receiving a beta blocker at the time of the test, and 43% took them at some time during the year. The Norris index score (which considers age, prior MI, and x-ray abnormalities) was related to a 12% mortality if the score was less than 3 and 85% if the score was more than 12. Mortality was similar in those not tested for logistic reasons (8.2%). Using univariate analysis, exertional hypotension generated a risk ratio of 8, inability to complete the protocol a risk ratio of 8, and an excessive HR response a risk ratio of 4. Angina, PVCs, and ST depression were not found to be predictive. Only chi-square and t-tests were used.

Fioretti et al. from the Thorax Center in Rotterdam evaluated the relative merits of resting EF by radionuclide ventriculography and the predischarge exercise test for predicting prognosis in hospital survivors of MI. A symptom-limited bike test was performed with increments of 10 W per minute. The Frank leads were computer processed; 43% had abnormal ST-segment depression and approximately 40% were on beta blockers. The hospital mortality was 13%, and 19 additional patients out of 214 died in the subsequent follow-up (9%). Mortality was 33% for patients with an EF less than 20%, 19% for patients with an EF between 20 and 39, and 3% for patients with an EF greater than 40%. Mortality was high (23%) in 47 patients excluded from performing exercise tests because of heart failure or other limitations. The patients could be stratified further into intermediate low-risk groups according to an increase in systolic blood pressure during exercise. Maximal work load, angina, ST-segment changes, and PVCs were less predictive. After discharge, 14% of the patients had clinical signs or symptoms of heart failure and 38% had angina; 17 were treated with bypass surgery or angioplasty. They concluded that symptom-limited exercise testing is the method of choice since it provides more information for patient management. This study was later expanded to 405 patients, and similar results were obtained. Discriminant function analysis demonstrated that the combination of clinical and exercise variables gave better predictive accuracy than either used alone.

Krone et al. reported the experience of the Multicenter Post MI Research Group using low-level exercise testing after MI, in which 1,417 patients met their criteria and 866 consented. Of those who consented to be in the study, 77% performed the treadmill test. The protocol was done to 5 METs with V2, V5, and AVF monitored on an average of 15 days after MI. The grade was 0% for three minutes, 5% for the next three minutes, and 10% for the final three minutes. After one minute at one mile per hour, the speed was increased to 1.7 miles per hour for the final eight minutes. Of those who exceeded an SBP of 110 during testing, there was a 3% mortality versus 18% for those unable to do so. In those that had an absence of couplets, there was a 4% mortality, while it was 13% in those with couplets. In patients with a normal exercise blood pressure and no pulmonary congestion on the chest x-ray, there was a 1% mortality versus 13% in those with either abnormality. Most of the results are presented in univariate form, with Fisher's exact test evaluation. Further analysis of selected clinical and demographic variables using stepwise logistic regression demonstrated that exercise results significantly improved the prediction model for cardiac death.

In this same study population, Dwyer et al. reported the experience with nonfatal events in the year post acute MI. Radionuclide ventriculography and Holter monitoring were done on all subjects, and treadmill tests were performed in 76%. Thirty-two percent were readmitted (7% for bypass surgery) with a death rate of 14%. The relative risk of death in the first year after readmission was 2.6 times greater than for patients who did not have a readmission. Only an EF less than 40% and post-MI angina were predictive of readmission. Reinfarction was best predicted by predischarge angina which carried a risk ratio of 2.5. Failure to perform the exercise test was significantly associated as well with reinfarction, but none of the treadmill variables were discriminating. They concluded that urgent referral to cardiac catheterization and CABS because of an abnormal exercise test post MI does not seem warranted. This study used the approach of chi-square testing followed by multivariate stepwise logistic regression as described for Krone's study.

Handler from Guy's Hospital in London has reported his findings using submaximal predischarge exercise testing, in which 339 consecutive patients 66 years of age or less were considered. Thirteen percent died in the hospital, and 71 patients were not tested because of CHF, unstable angina, previous CABS, bundle branch block, locomotive limitations, refusal, or for logistic reasons. The cardiac event recorded was the most serious one during the follow-up period in the following order of severity: (1) death, (2) pulmonary edema, (3) recurrent MI, (4) CABS, and (5) angina. Data for cardiac death alone were given, but all other events were combined. ECG signals were analyzed using a microcomputer. ST-segment elevation and depression were considered, but location was not. Whether or not there was a history of prior MI was not considered. An increase in SBP of less than 10 mm Hg or a fall during the final work load were considered abnormal blood pressure responses. PVCs were considered abnormal if frequent (more than 10/min), multiformed, or paired. ST-segment depression of 0.1 mV downsloping or horizontal was considered an abnormal response for depression while a similar amount was used for elevation. Risk ratios for death and total events were univariately calculated. Abnormal ST-segment depression generated a risk ratio of 6 which was not significant and elevation a risk ratio of 10 which was significant. Combined elevation and depression had a risk ratio of 13, which was statistically significant. Elevation was more common in anterior MIs. An abnormal blood pressure response and ST-segment elevation also predicted heart failure. Killip classes 3 and 4 predicted congestive heart failure and death. The only statistical methods used were Student's t test and chi-square analysis.

From the UCSD SCOR comes a report prepared by Madsen that attempts to answer two important questions: Can an "ischemic" exercise test response and the exercise capacity be predicted from historical and clinical data available during hospitalization? Can patients at low or high risk of death or new MI be identified by the exercise test? To answer these questions, they analyzed data from 1,469 patients discharged after an acute MI from four hospitals. Of these patients, 466 or 32% underwent a treadmill test at discharge. The exercise test was an optional part of the SCOR multicenter study protocol. The main reasons for not performing an exercise test were advanced age, poor general condition, severe cardiac dysfunction, or complicating diseases. The 466 patients who underwent exercise testing had a lower frequency of clinical risk factors than patients who did not undergo exercise testing. Various treadmill protocols were used, but MET levels were calculated. Limiting conditions of exercise tests were angina in 16%, marked ST segment changes in 7%, fatigue in 44%, shortness of breath in 17%, claudication in 4%, and severe arrhythmias in 2%. If no symptoms developed, the patients continued exercise until they approached 75% of maximal age-adjusted heart rate. In the 9% of patients without limiting symptoms where the exercise test was stopped at a low heart rate, the test was considered indeterminate. Patients taking beta blockers were included if a heart rate greater than 100 beats per minute were achieved above 6 METs. Medications taken during the testing time included digoxin in 26% and beta blockers in 53%. Patients with bundle branch block or LVH or those receiving digoxin therapy had test results considered indeterminate. Thus, 92 patients with indeterminate test results were excluded, leaving 374 patients. Among these patients, 295 were followed for one year; 19 died or had new MIs or both. Exercise test variables considered included (1) cardiac reasons for stopping exercise, (2) typical angina during the test, (3) exercise capacity in METs (with a cutpoint of 4 METs), (4) maximal heart rate, (5) abnormal SBP response (decrease or increase of less than 20 mm Hg), (6) ST-segment depression, (7) exercise-induced ST-segment elevation in leads without Q-waves and without ST-segment depression in other leads, (8) dysrhythmias (more than 6 PVC/min, ventricular, or supraventricular tachycardia), and (9) ischemic test response (exercise test-induced ST-segment depression and/or angina).

When attempting to predict who would have ischemic test responses, only the 374 patients with exercise tests satisfactory for analysis were considered. Four historical variables from hospitalization were chosen as predicting an ischemic exercise test response by discriminate analysis. These included previous angina, ST-segment depression at rest, beta-blocking agents on discharge, and age; however, prediction was poor. When attempting to predict who would have an exercise capacity of 4 METs or less, univariate analysis revealed a number of factors that were historically different. These included age, previous MI, angina, hypertension, heart failure, resting ST-segment changes, and EF. However, multivariate analysis found only age and ST-segment changes at rest to be significant. In the 295 patients followed one year with satisfactory exercise tests, among exercise test variables tested univariately, only exercise capacity in METs and the occurrence of exercise-induced ST-segment depression were important for predicting death and/or new MI within one year. A discriminate analysis using all exercise test variables selected only the exercise capacity in METs. Total correct classification was 75%. In the low-risk group of patients (72% of patients with an exercise capacity greater than 4 METs), fewer than 2% died or had a new MI within one year. In the high-risk group of patients (29% of patients with an exercise capacity less than or equal to 4 METs), 18% had a cardiac endpoint.

The Student's t-test was used to compare mean values and a chi-square test to compare incidences of discrete variables between groups. Stepwise discriminate function analysis was performed to evaluate the independent importance of clinical variables. The prediction results are based on the jackknife procedure. The results are presented as the percentage of correctly classified patients with predicted endpoints, percentage of correctly classified patients without an endpoint, and a percentage of the total number of patients correctly classified. Endpoints of death and reinfarction were combined for analysis.

They concluded that an ischemic exercise test response could not be reliably predicted from historical or clinical variables from the hospitalization. Patients likely to have good exercise capacity would be identified by using age and ST-segment changes at rest. Good exercise capacity is the most important exercise test variable for identifying those with a very low risk of death and new MI within a year. A group of patients at relatively high risk can be identified by a poor exercise capacity.

Jespersen and colleagues from two Danish hospitals have reported a series of 126 consecutive patients selected because they could exercise and had no evidence of prior MI, unstable angina pectoris, or severe heart failure, and were less than 71 years of age. The size of the population the patients were chosen from was not indicated. Their goal was to determine the prognostic value of ST-segment depression during a maximal exercise test performed in the third to fourth week after an acute MI. Eighteen of the patients were female. On the mean 24th day after MI, all patients underwent a maximal progressive bicycle test, exercising to an endpoint of limiting symptoms (i.e., increasing angina, severe dyspnea, exhaustion, or dizziness). Exercise testing was stopped because of arrhythmias in three patients and because of marked ST-segment depression in seven; no complications occurred. Maximal oxygen uptake was estimated from the bicycle work load. At discharge, 41 patients were receiving digoxin or beta blockers, and the medications were not discontinued before or after exercise testing. The patients were then seen at regular intervals in the outpatient clinic for one year. No secondary preventive medical treatment was established. Endpoints were major cardiac events, i.e., reinfarction, unstable angina, or sudden death. Group comparisons were carried out using the chi-square test with Yates correction and the level of significance was set at ≤.05. Cardiac event-free probability was estimated by the Kaplan-Meier method, and comparisons were done by a log-rank method.

Patients were grouped into those with (N = 46) or without (N = 80) exercise-induced ST-segment depression. The nine patients with ST-segment depression and subsequent cardiac events did not differ in any of their clinical or exercise test features from the patients without ST-segment depression. One patient underwent CABS who had ST-segment depression because of angina refractory to medical management. During the year of follow-up, there were nine major cardiac events, six being fatal, in the 46 patients who developed ST-segment depression. Only three cardiac events (all deaths) occurred in 80 patients without exercise-induced ST-segment depression. The subgroup with exercise-induced ST-segment depression had annual death rates and reinfarction of 13% and 17%, respectively, and the annual rate of cardiac death was 4% in the subgroup without ST-segment depression. The estimates of cardiac event-free probability showed a significantly worse prognosis for patients with ST-segment depression. Exercise-induced angina pectoris was not predictive for further cardiac events. There was no significant difference for rate pressure product, estimated VO_2, or arrhythmias in those with cardiac events. The predictive value of an abnormal exercise test (the percentage of patients with an abnormal test who had major cardiac events) was 20%, and the predictive value of a normal exercise test (the percentage of patients without ST-segment depression who did not have major cardiac events) was 96%.

SUMMARY OF PROGNOSTIC INDICATORS FROM EXERCISE TESTS

The inconsistencies found in these studies make it difficult to develop an algorithm for intervention in post-MI patients. One of the best means of selecting a high-risk group is to exclude an individual for clinical reasons from undergoing exercise testing. Possible biases due to this clinical selection process as well as the characteristics associated with being admitted to the academic centers from which these reports come must be considered. Following will be specific summaries grouped by each of the exercise test risk markers. Only studies reporting statistically significant results are explicitly cited. From the previous summaries of each study where the definitions for abnormal responses were given, it is apparent that often several different responses under each heading are being considered together by summarizing across studies (i.e., the thresholds for abnormal PVCs, exercise capacity, or BP response differ). In addition, not all of the exercise predictors were considered by the various investigators; such studies are indicated in Table 6–3 with an NR for "not reported" in the appropriate test response column.

The five exercise test variables suggested to have prognostic importance are summarized here and in Table 6–3. These include ST-segment depression (and sometimes elevation), exercise test-induced angina, poor exercise capacity or excessive heart rate response to a low work load, a blunted SBP response, and PVCs. Because they involved the same populations and institutions and usually obtained the same results, the following studies are grouped together: Theroux and Waters (Montreal Heart Institute); Sami, Davidson, and DeBusk (Stanford); Hunt and Srinivasan (Royal Melbourne Hospital), Krone and Dwyer (Multicenter Post MI Group), and Fioretti (1984 and 1985, Thorax Center). Thus, the results from a total of 24 centers are considered.

Exercise-Induced ST-Segment Shifts.   Kentala found T-wave inversion appeared earlier and was greater among patients who died suddenly compared to patients with no sudden deaths during a six-year follow-up period. However, ST depression was found to have little predictive power using linear discriminant analysis. In Smith's study of only 62 patients tested to 60% of the age-predicted maximal heart rate, patients who developed ST-segment depression were six times as likely to die or have a new MI than those without ST-segment depression. Hunt et al. found a positive association of ST-segment depression with death. Srinivasan et al., in an expanded study, found a sixfold increase in risk of dying with flat ST-segment depression of 0.1 mV or more.

Markiewicz et al. performed treadmill tests from 3 to 11 weeks after MI in 46 men, and ST depression (at least 0.1 mV) predicted later coronary events during a mean 18 month follow-up. All seven patients with events had ST depression. Sami et al. found that ST-segment depression of 0.2 mV or more was very predictive for cardiac arrest and led to CABS during the two-year follow-up. Only 35% of patients without an event had this amount of ST-segment depression. Cardiac arrest or recurrent MI at three weeks post-MI occurred in 40% of those with 0.2 mV ST depression and in only 5% of patients who had neither PVCs nor ST depression (eight times the risk). In patients with ST depression of 0.1 to 0.19 mV and in patients with PVCs only, 25% had these events. Davidson and DeBusk used multiple logistic analysis to show that ST-segment depression, equal to or greater than 0.2 mV, was the most valuable predictor for the two-year follow-up period. The two-year event rate of deaths and new MIs was 25% for 23 patients with this amount of ST-segment depression compared with 13% for 172 patients without it. DeBusk found ST-segment depression of 0.2 mV or more to carry a relative risk of eight times using stepwise discriminant analysis.

Theroux et al. found that ST-segment depression of 0.1 mV or more in CM5 was predictive of later death. Waters et al. expanded this series of patients and demonstrated similar results. ST-segment elevation had the same risk as ST depression, and so they were considered together.

Starling found that ST-segment depression of 0.1 mV or more was a strong predictor of later cardiac events (cardiac death, unstable angina, and new MI). The event rate was significantly higher for patients with ST-segment depression (60%) compared to patients without exercise-induced abnormalities (15%). However, if only death or reinfarction were considered, ST-segment changes did not predict increased risk. A risk ratio of four was reported by Velasco et al. with a 32% three-year mortality among 28 patients with ST-segment depression compared to 8% among 172 patients without it. Jespersen found ST depression to be highly predictive.

Thus, 7 out of the 24 centers found ST-segment depression to be significantly predictive of subsequent death; an additional five centers reported a positive but insignificant association. Seven centers reported a null effect with 5 of the 23 failing to report data on ST-segment depression.

ST Elevation.   Sullivan et al. evaluated the prognostic importance of exercise-induced ST-segment elevation in 64 patients who underwent submaximal exercise testing a mean of 11 days after an acute infarct. Follow-up was for one year. The presence of exercise-induced ST-segment elevation was the only exercise test variable that predicted cardiac death. DeFeyter et al. found that ST-segment depression indicated MVD, whereas ST-segment elevation indicated advanced left ventricular wall motion abnormalities and a low EF. Both shifts indicated that both MVD and advanced LV wall motion abnormalities existed. In Water's study, ST-segment elevation generated the same univariate risk as did depression, and so they were considered together. However, location of the ST shift was not specified. Saunamaki and Andersen considered ST-segment depression and elevation separately but did not specify location. In their study, the ST responses were found to have little prognostic value. Handler found ST-segment elevation to generate a risk ratio of 10 which was significant. Combined elevation and depression had a risk ratio of 13 which was significant. Elevation was more common in anterior MIs. ST-segment elevation also predicted heart failure.

Exercise-Induced Arrhythmias.   Granath et al. found the appearance of PVCs to generate a risk ratio of 2. Exercise-induced PVCs proved to be of higher prognostic significance than those recorded at rest. Weld et al. found PVCs in 43% of his patients and that during the one-year follow-up, they had two times the cardiac death rate than those without PVCs. Empirically, Saunamaki found complex exercise-induced PVCs to indicate a high-risk group. Madsen demonstrated that discriminant analysis led to selection of exercise test induced PVCs as risk predictors.

Thus, only four out of 24 centers reported exercise test-induced PVCs to indicate a significant increase in risk. Five centers did not include results regarding PVCs; six centers reported null or negative associations of PVCs with mortality.

Exercise Capacity.   Weld et al., utilizing multiple logistic regression analysis, found that exercise capacity was significantly associated with one-year cardiac mortality. Patients unable to reach an exercise capacity of four METs had a relative risk of 19. The prognostic importance of functional capacity was also reported by Davidson and DeBusk who included a maximum work load below four METs in multivariate analysis, although this was not confirmed by the two other reports from Stanford. Madsen used a multivariate analysis of exercise variables from a maximum symptom-limited bicycle test three weeks after MI in 205 patients and found that the most important variable was the duration of exercise. Williams et al. found a poor exercise tolerance along with three clinical variables to be predictive of death. Jennings found a tachycardia at a low work load to be predictive of cardiac events. Fioretti included functional capacity in his discriminant analysis derived algorithm for prediction. Krone, Handler, and Madsen (UCSD) all reported a three- to nine-fold increase in risk associated with a low exercise capacity.

Thus, eight centers out of 24 reported that a low exercise capacity and/or an excessive HR response to exercise indicated a high-risk group. Four additional centers reported nonsignificant positive associations, Stanford reported a positive association in only one of three studies, while 10 of the 24 centers failed to report sufficient data on this variable to assess its effect.

Exercise-Induced Angina.   Hunt et al. found that angina during an exercise test was associated with four times the increased risk of dying within one year. Velasco et al. found a 29% mortality among patients with angina versus 9% among patients free of angina. Jelinek et al. and Krone et al. reported that angina increased the risk of death two- to threefold. Thus, only four of 24 centers reported exercise test-induced angina to indicate a significantly increased risk group. Eight centers failed to report angina data. Seven of the remaining 11 reported nonsignificant positive associations.

Blood Pressure Response to Exercise.   Madsen found a small increase in the double product (heart rate times systolic blood pressure) to result in a low probability of survival after five years. An increase in double product from rest to maximum exercise of less than 1,500 implied a 59% probability of survival compared to 74% for patients with a greater increase in double product. Weld found a hypotensive response to generate a risk ratio of 5 times. Jennings and Krone found a risk of 8 times, and Waters found it to be a significant predictor. Saunamaki empirically chose limits based on the change in double product from rest to exercise (less than 2,500 mm Hg/min). This was very successful using survival curve analysis in discriminating high- and low-risk groups. Fioretti found that a limited increase during exercise in SBP (less than 30 mm Hg) was the only significant factor picked using multiple discriminant analysis. Handler found an abnormal BP response to generate a risk ratio of 10.

Thus, eight of 24 centers found that inadequate or abnormal SBP response to exercise significantly identified a high-risk group; 11 of the centers failed to report data, and four of the remaining six reported a nonsignificant positive association.

COMPARISON OF EXERCISE DATA TO CLINICAL DATA

An important consideration is, whether the exercise test gives more predictive information than the standard clinical risk predictors. Attempts to establish risk have included scores based on clinical features of the MI and historical information such as the Norris and Peel indices. There are reasons other than prognostication for performing exercise testing, but given the need to cost account, all possible justification for performing a procedure is needed.

Kentala and associates assessed clinical parameters including a careful history of prior activity level. The prognostic power of clinical and ECG variables recorded soon after MI and in connection with the exercise test were analyzed by stepwise multiple discriminant analysis. They found that both clinical and exercise variables were important. Patients dying within two years had a low exercise systolic BP. With longer follow-up, the exercise BP had a weaker impact. At the four- and six-year points, an abnormal resting terminal P-wave was the best predictor of poor prognosis. This probably identified a group with mild heart failure. For patients who suddenly died after two years, the T-wave changes after exercise, which possibly indicated subendocardial injury, were common. Patients with a high level of physical activity before their MI were less prone to die suddenly. Of the many factors considered, an abnormal apical impulse, T-wave inversion after exercise, prior CPR, sedentary life-style before infarction, and occurrence of PVCs during exercise were of discriminatory value in relation to sudden death.

Granath et al. found that analysis of clinical data in the CCU failed to produce any differences between survivors and those who died, although there were more deaths among those patients who had a previous MI. Saunamaki and Andersen demonstrated that exercise testing variables including PVCs and a poor SBP-HR change in response to exercise still were able to predict risk within the strata of CHF, prior MI, and anterior MI. The exercise variables outperformed these important clinical parameters. Weld found the exercise test variables of duration, PVCs, and ST-segment depression to be ranked in that order ahead of the clinical variables of x-ray vascular congestion, prior MI, and x-ray cardiomegaly in predictive value.

De Feyter was unable to identify from treadmill markers a higher risk group whereas three-vessel disease or a left ventricular EF of 30% or less did. Madsen and Gilpin found that in those who underwent testing, clinical variables were better able to predict outcome than in the nontested group. The most important exercise test variables were exercise duration and PVCs; however, they improved prediction of reinfarction but not death. Though exercise test variables were selected by discriminant analysis, the correct total classification of deaths and survivors was not improved. The total correct prediction was 71% for clinical data used alone, 67% for exercise data alone, and 71% for both combined.

DeBusk et al. found that prior MI or angina, or recurrence of pain in the CCU, identified the 10% of patients with the highest rate of reinfarction and death within six months (18%). Clinical contradictions to exercise testing identified another 40% with an intermediate risk (6.4%). In those who underwent treadmill testing, ST-segment depression and low-peak work load were selected before any clinical variables or ambulatory ECG data in the logistic regression analysis. Gibson et al. found no difference in univariate comparison of clinical variables between those with or without events; even EF was similar.

Norris found that total cardiac mortality was best predicted by EF and by an index dependent on age, history of MI, and chest x-ray. Neither the severity of coronary lesions nor the results of exercise testing predicted mortality. Reinfarction could not be predicted by any clinical exercise test or angiographic variable. William et al. considered the relative prognostic merits of 15 clinical and 10 predischarge exercise test variables in 226 patients. The predictors of death were found to be resting ST depression, a high CPK, a poor exercise tolerance, and a history of prior MI.

Jennings et al. found that the Norris index score (age, prior MI, x-ray abnormalities) of less than 3 was associated with a 12% mortality and a score of more than 12 with a mortality of 85%. Fioretti et al. evaluated the relative merits of resting EF by radionuclide ventriculography and the predischarge exercise test. Mortality was 33% for patients with an EF less than 20%, 19% for patients with EF between the 20 and 39, and 3% for patients with an EF greater than 40%. Mortality was high (23%) in 47 patients excluded from performing exercise tests because of heart failure or other limitations.

Krone et al. found that among those not able to take a treadmill test, there was a 14% mortality compared to 5% in those who were able to take it. In patients with a normal exercise blood pressure and no pulmonary congestion on the chest x-ray, there was a 1% mortality versus 13% in those with either abnormality. In this same population, Dwyer et al. reported the experience with nonfatal events in the year post MI. Thirty-two percent were readmitted (7% for CABS) with a death rate of 14% and a risk ratio of 2.6. Only an EF less than 40% and post-MI angina were predictive of readmission. Reinfarction was best predicted by predischarge angina. Failure to perform the exercise test was significantly associated with these events, but none of the treadmill variables were discriminating.

Waters et al. found that predictors by the Cox regression model were different in the first and the second year of follow-up. During the first year, ST-segment shift in either direction, a flat blood pressure response, or angina within 48 hours after admission were predictors ("markers of ischemia"). During the second year, a history of prior MI, the QRS score, or PVCs were independent risk predictors ("markers of LV dysfunction").

In summary, the results are mixed regarding whether the exercise test gives information that can predict death and reinfarction better than the clinical features.

CLINICAL DESIGN FEATURES

The column headings used in Table 6–3, and separately listed in Table 6–4, are the important features of the study design that could affect the findings. Following is a discussion of these features.

Exercise Protocol.   Bike protocols, especially a supine protocol like Velasco used, can give different responses than a treadmill. Most protocols were continuous, but some were not progressive in work load increments. The standard Bruce protocol starts at a relatively high work load (4–5 METs). Heart rate responses at submaximal levels can be affected by the protocol as well as beta blockade, fitness, and anxiety.

Endpoints of Exercise Test.   If stopped at a certain amount of ST-segment shift, MET level, or heart rate, this response could not be considered a continuous variable, nor could a higher value, which might be more

TABLE 6–4.
Methodologic Characteristics That Could Differ Between the Studies

Patients excluded
Entrance criteria
Age range, gender
Infarct mix (i.e., non-Q-wave, inferior/anterior/lateral Q-wave)
Patients with prior MI and those with complications included or not
Prior coronary artery bypass surgery
History of CHF and angina
MI size
Follow-up thoroughness and length
Percentage of patients undergoing CABS during follow-up
Cardiac events (problems with using CABS as an endpoint)
Mortality during follow-up (are they a high or low risk group)
Reinfarction rate
Exercise protocol
Time post-MI test performed
Endpoints of test
Leads monitored
Medications taken after discharge from hospital and at time of exercise test
Test responses considered (PVCs, ST, BP, exercise capacity, angina)
Statistical methods

discriminating, be reached. However, while it appears to be in good judgment not to exceed 5 METs or a heart rate of 130 prior to discharge, the differences in protocols lead to problems in analysis and interpretation. Early ambulation is important, but strenuous exercise should be avoided until healing of the myocardial scar is completed. Therefore, maximal testing seems more reasonable to postpone until when the patient is to return to full activities (one to two months post-MI).

ECG Leads Monitored.   Use of different electrode placements makes comparison between studies difficult. Bipolar leads, particularily CM5, give an isolated view of the electrical activity of the heart that can differ greatly even from V5. CM5 exaggerates ST slope, and depression and elevation in it means something different than in other leads. ST-segment elevation in V1–V4 in anterior Q-wave MIs is "normal," but when it extends laterally to CM5 or V5, it may mean a large dangerous aneurysm. Large anterolateral MIs with IVCD may well behave like LBBB and be associated with large ST shifts not due to ischemia but due to the underlying damage. ST-segment elevation laterally associated with a subendocardial or inferior wall MI most likely means dangerous ischemia while further elevation over the inferior Q-wave is normal. All of these hypothetical explanations for ST shifts due to pathophysiological interactions with the underlying MI make it difficult to characterize ST depression or elevation simply as normal or abnormal.

Time Post-MI When Exercise Test Was Performed.   "Stunned" myocardium and deconditioning affect predischarge testing more than they affect hemodynamic responses later. ST-segment responses appear more labile early post-MI. The responses differ at various times post-MI as well, with a spontaneous improvement in hemodynamics occurring by two months. The spontaneous improvement in both EF and functional capacity but their failure to correlate with each other makes them difficult to interpret. The studies that included exercise testing at multiple times found the same responses to have a different predictive value at the specific times the tests were performed. There is a spontaneous improvement during the first year post-MI in the blunted blood pressure response to exercise that occurs particularly in large anterior MIs.

MI Mix (i.e., Q-Wave Location).   Each has a different prognosis and different "normal" response to exercise. Exercise predictors may be different in each type. There has been a report of heart rate impairment in response to exercise in inferior wall MIs. An RV infarction accompanying an inferior MI has not been found to affect the hemodynamic response to exercise testing.

Inclusion of Non-Q-Wave MIs.   After much controversy regarding the risk of having a "subendocardial" MI, a study from the Mayo Clinic appears to clarify the situation. From 1960 to 1979, 1,221 residents of Rochester, Minnesota, had an MI as the first manifestation of CHD; 784 had a transmural (Q-wave) and 353 had a non-Q-wave MI. The 30-day fatality rate was 18% among transmural and 9% in subendocardial MIs. No significant difference was found in the rates of reinfarction, CABS, or mortality over the next five years. CHF was more common among patients with transmural MIs, and angina was more common among patients with non-Q-wave MIs.

Few previous studies have reported exercise test results in post-MI patients with Q-waves versus those without Q-waves. Koppes et al. did not find any difference with respect to estimated oxygen uptake, maximum heart rate, or rate pressure product in the two groups. Starling et al. included 28 patients with subendocardial MI. Differences in treadmill responses were not reported, and the incidence of cardiac events during 11 months of follow-up was the same in the two groups. Schwartz et al. found that 15 patients with non-Q-wave MIs reached a greater maximum work load, were more often symptom-limited on exercise (fatigue, dyspnea, chest pain), more often showed ST-segment depression and less often ST-segment elevation compared with 33 patients with transmural MI. Madsen and Gilpin reported the results from exercise testing of 456 post-MI patients including 27 patients with subendocardial MIs. In the symptom-limited maximum bicycle exercise test, these patients had a lower maximum heart rate (123 beats per minute, compared to 133 for patients with transmural MI), and more often had to stop the test because of angina (33% versus 19%). The one-year mortality was not significantly different in the two groups. DeFeyter et al. calculated the sensitivity and specificity of ST-segment depression for multivessel disease separately for their patients with non-Q-wave MIs. This yielded the highest values they found for any of their MI type subgroups.

Sia et al. in Australia evaluated early symptom-limited maximal exercise tests in predicting coronary anatomy, left ventricular ejection fraction, and hemodynamics in 64 patients after an acute non-Q-wave MI. Ten of the patients were women, 28% had prior MIs, 11% were on beta blockers, and 83% were on calcium antagonists. Exercise tests and cardiac catheterization were performed at a median of six and seven days, respectively, after the MI. Forty-one percent of the patients had a negative exercise test response (no angina, less than 0.1 mV of ST depression and normal blood pressure responses). Twenty-five percent had a positive response (0.1 to .19 mV of ST depression or angina); 34% had a "strongly positive" exercise test response (at least 2 mm of ST depression or a 10 mm Hg drop in SBP). A negative response predicted the absence of three-vessel disease (at least 70% stenosis) or critical stenoses (at least 90% stenosis) involving major coronary arteries (negative predictive accuracy 92%), whereas a strongly positive response predicted their presence (positive predictive value 77%, specificity 88%).

Because the number of exercise tested patients with non-Q-wave MIs has been rather small, more information is necessary to ascertain these patients' reactions to exercise after MI and the prognostic implications of the exercise test. It is possible that the exercise test results in these patients, especially ST-segment changes and SBP response, would be important in identifying an uncomplicated subgroup in contrast to patients with more severe ischemia with a high risk of subsequent transmural MI.

Thoroughness and Length of Follow-up.   Those lost to follow-up most likely have a higher percentage of deaths. Also, follow-up affects analysis if censored data cannot be handled adequately with the statistical program. Mortality changes over time and the impact of the predictors changes.

Percentage of Patients Undergoing CABS During Follow-up. CABS could alter mortality and affect outcome prediction. Also, patients with ischemic predictors would be selected to have this procedure more frequently.

Cardiac Events Considered as Endpoints.   The only hard endpoints that should be considered, from an epidemiological point of view, are death and reinfarction. Separation or distinction of sudden death makes little sense and may confuse the analysis, particularly if those with sudden death are compared to all others (including nonsudden cardiac death). Noncardiac deaths are often difficult to distinguish and lead to biased results but may play a confusing role, particularly in older populations. CABS is not a valid endpoint and should be considered censored outcome. It is clearly related to certain exercise test results that physicians feel motivated to "fix" with that procedure. "Instability" or progression of symptoms (CHF or angina) are soft endpoints that cannot be used for epidemiological purposes.

Mortality During Follow-up.   If there is a low mortality rate, more patients are needed to find a statistical difference between those with or without certain variables. Some studies have compensated for this by using soft endpoints and combining endpoints.

Prior MI Patients Included or Not.   Prior MI is an important predictive variable that is dependent upon the severity of the prior MI or MIs. Patients with prior large MIs are biased toward being admitted with non-Q-wave MIs since another transmural MI increases their likelihood of dying prior to hospitalization. Few studies have tried to account for the number or severity of prior MIs.

History of or Tests Indicating CHF, Angina, or Arrhythmias Prior to or Associated With the MI.   Historical features of prior coronary disease and signs and/or symptoms of major function, perfusion, or electrical abnormalities at the time of admission are important prognostic indicators and must be considered. It could be hypothesized that exercise testing has predictive power in high-risk patients (Hunt, Srinivasan) and in low-risk patients (Stanford), but when they are considered together, confounding factors and interactions may cancel out to show little impact on predicting prognosis. It appears that these features often lead physicians to exclude patients from testing, explaining why exclusion has such a high predictive value for death.

Exclusion Criteria.   Clearly, clinical judgment applied to the post-MI population to exclude patients from exercise testing identifies the highest risk group. Though this process considers complicating illnesses and age, cardiac dysfunction and ischemia are considered as well. Because of this, alternate testing methods that have been compared favorably to exercise testing have included right atrial pacing and electrophysiologic stimulation studies.

Age Range and Gender.   Women are thought to have a higher MI mortality and certainly are known to respond differently than men to exercise testing. Because of this, they should be considered separately, but the studies do not contain a sufficient number for valid analysis. Death rates are directly related to age.

Medications Taken After Discharge From Hospital and at the Time of the Test.   Digoxin causes ST depression but is usually taken for CHF, thus implicating an ischemic etiology for a potential death due to dysfunction. Digoxin administration post-MI may actually be an independent risk predictor and act by predisposing to ventricular dysrhythmias. Beta blockers affect BP and heart rate response and improve survival.

STATISTICAL CRITIQUE OF THE PROGNOSTIC STUDIES

The following is a discussion of issues involving the design and analysis of these studies. It is divided into general comments, specific design critiques, analysis critiques, potentially important relevant issues not generally considered, and meta-analysis comments.

General Comments.   Several general problems are apparent across many of the studies. The purpose of a specific study is not always clear; there is confusion between the desire to develop a prediction algorithm that will be of practical clinical use in patient treatment, and the desire to demonstrate an association of exercise testing responses to subsequent cardiac events in any form. Development of a prediction algorithm requires an approach to validation that is different from the testing of the statistical significance of an effect, as is done in many of the studies. Although effect size estimation is probably the most clinically relevant procedure, most of the studies report only significance test results, perhaps with some means or frequency differences cited. None of the studies reported effect size estimates with confidence intervals, even though this is the well-established method of reporting estimation results.

If investigators (and journal editors) insist on using hypothesis testing in studies that should be estimation problems, they should also report power computations for any negative results. Lack of this computation makes it difficult to judge whether a nonsignificant test is a likely result of a study design with low power to detect significant differences rather than an accurate reflection of no association between the population parameters.

Finally, many of the studies reviewed failed to provide enough details about the data to allow independent evaluation of the investigators' conclusions. Such details are especially necessary in order to compare results across different studies. Recomputation of effects may be required to compare studies that have reported results in different formats. The number of "?" appearing in the exercise test risk markers column of Table 6–3 illustrates how often data reported were insufficient to compute even the direction of the associations in the study (whether or not the association is "significant").

From the data analyst's view, existing studies share common problems both in design and in analysis performed. Not all of the problems occur in all of the studies, and not all in any one study, but the prevalence of certain difficulties is high enough to be of general concern.

Design Problems.   Common areas of difficulty include selection biases, a relatively rare outcome of interest, use of multiple endpoints, and unequal follow-up times. Many of the studies fail to be specific enough about the target population of interest. Selection biases in the patients studied may be too severe for the results to be considered representative of the general population. However, if the limited target population is carefully specified, other investigators can use the additional information gained from those patients in designing further research even if the results are not generally applicable. Evaluation of possible biases requires information on patients who were eligible for the study but declined to participate, or who dropped out of the study after their initial entry. A few of the investigators have reported on such nonparticipants or follow-up losses, but many do not report more than the number of individuals involved.

The most desirable endpoint for analyses in these studies is death because it is the most well-defined endpoint, even though some noncardiac deaths may be included in the results. However, this is a relatively rare outcome, requiring that large numbers of patients be tested and followed. Failure to include enough patients in a study can lead to reduced precision of estimates or low power to detect differences because of low effective sample size; effective sample size is limited by the number of deaths in the study group. One approach to dealing with small numbers of deaths is the use of multiple endpoints, often combined. However, this practice may obscure underlying relationships for several reasons. Endpoints other than death, such as angina, cannot be well enough defined to avoid extensive misclassification errors. A potentially more serious issue when endpoints are combined is independent of the precision of the endpoint measurement. Different endpoints may be related to different mechanisms and thus may have different associations with the test markers. Such differences will confound any attempt to measure associations using combined endpoints. Perhaps the worst pitfall is the use of an endpoint to assess associations that may be influenced by the exercise test result; studies that have included CABS as an endpoint have fallen prey to this trap.

Finally, the problem of unequal time periods in follow-up of patients cannot be ignored. This problem can be circumvented in the design of a study by using a limited time period for entry into the study, with follow-up that will allow the study to be completed with sufficient events. This approach requires that the follow-up time be limited enough to minimize loss-to-follow-up problems. Adjustments for unequal follow-up time can also be made in the analysis phase of the study, but these were not used in most of the studies.

Analysis Problems.   Problems in the analysis phase of the reported research were primarily related to the exclusive use of univariate test statistics and to attempts (or nonattempts) to deal with unequal follow-up. This area of research is so complex that investigators cannot use only univariate statistical analysis and hope to draw accurate conclusions. Many of the predictor variables being evaluated are interrelated. Thus, confounding of effects is likely to be present. The most probable error caused by such confounding is concluding that an association exists between an explanatory variable and the outcome variable when the association is spurious due to associations of each of the variables with a third variable. Similarly, estimates of effect size based on univariate analysis can be misleading in the presence of confounding variables.

Conclusions drawn without regard to the interrelationships of the variables are also more susceptible to errors due to the specific study sample and its particular combination of clinical subsets. Generalization to other patient groups is more questionable than would otherwise be the case. It is important to at least consider other possible explanations for any associations claimed.

Only one-fourth of the research centers reported any use of multivariate techniques. Computer programs for such analyses were certainly widely available after 1980; only 5 of the 24 centers have reports limited to before 1981, when access to such analysis tools may have been more difficult. None of the studies reported multivariate estimates of effect, even though the effect estimate is at least as sensitive to error from exclusive univariate analysis as significance tests. It is true that multivariate techniques often have stricter assumptions than some of the univariate techniques available, and should not be used without initial screening with univariate analysis. Even if univariate estimates are given for comparison to other studies, the multivariate results should be reported so that the extent of adjustment necessary for interrelationships can be assessed.

Most of the studies have reported results of various hypothesis tests, as noted earlier. However, there is no indication that any adjustment has been made in the alpha levels (or p values) to account for multiple comparisons. In many of the studies, the comparisons could have been preplanned and easily adjusted for this problem. Even in "data-dredging" approaches, such adjustments can be made in several commonly acceptable ways. Failure to address this problem greatly increases the chance of accepting spurious results as statistically valid.

The other major analysis issue is the problem of unequal follow-up. Unequal follow-up that is not controlled in the design of a study must be handled in the analysis of the data. Unequal follow-up of patients can be treated as censored data. A typical approach in biomedical research for analysis of censored time-to-response data is to use survival analysis techniques. This approach was used in several of the more recent studies. However, a fundamental assumption of most survival techniques is that the censoring is random with respect to the outcome of interest. This assumption cannot be evaluated without reporting on those patients who were lost to follow-up, either because of dropping out of the study or because of lack of complete follow-up due to late entry into the study. Information on those who have dropped out could be gathered by death certificate searches or other techniques; reports on such persons are often missing from the studies reviewed. Including patients who are censored, observations because of short follow-up time must be considered carefully since the risk of subsequent cardiac events is known to change with time. Multivariate approaches to survival analysis are available using proportional hazard regression models or other hazard functions. However, these models may be relatively insensitive to modelling of interactions among the variables. In addition, the results may not be readily interpretable in terms useful to clinicians.

Other approaches to the problem of censored data are possible. One solution often used in epidemiological research is computations in the form of events/person-time, or person-time incidence. Another approach that avoids the inclusion of short-term follow-up patients is to stop entry into the study early enough so that all patients available can be followed for a fixed time. A limited, fixed time of follow-up can also help reduce the number of dropouts, since the likelihood of losing a patient from the study increases with time. One approach to be avoided that was used in several of the studies is to merely count events in various subgroups without regard to differences in follow-up time. Data reported in such a way is essentially meaningless.

Survival analysis is appropriate when outcome measurements represent the time to occurrence of some event (i.e., death or reinfarction). If differences in important covariates or prognostic variables exist at entry between the groups to be compared, the investigator must be concerned with the analysis of the survival experience as influenced by that difference. In order to adjust for these differences in prognostic variables, stratified analysis or a covariance type of survival analysis could be done. If there are many covariates, the number of strata can quickly become large, with few subjects in each. Moreover, if a covariate is continuous, it must be divided into intervals and each interval assigned to a score or rank before it can be used in a stratified analysis. Cox proposed a regression model that allows for analysis of censored survival data adjusting for continuous as well as discrete covariates, thus avoiding these two problems. This model, also called the proportional hazards model, assumes that the hazard rate or "force of mortality" can be expressed as a product of two terms. Available statistical packages allow for incomplete data; that is, there are cases for which the response is not observed but the data (time in study) are included in the analysis. This could occur in the study of survival where an individual may remain alive at the close of the observation period or may drop out before the end. The Cox survival analysis allows for covariates that can be selected in a stepwise fashion. The covariates or prognostic factors usually represent either inherent differences among the study subjects or constitute a set of one or more indicator variables representing different groups. The covariates may also describe changes in a patient's prognostic status as a function of time. The Cox proportional hazards regression model presumes death rates may be modeled as log-linear functions of the covariates. A regression coefficient is estimated that relates the effect of each covariate to the survival function.

The Cox model is currently favored, but few investigators have compared the various techniques in one data set. Madsen et al. compared two software versions of the Cox multivariate analysis, stepwise discriminant analysis, and recursive partitioning. They concluded that all four techniques gave equally precise prognostic evaluations but that recursive partitioning was easier to use and the Cox models were more accurate. The data set was a post-MI population. Gilpin et al. at UCSD evaluated several multivariate statistical methods in two different hospital populations to predict 30-day mortality and survival following MI. The methods evaluated were linear discriminant analysis, logistic regression, recursive partitioning, and nearest neighbor. Variables used were identified as predictive univariately from the base hospital and were obtained during the first 24 hours. Linear discriminant analysis available in BMDP assumes normality among the predictor variables whereas logistic regression is based on the assumption that the log of the classification function is a linear function of the fitted coefficients. Recursive partitioning makes no assumption regarding normality and can detect interactions among variables and handle missing data. The nearest neighbor procedure is based on the concept that in the multidimensional space defined by the variables, a patient would likely have the same outcome as another patient in that space. It cannot detect interaction or assign importance. Linear discriminant analysis, logistic regression, or recursive partitioning all performed similarly within a given population, although each used the information contained in the prognostic variables differently. Application between different populations of prediction schemes based on linear discriminant analysis and logistic regression was shown to be feasible, but prior validation is essential.

Potentially Important Relevant Issues.   There are two issues intrinsic to this area of medical research that should be addressed when evaluating patients post MI for recurrent events. These are (1) biological interaction of some of the markers and (2) temporal changes in risk during the post-MI period. They may explain some of the inconsistencies in the studies to date. Comments were made by some of the investigators regarding one or both of these issues, but the studies in general failed to account for the potential analysis difficulties.

Biological Interaction. The term "biological interaction" expresses the idea that certain exercise test responses may have different meanings in different clinical subsets of patients. This in effect leads to a type of misclassification error when the subsets are combined.

None of the statistical approaches used in the reported studies accounted for biological interaction. Examples of interaction are the following. Patients with extensive anterior MI, often with ST-segment elevation in the anterior leads, have ST-segment shifts that behave like left bundle branch block. Therefore, the ST segment response to exercise is not an indicator of ischemia. However, ST-segment shifts are valid predictors of ischemia in patients with inferior/posterior, a first subendocardial, or a small anterior or septal MI. ST-segment elevation in patients with Q-waves means something different than in patients with a first subendocardial MI. The blood pressure response in patients with large anterior MIs or in patients with multiple MIs means something different than in other patients. A blunted blood pressure response in patients with inferior or non-Q-wave MIs is probably due to ischemia while in those with large or multiple MIs, it is most likely due to left ventricular damage. A very important form of interaction is that of a prior MI both in how it affects the ECG and ventricular function.

Interaction can be accounted for by incorporating such interaction into a model or by stratifying the population into those with and without the clinical variables that interact with exercise test results. The failure to account for these interactions could explain why certain of the exercise test variables have been found to be meaningful in some studies but not in others. The results would largely depend on the underlying populations. They may well be self-selected or stratified for certain underlying clinical features.

Biological interaction could be built into the analysis by considering the responses as markers for either mechanical or ischemic abnormalities. This may be better than stratification since the number of patients is not reduced for analysis. For ST-segment analysis, ST-segment depression should be specified as (1) mechanical or reciprocal depression when it occurs in patients with large anterior or anterolateral MIs and/or exercise-induced ST elevation anteriorly, and in patients with LVH and strain, LBBB, and WPW, or (2) ischemic ST depression when it occurs in any other patients. ST-segment elevation should be specified as (1) mechanical elevation occurring over inferior Q-waves and anterior Q-waves separately, or (2) ischemic elevation when occurring in subendocardial MI patients without old Q-waves present or elevation in Q-wave MIs in a location other than over the Q-wave.

A systolic BP response that is flat, has a drop of 10 mm Hg below baseline, or a drop of 20 mm Hg at a point during exercise after a normal rise should be considered as (1) mechanical BP abnormality if not associated with angina and/or an ischemic ST depression or elevation as specified above, or (2) ischemic BP abnormality if associated with angina and/or ischemic ST responses.

For classifying exercise capacity, the response could be considered as (1) mechanical exercise capacity abnormality if 4 METs or less without angina and/or ischemic ST response as above, or (2) ischemic exercise capacity abnormality if 4 METs or less with angina and/or ischemic ST responses as above. For the maximal treadmill at one month to six weeks, the response should be considered (1) mechanically abnormal if 6 METs or less without angina and/or ischemic ST response as above, or (2) ischemically abnormal if 6 METs or less with angina and/or ischemic ST responses as above. PVCs should be classified in the same manner.

Biological interactions of the type described should be taken into account in both the design and analysis of studies of exercise test risk markers in post-MI data. Failure to consider the patients as exhibiting a possible mixture of effects may result in estimates that can be thought of as some kind of grand mean or average effect. This may obscure important true relationships to the extent that biological interaction occurs and results in statistical interactions. Biological explanations of analysis findings should also be considered to help protect the investigator against spurious findings. This is often done by default in the studies reviewed or by selection of the variables to be included in the analysis. Evaluation of results and development of prediction algorithms should never be left solely to the computer.

Another approach to account for interaction would be to stratify by clinical subsets. This could be done as follows with multiple discriminate analysis performed in each subset. For ST analysis: (1) in patients *without* CHF, shock, intraventricular conduction defects, large anterior MIs; and (2) in all others. For SBP response: (1) in those with large infarcts and/or large prior MIs, shock and/or CHF; and (2) in all others. For exercise capacity analysis: (1) in those limited by angina and/or ST changes; and (2) in those not limited by angina or ischemic ST changes. For PVCs: (1) in those with large MIs, large prior MIs, CHF, and/or shock; (2) in those with ischemia by signs or symptoms; and (3) in all others.

Temporal Changes in Risk. It is well-documented that changes in the risk of subsequent cardiac events occurs within the first year post MI. Such underlying changes in the hazard function suggest that there may be temporal changes in the effects of any related risk markers. Evaluation of this effect requires time-dependent modelling or conditional analysis with respect to time. Waters et al. are the only investigators to have addressed this problem. One expected effect of not considering the temporal changes in risk is that estimates of effect size may be biased toward the null over intervals that span several risk periods.

Meta-Analysis Considerations. Meta-analysis is a statistical approach to develop a consensus from an existing body of research. It is a quantitative approach to reviewing research using a variety of statistical techniques for sorting, classifying, and summarizing information from the findings of many studies. It is also the application of research methodology to the characteristics and findings of studies. This includes problem selection, hypothesis formulation, the definition and measurement of constructs and variables, sampling, and data analysis.

The application of meta-analysis to a body of research involves three stages. First, a complete literature search is conducted that is analogous to the collection of data in an experimental study. Second, the important characteristics and findings of relevant studies are classified. Third, statistical techniques are applied to the compiled data. This last stage can involve descriptive, correlational, and inferential statistical analysis. The statistical techniques applied here are sign testing, correlations, and weighted regression analysis. Sign testing is a statistical test that evaluates the proportions of findings and determines if they are related by more than chance.

While scientific truth relies on reproducibility, clinical studies often do not agree due to the effect of confounding variables that at times can be accounted for by statistical techniques. When applying meta-analysis, it became apparent that an electronic spreadsheet facilitated the process. After word processing, electronic spreadsheets are the most common software used in microcomputers. The first of these was VisiCalc (1979), and its introduction was the greatest impetus for the use of personal computers in the office. These programs create a matrix of cells indexed by column and row headings. The cells can be adjusted for size and data presentation. Once data is entered, it can be moved, deleted, copied, sorted, and subjected to mathematical manipulation. However useful these programs have been in business, there has been little application in medicine.

To identify the studies previously presented, Med-line was searched using the key words "exercise testing" and "myocardial infarction." Studies were included if they attempted to evaluate the relationship between exercise test variables and cardiac events during a follow-up period and were published before 1986.

The review data was entered into the spreadsheet and tables directly printed from the program. The spreadsheet program allowed for very flexible data entry. Column and row headings were specified without excessive care for priority, appearance, or order since data ranges could be easily moved, ordered alphabetically or numerically, copied, or deleted. Graphic capabilities made it possible to present the data in various graphic formats (pies, bar, and x-y plots) and to visualize the relationships between data in columns and/or rows. Facile identification and separation of subgroups was possible; the latter being the second step in the application of meta-analysis.

Initial analysis consisted of searching and sorting findings within the spreadsheet. Studies were categorized by predischarge testing (arbitrarily set at less than three weeks post-MI) and postdischarge testing (three weeks or greater) and placed in Table 6–5. The studies were then subgrouped to see if differences were due to maximal or submaximal endpoints for exercise testing and placed in Table 6–6. Other exploratory subgroupings included examining American studies versus studies from other countries and selection of the "best" studies. Subset analysis by whether or not women or patients with prior or non-Q-wave MIs were included was limited by the small number of studies that used these features as exclusion criteria as well as by the surprising number of studies that did not make this information available. The same could be said for analyzing the data regarding cardiac medications. Therefore, the percentages of these clinical features were correlated and regressed against the risk ratios found for the exercise risk markers.

Due to the varied statistical treatments used by the studies analyzed, as well as the lack of complete reporting by some investigators, exercise responses were associated with relative risk by both quantified uni- or multivariate analysis or by unquantified multivariate analysis. Risk ratios from the former were used in regression and correlation analysis whether or not the reported value was statistically significant. All values were plotted in x-y graphs. For plotting purposes, if the risk ratios were not available, arbitrary values of positive or

TABLE 6–5.
Studies Using Exercise Testing in Post-Myocardial Infarction Populations With Follow-up Divided Into Those Done Before Three Weeks and Those Done Three Weeks or More After the MI

INVESTIGATOR		ENDPOINT	EXERCISE TEST RISK MARKERS				
			BP	PVCs	EXCAP	ANGINA	ST
Predischarge (13 institutional studies)							
7	MHI	sub	+*	+	+	NR	8×*
9	Starling	sub	5×	2×	NR	4×	4×
10	Weld	sub	5×*	2×*	19×*	2×	2×
12	Velasco	sub	3×	2×	NR	3×*	4×*
14	Jelinek	max	−	NR	+	2×*	1
15	Madsen	max	+*	+*	+*	?	1
16	Gibson	sub	NR	NR	NR	+	+
18	Williams	sub	2×	−	2×*	2×	1
19	Jennings	sub	8×*	1	8×*	?	1
20	Fioretti	max	+*	+	+*	1	−
21	MCPMIgrp	sub	8×*	2×	3×*	3×*	1
22	Handler	sub	5×*	1	8×*	1	2×
23	SCOR	sub	1	2×	9×*	2×	3×
No. significant out of 13			7	2	8	3	2
No. reporting positively			10	8	10	7	7
No. reporting analysis			12	12	10	12	13
Postdischarge (11 institutional studies)							
1	Ericsson	sub	NR	4×	?	?	NR
2	Kentala	max	+	+	NR	NR	+*
3	Granath	sub	NR	2×*	2×	2×	NR
4	Smith	sub	NR	−	NR	NR	6×*
5	Hunt	sub	NR	1	NR	4×*	3×*
6	Stanford	max	NR	NR	+*	1	8×*
8	Koppes	max	?	?	?	?	?
11	Saunamaki	max	3×*	2×*	NR	NR	1
13	DeFeyter	max	NR	3×	+	2×	1
17	Norris	max	NR	NR	?	?	1
24	Jespersen	max	1	1	1	1	3×*
No. significant out of 11			1	2	1	1	5
No. reporting positively			2	5	3	3	5
No. reporting analysis			4	9	7	8	9

*Statistically significant.

negative 1.6 and 1.3 are used for significant and nonsignificant multivariate ratios, respectively.

Initial data analysis consisted of the construction of a correlation matrix consisting of Pearson product moment correlations for the risk ratios of the five exercise test responses with each of the following clinical variables: percent tested, percent females, percent of prior MI, percent with each Q-wave location, percent on digoxin, percent on a beta-blocking agent, percent subsequent mortality if tested, and percent mortality if not tested. Subsequently, if the correlation was greater than 0.30 between an exercise test response risk ratio and one of the above, they were selected for regression analysis. Regression was performed on each pair selected. In order to adjust for differences in sample size between studies (i.e., the results of a study with only 60 subjects should not have the same effect on decision analysis as a study with 120 patients), regression analysis was weighted by the number of patients exercise tested in each study. Resulting f-values were tested for confidence levels. Regression equations associated with a p-value equal to or less than 0.10 are reported. The correlations are listed on Table 6–7.

TABLE 6–6.
Studies Using Exercise Testing in Post-Myocardial Infarction Populations With Follow-up Divided Into Those With Exercise Testing Performed Submaximally and Maximally

INVESTIGATORS	EXERCISE TEST RISK MARKERS				
	BP	PVCs	EXCAP	ANGINA	ST
Submaximal Testing (14 institutional studies)					
1 Ericsson	NR	4×	?	?	NR
3 Granath	NR	2×*	2×	2×	NR
4 Smith	NR	–	NR	NR	6×*
5 Hunt	NR	1	NR	4×*	3×*
7 MHI	+*	+	+	NR	8×*
9 Starling	5×	2×	NR	4×	4×
10 Weld	5×*	2×*	19×*	2×	2×
12 Velasco	3×	2×	NR	3×*	4×*
16 Gibson	NR	NR	NR	+	+
18 Williams	2×	–	2×*	2×	1
19 Jennings	8×*	1	8×*	?	1
21 MCPMIgrp	8×*	2×	3×*	3×*	1
22 Handler	5×*	1	8×*	1	2×
23 SCOR	1	2×	9×*	2×	3×
No. significant out of 14	5	2	6	3	4
No. reporting positively	8	8	8	8	9
No. reporting analysis	9	13	9	10	12
Maximal Testing (10 institutional studies)					
2 Kentala	+	+	NR	NR	+*
6 Stanford	NR	NR	+*	1	8×*
8 Koppes	?	?	?	?	?
11 Saunamaki	3×*	2×*	NR	NR	1
13 DeFeyter	NR	3×	+	2×	1
14 Jelinek	–	NR	+	2×*	1
15 Madsen	+*	+*	+*	?	1
17 Norris	NR	NR	?	?	1
20 Fioretti	+*	+	+*	1	–
24 Jespersen	1	1	1	1	3×*
No. significant out of 10	3	2	3	1	3
No. reporting positively	4	5	5	2	3
No. reporting analysis	7	7	8	8	10

*Statistically significant.

TABLE 6–7.
Exercise Testing: Correlation Matrix

	% EX TESTED	% WOMEN	% PRIOR MI	% SE MI	% AMI	% IPMI	% ON DIG	% ON BB	MORTALITY IF ET DONE	MORTALITY IF NOT DONE	BP	EXERCISE TEST RISK MARKERS PVC	EXERCISE TEST RISK MARKERS EXCAP	EXERCISE TEST RISK MARKERS ANGINA
% women	.23													
% prior MI	.01	.37												
% SEMI	.51	.22	.04											
% ANTMI	−.39	−.15	.44	−.57										
% IPMI	−.32	−.45	.05	−.67	.07									
% Dig	.15	.04	.29	.25	−.06	−.21								
% BB	−.17	.22	.31	.35	.24	−.17	.10							
Mort if ET	.09	−.15		−.12	.08	.14	.39	−.26						
Mort no ET	.60*	.21	−.01	.39	.14	−.61	.33	.21	.38					
BP	−.13	.14	.42	−.08	.60	.18	−.03	.21	−.15	−.31				
PVC	.20	−.21	.38	−.53	.28	.09	.16	−.33	−.08	−.99	−.10			
ExCap	.04	.25	.28	−.65	.41	.46	.50	.00	−.15	−.45	.20	.23		
Angina	−.40	−.34	.14	−.39	.26	.19	.40	.34	.15	−.73*	.43	.48	.01	
ST	−.28	−.49*	.04	−.37	.20	.64*	−.35	−.33	−.18	−.68*	−.40	−.09	.13	.42

Key: % Ex tested—% of study population that underwent exercise test. % Women included in the study; MI %—the percentage of the types of MIs, which included: PR—prior MI; A—anterior Q-wave MI; I—inferior and/or posterior MI; SE—subendocardial or non-Q-wave MIs. % on . . .—the percentage of patients on digoxin (Dig) or a beta blocker (BB) at the time of treadmill testing. Mortality if ET done—in patients who underwent exercise testing; if not done—mortality in those excluded from exercise testing. BP—abnormal SBP response; PVCs—abnormal PVCs; ExCap—abnormally low exercise capacity; Angina—induced by test; ST—abnormal ST-segment response (usually only depression); *—statistically significant.

Figure 6–1 illustrates the number of patients in each study and the proportion who underwent exercise testing. Figure 6–2 compares the mortality rates in patients tested versus those not exercise tested in the studies reporting mortality information in both groups.

As part of meta-analysis, sign testing was applied to the findings in Table 6–3. Since it is not possible to ascertain the directions of the nonsignificant associations listed as "?" in Table 6–3, meta-analysis conclusions must be tentative. Some researchers probably did not evaluate markers that are not reported (NR), but others are likely to have failed to report null or negative findings. The most generous evaluation would be to omit studies that did not report results for a particular marker; the most conservative approach would be to include these studies and to assume that any unreported results were not positive associations. Results are presented for both situations with upper and lower bounds on the overall published results on exercise test markers as predictors of death.

If there were not a true underlying association of a risk marker with death, we would expect that 50% of studies would report positive association based on chance. "Statistical significance" is not considered here; only the directions of the *observed* associations. Using only studies with any reported effect as the denominator, the generous estimates of the percentages of positive associations reported for BP (12 centers reporting positive associations, 15 centers presenting any results for BP), PVCs (13/20), ExCap (12/14), angina (11/

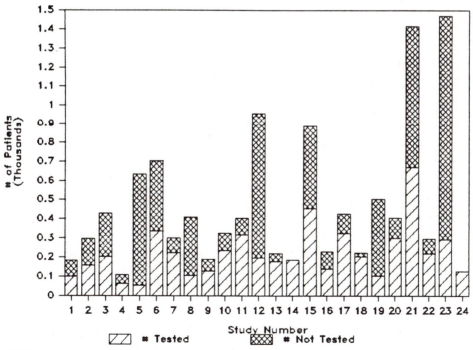

FIG 6–1.
Number in population and proportion exercise tested.

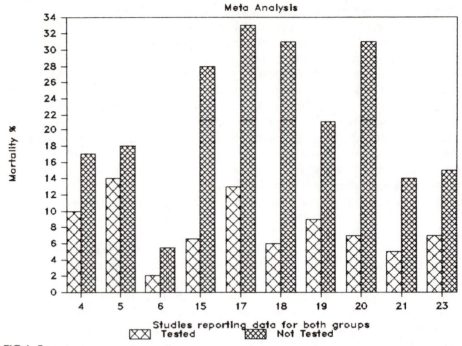

FIG 6–2.
Mortality in those exercise tested and in those excluded from testing in the studies giving data for both groups.

16), and ST (12/19) are 80%, 65%, 86%, 69%, and 63%, respectively. Only the *BP* and *exercise capacity* proportions are significantly different from chance by a sign test. The conservative estimates using all 24 studies as the denominator are 50%, 54%, 50%, 46%, and 50%, respectively. None of these are different from chance. Considering probable publishing bias against negative findings, the true situations are likely to be closer to the conservative computations than to the generous ones.

Subgrouping by predischarge testing (arbitrarily set at less than three weeks post-MI) and postdischarge testing (three weeks or greater) yielded the findings in Table 6–5. Note that all of the predictors except for ST shifts were reported positively more than 50% of the time during predischarge testing and not during postdischarge testing. To see if these differences were due to maximal or submaximal endpoints for exercise testing, Table 6–6 was constructed. Though during submaximal testing the exercise predictors were more likely to be associated with positivity than maximal testing, the finding was not as strong.

Subgrouping the studies by whether they were performed pre- or postdischarge (as done in Table 6–5) shows that the highest rate of positive predictors and the highest risk ratios occur with predischarge testing. Using only studies of predischarge exercise testing with any reported effect as the denominator, the generous estimates of the percentages of positive associations reported for BP (10 centers reporting positive associations/12 centers presenting any results for BP), PVCs (8/12), ExCap (10/10), angina (7/12), and ST (7/13) are 83%, 67%, 100%, 58%, and 54%, respectively. Only the BP and ExCap were significant, but none of the exercise test responses were significant for testing done postdischarge (50%, 56%, 43%, 38%, and 56%, respectively). In Table 6–6, the studies are divided into those that used maximal and those that used submaximal endpoints for exercise testing. Using only studies of submaximal exercise testing with any reported effect as the denominator, the generous estimates of the percentages of positive associations reported for BP (8 centers reporting positive associations/9 centers presenting any results for BP), PVCs (8/13), ExCap (8/9), angina (8/10), and ST (9/12) are 89%, 63%, 89%, 80%, and 75%, respectively. All exercise responses except for PVCs were significantly associated with a poor outcome with submaximal testing, and none of the exercise test responses with maximal testing were significant (57%, 71%, 63%, 25%, and 30%, respectively). Other exploratory subgroupings including American studies versus studies from other countries and selection of the "best" studies failed to identify test performance differences.

Under the criteria described for inclusion for regression analysis, 24 pairs of variables qualified for additional analysis. Of these pairs, only the following had weighted regressions with p values <.10: (1) percent mortality in those not tested was negatively related to ST (p = .06) and to angina (p = .10) risk ratios; (2) ST risk ratio was negatively related to the percent taking digoxin (p = .10). Additionally, ST risk ratio was negatively related to percent females in the studies and positively to the percent with inferior-posterior MIs, both with high confidence levels: p = .03 and .01, respectively. Lastly, the relationship between percent tested and percent mortality in those tested was examined; as the proportion of patients tested increased, mortality increased in those not tested. This relationship is significant at the .05 level of confidence. The most important relationships are presented in Figures 6–3, 6–4, and 6–5, which were directly produced by the graphic software.

Since meta-analysis tries to consider information from a pool of data (but at the study level, without actually pooling data), problems arise in comparing results from studies with different protocols. Differences in types of exercise tests, ECG leads used, and others increase the difficulties of summarizing the research by meta-analysis, particularly since effect sizes cannot be calculated from the data reported in many of the studies. Even though all of the published studies are considered, there is probably a serious publishing bias both by authors and editors toward excluding negative results. This occurs at two levels: completely negative studies may not get submitted or published and complete data on all risk markers evaluated may not be reported. Often not even the direction of a possible effect can be computed for a particular exercise test result.

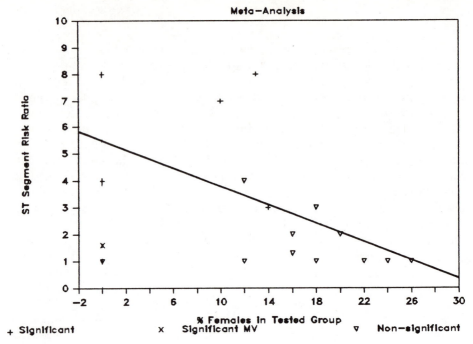

FIG 6–3.
Percent of women plotted against risk ratios for exercise-induced ST shifts in the studies.

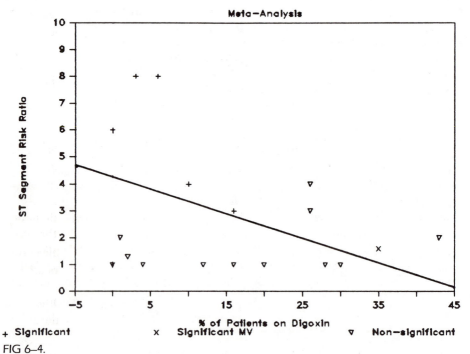

FIG 6–4.
Percent of patients taking digoxin plotted against the risk ratios for exercise-induced ST shifts in the studies.

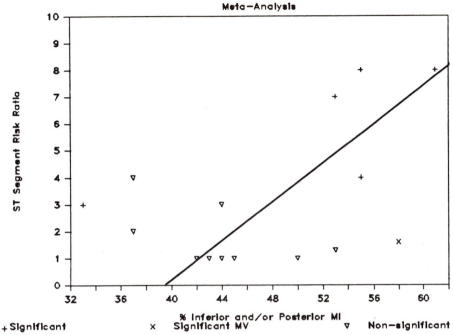

FIG 6–5.
Percent of patients with inferior-posterior Q wave MIs plotted against the risk ratios
for exercise-induced ST shifts in the studies.

SUMMARY

The benefits of performing an exercise test in MI patients are listed in Table 6–8. It
appears that submitting patients to exercise testing can expedite and optimize their
discharge from the hospital. Ventricular arrhythmias not present at rest can be provoked during exercise. The patient's reaction to physical exercise, the work capacity,
and limiting factors at the time of discharge can be assessed by the exercise test. An
exercise test prior to discharge is important for giving a patient guidelines for exercise
at home, reassuring him of his physical status, and determining his risk of complications. This provides a safe basis for advising the patient to resume or increase his or
her activity level and return to work. The test can demonstrate to the patient, the
relatives, and employer the effect of the MI on the capacity for physical performance.
Psychologically, it can cause an improvement in the patient's self-confidence by making the patient less anxious about daily physical activities. The test has been helpful
in reassuring spouses of post-MI patients of their physical capabilities. The psychological impact of performing well on the exercise test is impressive. Many patients increase their activity and actually rehabilitate themselves after being encouraged and
reassured by their response to this test. Its value for prognostication is less certain.

The angiographic studies correlating results with post-MI exercise testing involved
populations that were very selected. They particularly contain a higher prevalence of
patients with angina who are more likely to undergo angiography. In some studies, an
abnormal test result was considered to be angina and/or ST depression, and the results

TABLE 6–8.
Benefits of Exercise Testing Post Myocardial Infarction

Predischarge Submaximal Test

Setting safe exercise levels (exercise prescription)
Optimizing discharge
Altering medical therapy
Triaging for intensity of follow-up
First step in rehabilitation—assurance, encouragement
Reassuring spouse
Recognizing exercise-induced ischemia and dysrhythmias

Maximal Test for Return to Normal Activities

Determining limitations
Prognostication
Reassuring employers
Determining level of disability
Triaging for invasive studies
Deciding upon medications
Exercise prescription
Continued rehabilitation

for each response could not be separated. Few of these studies considered the other exercise test responses that have been associated with a poor prognosis. Review of the studies demonstrated a limited sensitivity and specificity for identification of patients with multivessel disease (MVD). Certainly the sensitivity for detecting those with left main and triple-vessel disease is higher but not 100%. On the other hand, the poor specificity could lead to more angiography than is necessary. This leads to unnecessary CABS since there is always the tendency to "do something," albeit the absence of data that survival is improved. Future studies must be designed that attempt to identify the angiographic subgroup post MI that would have improved survival if submitted to CABG or PTCA.

One consistent finding in the review of the 24 post-MI exercise test studies that included a follow-up for cardiac endpoints is that patients who met whatever criteria were set forth for exercise testing were at lower risk than patients not tested. This finding supports the clinical judgment of the skilled clinician. In the complete data set from the review, only an abnormal SBP response or a low exercise capacity were significantly associated with a poor outcome using the generous criteria. An argument could be made that neither an abnormal BP response nor a low exercise capacity are directly linked to the basic pathophysiological determinants of a poor prognosis. An abnormal BP response could indicate indirectly that much myocardium was lost due to prior MIs, a large anterior MI, or to dysfunction due to ischemia. A poor exercise capacity could be linked to a complicated MI that kept the patient bedridden longer than an uncomplicated MI. When the studies were subgrouped by whether testing was done pre- or postdischarge, a high proportion of predischarge test results indicated a poor outcome. This may mean that the risk predictors from exercise testing can only identify patients that die early post MI, i.e., before later testing can be done. Submaximal testing resulted in the highest proportion of positive associations and the highest risk ratios. This may mean that abnormal responses at higher work loads are not as predictive as those at lower work loads.

The correlations and regression analysis of risk ratios of the test responses to the prevalence of clinical features lead to other interesting hypotheses (Table 6–7). Surprisingly, the highest correlations for the exercise test risk markers were obtained with the mortality rate in the patients excluded from testing. The negative correlations indicate that the higher the mortality in those excluded, the less able are the exercise test responses to identify a high-risk group. Mortality in those excluded correlates directly with the percent exercise tested; the greater the percent tested out of an MI population, the higher the risk for death in those excluded. However, neither the percent tested nor the mortality in those tested correlated well with the exercise test results. Therefore, the more skilled the clinician is at selecting a high-risk group and excluding them from exercise testing, the poorer the exercise test functions for identifying high-risk patients because of the characteristics of the population who remain to be tested. One hypothesis from these results is that the exercise test is most useful for risk stratification in a setting where good clinicians are not available.

Other significant weighted regressions included the relationships between the risk ratios for ST-segment shifts and percent women, percent of patients receiving digoxin, and percent of patients recovering from an inferior-posterior Q-wave MI (Figures 6–3, 6–4, and 6–5). The first two were negative correlations, and so the ST response generated a higher risk in studies that included a lower percentage of women or a lower percentage of patients receiving digoxin. In studies that included a higher percentage of patients with inferior MIs, the ST-segment response was better able to identify a high-risk group.

The following were not statistically significant but had high correlations. The risk ratio for an abnormal BP response and a poor exercise capacity is higher when more patients with anterior Q-wave MIs are tested. The risk ratio for all exercise test responses except BP are low in patients with non-Q-wave MIs. This is most likely due to the association of prior MIs in these patients.

It could be hypothesized that the ST-segment response functions as a risk predictor in male patients not taking digoxin. Also, the ST-segment response functions well as a risk predictor in patients with inferior Q-wave MIs and not in patients with anterior Q-wave MIs. It has recently been shown that ST-segment depression indicates ischemia as detected by thallium scintigraphy in patients with inferior but not anterior Q-wave MIs. The poor response of the exercise test in studies with a high percentage of non-Q-wave MIs was probably due to the same association with prior MIs that confused the results of studies of the prognosis of non-Q-wave MIs. A high priority should be given to determining if the exercise test is the best method of identifying which of the non-Q-wave MI patients has "uncompleted" MIs.

Who should undergo coronary angiography post MI for consideration of CABS to improve survival? By working backward through known associations and relationships, the clinical description of the high-risk patient who potentially could have improved survival with CABS can be derived. The randomized trials of CABS have demonstrated that patients with triple-vessel or left main disease with an EF of 30% to 50% have improved survival with surgery as compared to medical therapy. Although coronary heart disease can cause myocardial fibrosis and decreased ventricular function without overt MIs by signs or symptoms, this is unusual. Studies have shown 15% to 25% of MIs are silent, but in these cases the diagnosis was made by the electrocardiogram. The clinical picture, either by history or by ECG, that would result in an EF from 30% to 50% would include patients with large anterior MIs, a history or ECG pattern of multiple MIs, transmural MIs followed by subendocardial MIs, or a history of transient congestive heart failure with an MI. In addition, physical findings of ventricular dyskinesia or cardiomegaly on palpation would support this. Thus, clinical and electrocardiographic features predict those with decreased ventricular function. Noninvasive testing (i.e., radionuclide ventriculography and echocardiography) could also be utilized. Although its sensitivity is decreased in one- or two-vessel disease, the exercise ECG is approximately 90% sensitive for triple-vessel or left main disease. Angina is also common in this group of patients. Therefore, the following profile identifies the high-risk patient after an MI who should undergo coronary angiography: the patient with a history or ECG findings of a large anterior MI, and/or multiple MIs, and/or abnormal precordial movements, and/or a history of transient congestive heart failure, and signs and symptoms of severe myocardial ischemia on the exercise test. Severe ischemia is characterized by the occurrence of ST-segment depression and/or angina at a double product less than 20,000 and less than 5 METs exercise capacity. If there are no contraindications to CABS in these patients, they should be considered for coronary angiography. Post-MI patients who should be considered for reasons other than improved survival are those whose angina is not controlled satisfactorily with medications and those in whom either the diagnosis of MI or the etiology of chest pain post-MI is uncertain. This "logical" algorithm requires validation.

Radionuclide Testing.   The conclusion from review of exercise nuclear cardiological studies is that they do not appear to offer a definite advantage over routine exercise testing. Certainly, the mixed results obtained using the nuclear techniques are not anywhere as extensive as the data reviewed for standard methods of exercise testing. In addition, they are not superior methodologically and suffer from the same design problems.

Higher Technology.   Certain tests may give a more direct measurement that otherwise is dependent upon multiple pieces of clinical information. By being more direct, this test result may avoid the problems with interaction and, though being more expensive than standard clinical measures, be justified because it simplifies prediction. An example of this may be the radionuclide ejection fraction (EF). An important marker of prognosis is how much myocardium is left. This is determined by prior MIs, other heart disease, the size of the current MI, and whether congestive heart failure or cardiogenic shock occurs. In one simple measurement, the radionuclide ejection fraction may give this information directly rather than the indirect sum of the clinical markers that often have many interactions. However, radionuclide EF can be complicated by the fact that myocardium may be stunned initially and subsequently improve and by inaccuracies in its measurements. Exercise EF hypothetically could combine the impact of ischemia with damage due to scarring, but there is only conflicting and limited data suggesting that it has more predictive power than routine exercise testing.

Design of Future Studies.   Prior studies using standard exercise testing have not been successful because interactions between the clinical characteristics and the exercise responses have not been considered. Also, the pathophysiological determinants of risk have not been properly related to exercise test responses. Exercise test responses function differently as risk predictors in the various clinical subsets of post-MI patients; that is, they interact with clinical markers. The most important interactions could be accounted for by classifying exercise test responses as being due to either myocardial dysfunction or ischemia, which are the pathophysiological basis for patient outcome. In order to clarify this problem, clinical and exercise test data must be analyzed considering temporal changes in both endpoints and predictive power, interaction of clinical and exercise test variables, censored data problems, survival analyses, and multivariate modelling techniques. Using these techniques, it would be possible to determine whether exercise testing adds to the predictive power of the clinical variables and if so, which of the sets of data provides the greatest discrimination. An algorithm based on clinical and exercise test data could be developed to optimize the care of patients who have sustained an acute myocardial infarction. Simplified multivariate equations that incorporate clinically relevant sets of information could be developed for prediction of risk.

An important form of interaction is that of a prior MI, both in how it affects the ECG and ventricular function. Recursive partitioning is one form of multivariate analysis that considers interaction and should be applied in future studies. Further refinement of the design and analyses of studies in this research area may help to finally resolve some of the issues discussed here. In particular, various exercise test markers may be important in certain subsets of patients. Validation of any algorithms developed should be done on subsequent "test" sets of patients. Reports of classification errors only on the "training" set used to develop the algorithm are not sufficient to evaluate the usefulness of the prediction procedure.

BIBLIOGRAPHY

Adams K, Perry JR, Popio K, et al: Positive treadmill stress tests post myocardial infarction in patients with single-vessel coronary disease. *Am Heart J* 1985;109:251–258.

Ahnve S, Gilpin E, Madsen E, et al: Prognostic importance of QTc interval at discharge after acute myocardial infarction: A multicenter study of 865 patients. *Am Heart J* 1984;108:395–400.

Ahnve S, Savvides M, Abouantoun S, et al: Can ischemia be recognized when Q-waves are present on the resting electrocardiogram? *Am Heart J* 1986;110:1016–1020.

Akhras F, Upward J, Keates J, et al: Early exercise testing and elective coronary artery bypass surgery after uncomplicated myocardial infarction. Effect on morbidity and mortality. *Br Heart J* 1984;52:413–417.

Angelhed J-E, Thorvald IB, Ejdeback J, et al: Computer aided exercise electrocardiographic testing and coronary arteriography in patients with angina pectoris and with myocardial infarction. *Br Heart J* 1984;52:140–146.

Atterhog J-H, Ekelund L-G, Kaijser L: Electrocardiographic abnormalities during exercise 3 weeks to 18 months after anterior myocardial infarction. *Br Heart J* 1971;33:871–877.

Bamrah VS, Ryan PA, Ptacin MJ, et al: Value of exercise electrocardiography to predict additional jeopardized myocardial regions remote from site of previous myocardial infarction. *Clin Cardiol* 1985;8:391–398.

Baron DB, Licht JR, Ellestad MH: Status of exercise stress testing after myocardial infarction. *Arch Intern Med* 1984;144:595–601.

Bhatnagar SK, Hudak A, Al-Yusuf AR: Left ventricular thrombosis, wall motion abnormalities, and blood viscosity changes after first transmural anterior myocardial infarction. *Chest* 1985;88:40–44.

Bhatnagar SK, Moussa MAA, Al-Yusuf AR: The role of prehospital discharge two-dimensional echocardiography in determining the prognosis of survivors of first myocardial infarction. *Am Heart J* 1985;109:472–477.

Borer JS, Rosing DR, Miller RH, et al: Natural history of LVEF during one year after acute MI: comparison with clinical, ECG, and biochemical determinations. *Am J Cardiol* 1980;46:1–12.

Boschat J, Rigaud M, Bardet J, et al: Treadmill exercise testing and coronary cineangiography following first myocardial infarction. *J Cardiac Rehabil* 1981;1:206–211.

Brush JE, Brand DA, Acampora D, et al: Use of the initial electrocardiogram to predict in-hospital complications of acute myocardial infarction. *N Engl J Med* 1985;312:1137–1141.

Cain HD, Frasher WG, Stivelman R: Graded activity program for safe return to self-care after myocardial infarction. *JAMA* 1961;177:111–120.

Castellanet MJ, Greenberg PS, Ellestad MH: Comparison of S-T segment changes on exercise testing with angiographic findings in patients with prior myocardial infarction. *Am J Cardiol* 1978;42:29–35.

Chaitman BR, Waters DD, Corbara F, et al: Prediction of multivessel disease after inferior myocardial infarction. *Circulation* 1978;57:1085–1090.

Cobelli F, Opasich C, Griffo R, et al: Short-term reproducibility of ergometric parameters in functional stress test after recent myocardial infarction. *Cardiology* 1983;70:161–170.

Cohn PF: The role of noninvasive cardiac testing after an uncomplicated myocardial infarction. *N Engl J Med* 1983;309:90–93.

Connolly DC, Elveback LR: Coronary heart disease in residents of Rochester, Minnesota. VI. Hospital and posthospital course of patients with transmural and subendocardial myocardial infarction. *Mayo Clin Proc* 1985;60:375–381.

Crean PA, Waters DD, Bosch X, et al: Angiographic findings after myocardial infarction in patients with previous bypass surgery: explanations for smaller infarcts in this group compared with control patients. *Circulation* 1985;71:693–698.

Davidson DM, DeBusk RF: Prognostic value of a single exercise test 3 weeks after uncomplicated myocardial infarction. *Circulation* 1980;61:236–241.

De Feyter PJ, van den Brand M, Serruys PW, et al: Early angiography after myocardial infarction: What have we learned? *Am Heart J* 1985;109:194–199.

De Feyter PJ, vanEenige MJ, Dighton DH, et al: Exercise testing early after myocardial infarction: Detection of multivessel coronary arterial disease and extent of left ventricular dysfunction six to eight weeks after infarction using a 12-lead exercise electrocardiogram. *Chest* 1983;83:853–859.

De Feyter PJ, van Eenige MJ, Dighton DH, et al: Prognostic value of exercise testing, coronary angiography and left ventriculography 6–8 weeks after myocardial infarction. *Circulation* 1982;66:527–536.

DeBusk RF, Dennis CA: "Submaximal" predischarge exercise testing after acute myocardial infarction: Who needs it? *Am J Cardiol* 1985;55:499–500.

DeBusk RF, Kraemer HC, Nash E, et al: Stepwise risk stratification after acute MI. *Am J Cardiol* 1983;52:1161–1166.

Deckers JW, Fioretti P, Brower RW, et al: Ineligibility for predischarge exercise testing after myocardial infarction in the elderly: Implications for prognosis. *Eur Heart J* 1984;5:97–100.

Deering TF, Weiner DA: Prognosis of patients with coronary artery disease. *J Cardiopulmonary Rehabil* 1985;5:325–331.

Denniss AR, Baaijens H, Cody DV, et al: Value of programmed stimulation and exercise testing in predicting one-year mortality after acute myocardial infarction. *Am J Cardiol* 1985;56:213–220.

Dillahunt PH, Miller AB: Early treadmill testing after myocardial infarction. *Chest* 1979;76:150–155.

Dwyer EM, McMaster P, Greenberg H: Nonfatal cardiac events and recurrent infarction in the year after acute myocardial infarction. *J Am Coll Cardiol* 1984;4:695–702.

Epstein S, Palmeri ST, Patterson RE: Evaluation of patients after acute myocardial infarction: Indications for cardiac catheterization and surgical intervention. *N Engl J Med* 1982;307:1487–1492.

Ericsson M, Granath A, Ohlsen P, et al: Arrhythmias and symptoms during treadmill testing three weeks after myocardial infarction in 100 patients. *Br Heart J* 1973;35:787–790.

Ewart CK, Taylor CB, Reese LB, et al: Effects of early postmyocardial infarction exercise testing on self-perception and subsequent physical activity. *Am J Cardiol* 1983;51:1076–1080.

Fioretti P, Brower RW, Simoons ML, et al: Relative value of clinical variables, bicycle ergometry, rest radionuclide ventriculography, and 24 hour ambulatory electrocardiographic monitoring at discharge to predict 1 year survival after myocardial infarction. *J Am Coll Cardiol* 1986;8:40–49.

Fioretti P, Brower RW, Simoons ML, et al: Prediction of mortality during the first year after acute myocardial infarction from clinical variables and stress test at hospital discharge. *Am J Cardiol* 1985;55:1313–1318.

Fioretti P, Brower RW, Simoons ML, et al: Prediction of mortality in hospital survivors of myocardial infarction. Comparison of predischarge exercise testing and radionuclide ventriculography at rest. *Br Heart J* 1984;52:292–298.

Fioretti P, Deckers JW, Brower RW, et al: Predischarge stress test after myocardial infarction in old age: results and prognostic value. *Eur Heart J* 1984;5:101–104.

Froelicher VF, Perdue S, Atwood JE, et al: Exercise testing of patients recovering from myocardial infarction. *Curr Probl Cardiol* 1986;11:370–444.

Froelicher VF, Wolthius R, Keiser N, et al: Comparison of several bipolar leads to V5. *Chest* 1976;70:611–616.

Fuller CM, Raizner AE, Verani MS, et al: Early post-myocardial infarction treadmill stress testing: An accurate predictor of multivessel coronary disease and subsequent cardiac events. *Ann Intern Med* 1981;94:734–739.

Gash AK, Warner HF, Zadrozny JH, et al: Electrocardiographic ST-T wave patterns, extent of coronary artery disease, and left ventricular performance following non-Q-wave myocardial infarction. *Cathet Cardiovasc Diagn* 1985;11:223–33.

Gewirtz H, Horacek BM, Wolf HK, et al: Mechanism of persistent S-T segment elevation after anterior myocardial infarction. *Am J Cardiol* 1979;44:1269–1275.

Gibson RS, Watson DD, Craddock GB, et al: Prediction of cardiac events after uncomplicated myocardial infarction: A prospective study comparing predischarge exercise thallium-201 scintigraphy and coronary angiography. *Circulation* 1983;68:321–336.

Gilpin E, Olshen R, Henning H, et al: Risk prediction after myocardial infarction: Comparison of three multivariate methodologies. *Cardiology* 1983;70:73–84.

Glass GV, McGaw B, Smith ML: Meta-analysis in social research. Beverly Hills, Sage Publications, 1981.

Goldschlager N: Treadmill exercise testing soon after acute myocardial infarction. *Cardiovasc Rev Rep* 1980;1(5):397–400.

Granath A, Sodermark T, Winge T, et al: Early work load tests for evaluation of long-term prognosis of acute myocardial infarction. *Br Heart J* 1977;39:758–763.

Haines DE, Beller GA, Watson DD, et al: A prospective clinical, scintigraphic, angiographic and functional evaluation of patients after inferior mycoardial infarction with and without right ventricular dysfunction. *J Am Coll Cardiol* 1985;6:995–1003.

Hamm LF, Stull A, Crow RS: Exercise testing early after myocardial infarction: historic perspective and current uses. *Prog Cardiovasc Dis* 1986;28:463–476.

Hamm LF, Stull GA, Ainsworth B, et al: Short- and long-term prognostic value of graded exercise testing soon after myocardial infarction. *J Am Phys Ther Assoc* 1986;66:334–339.

Handler CE: Exercise testing to identify high-risk patients after myocardial infarction. *J R Coll Physicians Lond* 1984;18:124–127.

Handler CE: Submaximal predischarge exercise testing after myocardial infarction: Prognostic value and limitations. *Eur Heart J* 1985;6:510–517.

Handler CE, Sowton E: Diurnal variation and reproducibility of predischarge submaximal exercise testing after myocardial infarction. *Br Heart J* 1984;52:299–303.

Handler CE, Sowton E: A comparison of the Naughton and modified Bruce treadmill exercise protocols in their ability to detect ischaemic abnormalities six weeks after myocardial infarction. *Eur Heart J* 1984;5:752–755.

Handler CE, Sowton E: Diurnal variation in symptom-limited exercise test responses six weeks after myocardial infarction. *Eur Heart J* 1985;6:444–450.

Handler CE, Sowton E: Stress testing predischarge and six weeks after myocardial infarction to compare submaximal and maximal exercise predischarge and to assess the reproducibility of induced abnormalities. *Int J Cardiol* 1985;9:173–187.

Haskell WL, DeBusk R: Cardiovascular responses to repeated treadmill exercise testing soon after myocardial infarction. *Circulation* 1979;60:1247–1251.

Haskell WL, Savin W, Oldridge N, et al: Factors influencing estimated oxygen uptake during exercise testing soon after myocardial infarction. *Am J Cardiol* 1982;50:299–304.

Hunt D, Hamer A, Duffield A, et al: Predictors of reinfarction and sudden death in a high-risk group of acute myocardial infarction survivors. *Lancet* 1979;1:233–236.

Ibsen H, Kjoller E, Styperek J, et al: Routine exercise ECG three weeks after acute myocardial infarction. *Acta Med Scand* 1975;198:463–469.

Jaarsma W, Visser CA, Funke AJ, et al: Usefulnes of two-dimensional exercise echocardiography shortly after myocardial infarction. *Am J Cardiol* 1986;57:86–90.

Jelinek VM: Exercise testing after myocardial infarction. *Aust NZ J Med* 1985;15:392–395.

Jelinek VM, McDonald IG, Ryan WF, et al: Assessment of cardiac risk 10 days after uncomplicated myocardial infarction. *Br Med J* 1982;284:227–230.

Jelinek VM, Ziffer RW, McDonald IG, et al: Early exercise testing and mobilization after myocardial infarction. *Med J Aust* 1977;2:589–593.

Jennings K, Reid DS, Hawkins T, et al: Role of exercise testing early after myocardial infarction in identifying candidates for coronary surgery. *Br Med J* 1984;288:185–187.

Jespersen CM, Kassis E, Edeling CJ, et al: The prognostic value of maximal exercise testing soon after first MI. *Eur Heart J* 1985;6:769–772.

Kelbaek H, Eskildsen P, Hansen PF, et al: Spontaneous and/or training-induced haemodynamic changes after myocardial infarction. *Int J Cardiol* 1981;1:205–213.

Kelly D: Clinical decisions in patients following myocardial infarction. *Curr Probl Cardiol* 1985;10:1–45.

Kentala E: Physical fitness and feasibility of physical rehabilitation after myocardial infarction in men of working age. *Ann Clin Res* 1972;(Suppl)4:9.

Kentala E, Pyorala K, Heikkila J, et al: Factors related to long-term prognosis following acute myocardial infarction: Importance of left ventricular function. *Scand J Rehabil Med* 1975;7:118–124.

Kentala E, Repo UK: Sudden death after myocardial infarction and T-wave changes in connection with exercise testing. *Ann Clin Res* 1983;15:109–112.

Kentala E, Sarna S: Sudden death and factors related to long-term prognosis following acute myocardial infarction. *Scand J Rehabil* 1976;8:27–32.

Koppes GM, Kruyer W, Beckmann CH, et al: Response to exercise early after uncomplicated acute myocardial infarction in patients receiving no medication: Long-term follow-up. *Am J Cardiol* 1980;46:764–769.

Kramer N, Susmano A, Shekelle RB: The "false negative" treadmill exercise test and left ventricular dysfunction. *Circulation* 1978;57:763–768.

Krone RJ, Gillespie JA, Weld FM, et al: Low-level exercise testing after myocardial infarction: Usefulness in enhancing clinical risk stratification. *Circulation* 1985;71:80–89.

Lindvall K, Erhardt LR, Lundman T, et al: Early mobilization and discharge of patients with acute myocardial infarction. *Acta Med Scand* 1979;206:169–175.

Luria MH, Debanne SM, Osman MI: Long-term follow-up after recovery from acute myocardial infarction. *Arch Intern Med* 1985;145:1592–1595.

Madsen EB, Gilpin E: How much prognostic information do exercise test data add to clinical data after acute myocardial infarction. *Int J Cardiol* 1983;4:15–27.

Madsen EB, Gilpin E: Prognostic value of exercise test variables after myocardial infarction. *J Cardiol Rehabil* 1983;3:481–488.

Madsen EB, Gilpin E, Ahnve S, et al: Prediction of functional capacity and use of exercise testing for predicting risk after acute myocardial infarction. *Am J Cardiol* 1985;56:839–845.

Madsen EB, Gilpin E, Henning H: Short-term prognosis in acute myocardial infarction: Evaluation of different prediction methods. *Am Heart J* 1984;107:1241–1251.

Madsen EB, Gilpin E, Henning H, et al: Prediction of late mortality after myocardial infarction from variables measured at different times during hospitalization. *Am J Cardiol* 1984;53:47–54.

Madsen EB, Hougaard P, Gilpin E: Dynamic evaluation of prognosis from time-dependent variables in acute myocardial infarction. *Am J Cardiol* 1983;51:1579–1583.

Maisel AS, Ahnve S, Gilpin E, et al: Prognosis after extension of myocardial infarct: The role of Q-wave or non-Q-wave infarction. *Circulation* 1985;71:211–217.

Maisel AS, Gilpin E, Hoit B, et al: Survival after hospital discharge in matched populations with inferior or anterior myocardial infarction. *J Am Coll Cardiol* 1985;6:731–736.

Maisel AS, Scott N, Gilpin E, et al: Complex ventricular arrhythmias in patients with Q-wave versus non-Q-wave myocardial infarction. *Circulation* 1985;72:963–970.

Markiewicz W, Houston N, DeBusk RF: Exercise testing soon after myocardial infarction. *Circulation* 1977;56:26–31.

May GS, Eberlein KA, Furberg CD, et al: Secondary prevention after myocardial infarction: A review of long-term trials. *Prog Cardiovasc Dis* 1982;24:331–352.

May GS, Furberg CD, Eberlein KA, et al: Secondary prevention after myocardial infarction: A review of short-term acute phase trials. *Prog Cardiovasc Dis* 1983;25:335–359.

McKirnan MD, Sullivan M, Jensen D, et al: Treadmill performance and cardiac function in selected patients with coronary heart disease. *J Am Coll Cardiol* 1984;3:253–261.

Mirvis DM, Wilson JL, Ramanthan KB: Effects of experimental myocardial infarction on the ST-segment response to tachycardia. *J Am Coll Cardiol* 1985;6:665–673.

Morris DD, Rozanski A, Berman DS, et al: Noninvasive prediction of the angiographic extent of coronary artery disease after myocardial infarction: comparison of clinical bicycle exercise, electrocardiographic and ventriculographic parameters. *Circulation* 1984;70:192–201.

Niederberger M: Values and limitations of exercise testing after myocardial infarction (monograph). Wien, Verlag Bruder Hollinek, 1977, pp 3–45.

Norris RM, Barnaby PF, Brandt PWT, et al: Prognosis after recovery from first acute myocardial infarction: Determinants of reinfarction and sudden death. *Am J Cardiol* 1984;53:408–413.

Norris RM, Mercer CJ, Deeming LW, et al: Coronary prognostic index for predicting survival after recovery from acute myocardial infarction. *Lancet* 1970;2:485–488.

Paine TD, Dye LE, Roitman DI, et al: Relation of graded exercise test findings after myocardial infarction to extent of coronary artery disease and left ventricular dysfunction. *Am J Cardiol* 1978;42:716–723.

Pardaens J, Lesaffre E, Willems JL, et al: Multivariate survival analysis for the assessment of prognostic factors and risk categories after recovery from acute myocardial infarction: the Belgian situation. *Am J Epidemiol* 1985;122:805–819.

Podczeck A, Frohner K, Foderler G, et al: Exercise testing in patients over 65 years of age after the first myocardial infarction. *Eur Heart J* 1984;5:89–92.

Pool J, Scheffer MG, Simoons ML, et al: Clinical value of exercise testing in elderly patients. *Eur Heart J* 1984;Suppl E:47–50.

Project Coronary Drug Group Research: The prognostic importance of the electrocardiogram after myocardial infarction. *Ann Intern Med* 1982;77:677–689.

Project Coronary Drug Group Research: The natural history of coronary heart disease: prognostic factors after recovery from myocardial infarction in 2,789 men. *Circulation* 1982;66:401–414.

Roberts JM, Sullivan M, Froelicher VF, et al: Predicting oxygen uptake from treadmill testing in normal subjects and coronary artery disease patients. *Am Heart J* 1984;108:1454–1460.

Roy D, Marchand E, Theroux P, et al: Programmed ventricular stimulation in survivors of an acute myocardial infarction. *Circulation* 1985;72:487–494.

Sami M, Kraemer H, DeBusk RF: The prognostic significance of serial exercise testing after myocardial infarction. *Circulation* 1979;60:1238–1246.

Sammel NL, Wilson RL, Norris RM, et al: Angiocardiography and exercise testing at one month after a first myocardial infarction. *Aust NZ J Med* 1980;10:182–187.

Sanz G, Castaner A, Betriu A, et al: Determinants of prognosis in survivors of myocardial infarction: A prospective clinical angiographic study. *N Engl J Med* 1982;306:1065–1070.

Saunamaki KI: The role of exercise testing soon after acute myocardial infarction. *Int Rehabil Med* 1983;5:192–196.

Saunamaki KI: Early post-myocardial infarction exercise testing in subjects 70 years or more of age: Functional and prognostic evaluation. *Eur Heart J* 1984;5:93–96.

Saunamaki KI, Andersen JD: Early exercise test in the assessment of long-term prognosis after acute myocardial infarction. *Acta Med Scand* 1981;209:185–191.

Saunamaki KI, Andersen JD: Post-myocardial infarction exercise testing: Clinical significance of a left ventricular function index and ventricular arrhythmias, a prospective study. *Acta Med Scand* 1985;218:277–278.

Saunamaki KI, Anderson JD: Early exercise test vs. clinical variables in the long-term prognostic management after myocardial infarction. *Acta Med Scand* 1982;212:47–52.

Saunamaki KI, Anderson JD: Prognostic significance of the ST-segment response during exercise testing shortly after acute myocardial infarction. Comparisons with other exercise variables. *Eur Heart J* 1983;4:752–760.

Schwartz KM, Turner JD, Sheffield LT, et al: Limited exercise testing soon after myocardial infarction: Correlation with early coronary and left ventricular angiography. *Ann Intern Med* 1981;94:727–734.

Shephard RJ: Exercise testing after myocardial infarction: A critical perspective. *Prac Cardiol* 1983;9:197–220.

Sia STB, MacDonald PS, Horowitz JD, et al: Usefulness of early exercise testing after non-Q-wave myocardial infarction in predicting prognosis. *Am J Cardiol* 1986;57:738–744.

Sivarajan ES, Bruce RA, Lindskog BD, et al: Treadmill test responses to an early exercise program after myocardial infarction: A randomized study. *Circulation* 1982;65:1420–1428.

Smith JW, Dennis CA, Gassmann A, et al: Exercise testing three weeks after myocardial infarction. *Chest* 1979;75:12–16.

Srinivasan M, Young A, Baker G, et al: The value of postcardiac infarction exercise stress testing: Identification of a group at high risk. *Med J Aust* 1981;2:466–467.

Starling MR, Crawford MH, Kennedy GT, et al: Exercise testing early after myocardial infarction: Predictive value of subsequent unstable angina and death. *Am J Cardiol* 1980;46:909–914.

Starling MR, Crawford MH, Kennedy GT, et al: Treadmill exercise tests predischarge and six weeks post-myocardial infarction to detect abnormalities of known prognostic value. *Ann Intern Med* 1981;94:721–727.

Starling MR, Crawford MH, O'Rourke RA: Superiority of selected treadmill exercise protocols predischarge and six weeks postinfarction for detecting ischemic abnormalities. *Am Heart J* 1982;104:1054–1059.

Starling MR, Crawford MH, Richards KL, et al: Predictive value of early postmyocardial infarction modified treadmill exercise testing in multivessel coronary artery disease detection. *Am Heart J* 1981;102:169–175.

Starling MR, Kennedy GT, Crawford MH, et al: Comparative predictive value of ST-segment depression or angina during early and repeat postinfarction exercise tests. *Chest* 1984;86:845–849.

Sullivan ID, Davies DW, Sowton E: Submaximal exercise testing early after myocardial infarction: Prognostic importance of exercise induced ST-segment elevation. *Br Heart J* 1984;52:147–153.

Tavazzi L, Giordano A: Exercise haemodynamics in patients over 65 years of age with recent myocardial infarction. *Eur Heart J* 1984;5:85–87.

Taylor CB, Bandura A, Ewart CK, et al: Exercise testing to enhance wives' confidence in their husbands' cardiac capability soon after clinically uncomplicated acute myocardial infarction. *Am J Cardiol* 1985;55:635–638.

Teo KK, Hsu L, Ramanaden I, et al: Cardiovascular responses to early exercise in inferior wall ST acute myocardial infarction. *Am J Cardiol* 1985;55:1277–1281.

Theroux P, Marpole DGF, Bourassa MG: Exercise stress testing in the post-myocardial infarction patient. *Am J Cardiol* 1983;52:664–667.

Theroux P, Waters DD, Halphen C, et al: Prognostic value of exercise testing soon after myocardial infarction. *N Engl J Med* 1979;301:341–345.

Torkelson LO: Rehabilitation of the patient with acute myocardial infarction. *J Chron Dis* 1964;17:685–704.

Tran ZV, Weltman A: Differential effects of exercise serum lipid and lipoprotein levels seen with changes in body weight. *JAMA* 1985;254:919–924.

Tzivoni D, Gottlieb S, Keren A, et al: Early right atrial pacing after myocardial infarction. I. Comparison with early treadmill testing. *Am J Cardiol* 1984;53:414–417.

van der Wall EE, Eenige van MJ, Visser FC, et al: Thallium-201 exercise testing in patients 6–8 weeks after myocardial infarction: Limited value for the detection of multivessel disease. *Eur Heart J* 1985;6:29–36.

Veenbrink WG, Van Der Werf T, Westerhof PW, et al: Is there an indication for coronary angiography in patients under 60 years of age with no or minimal angina pectoris after a first myocardial infarction? *Br Heart J* 1985;53:30–35.

Velasco J, Tormo V, Ferrer LM, et al: Early exercise test for evaluation of long-term prognosis after uncomplicated myocardial infarction. *Eur Heart J* 1981;2:401–407.

Waters DA, Bosch X, Bouchard A, et al: Comparison of clinical variables and variables derived from a limited predischarge exercise test as predictors of early and late mortality after myocardial infarction. *J Am Coll Cardiol* 1985;5:1–8.

Weiner DA: Prognostic value of exercise testing early after myocardial infarction. *J Cardiac Rehabil* 1983;3:114–122.

Weiner DA, McCabe C, Klein MD, et al: ST-segment changes post-infarction: Predictive value for multivessel coronary disease and left ventricular aneurysm. *Circulation* 1978;58:887–891.

Weld FM: Exercise testing after myocardial infarction. *J Cardiac Rehabil* 1985;5:20–27.

Weld FM, Chu K-L, Bigger JT, et al: Risk stratification with low-level exercise testing two weeks after acute myocardial infarction. *Circulation* 1981;64:306–314.

Wenger NK, Hellerstein HK, Blackburn H, et al: Uncomplicated myocardial infarction. *JAMA* 1973;224:511–514.

Williams WL, Nair RC, Higginson LA, et al: Comparison of clinical and treadmill variables for the prediction of outcome after myocardial infarction. *J Am Coll Cardiol* 1984;4:477–486.

Wohl AJ, Lewis HR, Campbell W, et al: Cardiovascular function during early recovery from acute myocardial infarction. *Circulation* 1977;56:931–937.

Zohman LR, Young JL, Kattus AA: Treadmill walking protocol for the diagnostic evaluation and exercise programming of cardiac patients. *Am J Cardiol* 1983;51:1081–1086.

7 SPECIAL APPLICATIONS: SCREENING APPARENTLY HEALTHY INDIVIDUALS

Screening can be defined as the presumptive identification of unrecognized disease by the utilization of procedures that can be applied rapidly. The relative value of techniques for identifying individuals who have asymptomatic or latent coronary heart disease (CHD) should be assessed in order to optimally and cost effectively direct secondary preventive efforts toward those with disease. After technological advances, interventional invasive catheterization could also be applied in individuals with silent disease if the benefits can be proven to outweigh the risks.

Eight criteria have been proposed for the selection of a screening procedure: (1) the procedure is acceptable and appropriate; (2) the quantity and/or quality of life can be favorably altered; (3) the results of intervention outweigh any adverse effects; (4) the target disease has an asymptomatic period during which its outcome can be altered; (5) acceptable treatments are available; (6) the prevalence and seriousness of the disease justify the costs of intervention; (7) the procedure is relatively easy and inexpensive; and, (8) sufficient resources are available. In addition, seven guides have been recommended for deciding whether a community screening program does more harm than good: (1) has the program's effectiveness been demonstrated in a randomized trial, and if so, (2) are efficacious treatments available? (3) does the current burden of suffering warrant screening? (4) is there a good screening test? (5) does the program reach those who could benefit from it? (6) can the health care system cope with the screening program? (7) will those who had a positive screening comply with subsequent advice and interventions?

Since it will be some time before the primary prevention of coronary heart disease is a reality, it is advisable to evaluate screening methods for detection prior to death or disability. As will be presented, risk-factor screening and resting techniques including the ECG have limited sensitivity, and so exercise testing, which brings out abnormalities not present at rest, deserves consideration. Various techniques have been recommended to improve the sensitivity and specificity of exercise testing such as new computerized and noncom-

266

puterized electrocardiographic criteria, other exercise test responses, cardiac radionuclide procedures, systolic time intervals, cardiokymography, cardiac fluoroscopy, digital radiographic imaging, and the computerized application of Bayesian statistics using risk factors and risk markers. These techniques may improve attempts to screen for latent coronary heart disease. Limited data suggest that angiographically documented asymptomatic coronary disease has a relatively good prognosis compared with symptomatic disease; it rarely should lead to coronary artery bypass surgery. Individuals identified by screening should be prime targets for behavior modification with the hope of avoiding the usual course of this disease.

Screening has also been recommended for evaluating asymptomatic individuals in whom sudden incapacitation could compromise public safety. Such individuals include pilots, firemen, and policemen. Others who possibly should be screened are railroad engineers, air traffic controllers, and drivers of large commercial vehicles. Because an exercise program does present a risk to sedentary, coronary prone middle-aged men, it may be prudent to evaluate such individuals with screening prior to prescribing an exercise program.

SENSITIVITY/SPECIFICITY

In order to evaluate the value of any screening test, sensitivity, specificity, predictive value, and relative risk must be demonstrated. Sensitivity is the percentage of times a test gives an abnormal response when those with disease are tested. Specificity is the percentage of times a test gives a normal response when those without disease are tested—a definition different from the conventional use of the word "specific." These two values are inversely related and are determined by the discriminant values or cut-points chosen for the test that separate abnormals from normals. The predictive value of an abnormal test is the percentage of individuals with an abnormal test who have disease. The relative risk of an abnormal test response is the relative chance of having disease if the test is abnormal compared to having disease if the test is normal. The values for these last two terms depend on the prevalence of disease in the population being tested.

A basic step in applying any testing procedure for the separation of normal subjects from patients with a disease is to determine a test value that best separates the two groups. One problem is that there is usually a considerable overlap of measurement values of a test in the groups with and without disease. Consider two bell-shaped normal distribution curves, one representing a normal population and the other representing a population with disease, with a certain amount of overlap of the two curves (see Figure 1 in Chapter 5). Along the vertical axis is the number of patients and along the horizontal axis could be the value for such measurements as Q-wave size, exercise-induced ST-segment depression, or creatinine kinase. The optimal test would be able to achieve the most marked separation of these two bell-shaped curves and minimize the overlap. Unfortunately, most tests have a considerable overlap of the range of measurements for the normal population and for those with heart disease. Therefore, problems arise when a certain value is used to separate these two groups (i.e., Q-wave amplitude or width, 0.1 mV of ST-segment depression, a 10 mm Hg drop in systolic blood pressure, less than 5 METs exercise capacity, three ventricular beats). If the value is set far to the right (i.e., 0.2 mV of ST-segment depression) in order to classify nearly all the normal subjects as being free of disease, the test will have a high specificity. However, a substantial number of those with disease will be called normal. If a value is chosen far to the left (i.e., .05 mV ST-segment depression) that classifies nearly all those with disease as being abnormal, giving the test a high sensitivity, then many normal subjects are identified as abnormal. If a cut-point value is chosen that equally mislabels the normal subjects and those with disease, the test will have its highest predictive accuracy.

There may be reasons for wanting to adjust a test to have a relatively higher sensitivity or relatively higher specificity than possible when predictive accuracy is optimal. For instance, sensitivity should be highest in the emergency room and the specificity the highest when doing insurance exams. Remember that sensitivity and specificity are inversely related. That is, when sensitivity is the highest, specificity is the lowest, and vice versa. Any test has a range of inversely related sensitivities and specificities that can be chosen by selecting a certain discriminant or diagnostic value. Attempts have been made to use a series of tests to improve diagnostic power, but test interaction is complex. Usually the highest sensitivity and the lowest specificity of the tests represent their combined performance.

THE RESTING ECG AS A SCREENING TECHNIQUE

As part of the Copenhagen City Heart Study, nearly 20,000 men and women, 20 years of age or older, had a resting 12-lead ECG performed. The Minnesota Code was used to classify the electrocardiograms. The prevalence of all electrocardiographic findings, with the exception of axis deviation, high amplitude R-waves, minor Q-wave abnormalities, and prolonged or short PR interval, was very low (below the age of 40 in men and 50 in women). Rates for Q-wave abnormalities, left axis deviation, ST depression, premature beats, and atrial fibrillation increased with age and were higher for men than for women. A strong association between total mortality and major ST depression and T-wave abnormalities, Q-wave patterns, and left bundle branch block existed. During a period from 1976 to 1980, 489 subjects died, but there were only a few deaths in those under the age of 50. Due to this and because the prevalence of ECG abnormalities was low in the young, relative risk was only significant in those 50 or older. Over 50% of the deaths were due to noncardiovascular specific deaths. The relative risk of ST-segment depression was as high as five times. Some Q-wave abnormalities carried a relative risk of about three times.

Rose and colleagues performed electrocardiograms (limb leads only) on 8,403 male civil servants aged 40 to 64 using the Minnesota Code. Coronary heart disease mortality rates were established over the ensuing five years (657 men died). Q-waves, left axis deviation, ST depression, T-wave changes, ventricular conduction defects, and atrial fibrillation were related to mortality. However, there was little significance to increased R-wave amplitude, QT interval, premature beats, or heart rate extremes. Among the 6% of men with patterns suggesting ischemia, the subsequent coronary heart disease mortality was little more than 1% per year and even lower in those who were asymptomatic when screened. However, a five times risk ratio was found.

As part of the Busselton City, Australia study, 2,119 unselected subjects had a 12-lead ECG performed and coded according to the Minnesota Code. In addition, all subjects completed the Rose chest pain questionnaire. Subjects were between the ages of 40 and 79, and included both male and female. Between 1967 and 1979, mortality in this group was determined, and the 13-year mortality from cardiovascular disease was significantly higher in those with an initial ECG that showed Q-wave and QS patterns, left axis deviation, ST-segment depression and T-wave abnormalities, atrial fibrillation, or premature ventricular beats. In subjects free of angina and other ECG abnormalities, ventricular extra systoles were associated with a significantly higher mortality from cardiovascular disease compared with controls. Q-wave patterns had the highest risk ratio (3.7 times), whereas the other abnormalities had about a 2 times risk ratio.

As part of the Manitoba Study, a cohort of 3,983 men with a mean age of 30 years at entry, were followed with annual examinations including ECGs since 1948. During the 30-year observation period, 70 cases of sudden death occurred in men without previous clinical manifestations of heart disease. The prevalence of ECG abnormalities before sudden death was 71%. The frequencies of these abnormalities was 31% for major ST and T-wave abnormalities, 16% for ventricular extra beats, 13% for left ventricular hypertrophy, and 7% for left bundle branch block. LBBB had a 14 times risk for sudden death, while ST and T-wave abnormalities, increased R-wave, and premature beats had relative risks as high as five. This was a serial ECG study with ECGs obtained usually each year, and specificity was not determined.

In 2,000 Framingham Study participants, the 12-lead ECG failed to correctly classify over half of the persons with clinically definite heart disease. The sensitivity was about 50% and specificity 90%. The utility of the ECG for assessing prior infarction can be evaluated by comparing results with postmortem findings or by comparing results with survivors of a previously documented infarction. Levine and Phillips found that only 20% of old infarcts found at autopsy were correctly identified by the antemortem ECG. ECG abnormalities may not persist in patients with a previously documented myocardial infarction. In the Framingham Study, 18% of the infarction patients had no ECG abnormalities on subsequent examination. Other studies have reported a 10% to 15% loss of diagnostic Q-waves in the year post MI. However, the ECG has a much stronger prognostic value in survivors of a coronary heart disease event than in apparently healthy populations.

ANGIOGRAPHIC FINDINGS IN ASYMPTOMATIC MEN WITH RESTING ECG ABNORMALITIES

USAFSAM.   Cardiac catheterization was used to evaluate 298 asymptomatic, apparently healthy air crewmen with ECG abnormalities. These men were identified from annual ECGs and exercise tests used to screen them for latent heart disease. Data from 27 additional symptomatic air crewmen who underwent cardiac catheterization because of mild angina pectoris were also included. The men were grouped according to the major reason for cardiac catheterization. The order of groups by increasing prevalence of significant coronary artery disease (CAD) was as follows: abnormal treadmill in a labile lead (4% prevalence of CAD), supraventricular tachycardia (14%), right bundle branch block (20%), left bundle branch block (24%), abnormal exercise-induced ST depression (31%), ventricular irritability (38%), probable infarct (56%), and angina (70%). Approximately 60% of the men were completely free of angiographic coronary disease. The ECG abnormalities studied had a poorer predictive value for coronary artery disease in asymptomatic apparently healthy men than in a hospital or clinical population. A hypothesis based on the USAFSAM data is that a first tier of serial screening with the resting ECG could identify a subpopulation that could be more effectively screened with the next tier of testing, i.e., exercise testing.

EXERCISE TESTING AS A SCREENING PROCEDURE

Economic Factors.   Hartley and colleagues reported an exercise testing program designed to examine large numbers of people effectively, conveniently, and inexpensively. This study was designed to evaluate the possible future application of exercise testing as a routine screening tool. A bicycle ergometer was used, and multilead testing was performed. More than 1,800 subjects were examined in three years. As many as 55 tests per day were performed at a cost of $60 to $70 each. Abnormalities uncovered were similar to those observed in other studies. The program was considered successful for rendering services conveniently, at low cost, and with accuracy.

Type of Test.   Maximal or near-maximal exercise tests are superior screening techniques compared with submaximal exercise tests. One shortcoming of submaximal testing is its relatively low sensitivity. Other shortcomings, specifically of a step test like the double Master's test, are that it cannot be used to evaluate exercise capacity and that the ECG is not monitored during exercise. There is a physiologic fallacy in adjusting the number of steps as determined by Master according to body weight. Rowell and colleagues have shown that the oxygen consumption per kilogram is much greater for light individuals than it is for heavy individuals when the number of steps performed is in accord with the Master's step tables. The work load can be near maximal for light persons whereas it is minimal for heavy subjects. A danger of the Master's test is that it is usually performed with the ECG monitored only in the postexercise period. There have been numerous anecdotal reports of patients who fibrillated during a double Master's test, and there is at least one published case.

The advantages of a progressive, continuous exercise test with ECG and blood pressure monitoring during the test have been discussed elsewhere. Numerous studies using such a test to screen asymptomatic individuals have been reported without subsequent follow-up data. Nevertheless, these studies have demonstrated that maximal testing is more sensitive and that abnormal responses correlate directly with other risk factors. These studies also show that women tend to have more false positive ECG responses than men.

FOLLOW-UP STUDIES THAT HAVE UTILIZED EXERCISE TESTING

Table 7–1 summarizes ten follow-up studies that utilized maximal or near-maximal exercise testing to screen asymptomatic individuals for latent coronary heart disease, and one that evaluated men and women with atypical chest pain. The populations in these studies were tested and followed for the coronary heart disease endpoints of angina, acute myocardial infarction, and sudden death. There has been controversy over whether in the absence of conventional risk factors, exercise testing provides additional prognostic in-

TABLE 7–1.
Screening Studies Using Exercise Testing With Follow-Up for Cardiac Events

RESEARCHER	NO.	FOLLOW-UP (YEARS)	% CAD	ABNORMAL EXERCISE TEST (%)	SENSITIVITY (%)	SPECIFICITY (%)	PV + (%)	RISK RATIO
Bruce	221	5	2.3	11	60	91	14	14×
Aronow	100	5	9.0	16	67	92	46	14×
Cummings	510	3	4.7	13	58	90	25	10×
Froelicher	1390	6	3.3	10	61	92	20	14×
Allen	356	5	9.6	23	41	79	17	2.4×
Bruce	2365	6	2.0	11	30	91	5	3.5×
MacIntyre	578	8	6.9	4	16	97	26	4×
McHenry	916	13	7.1	2.5	14	98	39	6×
	serial*			6.7	32	95	34	6.4×
Manca	947	5	5.0	18	67	84	18	10x
	508(w)*	5	1.6	28	88	73	5	15×
MRFIT	6217 (SI)*	6–8	1.7	12.7	17	88	2.2	1.4×
	6205 (UC)		1.9	12.2	34	88	5.2	3.7×
LRC	3630	8	2.2	5	28	96	12	6×
MEN TESTED ONCE	17218 (total)	7 (averages)	5	12	43	90	21	8x

*Excluded from total and averages because of repeat testing, women, intervention.
PV + = predictive value of an abnormal exercise test.

formation in normal men. Another concern is whether the knowledge of having an abnormal exercise test makes an individual more likely to report angina.

Bruce and colleagues studied 221 clinically normal men in Seattle who were 35 to 82 years of age. A CB5 bipolar lead was used, and 0.1 mV or more of ST-segment depression was the criterion for an abnormal response. The patients were monitored in the sitting position postexercise. Ten percent of them had abnormal ST-segment responses to the symptom-limited maximal treadmill test. They were followed for five years. The sensitivity was 60%, that is, of those who developed coronary heart disease over the follow-up period, 60% had an abnormal treadmill test when they entered the study. The specificity was 91%, that is, of those without coronary heart disease, 91% had a normal treadmill test. The probability of developing coronary artery disease with an abnormal treadmill test (the predictive value of an abnormal response) was 13.6%; of those who had an abnormal response, 13.6% developed coronary heart disease. The relative risk of developing coronary heart disease over the follow-up period was 13.6 times greater for those who had an abnormal ST-segment response to treadmill testing than for those who had a normal response.

Aronow and colleagues tested 100 normal men in Los Angeles, aged 38 to 64 years, and followed them for five years. Risk-factor analysis was not performed, but all subjects were normotensive. A V5 lead was used, and 0.1 mV or more of ST-segment depression was the criterion for an abnormal response. The patients were monitored in the supine position after exercise. Thirteen percent had an abnormal ST-segment response to near-maximal treadmill testing. The sensitivity for an abnormal response was 67%, the specificity was 92%, the predictive value was 46%, and the risk ratio was 13.6.

Cumming and colleagues reported their three-year follow-up for coronary heart disease endpoints in 510 asymptomatic men 40 to 65 years of age. Maximal or near-maximal effort was performed and a CM5 lead was monitored. The criterion for abnormal was 0.2 mV or more of ST-segment depression and the patients were monitored in the supine position postexercise. Twelve percent had an initial abnormal response to a bicycle exercise test. Subjects with an abnormal response had a higher prevalence of hypertension and hypercholesterolemia. The sensitivity of the test was 58%, the specificity was 90%, the predictive value was 25%, and the risk ratio was 10.

At USAFSAM, 1,390 asymptomatic men 20 to 54 years of age who did not have any of the known causes for false positive treadmill tests were screened for latent coronary heart disease by maximal treadmill testing and followed for a mean of 6.3 years. A CC5 lead was mainly used, but additional leads were obtained in the supine position postexercise. The criterion for abnormal was 0.1 mV or more horizontal or downsloping ST-segment depression. Ten percent of these men had abnormal treadmill tests. The sensitivity of the test was 61%, the specificity was 92%, the predictive value was 20%, and the risk ratio for an abnormal response was 14.3.

In Italy, Manca and colleagues studied 947 men and 508 women who were referred for exercise testing because of atypical chest pain. Those with typical symptoms of angina pectoris, valvular disease, hypertension, bundle branch block, dysrhythmias, Wolff-Parkinson-White syndrome, left ventricular hypertrophy with strain, significant resting repolarization abnormalities, and previous myocardial infarction were excluded. No patient received drugs such as digitalis, beta blockers, antidysrhythmics, or diuretics in the two weeks preceding exercise testing. Exercise was carried out after routine hyperventilation, using a supine bicycle, until at least 85% of the predicted maximal heart rate was reached. The conventional 12 electrocardiographic leads were recorded during and after the exercise test. The criterion for an abnormal response was 0.1 mV or more of horizontal or downsloping ST-segment depression. Eighteen percent of the men and 28% of the women had an abnormal electrocardiographic response. The endpoints for coronary disease were myocardial infarction or sudden death, and there was a mean follow-up of 5.2 years. The overall incidence of coronary disease was 5% in the men and 1.6% in the women. The sensitivity was 67% in the men versus 88% in the women. The specificity of the test in the men was 84% versus 73% in the women. The predictive value of a positive test was 18% in men, but only 5% in women. Men with positive tests had a relative risk of 10 for developing clinical manifestations of coronary heart disease; the relative risk for women with positive tests was 15. This study clearly shows how predictive value is influenced by the prevalence of coronary heart disease in the population under study, and that the specificity of the exercise test is lower in women.

Allen and colleagues recently reported a five-year follow-up of 888 asymptomatic men and women without known coronary heart disease who had initially undergone maximal treadmill testing. When tested, none of the subjects were on medications that would affect the electrocardiogram. None had pathologic Q-waves or other abnormalities. None had clinical evidence of pulmonary disease or vascular disease. No subject that was included developed serious dysrhythmias, conduction abnormalities, or chest pain in conjunction with the exercise test. Maximal treadmill testing was performed using the Ellestad protocol; leads CM5, V1, and a bipolar vertical lead were recorded. Subjects were exercised until they reached 100% of predicted maximal heart rate, fatigue, or marked dyspnea. Flat ST-segment depression of 0.1 mV or greater and downsloping of the ST-segment were considered a positive response. Subjects with major ST-segment changes at rest were excluded. If there were minor changes in the ST-segment before exercise, an additional 0.15 mV of depression at 80 msec from the J-point were required to indicate an abnormal exercise test. R-wave amplitude was measured for an average of six beats during a control period and immediately after exercise, and an increase or no change in the R-wave immediately after exercise compared with control was defined as an abnormal response. A decrease in R-wave amplitude was defined as a normal response. The original population included 1,077 subjects, and 888 (82.5%) were contacted for follow-up. Of the 113 subjects who initially had abnormal exercise tests, 105 were located (92.9%). There was a 1.1% incidence of coronary heart disease per year. Endpoints for coronary heart disease were angina pectoris, myocardial infarction, or sudden cardiac death.

TABLE 7–2.

Exercise Electrocardiographic Test Performance in Asymptomatic Men Less Than 40 Years of Age, With Differing Results

PRINCIPAL INVESTI- GATOR	N	AGE RANGE	INCIDENCE OF CHD	YEARS FOLLOW-UP	% WITH ABNORMAL EXERCISE TEST	SENSITIVITY	SPECIFICITY	PREDICTIVE VALUE	RELATIVE RISK*
Froelicher	563	30–39	1.4%	6.3	5.5	50%	95%	13%	17
Allen	221	<40	0.9%	5.0	3.6	0%	96%	0%	0

*Times that for normal subjects.
CHD = coronary heart disease.

Only 2 of 221 men 40 years of age or less developed heart disease end-points, and neither of the two had ST-segment abnormalities, abnormal R-wave response, or exercise duration of five minutes or less. Hence, in this study, abnormal results did not correlate with subsequent coronary heart disease in asymptomatic men 40 years of age or younger. These results contrast with those of the USAFSAM study of 563 men 30 to 39 years of age that found a 1.4% incidence of coronary disease. The exercise ECG was found to have a 50% sensitivity, 95% specificity, 13% predictive value, and a risk ratio of 17, and thus it still had value in this age range (Table 7–2).

Allen and colleagues concluded that the exercise test was only of value in men older than 40 years of age. For these men, subsequent coronary heart disease within five years was predicted by an abnormal ST-segment response, an increase or no change in R-wave, and an exercise duration of five minutes or less. The ST-segment, R-wave, and exercise duration criteria had sensitivities of 41%, 47%, and 26%, respectively. With the test results interpreted as abnormal when either ST or R-wave criteria were present, sensitivity was 65%. Adding exercise duration of five minutes or less as a third alternative criterion for a positive test did not change sensitivity. The performance of the exercise test responses is summarized in Table 7–3. When all three criteria were present, a sensitivity of 29% with a specificity of 100% was achieved. In men older than 40 years of age, the ST-segment criteria had the above mentioned sensitivity of 41%, specificity of 79%, predictive value of 17%, and risk ratio of 2.4. With the exception of predictive value, these values are strikingly lower than those found in earlier studies, including results previously presented by this group.

Of the 311 women whom Allen and colleagues followed, 10 developed coronary heart disease endpoints. The authors found that ST-segment depression and R-wave response did not correlate with subsequent development of coronary heart disease. Exercise duration of three minutes or less, however, proved to be a significant predictor of coronary heart disease. Four of 13 women with a low exercise time developed coronary heart disease. When used as a criterion for abnormal, exercise duration of three minutes or less in asymptomatic women had a sensitivity of 40%, specificity of 97%, predictive value of 31%, and risk ratio of 15. Limited follow-up of 80% of the original population and the low incidence of coronary disease endpoints in women

TABLE 7–3.
Performance of Exercise Test Variables and Risk Factors in Detecting Asymptomatic
Coronary Artery Disease

FIRST AUTHOR	ABNORMAL RESPONSE	SENSITIVITY (%)	SPECIFICITY (%)	PREDICTIVE VALUE	RISK RATIO
Allen	ST ↓	41	79	17	2
	RWA	47	78	19	3
	TM time < 5 min	27	96	43	6
	ST ↓ + RWA	40	86	27	5
	ST ↓ + TM time < 5 min	24	99	71	11
	RWA + TM time < 5 min	33	99	82	12
	ST ↓ + RWA + TM time < 5 min	29	100	100	17
Bruce	ST ↓	30	91	5	3.5
	Angina on TM	6	99	15	8
	TM time < 6 min	6	99	19	10
	HRI	19	93	7	4
	≥1 RF + ≥2 ExRP	19	—	46	18
Uhl	≥ 0.3mV ST	36	79	38	2
	Onset ST ↓ in stage I	33	64	23	1
	TM time < 10 min	46	92	67	4
	Persistent ST ↓ (6 min)	28	87	43	6
	RWA	28	87	42	2
	≥ 1 RF + ≥2 ExRP	55	86	84	4
	≥1 RF + ≥3 ExRP to detect multivessel disease	37	98	89	4.5

ExRP = exercise risk predictor; HRI = heart rate impairment; RF = risk factor; RWA = R-wave amplitude abnormality; ST ↓ = ST segment depression; TM = treadmill test.

and in men younger than 40 years of age are limitations of this study.

Bruce and colleagues recently reported a six-year follow-up of 2,365 clinically healthy men (mean age 45 years) who were exercise tested as part of the Seattle Heart Watch. They underwent symptom-limited maximal treadmill testing using neither ST depression nor target heart rates as endpoints of maximal exercise. The Bruce protocol was used, and the electrocardiogram was monitored with a bipolar CB5 lead. Conventional risk factors were assessed at the time of the initial examination in a subset of the population. Follow-up was obtained by questionnaire, with morbidity defined as hospital admission. Forty-seven men (2%) experienced coronary heart disease morbidity or mortality. Univariate analysis of the individual conventional risk factors (positive family history, hypertension, smoking, hypercholesterolemia) did not show a statistically significant increase in the five-year probability of primary coronary heart disease events. Only when the sum of risk factors in an individual were assessed did conventional risk factors become statistically significant in relation to the event rate. Four variables from treadmill testing were predictive: (1) exercise duration less than six minutes (which requires 6–7 METs, or multiples of resting oxygen requirement); (2) 0.1 mV ST depression during recovery; (3) greater than 10% heart rate impairment (defined as the percent reduction of age-adjusted maximal heart rate); and (4) chest pain during maximal exertion. The ST-segment criteria had a sensitivity of 30%, specificity of 89%, predictive value of 5.3%, and a risk ratio of 3.3. Angina and exercise duration each had sensitivities of about 6%. Heart rate impairment had a sensitivity of 19% and was otherwise comparable to ST-segment depression.

Table 7–3 summarizes the performance of the exercise test predictors. The presence of two or more of the exercise test predictors identified men in all age groups who were at increased risk. Furthermore, it was found that in the presence of one or more conventional risk factors and as the prevalence of exertional risk predictors rose from none to any three, the relative risk rose from 1 to 30. The group that had one or more conventional risk factors and two or more exertional risk predictors was found to have the highest five-year probability of primary coronary heart disease. In the absence of conventional risk factors, however, exercise testing in this study failed to provide additional prognostic information in normal men.

MacIntyre and colleagues performed maximal exercise tests on 548 fit, healthy middle-aged former aviators at the Naval Aerospace Medical Laboratory. To be included, subjects had to have no clinical evidence of heart or lung disease as determined by history, physical examination, chest x-ray, and a completely normal resting electrocardiogram. Leads X, Y, Z, and V5 were analyzed only after exercise for 0.1 mV or more of horizontal depression 80 msec after QRS end. Criteria for coronary disease after an eight-year follow-up were sudden death, myocardial infarction, coronary artery bypass surgery or angina. The predictive value of the test was not significantly greater in those with the cardinal risk factors. An abnormal exercise electrocardiogram generated a higher risk ratio than the risk factors.

McHenry et al. reported the results of an 8- to 15-year follow-up of 916 apparently healthy men between the ages of 27 and 55 (mean 37 years) who underwent serial medical and exercise test evaluations. In 1968, the Indiana University School of Medicine entered into an agreement with the Indiana State Police Department to provide employees with periodic medical evaluations including treadmill tests. This report covers their experience with the first male employees who underwent initial medical evaluations between July, 1968, and June, 1975, and includes a follow-up for all subjects through June, 1983. A CC5 lead was monitored and 0.1 mV or more horizontal or downsloping ST-segment depression during or after exercise was considered abnormal. A modified Balke protocol was used for all treadmill tests, and most were symptom-limited. Serial evaluations were planned at two- to five-year intervals, but about 15% of subjects elected not to return after their initial evaluation. During the initial evaluation, there were 23 subjects with an abnormal ST-segment response. During follow-up, there were nine coronary events in this group: eight cases of angina and one of sudden death. With serial testing, an additional 38 subjects experienced conversion to abnormal ST-segment response. During follow-up, there were 12 coronary events in this group; 10 cases of angina, 1 MI, and 1 "other." There were 833 subjects with normal ST-segment responses to exercise with all tests. In this group, there were 44 coronary events; 25 MIs, 7 sudden deaths and 12 cases of angina.

They concluded that an abnormal ST-segment response to exercise predicted angina pectoris but not other coronary events.

McHenry et al. did not present sensitivity/specificity calculations but the data they reported enabled the calculations shown in Table 7–1. The surprisingly low sensitivity from initial testing is probably due to the long follow-up period. An abnormal test indicates obstructive coronary disease that was most likely not present initially in most subjects who developed endpoints but developed later during the 12 years. An analysis of the treadmill test performance at five years, a time frame similar to the prior studies reporting a higher sensitivity, would be most informative. Otherwise, this leaves the possibility that the treadmill test is much less sensitive in asymptomatic men than previously demonstrated.

They found that serial testing did not improve the predictive value of the test and that angina was the main cardiac event predicted. Sudden death was actually more common in the individuals with normal test results. The USAF-SAM study also had angina as its most common endpoint. This both supports the concept that the knowledge of an abnormal exercise test makes an individual more likely to report angina or to be diagnosed as having CAD.

The Multiple Risk Factor Intervention Trial (MRFIT), a coronary heart disease (CAD) primary prevention trial, examined the effect on CAD of a special intervention (SI) program to reduce cholesterol, HBP, and cigarette smoking in men 35 to 57 years old. Half of the 12,866 participants were randomly assigned to usual care (UC) in the community. During a six- to eight-year follow-up, the CAD mortality rate was 7% lower in the SI than in the UC group, a nonsignificant difference. A prior subgroup hypothesis proposed that men with an abnormal exercise ECG would particularly benefit from intervention. An abnormal ST integral measured by computer of 16 microV-sec, was observed in 12.5% of the men at baseline, and was associated with a 3 times risk of CAD death within the UC group. In the subgroup with a normal ECG, there was no significant SI-UC difference in the CAD mortality rate. In contrast, there was a 57% lower death rate among men in the SI group with an abnormal test compared with men in the UC group. The relative risks (SI/UC) in these two strata were significantly different. These findings suggest that men with elevated risk factors who have an abnormal exercise ECG benefit from risk factor reduction. This study and that of the Lipid Research Center (LRC) are certainly the largest and probably the most reliable for demonstrating the predictive accuracy of exercise testing in an asymptomatic population since only cardiac deaths were considered the endpoint as opposed to angina in most of the other studies.

EXERCISE TESTING WITH CORONARY ANGIOGRAPHY

Froelicher and colleagues used cardiac catheterization to evaluate 111 asymptomatic men with an abnormal ST depression in response to a treadmill test. Only one-third of the subjects had at least one lesion equal to or greater than

50% luminal narrowing of a major coronary artery. Table 7–4 summarizes the impact of the resting ECG on the predictive value of an abnormal exercise ECG response. Resting mild ST-segment depression, that appears on serial ECGs and persists, increases the predictive value of an abnormal exercise test. Borer and colleagues reported angiographic findings in 11 asymptomatic individuals with hyperlipidemia and an abnormal exercise test. Only 37% were found to have coronary artery occlusions.

Barnard and colleagues used near-maximal treadmill testing to screen randomly selected Los Angeles firefighters. Ten percent had abnormal exercise-induced ST depression despite few risk factors for coronary disease. Six men with an abnormal exercise test elected to undergo cardiac catheterization. One had severe three-vessel disease, and another had a 50% obstruction of the left circumflex coronary artery. The other four men had normal studies.

Uhl and colleagues have reported their findings in 255 asymptomatic men who underwent coronary angiography for an abnormal ST-segment response to exercise testing over a seven-year period at the USAFSAM. None of the clinical or ECG variables were able to detect those with significant diseases. The three exercise test responses with high likelihood ratio were (1) at least 0.3 mV depression, (2) persistence of ST depression six minutes postexercise, and (3) an estimated oxygen uptake of less than 9 METs. However, because of their low sensitivity and predictive value, it was necessary to combine them with risk factors. A combination of any risk factor and two exercise responses was highly predictive (89%) but insensitive (39%) for any coronary disease. However, this combination had a sensitivity of 55% and a predictive value of 84% for two- or three-vessel diseases. Table 7–3 summarizes these results.

Erikssen and colleagues reported angiographic findings in 105 men aged 40 to 59 of a working population with one or more of the following criteria: (1) a questionnaire for angina pectoris positive on interview or either, (2) typical angina, or (3) ST depression as responses to a near-maximal bicycle test. The exercise test had a predictive value of 84% if a slowly ascending ST-segment was included. The higher predictive value in this study may be due to the older age of their population and inclusion of men with angina. Of the 36 who were found to have normal coronary arteries, a seven-year follow-up re-

TABLE 7–4

The Predictive Value of an Abnormal Exercise Electrocardiogram in 111 Aircrewmen Grouped According to Their Annual Resting Electrocardiographic Findings

ANNUAL RESTING ELECTROCARDIOGRAM	N	MEAN AGE	% WITH SIGNIFICANT ANGIOGRAPHIC CAD
Normal	34	44	24
Previous NSSTWC but current ECG normal	21	43	24
Low amplitude T-waves	24	42	25
ST segment abnormal	32	44	47

vealed that three died of sudden death, four received a diagnosis of cardiomyopathy, and one developed aortic valve disease. They had a relative decline in their physical performance over the follow-up period. Thallium
studies were normal, but the radionuclide ventriculogram revealed a subnor-
mal increase in ejection fraction during exercise in half of them.

Kemp et al. evaluated seven-year survival in patients having normal or near
normal coronary arteriograms using data from the CASS registry of 21,487
consecutive coronary arteriograms taken in 15 clinical sites. Of these, 4,051
arteriograms were normal or near normal, and the patients had normal left
ventricular function as judged by absence of a history of congestive heart failure, no reported segmental wall motion abnormality, and an ejection fraction
of at least 50%; 3,136 arteriograms were entirely normal, and the remaining
915 revealed mild disease with less than 50% stenosis in one or more segments. Of the total number, 843 patients had exercise tests and of these, 195
had abnormal ST depression. The seven-year survival rate was 96% for the
patients with a normal arteriogram and 92% for those whose study revealed
mild disease. They noted that the ECG response to exercise was a nonpredic-
tive variable. This is in contrast to the seven-year follow-up study of only 36
apparently healthy middle-aged men with a positive exercise test and normal
coronary arteriograms reported by Erikssen. Erikssen concluded that patients
with an abnormal exercise test could not be assured of a good prognosis on
the basis of a normal coronary arteriogram. The CASS data do not support
this conclusion. There were 195 subjects with abnormal ST-segment depression, and Kemp et al. were unable to show any predictive value of even
marked amounts of depression. If exercise-induced ST-segment depression is
due to ischemia in patients with normal coronaries, it is not related to a disease process that has an impact on mortality over seven years of follow-up.

In general, these angiographic studies confirm the low predictive value of
an abnormal exercise test response also found in the epidemiological studies
of populations with a low prevalence of CHD.

Labile ST Shifts.   Morris and McHenry have performed serial exercise tests on 900 presumably healthy men and identified 14 men with
labile ST-T changes with standing or hyperventilation and abnormal ST-segment depression at exercise. At seven-year follow-up, none had manifested a
coronary event while in 24 men with exercise-induced ST changes but no
labile ST-T wave phenomena preexercise, 10 (42%) had a coronary event.

Exercise-Induced Dysrhythmias.   Few studies in asymptomatic subjects have evaluated exercise-induced ventricular premature beats
for detecting coronary disease. In USAFSAM study of 1,390 men, only 39 men
(2.1%) of the population developed "ominous" dysrhythmias. The risk of developing coronary disease over six years of follow-up with these dysrhythmias was $3\times$; however, the predictive value was only 10%, and sensitivity
only 6.7%. In Piepgrass' study, 14 asymptomatic men developed ominous
ventricular dysrhythmias. Six underwent thallium scintigraphy, and the two

TABLE 7–5.

Ancillary Techniques Discussed That Have Been Used to Screen for Asymptomatic CHD

Thallium perfusion imaging
Radionuclide ventriculography during bicycle exercise and posttreadmill exercise
Cardiac fluoroscopy for coronary artery calcification (enhanced with digital subtraction angiography)
Cardiokymography
Total cholesterol/HDL ratio, conventional risk factors
ECG gated chest x-ray pre- and postexercise
Computerized multifactorial risk prediction using Bayesian statistics
Systolic time intervals during and after exercise
Digital subtraction angiography with intravenous injection of contrast to visualize the coronary arteries
Echocardiography (or Doppler) during and/or after exercise (even posttreadmill)

with abnormal scans were found to have coronary artery disease at catheterization. Thus, dysrhythmias induced by exercise testing have not been helpful in detecting latent coronary disease in apparently healthy men.

Techniques to Improve Screening.   Numerous techniques have been recommended to improve the sensitivity and specificity of exercise testing. Various computerized criteria for ischemia have been proposed, as well as new standard visual ST criteria. In addition, there are ancillary techniques that could possibly improve the discriminating power of the exercise test. These methods are listed in Table 7–5.

Electrocardiographic Criteria.   Lozner and Morganroth studied 37 subjects (10 asymptomatic and 27 symptomatic) who had undergone maximal treadmill testing and coronary angiography to determine whether the predictive value of ST-segment depression could be enhanced. These investigators felt that the predictive value for coronary artery disease could not be enhanced by increasing the degree of ST-segment depression for qualification as abnormal. However, if ST changes that persisted for longer than two minutes were interpreted as a positive test, then a more accurate identification of an abnormal response was possible.

Chahine evaluated the predictive value of an abnormal response by considering different exercise-induced patterns of ST-segment depression. Fifty consecutive symptomatic patients with abnormal ST-segment depression who displayed an evolutionary ST-segment pattern were compared with 50 similar patients with simple ST-segment depression. Those with the evolutionary ST depression showed upsloping or horizontal ST-segment depression followed by a downsloping pattern with complete or partial inversion of the T-wave and gradual return to its baseline. Those with simple ST-segment depression showed horizontal or downsloping ST-segment depression returning directly to baseline without any significant T-wave inversion. Correlation of ST depression with coronary angiography showed an overall predictive value of 90%, which improved to 94% after excluding 19 patients who were receiving digitalis. The predictive value improved to 98% when only the patients with evolutionary ST-segment depression were considered, in comparison with 82% in those with simple ST-segment depression. Hollenberg has applied his computerized treadmill score in an asymptomatic Army population with success.

Thallium Exercise Testing. Caralis and colleagues used thallium exercise testing and coronary angiography to evaluate asymptomatic individuals with abnormal ST-segment responses to exercise testing. Of 3,496 consecutive treadmill exercise tests performed primarily on asymptomatic individuals, 22 developed 0.2 mV or more of asymptomatic horizontal ST-segment depression. These individuals had physical examinations, routine laboratory studies, chest x-rays, and resting electrocardiograms, all of which were normal. Fifteen of these 22 patients agreed to be evaluated further with thallium and coronary angiography. These 15 included 13 men and 1 woman; the mean age was 52. Thallium was administered intravenously for separate rest and exercise myocardial studies. Myocardial imaging began 10 minutes after administration, and imaging in each of the views required 8 to 12 minutes. The rest and subsequent exercise studies were performed one week apart, and all of the resting studies were normal. The thallium was injected at peak bicycle exercise and patients were encouraged to keep a constant level of exercise for an additional one minute. Rest and exercise studies were examined together and considered positive for ischemia only if a new perfusion defect involved more than 15% of the left ventricular circumference. Of the 15 asymptomatic individuals with horizontal ST-segment depression on exercise testing, 5 had normal scans with exercise, and 10 developed new defects. The angiographic criterion for abnormal was based on 70% luminal narrowing. Four of the five individuals with normal exercise thallium images had normal coronary angiograms, and one had an abnormal angiogram. Of the 10 with abnormal exercise scans, nine had significant narrowing of two or more major coronary arteries, and one patient had essentially normal coronary vessels. Hence, once subjects were selected on the basis of an abnormal exercise test, the thallium exercise scans classified 13 of 15 patients properly.

Nolewajk and colleagues performed thallium treadmill tests on 58 asymptomatic men as part of a screening study. The risk for coronary heart disease was determined using the Framingham risk equation, based on age, cholesterol, systolic blood pressure, cigarette-smoking history, left ventricular hypertrophy on the electrocardiogram, and glucose intolerance. The risk calculation was greater in those with abnormal exercise studies compared with those who had normal studies. Five of the subjects had electrocardiographic left ventricular hypertrophy, six had abnormal exercise-induced ST depression, and six had abnormal thallium scans (five consistent with ischemia, one with scar). Three of the subjects with abnormal thallium studies underwent coronary angiography, and all had normal coronary arteries. Surprisingly, two of these had left bundle branch block (one with exercise only, the other at rest). The disappointment of these results was compounded by profound psychological stress to the individuals who were told they had "abnormal" results.

Uhl and colleagues performed thallium exercise tests on 119 air crewmen prior to undergoing coronary angiography because of abnormal treadmill tests or serial ECG changes. Of these, 41 men had significant angiographic disease (equal to or greater than 50% occlusion) for a predictive value of the ECG screening procedures of 21%. The sensitivity of the computer-enhanced thallium exercise test was 95%, as compared with 68% for analog polaroid interpretation, and its specificity was 90%. There were mixed results in the 10 men who had minimal angiographic disease (less than 50% occlusion); 10 had abnormal scans and 5 had normal scans. The high sensitivity and specificity of the computer-enhanced thallium exercise test in this population of apparently healthy men is a strong support for its use as a second line screening procedure. If both an abnormal exercise electrocardiogram and abnormal perfusion scintigram had been required before angiography was performed, 136 of those free of coronary disease would not have needed to undergo angiography.

RADIONUCLIDE LEFT VENTRICULAR ANGIOGRAPHY DURING EXERCISE

Borer and associates reported their study of 10 men and 1 woman, all of whom had coronary heart disease and normal resting left ventricular function confirmed by angiography. Fourteen normal subjects were also studied. Gated radionuclide angiography was performed in the supine position at rest and during exercise. Imaging was performed during exercise for at least two minutes of near-maximal effort. From resting values, ejection fraction increased during exercise in all normal subjects, with the increase ranging from 7% to 30%. In patients with coronary disease, ejection fraction during exercise diminished in all but one patient, and in that patient it remained unchanged. At least one new region of left ventricular dysfunction developed during exercise in each of the patients with coronary heart disease.

The only reported application of exercise radionuclide angiograms to detect coronary artery disease in asymptomatic men compared global ejection fraction changes to visual evaluation of segmental wall motion and the visual interpretation of thallium scintigraphy in 32 men. The thallium study had a better sensitivity (92%) than did global (85%) or regional (62%) abnormalities by radionuclide angiograms without loss of specificity (95% versus 85% and 95%, respectively). However, most studies have shown exercise ventriculography to have a much poorer specificity, making it unacceptable for screening.

At the University of California, San Diego, we developed an approach using radionuclide angiography to increase the sensitivity and specificity of treadmill testing. Tagged technetium was administered intravenously in order to perform sequential left ventricular ventriculography in 10 coronary heart disease patients and 8 normal subjects. All 18 subjects underwent maximal treadmill testing. Ejection fractions were measured at 2 to 4, 4 to 6, and 8 to 10 minutes of recovery. At 8 to 10 minutes of recovery, all normal subjects but none of the coronary heart disease patients had higher ejection fractions than they did at rest. The addition of regional wall motion analysis after treadmill testing could add further discriminant value. Posttreadmill analysis could be more sensitive than the supine bicycle technique because of the higher work load achieved, and an increase in specificity could possibly be obtained over standard ST-segment analysis by detecting regional wall motion abnormalities.

Cardiokymography. The cardiokymograph is an electronic device that produces a representation of regional left ventricular wall motion noninvasively. It generates an electromagnetic field, and motion within the field causes a change in the frequency of an oscillator. A change in frequency is converted into a change in voltage proportional to the motion. The cardiokymograph produces a recording similar to the apexcardiogram and the kinetocardiogram. The advantage of the cardiokymograph is that it records absolute cardiac motion without chest motion, thus eliminating the distortion problem inherent in both the apexcardiogram and the kinetocardiogram. There is considerable tissue penetration, so the cardiokymograph responds to deeper cardiac motion as well as precordial surface movement. Cardiokymographic recordings have been shown to be predictive of ventriculographic wall motion abnormalities.

Silverberg and colleagues reported their use of the cardiokymograph after exercise in 157 patients, including 27 apparently healthy volunteers and 130 patients with suspected coronary heart disease who underwent coronary angiography. The subjects performed a progressive symptom-limited maximal treadmill test. The cardiokymograph was recorded within two minutes of termination of exercise, and every minute thereafter for 10 minutes. Two sets of empiric criteria for an abnormal cardiokymographic pattern were defined in relation to known effects of ischemia on regional wall motion. The first abnormality was defined as paradoxical systolic outward motion. The second abnormality was defined as development of total absence of inward motion, a resultant holosystolic outward motion, or systolic outward motion occurring for less than the entire period of ejection but not preceded by inward motion. For detecting coronary heart disease in atypical chest pain patients, the cardiokymogram had a higher sensitivity, specificity, and predictive value than did the electrocardiogram. However, no statistical difference existed between the electrocardiogram and the cardiokymogram in asymptomatic patients. This may be explained by the distribution of disease in this study: patients with atypical chest pain had a 30% prevalence of disease, and asymptomatic patients had a 64% prevalence of angiographic coronary artery disease. Exercise-induced cardiokymographic abnormalities persisted longer during recovery than electrocardiographic changes. Although the cardiokymogram had higher sensitivity and specificity than the electrocardiogram for the detection of coronary disease in patients with atypical chest pain, the results could be due to the population sample selected for this study.

Alexander et al. utilized cardiokymography as part of a serial testing evaluation of 287 asymptomatic subjects. Type II cardiokymographic abnormalities occurred in 10 subjects, 5 of whom had coronary disease. The resultant sensitivity of 63% and specificity of 74% and predictive value of 50% was more effective than horizontal ST-segment depression (25%, 89%, and 50%, respectively) and was the second best single screening test (thallium scintigraphy was best).

A multicenter study (Weiner et al.) has demonstrated the diagnostic accuracy of cardiokymography recorded two to three minutes after exercise in 617 patients undergoing cardiac catheterization. Of these patients, 29% had prior MI. There were 12 participating centers using a standardized protocol. Adequate CKG tracings, which were obtained in 82% of patients, were dependent on the skill of the operator and on certain patient characteristics. Of the 327 patients without prior MI who had technically adequate CKG and electrocardiographic tracings, 166 (51%) had coronary disease. Both the sensitivity and specificity of CKG (71% and 88%, respectively) were significantly greater than the values for the exercise ECG (61% and 76%, respectively). Coronary artery disease and multivessel disease were present in 98% and 68%, respectively, of the 70 patients with both abnormal CKG and ECG results, and in 15% and 5%, respectively, of the 132 patients with both studies normal. The CKG was most helpful in those patients in whom the posttest probability of coronary disease was between 21% and 72% after the exercise ECG. In these patients, an abnormal concordantly positive CKG result increased the probability of coronary disease to between 67% and 100%, while a normal response decreased it to between 12% and 15%. In the subgroup of 102 patients undergoing concomitant exercise thallium testing, the sensitivity and specificity for the thallium scintigraphy (81% and 80%, respectively) were similar to the values for CKG (72% and 84%, respectively).

To determine which subgroup of patients derive the most benefit from testing, they categorized the chest pain complaints of the 327 patients without prior MI undergoing testing for the purpose of diagnosis into four symptom groups. (1) Typical angina: A history of typical angina pectoris in men was predictive of both coronary artery disease (85%) and multivessel disease (51%). An abnormal exercise ECG increased the probability of coronary disease to 94%. In these patients, an abnormal CKG only slightly increased the probability of coronary disease (to 95%), whereas a normal CKG was still associated with a high probability. (2) Atypical angina: 51% of these men and 33% of these women had coronary artery disease. An abnormal exercise ECG increased the probability of coronary disease to 90% in men and to 86% in women, while a negative result was associated with a probability of 27% in men and 25% in women. A normal exercise ECG in patients with atypical angina was still associated with a 37% probability of coronary disease in men and a 20% probability in women. In these patients, when the CKG was normal, the probability of coronary disease (15% in men and 12% in women) and of multivessel disease (5% in men and 3% in women) was very low. (3) Nonischemic chest pain: of 43 patients, 24% had coronary disease and 7% had multivessel disease. An abnormal ST response resulted in a 45% probability of coronary disease, while a negative ECG result was associated with a 17% probability. In the 14 patients with an abnormal exercise ECG, a positive CKG response increased the probability of coronary disease to 80%. In the 30 patients with negative ECG, a negative CKG response, which was present in 26 patients, lowered the probability to 8% and none had multivessel disease. (4) Unfortunately, there were too few individuals for analysis in the asymptomatic group. This study confirms that the CKG performed during exercise testing improves the diagnostic accuracy of the ECG response and is a cost-effective indicator of myocardial ischemia.

Coronary Artery Calcification on Fluoroscopic Examination. Kelly and Langou reported the use of cardiac fluoroscopy as a prescreening tool in asymptomatic men prior to exercise testing. In one study, 129 healthy men (average age 49) were evaluated with cardiac fluoroscopy to detect coronary artery calcification, followed by a submaximal exercise test. Of the 108 subjects who completed the exercise test, 37 (34%) had at least one fluoroscopically detected calcified coronary artery. Of this group of subjects with positive fluoroscopic findings, 13 (35%) had an abnormal ST-segment response to the exercise test. Of the 68 subjects with normal fluoroscopy, only 3 (4%) had an abnormal exercise response. Consequently, those with calcification of at least one coronary artery had a ninefold increased risk of having an abnormal exercise electrocardiographic test. Of the 16 subjects with an abnormal exercise test, 81% had calcification of at least one coronary artery. The location of the calcific deposit conferred greater risk for exercise-induced ischemic changes than did multivessel involvement. Forty-seven percent of men with calcification in the left anterior descending coronary artery had an abnormal exercise electrocardiogram versus 33% and 16% of persons with left circumflex and right coronary artery calcifications, respectively.

In a second study, the 13 men who had both coronary artery calcification and an abnormal exercise test had coronary angiography. They had a mean age of 44, none had any symptoms or signs of coronary disease, and all had a normal resting electrocardiogram. Coronary artery calcification was first detected by fluoroscopy in a single artery in 10 men, in two arteries in two men, and in three arteries in one man. On angiography, coronary artery disease was considered clinically significant if there was greater than 50% luminal narrowing in any major coronary branch. Coronary arteriography revealed 12 men with clinically significant coronary artery disease: single-vessel disease in four, double in five, and triple in three men. One man had only a minor lesion. On a three-year follow-up in these 13 patients, 3 had developed typical angina and 1 had developed a Q-wave MI. The results of this study suggest that the combination of coronary artery calcification and an abnormal exercise test is highly predictive of coronary heart disease. However, the sensitivity and specificity of the combination of these procedures remains to be clarified. Did the three subjects with an abnormal exercise test and no fluoroscopically detected coronary artery calcification have angiographic disease? What of the

24 individuals with coronary artery calcification and a normal exercise electrocardiogram?

In the study of Alexander et al., fluoroscopic evaluation of 26 asymptomatic subjects who had abnormal exercise tests or ominous exercise-induced arrhythmias failed to reveal calcification in any of them including the eight with proven coronary disease. Perhaps coronary calcifications are detectable only in patients with long-standing coronary disease, i.e., older subjects.

Detrano has used digitally enhanced fluoroscopy to visualize coronary artery calcifications. Initial results suggest that it may have its greatest predictive accuracy in younger individuals.

Lipid Screening.   Total cholesterol to high-density lipoprotein cholesterol (TC-HDL) ratios have been shown to be directly correlated with coronary heart disease risk. In a study by Williams and colleagues on 2,568 asymptomatic men, a TC-HDL ratio of four correlated with a very low coronary heart disease conventional risk factor rating, and a TC-HDL ratio of eight was correlated with very high risk for coronary heart disease.

Uhl and colleagues measured fasting total cholesterol and high-density lipoproteins in 572 asymptomatic air crewmen. Of these, 132 had an abnormal treadmill test and underwent coronary angiography. Coronary disease defined as a lesion of 50% or greater diameter narrowing was found in 16, with the rest having minimal (N = 14) or no coronary artery disease (N = 102). The 14 men with minimal coronary artery disease had TC-HDL ratios that differed from the normals (P < .001). Two of the 16 with angiographic coronary artery disease had TC-HDL ratios of less than six, whereas four of the 102 angiographic normal subjects had a ratio of greater than six. Only 42 of 440 (9.5%) with a normal treadmill test had a TC-HDL ratio greater than six; 87% of those with coronary heart disease had TC-HDL ratios greater than six. This ratio generated a risk of 172. A limitation of this study is that true sensitivity cannot be determined because only those with an abnormal treadmill test underwent coronary angiography.

At the USAFSAM, 255 totally asymptomatic men underwent cardiac catheterization because of at least 0.1 mV of ST depression. Sixty-five men had at least 50% coronary artery narrowing. Thus, the predictive value of ST-segment changes was only 24%. Five risk factors were studied (smoking, hypertension, hypercholesterolemia, family history, and glucose intolerance), and univariate analysis did not increase the predictive value. However, 41 men had no abnormal risk factors, and the odds ratio was over 3:1 with hypercholesterolemia alone or the presence of three risk factors. The presence of at least one risk factor and two or more exercise variables identified as predictive (including 0.3 mV of ST depression early, persistent ST depression postexercise, or exercise duration under 10 minutes) identified over half the cases of two- or three-vessel disease with a predictive value of 84%.

Gated Chest X-Rays.   Dinsmore and colleagues reported the use of electrocardiographically triggered chest x-rays to diagnose coronary heart disease. A bicycle ergometer was pedaled directly in front of an x-ray film cassette, and chest x-rays were taken at rest and at peak exercise. Wall motion abnormalities, volume change, and pulmonary hypertension were criteria for ischemia.

Computer Probability Estimates. Diamond and Forrester have reviewed the literature to estimate pretest likelihood of disease by age, sex, symptoms, and the Framingham risk equation (based on blood pressure, smoking, glucose intolerance, resting electrocardiogram, and cholesterol). In addition, they have considered the sensitivity and specificity of four diagnostic tests (the exercise test, cardiokymography, thallium, and cardiac fluoroscopy) and applied Bayes' theorem. This information has been assimilated in a computer program written in basic that can be used to determine probabilities of coronary disease for a given individual after entry of any of the above data. CADENZA is the acronym for this program and it is commercially available (Cardiokinetics, Seattle).

Essentially, they derived a system of decision analysis that prescreens individual patients before they undergo more expensive tests. This enhances the predictive value of these noninvasive tests by selecting a subgroup with a greater pretest likelihood of disease (perhaps with a 15%–40% prevalence) so that the posttest probability of an abnormal test will be raised to 60%–80%.

The biggest weakness of this approach is that the sensitivities and specificities of the secondary tests is not certain, and it is uncertain how they interact because of similar inadequacies. In addition, a step approach that uses risk markers to identify a high-risk group excludes the majority of individuals who will eventually get coronary disease. This approach concentrates the preventive impact on the small, high-risk group while ignoring the majority of individuals in the moderate risk range who will contribute larger numbers but at a lesser rate to disease endpoints.

Hlatky et al. attempted to validate two available methods of probability calculation by comparing their diagnostic accuracy with that of cardiologists. Ninety-one cardiologists evaluated the clinical summaries of eight randomly selected patients. For each patient, the cardiologist assessed the probability of coronary heart disease after reviewing the clinical history, physical examination, and laboratory data, including an exercise test. The probability of coronary disease was also obtained for each patient using identical information from (1) a published table of data based on age, sex, symptoms, and degree of ST-segment change during exercise, and (2) Cadenza using the age, sex, risk factors, rest electrocardiogram and multiple exercise measurements. With the coronary angiogram as the standard, average diagnostic accuracy was best for the computer program. One wonders how helpful the computer program would be for noncardiologists and what the findings would have been if more than just eight patients and more apparently healthy individuals had been included.

Systolic Time Intervals. Spodick and colleagues reported that systolic time intervals measured using ear densitography during exercise appear to prove the sensitivity and specificity of the exercise test. These workers recorded ear densitograms using a photoelectric earpiece attached to the pinna of the ear which enables measurements of the preejection period (PEP) and left ventricular ejection time (LVET). Ten patients with coronary heart disease were compared with 17 normal men. Despite nearly identical heart rate and blood pressure responses, men with coronary heart disease had a significantly greater reduction of preejection period at one minute and four minutes during exercise as well as a greater decrease in the PEP-LVET ratio. The investigators believed that the early fall in the PEP-LVET ratio represented limited functional reserve, and the subsequent increase was consistent with functional deterioration. Louis and colleagues noted prolongation of left ventricular ejection time postexercise and suggested that this enhanced the diagnostic power of the exercise test. These approaches need further evaluation to determine if they have additional value compared with standard exercise measurements.

PROGNOSIS IN ASYMPTOMATIC PATIENTS WITH ANGIOGRAPHIC CAD

Hammermeister and colleagues reported the effects of coronary artery bypass surgery on asymptomatic or mildly symptomatic angina patients who were studied as part of the Seattle Heart Watch. The report was based on 227 medically treated and 392 surgically treated patients who were nonrandomly assigned to medical or surgical therapy. Cox's regression analysis was used to correct for the differences in baseline characteristics. Patients with three-vessel disease who underwent surgery had significantly improved survival, but surgically treated patients with one-vessel disease and two-vessel disease did not. The results of this study suggest that surgery may be indicated in the asymptomatic or mildly symptomatic patient with three-vessel disease, moderate impairment of left ventricular function (ejection fraction 31% to 50%), good distal vessels, and no other major medical illness. Asymptomatic patients with normal left ventricular function (ejection fraction greater than 51%) had an excellent prognosis regardless of the treatment.

Hickman and colleagues at USAFSAM followed for five years 90 men aged 45 to 54 years with asymptomatic angiographic coronary disease without previous MI. Sixteen patients developed angina, four had myocardial infarctions, and two died suddenly. The events were not significantly different in those with one-, two-, or three-vessel disease. They concluded that in asymptomatic patients with angiographic coronary disease, the five-year prognosis was good even in those with high-risk lesions. Conventional risk factors predicted risk more than the angiographic severity of disease did. Angina, a soft endpoint, was the most common initial event.

Kent et al. have reported 147 asymptomatic or mildly symptomatic patients with coronary heart disease who were followed prospectively for an average of two years. None had significant one-vessel, 31% had two-vessel, and 41% had three-vessel coronary disease. The ejection fraction was 55% or greater in

70% of the patients. Thirty-five percent of the patients had a normal electro-cardiogram, while 30% had evidence of a previous myocardial infarction. During the follow-up period there were eight deaths. There was an annual mortality of 3% for the entire group, 1.5% for patients with single- and dou-ble-vessel disease, and 6% for those with triple-vessel disease. In those with triple-vessel disease, exercise testing enabled better identification of high- and low-risk groups. In spite of a history of mild symptoms, 25% of the patients with triple-vessel disease exhibited poor exercise tolerance; of these, 40% ei-ther died (for an annual mortality of 9%) or had progressive symptoms re-quiring an operation. In those with good exercise capacity, only 22% died or had progressive symptoms, giving an annual mortality of 4%. The prognosis is excellent in patients with no or mild symptoms with one- or two-vessel disease. In those with three-vessel disease and with good exercise capacity, there was an annual mortality of 4% versus 9% in those with three-vessel disease and poor exercise capacity.

SERIAL TESTING PROCEDURES TO DETECT CORONARY ARTERY DISEASE

A program of serial testing to detect latent coronary heart disease has been completed by the U.S. Army. Screening was considered necessary before ini-tiating a mandatory exercise program for all personnel older than 40 years. The screening tests were applied in a sequential manner in an attempt to eliminate low-risk patients from further testing and to enhance the pretest likelihood of disease in the remaining subset. An initial history, physical ex-amination, and rest electrocardiogram were performed on 285 men and 2 women over 40 years of age (mean age 44). A fasting biochemical profile was obtained, and a risk factor index based on the Framingham data base was calculated. All subjects underwent maximal symptom-limited exercise test-ing. All were encouraged to exercise to exhaustion and the average oxygen consumption was 38.5 ml/kg per min (range 25 to 64). Pre- and postexercise CKGs were performed. A risk factor index over 5.0 was considered abnormal. Unfortunately, the ratio of total cholesterol to high-density lipoprotein choles-terol was not studied. An abnormal ST-segment response occurred in 4 men; an "abnormal nondiagnostic" response, defined as upsloping ST changes, oc-curred in 15 men. Six men had frequent exercise-induced PVCs. These 26 men underwent cardiac fluoroscopy and thallium scintigraphy. Seven men had abnormal thallium scintigraphic findings, six underwent cardiac catheter-ization, and one died of MI. One man with a low-risk index and normal tread-mill test, cardiokymogram, and fluoroscopic findings had a MI after six months of follow-up. The performance of these various tests is presented in Table 7–6. No patient had coronary calcification. An abnormal ST-segment response was insensitive and not highly predictive of coronary disease. Car-diokymography had a 63% sensitivity, a 74% specificity, a predictive value of 50%, and was the most accurate individual test. Risk factor analysis was not

TABLE 7–6.
Performance of Stratified Risk Analysis in Predicting Coronary Artery
Disease in Apparently Healthy Persons

VARIABLE	NO. OF POSITIVE RESULTS	SENSITIVITY (%)	SPECIFICITY (%)	PREDICTIVE VALUE	ODDS RATIO
Risk index ≥ 5	11	12.5	53	18	0.16
2 or more RF	15	62.5	47	33	1.5
Abnormal TM	4	25	98	50	2.8
TM PVCs	21	75	21	29	0.8
Abnormal CKG	10	62.5	74	50	1.75
Two or more RF + abnormal CKG	96	50	89	67	8.5

CKG = cardiokymogram; PVCs = significant premature ventricular complexes; RF = conventional risk factors; TM = treadmill test.

predictive, and only when there were two or more risk factors and an abnormal cardiokymogram was screening accuracy improved.

SECONDARY PREVENTION AND TESTING

Hypothetically, if a method of secondary prevention were proven and available today, the following three-step approach to screening for asymptomatic coronary heart disease in men over 35 years old appears reasonable. First, chest pain history, risk factor analysis, and a resting electrocardiogram should be obtained. If any data collected place the individual at risk, the second step should be a maximal exercise test. If this test is interpreted as abnormal, based on ST-segment shifts and perhaps other abnormal responses, the third step should be utilization of thallium exercise scintigraphy, cardiac fluoroscopy, or cardiokymography. The lack of data on the diagnostic value of these tools in asymptomatic individuals prevents strict recommendations at this time. Good clinical judgment must be exercised to avoid producing "cardiac cripples" by mislabeling healthy people. The severity of the abnormal response must be considered. Most often it is appropriate to follow an asymptomatic individual with only abnormal ST-segment depression.

EXERCISE TESTING FOR EXERCISE PROGRAMS

There are several reasons for doing an exercise test prior to initiating an exercise program. The optimal exercise prescription, based on a percentage of an individual's maximal heart rate or oxygen consumption (50%–80%) or to exceed the gas exchange anaerobic threshold, can only be written after performing an exercise test. The best way to assess the risk of an adverse reaction during exercise is to observe the individual during exercise. The level of exercise training then can be set at a level below that at which adverse responses or symptoms occur. Some individuals motivated by popular misconceptions about the benefits of exercise may disregard their natural "warning systems" and push themselves into dangerous levels of ischemia.

An individual with a good exercise capacity and only 0.1 mV ST-segment depression at maximal exercise has a relatively low risk of cardiovascular events in the next several years compared to an individual with marked ST-segment depression at a low heart rate and/or systolic blood pressure. Most individuals with an abnormal test can be put safely into an exercise program if the level of intensity of the exercise at which the response occurs is considered. Such patients can be followed with risk factor modification rather than being excluded from exercise or their livelihood.

Exercise testing is indicated prior to entering an exercise program for individuals with a strong family history of coronary disease (i.e., family members aged less than 60 with a coronary event), the presence of increased risk factors (particularly serum cholesterol), or any symptoms suggestive of myocardial ischemia currently or in the past. In addition, there is a group of patients who self-select themselves for exercise testing. They may request the test even though they deny having any symptoms.

High Risk Selection.   A problem with using exercise testing only in those patients with identified abnormal risk factors is that a large number of patients with coronary artery disease would be excluded. Thus, this approach increases the pretest probability of coronary artery disease and improves the predictive value of an abnormal response, but leaves a large number of patients with potential coronary artery disease without the potential benefits of this screening technique. It has been hypothesized that this approach concentrates the preventive impact on the small, high-risk group but ignores the majority of individuals in the moderate risk range.

Further Testing.   A major problem with performing an exercise test in apparently healthy people is the difficulty associated with a "positive" response. The thallium test appears to have relatively high sensitivity (80%) and specificity (90%), but it requires experienced readers and a good laboratory. It is, however, superior to radionuclide ventriculography, which in some studies has had a specificity as low as 60%. In some patients, a clearly abnormal secondary study may ultimately require coronary arteriography to assess coronary anatomy. It is necessary to see if there is an overlap in calling false positives; i.e., the exercise electrocardiogram and thallium could be abnormal in women because of attenuation by breast tissue causing cold spots, and the X phenomena causing ST-segment depression. Also, thallium may be falsely positive for unknown reasons in mitral valve prolapse as is the exercise electrocardiogram. A low specificity (i.e., a high rate of false positivity) must be avoided in screening.

EXERCISE TESTING FOR SPECIAL SCREENING PURPOSES

Pilots.   Unfortunately, politics and economic factors are two of the strongest factors influencing the use of exercise testing in subjects with flying responsibilities. The pool of available pilots is obviously an important national resource. If there are many pilots available, society is more likely to be more strict with regulations regarding flying standards. Physicians must be concerned with public safety. Allowing an individual with an increased health risk to take responsibility for many other peoples' lives could result in a tragedy. The presence of a back-up pilot and the impact of modern technology on flying do not lessen the stresses of this occupation. There are numerous situations of very high stress, such as takeoffs and landings, where it might not be possible for another cockpit personnel to take over control of the aircraft, and a disaster not averted if the key pilot was to have a cardiac event. In general, pilots are a highly motivated, intelligent group of men who feel a high level of responsibility for the performance of their work. Flying is their livelihood, however, and most of them love it so dearly that they may conceal medical information that could endanger their flying status. In addition, the stress of work often leaves them unable to maintain a healthy lifestyle. The stress of altering one's circadian cycle and trying to navigate in and out of today's busy airports leaves many of them overweight, deconditioned, and smoking heavily. Whenever possible, health professionals should recommend that these men and women have the full benefits of modern preventive medicine, including the periodic assessment of physical work capacity, response to stress, and the probability of coronary atherosclerosis.

CONCLUSIONS

Several recent studies markedly change our understanding of the application of exercise testing as a screening tool. These were additional follow-up studies including one from the CASS population based on 195 individuals with abnormal exercise tests by ST depression criteria and normal coronary angiograms followed for seven years. No increased incidence of cardiac events was found, and so the concerns raised by Erikssen's findings in 36 individuals that such individuals were still at increased risk are not substantiated. The other new follow-up studies (MRFIT, Seattle Heart Watch, LRC and Indiana State Police) had different results than prior studies, mainly because hard cardiac endpoints rather than angina were required.

Careful review of the 10 prospective studies of exercise testing in asymptomatic individuals reveals that screening has serious limitations. First of all, most of the studies included angina in the incidence of coronary heart disease and had to use it as a cardiac disease endpoint. This led to a bias for individuals with abnormal tests to subsequently report angina or to be diagnosed as having angina. When only hard endpoints (death or MI) were used, as in MRFIT, LRC, or the Seattle Heart Watch, the results are very discouraging. The test could only identify one-third of the patients with hard events, and 95% of abnormal responders were false positives; that is, they did not die or have an MI. The iatrogenic problems resulting from screening must be considered.

These results in a population first screened for risk factors to increase the prevalence of disease argue strongly against the routine use of exercise testing as a screening tool.

Some individuals who eventually develop coronary disease will change on retesting from a normal to an abnormal response. However, McHenry has reported that a change from a negative to a positive test is no more predictive than is an initially abnormal test; an individual has been reported who changed from a normal to an abnormal test but was free of angiographically significant disease.

The predictive value of the abnormal maximal exercise electrocardiogram ranged from 5% to 46% in the studies reviewed. That is, 5% to 46% (average 22%) of the abnormal responders developed coronary heart disease over the follow-up period. Thus, more than three-quarters of the abnormal responders were false positives. Some of these individuals have coronary disease that has yet to manifest itself, but angiographic studies have supported this high false positive rate when using the exercise test in asymptomatic populations, and the CASS study indicates that such individuals have a good prognosis.

Exercise testing may prove to have value in asymptomatic populations other than for screening. Bruce and colleagues examined the motivational effects of maximal exercise testing for modifying risk factors and health habits. A questionnaire was sent to nearly 3,000 men 35 to 65 years of age who had undergone symptom-limited treadmill testing at least one year earlier. Individuals were asked if the treadmill test motivated them to stop smoking (if already a smoker), increase daily exercise, purposely lose weight, reduce the amount of dietary fat, or take medication for hypertension. There was a 69% response to this questionnaire, and 63% of the responders indicated that they had modified one or more risk factors and health habits and that they attributed this change to the exercise test. In fact, a greater percentage of patients with decreased exercise capacity, compared with normal subjects reported a modification of risk factors or health habits.

Given the current approaches competing for health care resources, it is best to screen only those who request it, those with abnormal risk factors, those with worrisome medical histories, or a family history of premature cardiovascular disease. It is difficult to choose a chronological age after which exercise testing is necessary as a screening technique prior to beginning an exercise program, since physiological age is important. In general, if the exercise is more strenuous than vigorous walking, most individuals over the age of 50 will benefit from such screening. The iatrogenic problems resulting from screening must be considered and the results of testing must be applied using the predictive model and Baysian statistics. Test results must be thought of as probability statements and not as absolutes. The recent data from treadmill screening studies convincingly demonstrate the inappropriateness of including exercise testing as part of routine health maintenance in apparently healthy individuals. If it is used to classify asymptomatic individuals as having or not having coronary artery disease, it is very ineffective and causes more problems (psychological, work and insurance status, cost for more tests) than good by misclassifying approximately 10% of those without CAD as having disease.

BIBLIOGRAPHY

Abinader EG: The effect of beta blockade on the abnormal exercise test in patients with mitral valve prolapse. *J Cardiac Rehabil* 1984;4:95–100.

Abinader EG, Shahar J: Exercise testing in mitral valve prolapse before and after beta blockade. *Br Heart J* 1982;48:130–133.

Allen WH, Aronow WS, Goodman P, et al: Five-year follow-up of maximal treadmill stress testing in asymptomatic men and women. *Circulation* 1980;62:522–531.

Almeida D, Stanford J, Lutz J et al: Chest pain with normal coronary arteries. *J Cardiopulmonary Rehabil* 1985;5:364–372.

Ando J, Yasuda H, Miyamoto A, et al: Myocardial perfusion and left ventricular performance during exercise-induced ST-segment depression in apparently healthy subjects. *Jpn Heart J* 1984;25:155–166.

Aronow WS, Cassidy J: Five year follow-up of double Master's test, maximal treadmill stress test, and resting and postexercise apexcardiogram in asymptomatic persons. *Circulation* 1975;52;616–622.

Barnard RJ, Gardner GW, Diaco NV: "Ischemic" heart disease in fire fighters with normal coronary arteries. *J Occupational Med* 1976;18:818–827.

Barnard RJ, Gardner GW, Diaco NV, et al: Near-maximal ECG stress testing and coronary artery disease risk factor analysis in Los Angeles City fire fighters. *J Occupational Med* 1975;18:818–827.

Barrett PA, Peter CT, Swan HJC et al: The frequency and prognostic significance of electrocardiographic abnormalities in clinically normal individuals. *Prog Cardiovasc Dis* 1981; 23:299–310.

Bengtsson C, Grimby G, Lindquist O, et al: Prognosis of women with exercise-induced ECG changes—results from a longitudinal population study. *Cardiology* 1981;68:9–27.

Blackburn H: The prognostic importance of the electrocardiogram after myocardial infarction. *Ann Intern Med* 1972;77:677–689.

Borer JS, Brensike JF, Redwood DR, et al: Limitations of the electrocardiographic response to exercise in predicting coronary artery disease. *N Engl J Med* 1975;193:367–375.

Breslow L, Sommers AR: The lifetime health monitoring program: A practical approach to preventive medicine. *N Engl J Med* 1977;296:601–606.

Bruce RA, DeRouen TA, Hossack KF: Pilot study examining the motivational effects of maximal exercise testing to modify risk factors and health habits. *Cardiology* 1980;66:111.

Bruce RA, Fisher LD, Hossack KF: Validation of exercise-enhanced risk assessment of coronary heart disease events: Longitudinal changes in incidence in Seattle community practice. *J Am Coll Cardiol* 1985;5:875–881.

Bruce RA, McDonough JR: Stress testing in screening for cardiovascular disease. *Bull NY Acad Med* 1969;45:1288–1295.

Burke JF, Morganroth J, Soffer J, et al: The cardiokymography exercise test compared to the thallium-201 perfusion exercise test in the diagnosis of coronary artery disease. *Am Heart J* 1984;107:718–724.

Cadman D, Chambers L, Feldman W, et al: Assessing the effectiveness of community screening programs. *JAMA* 1984;251:1580–1585.

Caralis DG, Bailey I, Kennedy HL, et al: Thallium-201 myocardial imaging in evaluation of asymptomatic individuals with ischemic ST segment depression on exercise electrocardiogram. *Br Heart J* 1979;42:562–571.

Carboni GP, Celli P, D'Ermo M, et al: Combined cardiac cinefluoroscopy, exercise testing and ambulatory ST-segment monitoring in the diagnosis of coronary artery disease; a report of 104 symptomatic patients. *Int J Cardiol* 1985;9:91–101.

Crow R, Grimm R, Prineas R, et al: Baseline rest electrocardiographic abnormalities, antihypertensive treatment and mortality in the multiple risk factor intervention trial. *Am J Cardiol* 1985;55:1–15.

Cullen K, Stenhouse NS, Wearne KL, et al: Electrocardiograms and 13-year cardiovascular mortality in Busselton study. *Br Heart J* 1982;47:209–212.

Cumming GR, Samm J, Borysyk L, et al: Electrocardiographic changes during exercise in asymptomatic men: three-year follow-up. *Can Med Assoc J* 1975;112:578–585.

Dawber TR, Kannel WB, Love DE, et al: The Framingham Study. *Circulation* 1952; 5:559–566.

Detrano R, Salcedo EE, Hobbs RE, et al: Cardiac cinefluoroscopy as an inexpensive aid in the diagnosis of coronary artery disease. *Am J Cardiol* 1986;57:1041–1046.

Diamond GA, Forrester JS: Analysis of probability as an aid in the clinical diagnosis of coronary artery disease. *N Engl J Med* 1979;300:1350–1359.

Dinsmore RE, Wernikoff RE, Miller SW, et al: Evaluation of left ventricular free wall asynergy due to coronary artery disease: use of an interlaced ECG-gated radiography system. *AJR* 1979;132:909–918.

Engelberg AL, Gibbons HL, Doege TC: A review of the medical standards for civilian airmen. *JAMA* 1986;255:1589–1599.

Epstein SE, Kent KM, Goldstein RE, et al: Strategy for evaluation of surgical treatment of the asymptomatic or mildly symptomatic patient with coronary artery disease. *Am J Cardiol* 1979;43:1015–1025.

Erikssen J, Amlie JP, Thaulow E, et al: PR interval in middle-aged men with overt and latent coronary heart disease compared to PR in angionegative and normal men of similar age. *Clin Cardiol* 1982;5:353–359.

Erikssen J, Dale J, Rottwelt K, et al: False suspicion of coronary heart disease: A seven-year follow-up study of 36 apparently healthy middle-aged men. *Circulation* 1983;68:490–497.

Erikssen J, Enge I, Forfang K, et al: False positive diagnostic tests and coronary angiographic findings in 105 presumably healthy males. *Circulation* 1976;54:371–376.

Erikssen J, Otterstad JE: Natural course of a prolonged PR interval and the relation between PR and incidence of coronary heart disease. A seven-year follow-up study of 1,832 apparently healthy men aged 40–59 years. *Clinc Cardiol* 1984;7:6–13.

Fleg JL, Lakatta EG: Prevalence and significance of postexercise hypotension in apparently healthy subjects. *Am J Cardiol* 1986;57:1380–1384.

Froelicher VF, Thomas M, Pillow C, et al: An epidemiological study of asymptomatic men screened with exercise testing for latent coronary heart disease. *Am J Cardiol* 1975;34:770–779.

Froelicher VF, Thompson AJ, Wolthuis R, et al: Angiographic findings in asymptomatic aircrewmen with electrocardiographic abnormalities. *Am J Cardiol* 1977;39:32–39.

Froom J, Boisseau V, Sherman A: Selective screening for lead poisoning in an urban teaching practice. *J Fam Pract* 1979;65:9–15.

Giagnoni E, Secchi MB, Wu SC, et al: Prognostic value of exercise EKG testing in asymptomatic normotensive subjects. *N Engl J Med* 1983;309:1085–1092.

Gordon D, Ekelund L, Karen J, et al: Predictive value of the exercise test for mortality in North American men: LRC follow up. *Circulation* 1986;74:252–261.

Hammermeister KE, DeRouen TA, Dodge HT: Effect of coronary surgery on survival in asymptomatic and minimally symptomatic patients. *Circulation* 1980;62:98.

Hartley LH, Herd JA, Day WC, et al: An exercise testing program for large populations. *JAMA* 1979;241:269–275.

Hickman JR, Uhl GS, Cook RL, et al: A natural history study of asymptomatic coronary disease. *Am J Cardiol* 1980;45:422–430.

Hjermann I, Holme I, VelveByre K, et al: Effect of diet and smoking intervention on the incidence of coronary heart disease. *Lancet* 1981;2:1305.

Hlatky M, Bovinick E, Brundage B: Diagnostic accuracy of cardiologists compared with probability calculations using Bayes' rule. *Am J Cardiol* 1982;49:192–197.

Hollenberg M, Zoltick JM, Go M, et al: Comparison of a quantitative treadmill exercise score with standard electrocardiographic criteria in screening asymptomatic young men for coronary artery disease. *N Engl J Med* 1985;313:600–606.

Hopkirk JAC, Uhl GS, Hickman JR, et al: Discriminant value of clinical and exercise variables in detecting significant coronary artery disease in asymptomatic men. *J Am Coll Cardiol* 1984;3:887–894.

Hopkirk JAC, Uhl GS, Hickman JR, et al: Limitation of exercise-induced R-wave amplitude changes in detecting coronary artery disease in asymptomatic men. *J Am Coll Cardiol* 1984;3:821.

Johnson RL, Bungo MW: The diagnostic accuracy of exercise electrocardiography—a review. *Aviat Space Environ Med* 1983;54:150–157.

Joy M, Trump DW: Significance of minor ST-segment and T-wave changes in the resting electrocardiogram of asymptomatic subjects. *Br Heart J* 1981;45:48–55.

Kelley MJ, Huang EK, Langou RA: Correlation of fluoroscopically detected coronary artery calcification with exercise stress testing in asymptomatic men. *Radiology* 1978;129:1–12.

Kemp HG, Kronmal RA, Vlietstra RE, et al: Seven-year survival of patients with normal and near normal coronary arteriograms: A CASS registry study. *J Am Coll Cardiol* 1986;7:479–483.

Kennedy HL, et al: Coronary artery disease in healthy subjects with frequent and complex ventricular ectopy. *Ann Intern Med* 1980;92:179–185.

Kent KM, Rosing DR, Ewels CJ, et al: Prognosis of asymptomatic or mildly symptomatic patients with coronary artery disease. *Am J Cardiol* 1982;49:1823–1831.

Langou RA, Huang EK, Kelley MJ, et al: Predictive accuracy of coronary artery calcification and abnormal exercise test for coronary artery disease in asymptomatic man. *Circulation* 1981;62:1196–1202.

Levine HD, Phillips E: The electrocardiogram and MI. *N Engl J Med* 1951;245:833–842.

Louis RP, Marrsh DG, Sherman JA, et al: Enhanced diagnostic power of exercise testing for myocardial ischemia by addition of post exercise left ventricular ejection time. *Am J Cardiol* 1977;39:767–775.

MacIntyre NR, Kunkler JR, Mitchell RE, et al: Eight-year follow-up of exercise electrocardiograms in healthy, middle-aged aviators. *Aviat Space Environ Med* 1981;52:256–259.

Manca C, Barilli AL, Dei Cas L, et al: Multivariate analysis of exercise ST depression and coronary risk factors in asymptomatic men. *Eur Heart J* 1982;3:2–8.

Manca C, Cas LD, Albertini D, et al: Different prognostic value of exercise electrocardiogram in men and women. *Cardiology* 1978;63:312–320.

McHenry PL, O'Donnell J, Morris SN, et al: The abnormal exercise electrocardiogram in apparently healthy men: A predictor of angina pectoris as an initial coronary event during long-term follow-up. *Circulation* 1984;70:547–551.

McHenry PL, Richmond HW, Weisenberger BL, et al: Evaluation of abnormal exercise electrocardiogram in apparently healthy subjects: Labile repolarization (ST-T) abnormalities as a cause of false positive responses. *Am J Cardiol* 1981;47:1152–1161.

MRFIT: Risk factor changes and mortality. *JAMA* 1982;248:1465.

MRFIT: Exercise electrocardiogram and coronary heart disease mortality in the multiple risk factor intervention trial. *Am J Cardiol* 1985;55:16–24.

Nolewajk AJ, Kostuk WJ, Howard J, et al: 201 Thallium stress myocardial imaging: An evaluation of 58 asymptomatic males. *Clin Cardiol* 1981;4:134–142.

Oliver MF: Strategies for preventing and screening for coronary heart disease. *Br Heart J* 1985;54:1–5.

Ostor E, Schnohr, Jensen G, et al: Electrocardiographic findings and their association with mortality in the Copenhagen City Heart Study. *Eur Heart J* 1981;2:317–328.

Rabkin SW: Electrocardiographic abnormalities in apparently healthy men and the risk of sudden death. *Drugs* 1984;28:28–45.

Rabkin SW, Mathewson FAL, Tate RB: The electrocardiogram in apparently healthy men and the risk of sudden death. *Br Heart J* 1982;47:546–552.

Rautaharju PM, Prineas RJ, Eifler WJ, et al: Prognostic value of exercise electrocardiogram in men at high risk of future coronary heart disease: Multiple risk factor intervention trial experience. *J Am Coll Cardiol* 1986;8:1–10.

Robertson WS, Feigenbaum H, Armstrong WF, et al: Exercise echocardiography: A clinically practical addition in the evaluation of coronary artery disease. *J Am Coll Cardiol* 1983; 2:1085–1091.

Rose G, Baxter PJ, Reid DD, et al: Prevalence and prognosis of electrocardiogram findings in middle-aged men. *Br Heart J* 1978;40:636–643.

Rubler S, Fisher VJ, Schreiber SS, et al: Left ventricular ejection times during exercise testing with scintigraphy. *Arch Intern Med* 1984;144:1386–1391.

Silverberg RA, Diamond GA, Vas R, et al: Noninvasive diagnosis of coronary artery disease: The cardiokymographic stress test. *Circulation* 1980;61:579–589.

Spirito P, Maron BJ, Bonow RO, et al: Prevalence and significance of an abnormal ST-segment response to exercise in a young athletic population. *Am J Cardiol* 1983;51:1663–1666.

Sugiura T, Doi Y, Haffty B, et al: Noninvasive assessment of left ventricular performance in patients with ischemic heart disease: Ear densitographic study during uninterrupted treadmill exercise. *Am J Cardiol* 1981;48:101–112.

Theroux P, Franklini D, Ros J, Jr, et al: Regional myocardial function during acute coronary artery occlusion and its modifications by pharmacologic agents in the dog. *Circ Res* 1974;35:896.

Thompson AJ, Froelicher VF, Longo MR, et al: Normal coronary angiography in an aircrewman with serial exercise test changes. *Aviat Space Environ Med* 1975;46:69–75.

Uhl GS, Hopkirk AC, Hickman JR, et al: Predictive implications of clinical and exercise variables in detecting significant coronary artery disease in asymptomatic men. *J Cardiac Rehabil* 1984;4:245–252.

Uhl GS, Kay TN, Hickman JR: Computer-enhanced thallium-scintigrams in asymptomatic men with abnormal exercise tests. *Am J Cardiol* 1981;48:1037–1046.

Uhl GS, Troxler RG, Hickman JR, et al: Angiographic correlation of coronary artery disease with high density lipoprotein cholesterol in asymptomatic men. *Am J Cardiol* 1981;48:903–911.

Vas R, Diamond GA, Silverberg RA, et al: Assessment of the functional significance of coronary artery disease with atrial pacing and cardiokymography. *Am J Cardiol* 1979;44:1283–1289.

Wasserman AG, Bren GB, Ross AM, et al: Prognostic implications of diagnostic Q-waves after myocardial infarction. *Circulation* 1982;65:1451–1460.

Weiner DA: Accuracy of cardiokymography during exercise testing: Results of a multicenter study. *J Am Coll Cardiol* 1985;6:502–509.

Williams P, Robinson D, Bailey A: High density lipoprotein and coronary risk factors in normal men. *Lancet* 1979;1:72–80.

Zoltick MJM, McAllister HA, Bedynek JL: The United States Army cardiovascular screening program. *J Cardiac Rehabil* 1984;4:530–535.

8 RADIONUCLIDE EXERCISE TESTING

Radionuclide imaging techniques have been added to exercise testing with the aim of complimenting or adding to the diagnostic and prognostic power of standard exercise testing. The two techniques commonly used are (1) imaging after exercise with a radionuclide that behaves metabolically like potassium, and (2) imaging during and after exercise using blood pooling agents. Before the methodology of these techniques is discussed, let us review radiation physics.

BASIC RADIATION PHYSICS

Each atom contains at its center a cluster of particles with a net positive charge called a nucleus. Some of these particles with positive charges are called protons and some of the uncharged particles are called neutrons. Neutrons can change into protons by emitting a beta particle. This transformation is called beta-ray decay. Outside the nucleus, the atom consists of a swarm of negatively charged electrons arranged in shells. The outer ring contains the chemically active valence electrons.

The position of an atom in the periodic table of chemical elements is determined by the number of electrons and protons that an atom contains. The atomic number of an atom is the number of protons in its nucleus. The mass of an atom mostly depends on the number of protons and neutrons in the nucleus.

The chemical elements differ from one another by the number of protons in their nuclei. Any individual atom, characterized by a particular atomic number and mass number, is called a nuclide. Atoms differing in atomic weight but not in atomic number (i.e., having the same number of protons) are referred to as isotopes, from Greek words meaning "same place," because they occupy the same place in the periodic table. Isotopes of each element differ mainly by the number of neutrons they contain. The word *isotope* is often used when nuclide is actually meant. We can certainly speak of one nuclide, but when referring to a single isotope, one might as well speak of one twin.

The neutrons play the role of glue holding the entire nucleus together in

298

spite of a very strong repulsion exerted by the positive protons. The most complicated nucleus known in nature is the common isotope of uranium (U-238). It contains 92 protons (giving it an atomic number of 92) and 92 electrons. The nucleus also contains 146 neutrons, giving it a mass number of 238. Uranium does not have a stable nuclear configuration. It can become less unstable by splitting off a helium nucleus (an alpha particle). This phenomenon is the basis of the alpha-ray radioactivity of the heavy elements.

Electrons are arranged in shells and in subshells, each of which is characterized by energy level and by number of electrons. The inner-shell electrons are more tightly bound than are the outer-shell electrons. When atoms are bombarded by high-energy particles or radiation, an electron may be knocked out of a neutral atom. The energy expended by electrons moving between shells can be emitted in two ways: either as electromagnetic radiation or as electrons themselves.

Radioactivity is the constant emission of penetrating and ionizing radiation. It is dependent on the spontaneous transformation within the nucleus of neutrons and protons or of their internal arrangement. Knowledge of the properties of the three types of radiation (alpha, beta, and gamma) is based on the effects of collisions of these ionizing radiations with electrons and nuclei. There are five types of transformations that can take place in the nucleus causing radioactivity: alpha decay, beta decay, electron capture, isomeric transition, and spontaneous fission.

Alpha decay is found only in the isotopes of heavy elements. The alpha ray ejected from the nucleus in this type of decay is a fast helium nucleus (i.e., two protons and two neutrons). For a given radionuclide, alpha rays are emitted in one or more monoenergetic groups. Alpha rays are the heaviest particles emitted from nuclei and have the greatest kinetic energy. Radium and radon are typical alpha ray emitters. All of the very heavy nuclides (atomic number greater than 83) have a prolonged radioactive decay in the form of spontaneous nuclear fission. This fission results in the release of alpha rays. All of the nuclides produced by nuclear fission are negatron beta-ray emitters.

Beta rays are high-speed electrons produced in radioactive transformations by one of two types of beta decay. The slightly more common type of beta ray is an ordinary negative electron called a negatron, and the other type consists of a positive electron called a positron. Because many nuclear reactors can only provide a source of neutrons, the most commonly used radionuclides are neutron-rich, negatron beta-ray emitters. The production of positron-emitting radionuclides usually requires a cyclotron or linear accelerator. These complex devices are particle accelerators and are located at only a few research facilities.

All proton-rich nuclides can accomplish a transformation of a proton into a neutron by capturing an electron. This capture results in a reduction of the atomic number and a change in the isotope's position in the periodic table. If the nuclear transformation leaves the decay product nucleus at an excited level, then gamma rays will be emitted. All radionuclides that transform by positron beta-ray emission or by electron capture (e.g., thallium) are man-made from particle accelerators. All the naturally occurring radioactive nuclides emit either alpha rays or negatron beta rays. Man-made radioactive nuclides not found in nature have the advantage for nuclear medicine of having short half-lives since they must be unstable if they do not exist in nature.

Gamma rays are emitted when there are shifts of neutrons or protons within the shells and subshells of the nucleus. Gamma rays originate in nuclei, whereas x-rays originate from the transformation of extranuclear electrons. Every radionuclide that emits gamma rays has its own particular gamma ray energy spectrum that characterizes it. There are a few cases in which an excited state in a nucleus is prolonged, when the gamma ray transition is delayed by minutes or hours rather than by microseconds. Because the ground level and the excited level have the same number of protons and neutrons, they are called nuclear isomers and the transition between them is called isomeric transition. Technetium 99m, which can be produced by commercial nuclear generators, emits gamma rays in this way.

Alpha or beta rays ionize some of the atoms that lie along their path as they travel through matter. Gamma rays and x-rays interact with matter and produce secondary electrons. Beta rays can travel roughly 100 times farther than alpha particles can. X-rays and gamma rays are electromagnetic radiations. They behave like a stream, called photons or quanta, rather than as waves. The modes of interaction of x-rays or gamma rays with matter include photoelectric interaction, Compton interaction, and pair-production interaction. The photoelectric interaction is with an atom and produces a single photoelectron. The Compton interaction takes place with an electron and produces both a Compton-recoil electron and a Compton-scatter photon. The pair-production interaction occurs with a nucleus and produces a pair of electrons—one positron and one negatron.

The basic unit of activity for all radionuclides is the curie (Ci). This activity unit is defined as 3.5×10^{10} disintegrating nuclei per second and is not a measure of the number of rays emitted. The energy of nuclear radiations is usually measured in electron volts (eV). The unit of absorbed radiation is the rad which is equal to 6.25×10^{13} eV per gram of exposed tissue. The rate of decay is a constant for each radionuclide. The so-called decay constant is the probability of disintegration per unit time and per atom. It can be shown that the mean life or average life for a large group of identical atoms is simply the reciprocal of the decay constant. Instead of the mean life, the rate of decay of any radionuclide can be described by its half-life, which is equal to the product of 0.693 and the mean life. Half-life is the time at which one-half of any initial amount of radioactive atoms remain undecayed.

The measurement of alpha activity does not play a role in nuclear medicine because the radioisotopes utilized emit only beta and gamma rays. The photoelectrons or Compton electrons originating from gamma-ray absorption or scatter produce ionization and excitation along their paths similar to that produced by beta rays of corresponding energies. Radiation-measuring devices depend upon effects mediated through the charged-particle path of ionization or excitation. There are three principal classes of such devices: a gas, a liquid, or a solid. Gas devices such as ion chambers and Geiger tubes are now only used for dosing applications. They have been largely replaced by liquid and crystal scintillation cameras or scintigraphs. An Anger camera uses one crystal; various other cameras use multiple crystals.

MYOCARDIAL IMAGING WITH
POTASSIUM-LIKE RADIONUCLIDES

The radionuclides that metabolically behave like potassium (including potassium 43, cesium 129, rubidium 81, and thallium 201) are expensive since they are produced by either a cyclotron or an accelerator. The optimal gamma-emitting potassium-like radionuclide would have its major energy peak in the range of technetium 99m (i.e., 140 keV) and, like technetium, be produced by commercial nuclear generators. With the exception of thallium 201, all of the potassium-like radionuclides have a relatively high energy spectrum of gamma-ray emission that requires special shielding and collimation of the scintillation camera for efficient imaging. Potassium 43 and rubidium 81 provide relatively poor myocardial-to-background ratios and have limited availability. Also, potassium 43 has a relatively high beta emission that leads to a high radiation dose for a patient. Cesium 129 is not extracted rapidly enough to detect transient ischemia. The lowest energy can be obtained from thallium 201 with imaging centered around 80 keV (actually, these are x-ray emissions from a mercury breakdown product of thallium).

The regional myocardial potassium-sodium ratio has been studied during acute coronary occlusion in animals. A fall from the normal ratio of five to less than three in the central ischemic zone occurs 15 minutes after occlusion. At 60 minutes, this ratio falls to less than two, and at 24 hours it is less than 0.5. Parallel changes or ones of lesser magnitude occur in border zones. Abnormalities in transmyocardial potassium flux have also been noted in humans during ischemia. The regional myocardial uptake of potassium-like radionuclides is based on regional myocardial blood flow and the myocardial extraction of these cations. Potassium is extracted efficiently by cardiac muscle. Following intracoronary injection, approximately 70% of the potassium is extracted.

Rubidium has a similar extraction compared to potassium, whereas thallium extraction is higher. Peak myocardial concentration of these radionuclides is generally reached within five minutes after intravenous injection. Cesium is cleared much more slowly, and peak myocardial uptake takes much longer. The myocardial biologic half-life of potassium is approximately one hour, and for cesium seven hours. Therefore, cesium cannot be used for exercise scintigraphy. Thallium also has a lesser hepatic and gastric uptake than either rubidium or potassium. The two major unfavorable physical properties of thallium are its half-life of 73 hours, which is much longer than required for clinical measurements. Its emissions are less energetic than gamma photons, which results in a higher likelihood of absorption and scatter within the body. These properties result in unnecessary radiation exposure and poor imaging characteristics. However, all things considered, thallium 201 is the best agent available because it produces diagnostic quality images on available scintillation cameras using standard collimation. It is produced by bombarding stable thallium 203 in a cyclotron.

Myocardial imaging with radioactive cations has been used to (1) diagnose and localize acute or prior myocardial infarctions, (2) diagnose and localize ischemia, (3) determine disease severity and prognosis, and (4) evaluate interventions. When patients are studied at rest, a reduction in regional activity corresponds to areas of scar most likely secondary to myocardial infarction. When radioactive cations are injected intravenously after the onset of angina pectoris or during exercise, a new region of decreased activity identifies an ischemic area secondary to an obstructed coronary artery. The radionuclide materials used for analysis of regional myocardial perfusion have been termed "cold spot" agents because the areas of decreased myocardial perfusion are identified by a decrease in regional radioactivity or a cold spot.

Exercise Methodology.   An intravenous line is inserted prior to exercise, and the patient is encouraged to exercise maximally to the point of angina or fatigue. At this point, thallium is injected into the infusion line. Exercise is continued for an additional minute to allow adequate distribution of the radionuclide even if the work load must be decreased. Imaging is begun as quickly as possible so that ischemia is not missed. Patients must exercise to a maximal effort for the test to have maximum sensitivity. Patients should be studied in multiple views: anterior, 45-degree, and 70-degree left anterior obliques. The 45-degree oblique view is of value in separating inferolateral from anteroseptal defects. The 45-degree anterior oblique view is especially valuable for quantitative techniques, and sometimes inferior wall defects are best seen in this view. The 60-degree left anterior oblique and the lateral views are commonly replaced with a single 70-degree left anterior oblique view. This maneuver helps to visualize transient ischemia by decreasing imaging time. Ischemia can be missed if imaging is delayed after exercise. Care should also be taken so that the diaphragm does not cause a pseudo-defect. The resting view is usually obtained when redistribution occurs four hours after the exercise study without requiring a second injection of thallium on another day. A defect at the time, however, can be due to severe ischemia instead of scar. Approximately 25% of patients with angina and no prior MI will have a defect still present at this time that fills in later. Repeat imaging 24 hours later will show if the defect has "reperfused," but imaging quality is poor, and long recording times are necessary because of decay. Immediate-delay films can be used to follow the rate of redistribution. Tomographic imaging requires more time and computer reconstruction of three-dimensional images.

Thallium Extraction.   Thallium uptake tends to underestimate the flow in conditions of hyperemia. Extraction will vary with the degree of flow and will increase as flow decreases. This phenomenon is not reflected by increased uptake in low-flow regions, since the amount of cation presented to the low-flow zone is decreased. Extraction or uptake patterns cannot be altered without changes in flow. For instance, the infusion of glucose and insulin leads to significant increases in the uptake of potassium and its analogs. Hypercapnea and respiratory acidosis are said to result in increased myocardial potassium accumulation. In an animal study, extraction of thallium by the myocardium was evaluated as a function of heart rate, coronary blood flow, hypoxia, changes in pH, and after administration of propranolol, insulin, and strophanthin. Under basal conditions, the extraction fraction measured 88% and was unchanged by pacing, alterations in pH, and administration of propranolol, insulin, and digitalis. Hypoxia caused a significant decrease in extraction fraction, to 78%. When coronary blood flow was increased in excess of the demand due to drugs, extraction fraction fell logarithmically. Thus, for clinical purposes, if an image were obtained immediately after thallium administration, the regional concentration in the myocardium would be representative of blood flow. In a study comparing thallium and radio-labeled microspheres, variable areas of ischemia were assessed in 16 closed-chest dogs. An excellent correlation between thallium and the microspheres with ischemic segments was found. The major limitation of thallium was the inconsistent detection of small perfusion defects. Figure 8–1 shows the relationship of the heart and coronary arteries to the thallium images.

Apical Thinning and Increased Uptake With Exercise. Forty-four normal subjects were studied at both rest and exercise by Zaret; homogeneous myocardial images were recorded. Decreased uptake in the apical region was found to be a normal variant. This result occurred in approximately 20% of normal subjects and is probably due to thinning of the apex of the heart. Thirteen healthy adults were studied by Cook and colleagues after administration of thallium, both at rest and at maximal exercise. On the rest scan, the left ventricular myocardium, liver, and spleen were seen. In two subjects with a resting tachycardia, the right ventricle was slightly visualized. When the nuclide was administered during exercise, the left ventricular activity was more homogeneous, and the left ventricle was better defined on the scan. The left ventricle-to-lung background activity ratio increased from 2.4 at rest to 3.4 during exercise. The right ventricle myocardium was seen on the exercise scan. Phantom studies showed that small lesions are best viewed either straight on or at a tangent. The usual dose of thallium given for cardiac scanning is 2 mCi. When studying healthy persons, the scanning period can be prolonged and the dose administered reduced to 1 mCi. Although the total body dose is low, the renal and gonadal doses should be a major consideration when studying normal volunteers or apparently healthy individuals.

Slow Washout. The classic hallmark of coronary artery disease (CAD) on an exercise thallium image is reduced initial myocardial uptake that fills in later, indicating a regional perfusion abnormality. Slow thallium myocardial clearance has been suggested as a second imaging marker of CAD even though other factors unrelated to coronary perfusion affect clearance rate. If initial uptake and clearance are useful variables in identifying CAD, their range in normals should be narrow. To clarify the range of normal

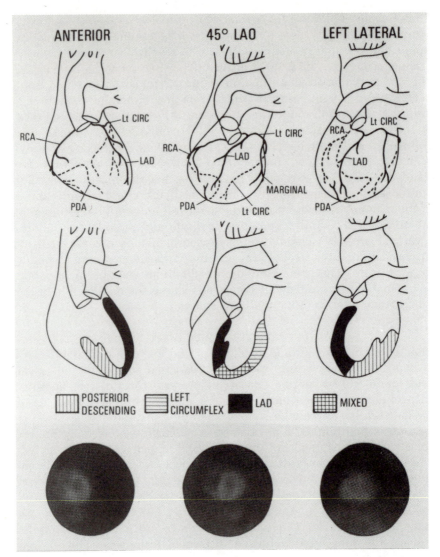

FIG 8–1.
Illustration of thallium scintigrams in relation to cardiac anatomy and coronary
artery distribution.

thallium clearance and its relationship to the level of exercise achieved, exercise thallium images in 89 normal subjects were analyzed by Kaul et al.
Analysis of variance using 10 clinical and exercise variables as covariates
showed that the slower clearance was related to a lower peak exercise heart
rate (HR). By linear regression analysis, a decrease in peak HR of 1 beat/min
was associated with a slower thallium clearance (longer half-life) of three
minutes. Using this formula, the clearance value in each patient was then
corrected for peak exercise heart rate by decreasing measured clearance by

0.05 hr multiplied by the amount of peak exercise heart rate which was below 183. There were no differences in the "corrected" clearance. Thus, thallium myocardial clearance after exercise is slower when peak exercise heart rate is lower. Therefore, thallium clearance rates (if uncorrected for peak exercise heart rate) should be used with caution for diagnosing CAD. None of the computer programs for analyzing thallium images take this into account.

Reverse Redistribution.   The observation has been made in several laboratories where the delayed or four-hour ("rest") thallium study shows defects not apparent just after exercise, or where perfusion defects seen with exercise worsened. This phenomenon has been called reverse redistribution and has been suggested to be due to significant coronary artery occlusion. Silberstein and DeVries found that the reverse redistribution phenomenon (apparent worsening of a stress-induced defect or appearance of a new area of relative hypoperfusion) does not always indicate CAD as previously suggested. Reverse redistribution does not correlate with the degree of CAD nor with the location of the stenosis. Multiple mechanisms are hypothesized wherein the "defect" may be located in the best or worst perfused area.

False Positives.   Bulkley and coworkers used exercise thallium scans in six normal volunteers and in five patients with systemic sarcoidosis and cardiac dysfunction. The scans were normal in the volunteers; segmental defects were found in the left ventricle compatible with infiltrative disease of the myocardium in three of the patients with sarcoidosis. Segmental myocardial infiltration by sarcoid was confirmed by autopsy in one of these patients and by an operation in another. They concluded that thallium myocardial perfusion defects can be secondary to myocardial sarcoidosis and other infiltrative disorders, and thus represent false positive responses.

REPRODUCIBILITY OF
THALLIUM INTERPRETATION

McLaughlin reported 76 thallium myocardial scans performed on 25 patients to assess reproducibility and the effects of varying levels of exercise on the results of imaging. Of 70 segments among the 14 patients assessed by two maximal exercise tests, 64 (91%) were reproducible. Only 51% of the defects present at maximal exercise were seen in the submaximal exercise study in 12 patients studied at two exercise levels. In terms of observer agreement, they noted total agreement of three observers in 60 of 76 studies. Only once was a defect seen without a significant lesion in the arteries supplying the area.

Trobaugh and colleagues have reported a multicenter study of observer variability, another term describing interobserver agreement or reliability. Two readers from different institutions interpreted a total of 100 resting scintigrams (50 from each institution) as normal, borderline, and abnormal. Exact agreement of all four observers in regard to these categories occurred in 44% of the studies; and in an additional 35% of the studies, three of the four observers agreed and the fourth observer differed by one grade of abnormality. Hence, in 79% of the studies, at least three of four observers agreed. The percentage of interobserver agreement is similar to other studies (Bailey 90% agreement; Verani 82%; Blood 90%; Ritchie 80%; and Lenaers 80%).

In Atwood's study at UCSD of thallium images, four experienced interpreters evaluated 100 analog thallium myocardial images on two occasions using a form designed to limit reader variability. A high intraobserver agreement (agreement by same observer at separate times) of 89%–93% was found when films were interpreted as normal or abnormal (a dichotomous decision). Interobserver agreement for a majority grouping of observers (three or four) was 75% for an abnormal and 68% for a normal interpretation. However, agreement ranged from 11%–79% when interpreters were asked to read the anatomic locations of defects. Posterior and lateral wall defects were interpreted with the least amount of agreement. The results summarized in Figure 8–2 indicate that caution must be taken when interpreting defect location. Using a scale of 1–10 to grade the severity of a defect, correlations of 0.82–0.86 were found when reading defects in the lateral and anterior projections. Higher correlations, from 0.86–0.94, were found in left anterior oblique views. The greatest intraobserver agreement occurred when the interpreters were asked for only an abnormal or normal response (a dichotomous interpretation). Intraobserver agreement averaged 91%, and interobserver agreement among at least three readers of abnormal scintigrams occurred in 77% of the studies. This increased consistency in dichotomous judgments is encouraging and has been found in other studies, but chance may well contribute to this phenomenon. The poorest intraobserver agreement was noted in the location of an abnormality. The septal area was the most reproducible and the lateral wall

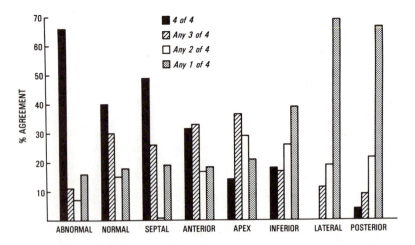

FIG 8–2.
Results of interobserver reliability in the reproducibility study of visual reading of thallium scintigrams.

the poorest. Part of the lack of observer agreement may also be due to inadequate definitions of terms as well as to normal variation. It appears that a reporting form that not only contains the usual written description and location of a lesion but also requires a shaded area or other drawing of a lesion on schematic representations is helpful. Use of reporting forms with specific criteria, multiple observers at one occasion, and/or computer processing may improve agreement.

Thallium Exercise Imaging with Angiographic Correlation. Clinical studies (summarized in Table 8–1) have evaluated the sensitivity and specificity of rest and exercise cold spot imaging, with coronary angiography as the diagnostic reference. Most of these studies also included the results of rest and exercise electrocardiography. Significant coronary artery disease was considered equal to or greater than 50% or 75% reduction of the luminal diameter of one or more of the three major coronary arteries; some of the investigators mentioned that similar results were obtained using either criteria. Most of the exercise tests were performed with only one ECG lead recorded, which lowered the sensitivity of exercise ECG. Usually, other diagnostic endpoints of exercise testing were not considered.

In one of the first studies, Berman and associates reported their results in 40 patients studied with rest and exercise rubidium 81 scans, exercise electrocardiography, and coronary angiography. During the exercise tests, leads I, II, aVF, and V5 were recorded. In 33 patients with significant coronary disease, the rubidium 81 scan was abnormal in 88% while 58% showed abnormal ST-segment depression. In seven patients with less than 50% narrowing, the scans showed no defects, but two of the seven had abnormal ST-segment depression.

Rosenblatt and coworkers performed rest and exercise thallium scans, single-lead exercise ECG, and coronary angiography on 15 patients with severe coronary disease, 12 patients with mild coronary disease, and 3 patients with normal coronary arteries. Forty percent of the patients with severe coronary artery disease had abnormal treadmill tests, whereas 93% had abnormal exercise scans. Correlation between scan defects and sites of coronary lesions was poor in patients with two- and three-vessel disease as compared with those with single-vessel disease. The one patient with a false negative scan had three-vessel disease. The scans of patients with diffuse disease were characterized by generalized poor uptake. The scans after exercise, however, exhibited greater uptake. Of the four patients without lesions exceeding 50% narrowing, one had both an abnormal ST-segment response to exercise and an abnormal myocardial scan. Another patient had an abnormal scan despite normal left ventricular contraction and minimal coronary disease. Three patients with chest pain but with normal coronaries and left ventriculograms had normal myocardial scans.

Bailey and colleagues studied 20 healthy subjects and 63 coronary artery disease patients using treadmill testing with thallium scans and simultaneously recorded 12-lead ECGs. The studies in the healthy subjects were all normal. Small inhomogeneities of uptake were frequent, but they were not

TABLE 8–1.
Exercise Thallium Studies With Angiographic Correlation Demonstrating
Sensitivity and Specificity

PRINCIPAL INVESTIGATOR	N	SENSITIVITY	SPECIFICITY	COMMENTS
Berman	40	88%	100%	Rubidium
Rosenblatt	30	93%	71%	Unprocessed analog images
Bailey	83	75%	100%	Manual quantification of analog images
McGowan	160	83%	82%	Potassium or rubidium
Ritchie	101	76%	92%	Unprocessed analog images
Collaborative study	190	78%	88%	Some images interpreted after 20%–25% background subtraction
Turner	64	68%	97%	Unprocessed Polaroid film; no MI patients
Verani	82	78%	97%	Unprocessed analog images; no delayed images obtained
Botvinick	65	85%	92%	Unprocessed analog images using rubidium
McCarthy	128	85%	79%	Five-point smooth, 30% background subtraction on Polaroid film
Zeppo	30	70%	—	Unprocessed Polaroid film; patients with 3-vessel disease only
Caldwell	52	85%	100%	Unprocessed Polaroid film
Jengo	58	93%	94%	Unprocessed Polaroid film
Uhl	100	75%	89%	Processed images; large sample of asymptomatic patients
Detrano	1,341	75%	85%	Average of 19 studies excluding MI patients, planar images
Kaul	325	95%	80%	Computer quantification, multivariate approach excluding basal segments

equal to 15% of the left ventricular circumference in any projection. None of
these subjects developed a new perfusion defect on the exercise image. When
the abnormal ECGs (Q-waves at rest or ST-segment depression during exercise
or both) and abnormal myocardial scans (perfusion defect at rest or a new
defect with exercise or both) in patients with coronary artery disease were
compared, the sensitivity for the ECG studies was 65% versus 75% for the

thallium scans. In those with single-vessel disease, the sensitivities were 46% versus 71%, in those with two-vessel disease 70% versus 65%, and in those with three-vessel disease 93% versus 93%. If the development of precordial chest pain with the exercise test was also considered an abnormal response, the sensitivity of the routine exercise test was similar to that of the exercise myocardial imaging. Two patients with left bundle branch block and coronary disease had abnormal scans. Eleven percent of the patients with significant coronary artery disease failed to develop chest pain, a scan defect, or ST-segment depression during exercise.

McGowan and coworkers reported 160 patients studied with rest and exercise imaging using potassium 43 or rubidium 81, a V5 lead, and coronary angiography. Fifty-one of 62 patients with insignificant coronary disease had normal scans, and 81 of 98 patients with significant coronary disease had abnormal scans.

Ritchie and colleagues reported 101 patients studied with rest and exercise imaging using thallium, a V5 lead, and coronary angiography. Of 25 patients with insignificant coronary disease, one had a resting defect and one had an exercise defect. Four of these had exercise-induced ST-segment depression. Among the 76 patients with significant coronary disease, 76% had a defect on either the rest or exercise thallium image. Forty-five percent of them had exercise-induced ST-segment depression. Of the patients with coronary disease, 91% had either an abnormal thallium study or an abnormal resting or exercise ECG. Image defects localized a coronary lesion in all patients with single-vessel disease. In patients with two- or three-vessel disease, the image defect was always associated with a lesion; however, other high-grade lesions were often present but image defects did not develop in these regions.

Botvinick and associates reported results in 65 patients studied with rest and exercise imaging using rubidium 81, a V5 lead, and coronary angiography. Thirty-four patients had significant coronary artery disease. Myocardial imaging had a sensitivity of 85% and a specificity of 92% while the exercise ECG had a sensitivity of 79% and a specificity of 64%. Thallium imaging was more sensitive in patients with one- and two-vessel disease while the exercise ECG was more sensitive in those with three-vessel disease. There were two patients with false positive myocardial scans who had documented anterior infarctions without significant coronary disease. The three false negative images occurred in one patient with one-vessel disease and well-established coronary collaterals, one patient with severe three-vessel disease, and one patient with a prior MI.

In a collaborative study involving six institutions, Ritchie and colleagues used myocardial imaging with thallium in patients with angina pectoris or acute myocardial infarction. Ninety of 111 patients (81%) with acute MI had image defects, compared with 71 (64%) who had new Q-waves. Patients with large infarctions and anterior infarcts were more commonly detected than were those with smaller or inferior infarcts. In patients presenting with angina pectoris, 42 patients had no coronary lesion with greater than 50% luminal narrowing, and five of them had an abnormal rest or exercise defect, a specificity of 88%. Among the 148 patients with significant coronary lesions, image defects occurred at rest or with exercise in 115. New exercise image defects were more common than was exercise ST-segment depression. False positive responses occurred in one patient with catheter-induced spasm, one with an isolated distal 40% narrowing left anterior descending lesion, and one with normal coronary arteries but with both angina and exercise-induced ST-segment depression. Exercise imaging was particularly useful in the patients with digitalis effect or left bundle branch block. Thirteen of 16 such patients had exercise thallium defects. Imaging also localized the site of ischemia.

Dunn and colleagues studied 76 consecutive patients with documented normal coronary arteries who had thallium exercise studies. The thallium scintigrams were normal in 79% and abnormal in 21%. Analysis of the locations of thallium defects in the 16 normal subjects with abnormal scintigrams revealed a pattern consistent with coronary disease in five (including four with an abnormal left ventricle) and a pattern that suggested soft tissue attenuation in nine (diaphragm, breast, or adipose tissue), while the other two had apical defects. Consistent defects were defined as: anteriorly, if seen in more than one projection and extending into the apical segment; inferiorly, if seen in more than one projection; and laterally, if associated with inferior defects. This manner of interpretation improved the specificity of the thallium test.

Thallium scanning and exercise electrocardiography have been said to complement each other by being strong in the situation of the other's weakness. Thallium was thought to be more sensitive in single-vessel disease because of the greater chance of contrast between poorly and well-perfused areas than in triple-vessel disease. The opposite situation would apply in exercise electrocardiography, which is clearly more sensitive in multivessel disease. Also, thallium studies were thought to be helpful in patients with chronotropic incompetence or with poor exercise tolerance. Studies have shown that false negative thallium scans usually occur in patients with inadequate heart rates and in those with single-vessel disease. Thus, it appears that both procedures have some similar limitations. Iskandrian and Segal evaluated the impact of exercise thallium studies in 71 patients who had inconclusive, or equivocal, exercise electrocardiograms. The thallium exercise test had a sensitivity of 79% and a specificity of 95% in these patients, and thus was comparable to the results in patients who had exercise electrocardiographic studies that were unequivocal.

Rigo and colleagues evaluated the diagnostic value of thallium exercise testing in 141 patients with angiographically proven coronary disease. One hundred had a previous myocardial infarction and 40 did not. In the patients without infarction, the sensitivity for detecting left anterior descending and right circumflex and left circumflex coronary artery occlusions was 66%, 53%, and 24%, respectively. In those without a previous infarction, the sensitivity for demonstrating disease in the artery corresponding to the site of infarction was 100% for the left anterior descending, 79% for the right circumflex, and 63% for the left circumflex coronary artery. In patients with a prior anterior infarction, concomitant right or left circumflex coronary artery lesions were detected in only one of 12 cases, while in those with a prior inferior infarct, the sensitivity for left anterior disease was 69%. Thallium exercise testing was useful for identifying multivessel disease in patients with previous inferior infarction, but had relatively no value in detecting right or left circumflex disease in patients with a prior anterior infarction and in patients without previous MI. Overall, in the group without previous MI, 76% had an abnormal exercise scintigram, and in the group with a previous MI, 96% had abnormal scintigrams at rest or during exercise.

Rehn and colleagues assessed thallium exercise testing for identifying left main coronary artery disease by studying 24 patients with left main disease and 80 patients with narrowing of other vessels. Ninety-two percent of those with left main disease had abnormal exercise scintigrams, but the patterns of perfusion defects were not specific.

Detrano reviewed previous studies and found 19 reporting the sensitivity and specificity of exercise thallium scintigraphy that fulfilled the following criteria: (1) patients with a history or ECG evidence of a myocardial infarction were not included in the study sample or, if included, the results for these patients were reported separately; (2) patients taking beta-blocking medications were neither excluded nor taken off their medications before their exercise test; and (3) planar (not tomographic) thallium imaging was used. Pooling the results of the 1,341 patients without myocardial infarction in these 19 investigations yielded a sensitivity of 75%, specificity of 85%, and a diagnostic accuracy of 80%. These results are similar to those obtained at the Cleveland Clinic for planar thallium imaging applied to subjects without myocardial infarction. Many of these studies are difficult to evaluate since the criteria for abnormal is not specified as being a fixed or a reversible defect or both. Also, they do not fulfill the criteria of adequacy as defined by Philbrick et al. in Chapter 4.

Computer Quantification.   Although quantification of exercise thallium images using computer algorithms has been previously reported, the relative value of different imaging variables for detection of CAD has not been analyzed in a large group of patients with cardiac catheterization. Regional initial thallium uptake, redistribution, and clearance on thallium study were measured in 325 patients (281 patients with and 44 patients without angiographic CAD) by Kaul et al. Half had ECG evidence of prior Q-wave MIs. Normal values were defined in 55 other clinically normal subjects. When five myocardial segments were analyzed in each view, the respective values for sensitivity and specificity were 95% and 50% for initial thallium uptake, 60% and 87% for redistribution, and 74% and 66% for clearance. Initial thallium uptake was the most sensitive but least specific, while redistribution was the least sensitive and most specific.

Using stepwise logistic regression analysis, the best correlate of CAD was initial thallium uptake. Addition of redistribution to a mathematical model of the probability of CAD did not alter sensitivity but increased specificity from 50% to 70%. Once initial uptake and redistribution were considered, myocardial thallium clearance provided no additional improvement in the correlation. Excluding the two basal segments in each view from the analysis increased the specificity from 70% to 80% without affecting sensitivity. Of the

15 patients (5%) with coronary disease not detected using this approach, none had left main disease and 10 (67%) had one-vessel disease. A combination of variables derived from quantification of exercise thallium images provided a superior sensitivity (95%) and specificity (80%) for the detection of coronary artery disease compared with the use of a single variable. If a cutpoint yielding a specificity comparable to visual analysis studies was used, a comparable sensitivity would be obtained.

Comparison of Exercise ECG and Thallium.   Previous studies evaluating the sensitivity and specificity of exercise electrocardiography, using coronary angiography or follow-up coronary events, have established its sensitivity to be 60% and its specificity to be 85%. This level of specificity was obtained by avoiding the conditions that can cause false positive responses. The low specificity of exercise electrocardiography in the studies performed for comparison with thallium scintigraphy was due to the inclusion of patients likely to have false positive exercise electrocardiographic responses. The greater sensitivity of exercise thallium imaging compared with ST-segment depression can be partially explained by the inclusion of patients with myocardial damage (i.e., they should have defects due to scarring).

THALLIUM EXERCISE TESTING POST-MI

The images of post-MI patients are complicated by the defect due to scarring; reproducibility problems make it difficult to distinguish peri-infarctional ischemia from the normal variability in sizing defects. Thallium scintigraphy was utilized by Turner et al. in 32 patients without complications post-MI. A treadmill test to 75% of the age-predicted maximum heart rate was done three weeks after MI. All patients also underwent coronary and left ventricular angiography. Among the 16 patients with greater than 70% stenosis of two or more vessels, nine (56%) had an abnormal exercise test response (angina or 0.1 mV or more ST-segment depression), 10 (63%) had a reversible scintigraphic defect consistent with an ischemic area, and 13 (81%) had either one of the two tests abnormal. The results were essentially the same for detecting areas of jeopardized myocardium (areas with normal or hypokinetic wall motion supplied by a stenotic artery).

In 42 post-MI patients undergoing submaximal exercise testing with thallium scintigraphy just before discharge, Gibson et al. found that multiple defects were the best predictors of multivessel disease (MVD) by utilizing discriminant function analysis of 23 clinical and laboratory variables. Of 16 patients with multiple scintigraphic defects in two or more scan segments, 14 had MVD, giving an 88% predictive accuracy. Of 11 patients with ST-segment depression of 0.1 mV or more, only five had MVD, but the remaining six all had one-vessel disease. This group has also reported 61 post-MI patients exercised to a target heart rate of 120. Increased lung uptake of thallium, which occurred in 22 patients, was related to a higher frequency of previous MI

(36% versus 13%), less global cardiac reserve as assessed by the NYHA or Killip classes, and frequent MVD (73% versus 17%). Increased lung uptake was related to failure to achieve the target heart rate because of dyspnea, fatigue, or angina (86% versus 36%) and a greater prevalence of exercise induced ST-segment depression. There were more anterior thallium defects, a lower EF at rest (40% versus 50%) and more abnormal left ventricular segments in these patients. Increased lung uptake of thallium during exercise appeared to be a marker of functionally important coronary artery disease with left ventricular dysfunction in the post-MI patient.

Van Der Wall et al. from Amsterdam compared the results of maximal exercise testing with ECG and thallium to coronary angiography. Their study included 176 patients 6–8 weeks post their first transmural MI. The exercise ECG was considered abnormal if at least 0.1 mV ST depression occurred, and the thallium scan was abnormal if a defect was seen in an area other than that of the scar. Of these patients, 44% had MVD; the ECG detected 64%, and only 31% were detected by thallium.

RADIONUCLIDE VENTRICULAR ANGIOGRAPHY DURING BICYCLE EXERCISE

Evaluation of left ventricular contraction and volume by qualitative and quantitative techniques has been a goal of cardiology. Until the advent of echocardiography and radionuclide angiography, these types of analyses were performed with direct injection of radiopaque contrast material into the left ventricle. Now, however, these two noninvasive methods can supply much of the data from contrast ventriculograms, and can be safely repeated.

Wall motion, ventricular function (ejection fraction), and ventricular volume can be derived from radionuclide angiograms by geometric or count-based techniques. Much of the original work in radionuclide imaging involved application of the traditional area-length formula to left ventricular images to derive left ventricular volumes and ejection fraction. Area-length calculations are difficult and depend on geometric assumptions. Thus, count-based methods for evaluation of left ventricular size and function have been developed. These techniques involve external imaging of the cardiac blood pool with an external imaging device, such as a probe or gamma scintillation camera.

Two methods of radionuclide analysis of left ventricular function have been utilized. First, the transit of a bolus of a radionuclide material as it passes through the central circulation is observed. In the second, the left ventricle is visualized using radioactive substances that circulate in the blood in a steady state. This equilibrium technique requires gating of multiple R-R intervals to produce a summed, composite cardiac cycle (Fig 8–3).

A variety of 99mTc-labeled radiopharmaceuticals may be used for these procedures. First-transit, or first-pass, studies can be done with any agent that is not filtered out by the lungs. Any pharmaceutical that can be injected in a

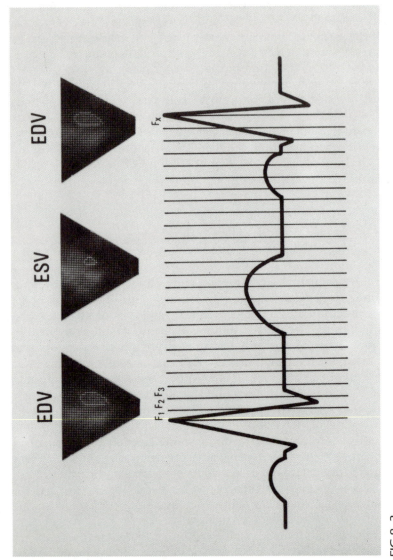

FIG 8–3.
Description of the process of multigated acquisition (MUGA) for radionuclide ventriculography.

bolus is suitable. If repeated studies are needed, two agents should be used: one is excreted by the kidneys and one extracted by the liver. For equilibrium studies, any blood pool imaging agent is suitable, including human serum albumin and in vitro or in vivo labeled red blood cells.

First-transit studies can be performed with standard single-crystal Anger cameras. The use of multicrystal cameras increases the count rate with loss of resolution. A dedicated nuclear computer system is needed to perform the analyses. Gated or equilibrium studies are usually performed with single-crystal cameras and dedicated computer systems.

The first-pass approach requires the evaluation of the radioactive bolus as it passes through the right and left ventricle. A variety of camera projections can be used, the requirements being that the left ventricle can be clearly seen and that the aorta and mitral valve plane can be located. Data are acquired in list or serial mode at a sampling frequency equal to or greater than 20 frames per second. Usually the right and left ventricular time-activity curves are separated. The computer operator then assigns a fixed left ventricular and background region of interest, from which a time-activity (volume) curve is generated. Ejection fraction can thus be calculated by averaging the end-diastolic and end-systolic data points. This technique has been shown to correlate well with contrast ventriculography. Gating must be used for imaging with a first-pass agent when using a single-crystal camera if wall motion and volume estimates are to be made.

The equilibrium techniques can be used after the blood pool imaging radionuclide passes through the heart numerous times and reaches a stable concentration in the circulation. An electrocardiographic gate is utilized to initialize time blocks in the cardiac cycle. The ECG gate is used to accumulate two frames, either end-diastole or end-systole (now more commonly), multiple frames throughout the entire cycle-based on short acquisition intervals phased from a fiducial point on the electrocardiogram. When multiple R-R intervals are summed and the resulting frames viewed in sequence, a cine format produces the illusion of ventricular contraction. The left ventricle can be assigned manually or with a variety of edge-detection algorithms. Ejection fraction and ventricular volume can be quantitated from the time-activity curves.

Using a single-crystal camera, the first-pass angiogram can reliably estimate both right and left ventricular ejection fractions. However, because the end-diastolic and end-systolic regions of interest have less than 200 counts per 0.04-second frame, visualization of the ventricular silhouette and wall motion analyses are difficult. Analysis of ventricular volume is even more difficult, although area-length methods have been successfully applied to first-pass angiograms derived from multicrystal cameras. First-pass ejection fractions can be obtained in the right anterior oblique position so that single plane wall motion analyses can be performed. Intervention studies require multiple injections, and wall motion analyses require higher doses of radionuclides.

Gated radionuclide studies, unlike first-pass techniques, cannot be performed in the right anterior oblique projection for the purpose of evaluating left ventricular function because the right ventricle overlies the left ventricle in this projection. Studies of ventricular function and wall motion must therefore be performed in the left anterior oblique projection, in which the right and left ventricle are clearly separated. Visual interpretation of the ventricular silhouette in this view is not as informative as the right anterior oblique view because the anterolateral and inferior walls are not well seen. Nonetheless, one dose of a radionuclide can produce multiple studies for up to four hours after injection. It has been thought that the right ventricle could best be evaluated by first-pass techniques, but equilibrium angiograms can also produce estimates of right ventricular ejection fraction and volume. The advantages and disadvantages of these two techniques are summarized in Table 8–2.

While attempts have been made to utilize the posttreadmill exercise period

TABLE 8–2.

Comparison of Two Noninvasive Techniques of Radionuclide Left Ventricular Angiography

The First-Pass (Transit) Technique

Disadvantages

1. Multiple injections are required for intervention studies, with time allowed between injections for clearance of the previously injected material.
2. This camera is immobile, expensive, delicate, and less commonly available. Some investigators have gated and used a standard camera. In general, a multicrystal scintillation camera is needed for regional wall motion studies.
3. Imaging cannot be done during exercise because of motion artifact. The radionuclide is injected during exercise immediately before stopping, and imaging is begun after stopping. This is a disadvantage since the ejection fraction can normalize quickly after exercise.
4. Volume measurements are less reproducible.

Advantages

1. Can be done in the right anterior oblique or anterior projections, enabling evaluation of wall motion of the anterior left ventricular wall.
2. Easier to account for interference from the right ventricle and left atrium.
3. Short data acquisition time (about 10 sec).
4. Can be performed with a scintillation probe ("nuclear stethoscope").

Gated Blood-Pool Studies

Disadvantages

1. The optimal pooling agent has not been demonstrated.
2. Requires left anterior oblique imaging to avoid the right ventricle, so regional wall motion abnormalities of the anterior left ventricular wall cannot be assessed while ejection fraction is measured.
3. The left atrium is difficult to account for during imaging.
4. Relatively long acquisition time (2 min or more) required for sufficient counts.
5. Correlation studies have suggested that ejection fraction is lower using this technique because of interference from the left atrium.

Advantages

1. After one injection, serial studies can be performed for four hours or longer.
2. Wall motion can be assessed using a conventional Anger scintillation camera.
3. Ejection fraction and volume can be followed through exercise and recovery after one injection of a radionuclide.
4. Ejection fraction and volume can be determined serially after treadmill testing.

to evaluate left ventricular performance, most investigators have utilized either supine or erect bicycle exercise. The investigations that evaluated the hemodynamic response to supine exercise using invasive techniques have shown that there is a marked difference between the body's response to acute exercise in the supine and erect positions. In normal subjects, stroke volume and end-diastolic volume do not change much during supine bicycle exercise from rest, while in the erect position, both increase during mild work and then plateau. When angina patients perform identical submaximal bicycle work loads, supine and erect, heart rate is higher in the supine position. Maximal work load is lower in the supine position and angina develops at a lower double product. In angina patients, left ventricular filling pressure is more likely to increase during exercise in the supine position than erect. Also, ST-segment depression is greater in the supine position.

Supine protocols for radionuclide imaging have consisted of two to four exercise levels, three or four minutes in duration, to fatigue or angina. They have been continuous and progressive. Usually scintigraphic data are obtained during the last few minutes of each stage to minimize heart rate variation while collecting the gated images. Erect exercise has been used in similar fashion, though mostly by investigations with multicrystal cameras. Arguments over which method is more suitable for diagnostic testing at present remain unresolved though one study found no difference in diagnostic value between the two positions. Although supine exercise is not as physiologic as erect exercise, it is technically easier to perform and is associated with increased venous return, cardiac dilation, and greater resting left ventricular wall stress. Positioning of the camera is extremely critical, and four-chamber separation should be achieved for optimal calculations; such separation is much easier to accomplish in supine patients.

The response of the left ventricle to acute exercise depends on the functional reserve of the left ventricle, myocardial perfusion, as well as the exercise performed. The following is a review of studies that have investigated the role of exercise in the evaluation of heart function using radionuclide left ventricular angiography.

Ejection Fraction Response to Exercise. Borer and colleagues studied 10 men and one woman with angiographic coronary artery disease and normal resting left ventricular function confirmed by angiography. Fourteen normal subjects were also studied. Gated radionuclide angiography was performed in the supine position at rest and during exercise. Human serum albumin labeled with 10 mCi of radioactive technetium was administered intravenously. A conventional Anger camera was oriented in a modified left anterior oblique position to isolate the left ventricle. Ejection fractions by this technique were consistently lower than those determined by contrast angiography, but there was a correlation coefficient of .86. Imaging was performed during exercise for at least two minutes at near-maximum effort. Ejection fraction increased from rest during exercise in all normal subjects, with the increase ranging from 7% to 30%. In patients with coronary disease, ejection fraction during exercise diminished in all but one patient, and in that patient it remained unchanged. At least one new region of left ventricular dysfunction developed during exercise in each of the patients with coronary artery disease.

Rerych and colleagues studied 30 normal volunteers (mean age 34 years) using the first-pass technique and maximal upright bicycle exercise. An increase of the ejection fractions from a resting value of 66% to 80% obtained at peak exercise was reported for mean values. Similar values were obtained by these same investigators when evaluating college swimmers before and after training. They found a rest to peak exercise ejection fraction increase from 73% to 87% before training, and a similar increase (67% to 86%) following training. Port and colleagues studied 12 subjects in the upright position during maximal exercise and found all subjects to increase exercise ejection fraction above the resting value. Bodendeimer and coworkers employed isometric handgrip exercise to evaluate 19 subjects without coronary artery disease. Although global function was found to be of limited value (only 3 of 19 patients increased exercise ejection fraction by more than 5%), the authors found assessment of relative changes in regional ejection fraction to be useful.

Conflicting results were reported by Foster and colleagues who studied the response of nine healthy male volunteers to maximal upright bicycle ergometry. Using the first-pass technique and progressive exercise, they found a mean ejection fraction increase from rest to peak exercise (67% to 73%) and decrease in one from 85% to 83%. In addition, all of these normal subjects decreased their peak ejection fraction when subjected to sudden strenuous exercise. The fact that the subjects were stressed to their true maximal effort, that the ejection fraction was obtained during the last minute of exercise (as opposed to immediately after), and that they started with high ejection fraction may possibly explain these results.

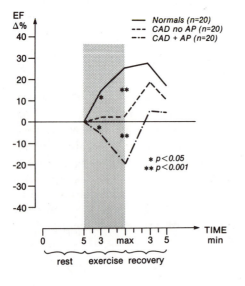

FIG 8–4.
The ejection fraction response to supine bike exercise measured with radionuclide ventriculography.

TABLE 8–3.
Results of Studies Using Exercise Radionuclide Ventriculography With Coronary
Angiographic Correlation

PRINCIPAL INVESTIGATOR	N	SENSITIVITY	SPECIFICITY	METHOD (1) AND CRITERIA (2) FOR NORMAL
Borer	25	100%	100%	(1) Gated (2) Exercise EF ≥ 7% above rest
Berger	73	87%	100%	(1) First pass (2) Wall motion, rest EF ≥ 55%, exercise EF > 5% above rest
Brady	89	93%	100%	(1) Gated (2) Exercise EF > rest
Pfisterer	40	95%	55%	(1) Gated (2) Rest EF > 50%, exercise EF ≥ 10% above rest
Caldwell	52	93%	54%	(1) Gated (2) Rest EF > 50%, exercise EF > 5% above rest
Jengo	58	98%	94%	(1) First pass (2) Wall motion, exercise EF > 10% above rest
Jones	387	90%	58%	(1) First pass (2) Rest EF > 50%, predicted exercise EF, end-systolic volume, wall motion
TOTAL	724	92%	70%	

EF = ejection fraction

Few studies have examined the ejection fraction response in coronary heart disease patients with respect to the nature or severity of their disease (angina, infarct, or vessels involved). Battler and coworkers reported that 20 patients with typical angina decreased their ejection fraction from a resting value of 57% to 47% at peak supine exercise. Only three patients failed to decrease their ejection fractions by more than three ejection fraction units. Similar results were obtained by Borer and coworkers in 44 patients who experienced chest pain during supine exercise. The resting mean left ventricular ejection fraction of 48% decreased to 39% during chest pain. Five of the 44 patients did show an increase in the exercise ejection fraction, and one remained unchanged. The remaining 38 patients decreased their exercise ejection fraction response.

Patients with angiographic evidence of coronary heart disease but without angina or infarction usually do not significantly increase peak exercise ejection fraction value from the resting value. Figure 8–4 is an illustration of this finding from a study by our group. Table 8–3 summarizes the studies that have investigated the sensitivity and specificity of exercise ventriculography for coronary heart disease using coronary angiography as the gold standard. One of the problems with comparing results is that the criteria for what is considered abnormal differ among these studies.

The Declining Specificity of Exercise Radionuclide Ventriculography. Rozanski et al. noted that although exercise radionuclide ventriculography was initially reported to be a highly specific test for CAD, later studies reported a high false positive rate. To verify this reversal, they analyzed the responses in 77 angiographically normal patients; 32 were studied from 1978 to 1979 (the early period), and 45 from 1980 to 1982 (the recent period). Most patients studied in the early period had normal responses (94% for EF and 84% for wall motion). In contrast, normal responses were less frequent in patients studied in the recent period (49% for EF and 36% for wall motion). The probability of coronary disease before testing was higher in these patients (38% vs. 7%, p<0.001). More patients studied in the recent period underwent RNV before angiography (78% vs. 22%, p<0.001), and more of these prior studies had abnormal results than those performed after angiography (55% vs. 6%, p<0.0001). Thus, two factors appeared responsible for the temporal decline in specificity: a change in the population being tested (pretest referral bias) and a preferential selection of patients with a positive test response for coronary angiography (posttest referral bias).

Detection of Wall Motion Abnormalities. Left ventricular contraction is a series of sequential contractions of muscle bundles, and abnormal contraction, which can be regional or global, is due to disorganization of the contraction sequence. Regional contraction or wall motion abnormalities are characteristically seen in patients with coronary heart disease and are due to disorganized contraction in a localized area. Asynergy is usually classified as hypokinesia (decreased motion), akinesia (no motion), or dyskinesia (bulging during systole). The exact relationship of these findings to pathologic aneurysms is uncertain. Regional contraction abnormalities can be found in more than one-half of all patients with coronary disease, and in more patients when midsystole or early systole are considered. In general, regional wall motion disturbances induced by exercise are due to inadequate coronary perfusion, and those present at rest are due to scar. However, some abnormalities present at rest can be reversed with nitroglycerin. Though such abnormalities are considered by some to be due to resting ischemia, their disappearance is most likely due to unloading of the LV. There is a progressively higher prevalence of asynergy with occlusion of more coronary vessels. However, asynergy is a dynamic event and may be induced by a variety of pharmacologic and physiologic interventions. The ability to analyze resting and stress-induced wall motion abnormalities should enhance the ability to discern the severity and location of coronary lesions.

Ventricular asynergy can be seen in any location, although the apex is the most common site. The prevalence of asynergy has not been altered by the addition of the left anterior oblique view, and biplane ventriculography is found to add only a small number of additional abnormally contracting zones to the right anterior oblique single plane view. However, visual interpretation of single plane left anterior oblique equilibrium radionuclide angiograms provide less information than do first-pass right anterior oblique radionuclide angiograms. Assessment of wall motion abnormalities has relied on visual interpretation of radionuclide images and computer programs for regional ejection fraction and phase analysis have been disappointing. These techniques rely on area or time analysis of pie-shaped wedges of the left ventriculogram. Regional ejection fractions correlate somewhat with regional wall motion abnormalities detected by contrast ventriculography, as do phase analysis abnormalities. It appears that regional wall motion abnormalities are not specific for coronary disease; that is, they can occur in other forms of heart disease. Also, in some views, the normal septum appears akinetic.

                    Digital Subtraction Angiography.   Digital subtraction angiography permits high resolution imaging of the left ventricle following an intravenous injection of contrast medium. The application of such techniques to left ventricular imaging at rest and after exercise should be an excellent means to validate or improve on radionuclide ventriculography. In order to test the clinical applicability of such a procedure, Detrano submitted 150 consecutive patients without myocardial infarction who were referred to Cleveland Clinic for coronary angiography to resting and exercise digital subtraction ventriculography. Digital ventriculograms were considered abnormal if a severe wall motion abnormality existed at rest or if worsening of segmental wall motion occurred after exercise. Global ventricular response to exercise was considered abnormal if the ventricular ejection fraction computed using the Dodge area length formula was less than 50% at rest or failed to increase after exercise. Seventy-eight (52%) of these subjects had at least one greater-than-50% obstruction of a major coronary artery. Thirty-six (24%) had such involvement in more than one major coronary vessel (multivessel disease). Sensitivities of these test responses were 76% and 68%, respectively.

    To compare the relative accuracies of exercise digital subtraction ventriculography and digital subtraction fluoroscopy with thallium scintigraphy, Detrano submitted 97 consecutive patients without myocardial infarction to all three tests on the day before their scheduled coronary angiograms. Forty-two patients had CAD (>50% diameter narrowing of one major artery). A fixed or reversible perfusion defect defined an abnormal thallium test while a segmental wall motion abnormality at rest or with exercise defined an abnormal digital ventriculogram. Any visualized coronary calcific deposit defined an abnormal digital fluorograph. The sensitivities of digital fluoroscopy (86%) and digital ventriculography (79%) were significantly higher than the sensitivity of thallium (62%, $p < 0.05$). The specificity of thallium (82%) was not significantly higher than that of either digital ventriculography (73%) or fluoroscopy (67%). The diagnostic accuracies of digital fluoroscopy, digital ventriculography, and thallium were 75%, 75%, and 73%, respectively. A logistic regression model demonstrated that thallium and digital fluoroscopy were more accurate in younger patients while digital ventriculography was more sensitive in hypertensives and in those not taking beta blockers. Thus, the choice of test should depend on disease prevalence, clinical variables (age, hypertension, sex), and the importance of functional information obtained for exercise testing.

PROGNOSTIC VALUE OF
RADIONUCLIDE VENTRICULOGRAPHY

Pryor et al. at Duke attempted to determine which variables obtained when performing exercise radionuclide ventriculography predict subsequent survival or total events (cardiovascular death or nonfatal MI). In their stable patients with symptomatic coronary artery disease (CAD), 52% had prior MIs. Univariable and multivariable analyses of six variables, including ejection fraction (EF) at rest and exercise, change in EF with exercise, development of ischemic chest pain or ECG changes, left ventricular (LV) wall motion abnormalities and exercise time were examined in 386 patients followed up to 4.5 years. Univariate analyses revealed that the exercise EF was the variable most closely associated with future events (p<0.01), followed by EF at rest, wall motion abnormalities, and exercise time. Multivariate analyses revealed that once the exercise EF was known, no other radionuclide variables contributed independent information about the likelihood of future events. Multivariate analyses also revealed that the exercise EF described much of the prognostic information of coronary anatomy. The radionuclide ventriculogram appears useful in predicting future events in patients with stable CAD, but they did not consider clinical or exercise test markers.

Bonow et al. at the NIH prospectively evaluated whether objective markers of exercise-induced ischemia would provide prognostic information in patients with coronary artery disease with preserved left ventricular function at rest (EF greater than 40%). They studied 117 patients by means of exercise ECG and radionuclide ventriculography; 66% complained of mild angina, and the rest were asymptomatic. No patient had stenosis of the left main coronary artery, but 40% had a prior MI. Mortality during subsequent medical therapy was significantly associated (by univariate life-table analysis) with three-vessel coronary artery disease and the magnitude of the EF during exercise. In patients with three-vessel disease who had both ST-segment depression of 0.1 mV or more and a decrease in EF during exercise, in addition to an exercise capacity of 120 W or less, the probability of four-year survival was only 71%. All deaths occurred in this subgroup. Objective evidence of left ventricular ischemia by ECG and/or exercise ventriculography during exercise and exercise capacity identified one subgroup of minimally symptomatic patients with three-vessel disease with an excellent prognosis and another subgroup at relatively high risk of dying.

Hammond investigated the relationship among four exercise-induced phenomena—angina, ST-segment depression, decrease in EF, and thallium perfusion defects—and determined their impact on aerobic capacity. One hundred fifty-six men (mean age 52 ± 8 years) with documented coronary heart disease were studied with radionuclide ventriculography during supine bicycle exercise, thallium scintigraphy and treadmill testing with computerized ECG and maximal oxygen uptake. Of 624 administered tests, 243 results (39%) were considered to indicate ischemia. The average number of abnormal tests was 1.6 per patient and, when considered as continuous variables, their

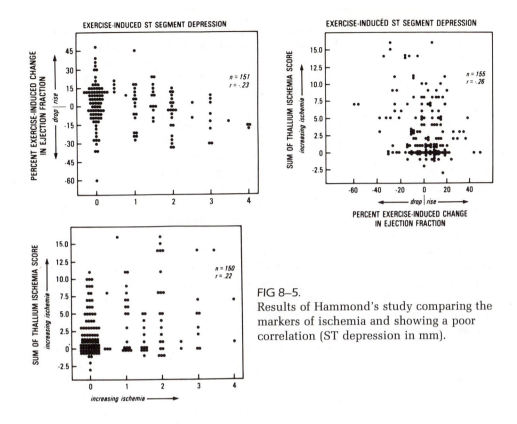

FIG 8–5.
Results of Hammond's study comparing the markers of ischemia and showing a poor correlation (ST depression in mm).

results correlated poorly as shown in Figure 8–5. Correlations did not improve when adjusting for heart rate achieved or by eliminating patients with coronary artery bypass surgery or myocardial infarction. Statistical methods of comparing degree of intertest agreement yielded surprisingly weak relations among the four tests of ischemia. Treadmill performance was markedly impaired by angina, but much less impaired by other indicators of ischemia. Unfortunately, the usual test responses implying ischemia have weak agreement when uniformly applied to patients with known coronary artery disease.

RADIONUCLIDE VENTRICULOGRAPHY POST-MI

Pulido et al. studied 27 patients two to three weeks post-MI. Submaximal supine bicycle exercise was performed to a heart rate of 125 using in vivo labeled red blood cells for gated blood pool scintigrams. Ejection fraction and wall motion abnormalities were assessed. The eight patients with Q-wave anterior MI had a significantly lower EF at rest (mean 44%) compared to the 13 patients with inferior MI (mean 61%). Furthermore, EF decreased considerably in seven of the eight patients with anterior MI during exercise while it did not change significantly in the other patients. Segmental wall motion abnormalities were reported in seven of the eight anterior MI patients at rest with four of them displaying more severe changes during exercise. Among the 13 inferior MI patients, only two had wall motion abnormalities at rest. These two and two more with normal resting images had exercise-induced abnormalities.

There is a large individual difference in the ejection fraction response in patients who have sustained a myocardial infarction due to differences in the size of the myocardial infarction number, severity of vessel involvement, and the presence of collateral circulation. In a group of 21 patients with documented myocardial infarctions, Jengo and coworkers reported that 14 decreased their ejection fraction response to upright bicycle exercise, five remained unchanged, and two increased. In agreement with these findings, Rerych and associates found that 9 of 13 patients decreased their exercise ejection fraction, 2 remained unchanged, and 2 increased. Borer also noted that among the coronary patients who had Q-waves, all had regional dysfunction. Most patients with angina pectoris decrease left ventricular ejection fraction response from rest to peak exercise. However, patients with myocardial infarction either decrease their ejection fraction during exercise or show no change, depending on the location and extent of their infarction.

Borer et al. studied 45 post-MI patients one day before discharge and repeated the studies 6–14 months after discharge. They did a submaximal supine exercise test in 45 patients to a heart rate of 115. EF was depressed at rest prior to discharge (mean 39%) and showed little change during the exercise test (mean 37%). EF was not correlated with the site of MI. All four patients who died within one year had a resting EF less than 35%. The measured EF at the later study during rest or exercise was not different from the early study. However, a subgroup of 17 patients with an EF above 40% in the first study showed a significant increase in EF in the later study. The radionuclide exercise test did not provide any additional information over the resting measurements.

Corbett et al. performed submaximal supine exercise test to a heart rate of 130 with gated left ventriculography 19 days after MI. Their patients were followed for a mean of nine months for cardiac death, recurrent MI, unstable or limiting angina, and persistent congestive heart failure. The sensitivity and the specificity of the ventriculography findings for predicting these events were (1) 95% and 96% for failure to increase EF by at least five units as well as for an increase in end-systolic volume of more than 5%; (2) 97% and 88% for failure of the ratio of systolic blood pressure to end-systolic volume to increase by more than 35%; and (3) 81% and 88% for a decrease in wall motion score during exercise. The corresponding findings for exercise-induced ECG abnormalities (ST-segment depression less than 0.05 mV and ST-segment elevation greater than 0.1 mV) were 54% and 58%. A stepwise discriminant analysis with inclusion of clinical variables showed that the change in EF with exercise and the end-systolic volume and the pressure/volume ratio were the most important predictors.

Hung et al. at Stanford evaluated 117 men three weeks after recent MI to determine the prognostic ability of exercise testing with thallium imaging, radionuclide ventriculography, and the routine treadmill. Although the population consisted predominantly of patients with inferior MIs (59%), anterior (27%) and non-Q-wave MI (14%) were included. Men 70 years of age or younger admitted to a university hospital or to Kaiser Permanente Hospitals with a diagnostic MI between 1979 and 1982 were considered for the study. Patients with complications were excluded. The selected patients had a mean age of 54, 23% had a history of angina, 2% had a prior MI, and 16% had recurrent ischemic chest pain in the CCU. Symptom-limited treadmill testing was performed with thallium imaging 21 days after MI. On the next day, symptom-limited exercise testing upright on a bike was performed for radionuclide ventriculography. Their follow-up endpoints over one year included hard medical events (N = 8) including one patient with sudden death, six patients with recurrent infarction, one with nonfatal ventricular fibrillation, and a group with "important events" (N = 14) including hospitalization for unstable angina in four patients, one with CHF, and nine for CABS. Using a Cox proportional hazards model, the following findings were predictive of a hard medical event: peak work load of 4 METs or less and a 5% fall in EF during submaximal effort. Exercise-induced angina or ST-segment depression, thallium defects, and EF were significantly predictive of combined events. A peak work load of 4 METs or less or a decrease in EF of 5% or more during submaximal effort identified 22 high-risk patients (20%) from 89 low-risk patients. They concluded that radionuclide ventriculography contributed independent prognostic information to that provided by treadmill testing and was superior to exercise thallium scintigraphy. Unfortunately, their endpoints were "too soft."

Morris et al. at Cedars Sinai in Los Angeles evaluated criteria for the prediction of MVD after MI using the clinical, ECG, and radionuclide ventriculography findings in 110 patients undergoing coronary angiography. Only 40 of the patients were asymptomatic, most of them being evaluated because of chest pain. Clinical or ECG abnormalities were observed in 41 of 97 patients with MVD (sensitivity 43%) and only 2 of 13 patients without MVD (specificity 85%). An EF rise of less than 5% had a sensitivity of 72% and a specificity of 62%. A fall in EF of 5% or more had a sensitivity of 39% and a specificity of 92% for MVD. Wall motion abnormalities in a remote area had a specificity of 55%. These investigators concluded that if a worsening of a remote wall motion abnormality and a fall in EF were combined, additional information over routine evaluation was gained (sensitivity 62%, specificity 75%).

Morris et al. from the Durham VAMC studied the value of rest and exercise radionuclide ventriculography (RNV) for predicting specific events including death, MI, and CCU admission for unstable chest pain, and medically refractory angina after MI in 106 consecutive survivors. Analysis of the RNV variables using the Cox model yielded significant associations of the time to death with ejection fraction at rest and during exercise. Both variables added significant prognostic information to the clinical assessment. The change in ejection fraction from rest to exercise predicted the time to CABS for medically refractory angina before and after adjustment for the clinical descriptors, but did not predict death or other nonfatal events. Significant correlations were found between RNV variables and a variety of clinical descriptors previously reported to have prognostic significance. Clinical and RNV variables that are measures of left ventricular function were predictive of subsequent mortality, while those that reflect residual potentially ischemic myocardium were predictive of subsequent nonfatal ischemic events. Rest and exercise RNV after MI appeared to provide significant prognostic information regarding specific events during follow-up independent to that provided by clinical assessment.

RIGHT VENTRICULAR EJECTION FRACTION RESPONSE TO EXERCISE

At UCSD, 20 normal subjects and 50 patients with coronary heart disease were studied using equilibrium radionuclide angiography. The resting right ventricular ejection fraction did not differ between these two groups (49% vs. 46%). Patients were then maximally exercised in the supine position. The normal subjects increased their ejection fraction from 49% at rest to 64% at peak exercise; those patients with right coronary occlusion either alone or with other vessel involvement showed no increase in right ventricular ejection fraction (46% to 45%). Those patients with coronary artery disease, but with no evidence of right coronary artery occlusion increased the right ventricular ejection fraction from a resting value of 46% to 53% at peak exercise. Right ventricular dysfunction was probably related to both local ischemia and an increased load due to left ventricular dysfunction.

At UCSD, 10 normal subjects and 37 patients with chronic obstructive lung disease were studied, some with and some without coronary disease, using first-pass radionuclide angiography. Despite a mean left ventricular ejection fraction above 51% in all three groups, the patients with severe chronic obstructive pulmonary disease without coronary heart disease and those with coronary disease had mean resting right ventricular ejection fractions of 46% and 43%, respectively. Berger and colleagues studied 36 patients with chronic obstructive pulmonary disease also using the first-pass technique and reported a wide variation in the resting right ventricular ejection fraction. More than half had normal values. All 10 chronic obstructive pulmonary disease patients with cor pulmonale had an abnormal resting right ventricular ejection fraction.

Matthay and colleagues evaluated the right and left ventricular ejection fraction responses to exercise in 24 chronic obstructive pulmonary disease patients. Twenty failed to increase their right ventricular ejection fraction more than five ejection fraction units above the resting value with exercise. Only 7 of these 24 patients demonstrated an abnormal exercise left ventricular ejection fraction. Workers at UCSD found a similar decrease in the exercise right ventricular ejection fraction in 11 patients with severe chronic obstructive lung disease (43% to 36% with exercise). Volume and pulmonary pressures were also assessed, and patients with severe chronic obstructive pulmonary disease often dilated the right ventricle and therefore decreased the ejection fraction with exercise. These changes correlated with pulmonary pressure. Olvey and coworkers studied the effects of oxygen administration on exercise function in 18 patients with chronic hypoxic lung disease. These investigators concluded that while oxygen does not alter right ventricular performance at rest, it can improve the function during exercise.

Pulmonary Blood Volume.   Okada and colleagues used multigated blood pool images at rest and during supine bicycle exercise to determine the pulmonary blood volume ratio in patients being evaluated with angiography for chest pain. The mean exercise-to-rest pulmonary blood volume ratio was lower for persons without coronary artery disease and for those with only right coronary artery disease, as compared to all others with coronary artery disease. A pulmonary blood volume rest-exercise ratio equal to or greater than 1.06, that is, an increase in pulmonary volume with exercise, had a sensitivity of 79% for coronary disease in their population.

Ejection Fraction Response in Valvular Heart Disease.   Radionuclide angiography has been used to evaluate patients with valvular heart disease. Employing the first-pass technique, flow patterns and transit times can be studied. Regurgitant fraction can be calculated from right and left ventricular stroke volume and counts. Using gated equilibrium, Borer and coworkers studied 34 patients with severe aortic regurgitation. Although 14 of the 21 symptomatic patients had a normal resting left ventricular ejection fraction, only one patient had a normal response to exercise. In the 22 asymptomatic patients, 21 had a normal resting left ventricular ejection fraction and only 13 responded normally to supine exercise. This technique could be useful for following ventricular function in patients with aortic regurgitation.

Determination of Left Ventricular Volume.   The determination of left ventricular volume provides a better understanding of the pathophysiology of heart disease than does ejection fraction alone. In clinical practice, left ventricular volume is of proven value as a prognostic index in patients with heart disease. The ability to assess left ventricular volume changes in response to exercise, drug administration, or other interventions is exciting because it impacts on wall tension, one of the major determinants of myocardial oxygen. Both noninvasive radionuclide approaches to visualizing the left ventricle can be used for volume assessment.

First-Pass Method.   The study of heart function using the first pass of a radionuclide bolus through the central circulation has been described. In brief, radioactivity in the left or right ventricle during the first circulation of a radionuclide tracer is proportional to the amount of blood in the chamber at any time. By sampling left ventricular radioactivity over time using a standard gamma camera and a dedicated computer, it is possible to obtain a time-activity curve for each heartbeat during several cardiac cycles. The time-activity curve is the radioactivity (counts over time) and usually contains three to eight heartbeats with peaks and valleys of counts until equilibrium occurs. After subtraction of the background activity, a time-activity curve with a high sampling rate (25 points per second) is obtained. It consists of a succession of peaks and valleys in which the peaks correspond to end-diastole and the valleys to end-systole. Images obtained at 25- to 50-msec intervals from several cardiac cycles of similar duration and characteristics are superimposed to obtain high-fidelity images that can be displayed in movie format for qualitative analysis of wall motion. Left ventricular volumes can then be obtained by planimetry of the end-diastolic frame images using a similar technique for contrast ventriculography. This method postulates that the left ventricular cavity can be represented by an ellipsoid. The same methodology can be applied to the radionuclide angiogram in the anteroposterior or right anterior oblique projection.

Rerych and coworkers used this method to derive cardiac output from the ejection fraction, left ventricular end-diastolic volume, and heart rate (cardiac output = EF × LVEDV × HR). The correlation coefficient between simultaneous dye cardiac output and calculated radionuclide cardiac output was .95. Resting and exercise values for the same patient were included in the correlation coefficient analysis, making this technique appear better than it really is.

A second method for calculating ventricular volume is the use of the first transient of the radionuclide through the central circulation. A simple calculation of cardiac output using this method is based on the indicator-dilution principle. In short, a curve similar to the one obtained using dye and a densitometer is generated by using a gamma camera to sample a radionuclide passing through the heart. The integration of the area under the curve is proportional to cardiac output and correlates well with the dye technique. It is possible to use the cardiac output and ejection fraction to derive left ventricular volume: LVEDV = cardiac output ÷ (EF × HR).

Equilibrium Multiple-Gated Blood Pool Imaging. This technique is based on the administration of technetium linked to human serum albumin or red cells that remains relatively stable in the circulation for a period of four to six hours. Stannous salt helps technetium bind to red cells. Using a standard gamma camera and a computer, the radioactivity in the left ventricle can be assessed throughout the cardiac cycle. Because the amount of radioactivity in one cycle is insufficient for imaging, the study requires the accumulation of counts through 300 or more heartbeats.

Once the radioactive substance has reached equilibrium in the blood pool, the study is performed in the following way. Using a fiducial point on the electrocardiogram, the R-R interval is divided into equal portions (12, 36, or more portions have been used), and the information from each corresponding portion of each cycle are added, forming composite images based on all 300 cycles. The movie format display of the images is used for the assessment of wall motion, and the count-rate changes through the cycle are used for constructing a time-activity curve. Ejection fraction is then obtained by the formula EF equals end-diastolic counts minus end-systolic counts (all background corrected values) divided by end-diastolic counts. End-diastole and end-systole are considered the highest and lowest values of the curve. If it is possible to convert counts to milliliters, the volume calculated by this method would be of great value because, in addition to being noninvasive, it is less influenced by the inherent errors of geometric assumptions. A review of several methods follows.

If the distribution of the radioactive tracer in the blood is homogeneous, the radioactivity per milliliter of a sample of peripheral blood may be used to calculate the counts in the left ventricle at any time during the cardiac cycle with the actual volume. Left ventricular volume equals total counts in the left ventricle (at a particular time of the heart cycle) divided by activity per milliliter of the blood sample. To make an appropriate conversion, several factors are important: (1) the time during which the reference blood sample and the left ventricle counts are obtained should be normalized; (2) the radioactive decay should be considered when there is a significant time difference between the sampling of peripheral blood and the performance of the radioactivity assay of the sample; and (3) attenuation factors must be considered.

The first two factors can be accounted for in calculating volume. The radioactivity (counts at end-diastole) is theoretically the same for all cycles processed; so if the time per frame (R-R interval in seconds divided by number of frames) and the number of heartbeats processed are known, the counts at end-diastole per single beat per unit of time can be easily calculated. The second factor involves a decay constant, assuming a half-life of six hours, and knowing the time between the blood sampling and counting.

The most controversial factor is attenuation. The reference blood sample should be counted at a similar distance from the camera as the left ventricle. Lung and soft tissue between the heart and the camera equally influence the amount of radioactivity arriving at the camera. The main factors influencing the amount of radioactivity seen by the camera include (1) the distance and (2) the kind of tissue interposed between the heart and the camera. Assuming a source at a distance d, separated from the camera by a tissue with attenuation characteristics defined by a coefficient r, the counts arriving at the camera (Cc) will be equal to the real counts (Cr) times e^{-rd}. For an ellipsoid source (the left ventricle), the distance will be shorter for the anterior portion of the ventricle compared with the most posterior portion. The radioactivity from the posterior regions of the left ventricle will have to cross the whole thickness of blood inside the left ventricle in addition to the soft tissue, so the left ventricular geometry plays a role in the calculation of ventricular volumes.

The complexity of the issue has resulted in two approaches to the problem, one that does not account for attenuation and a second that does. The background-corrected counts in the left ventricle are obtained from the time-activity curve using a semiautomated computer program or by manually assigning a region of interest around the left ventricle at end-diastole and end-systole. A blood sample (3 to 5 ml) is drawn in the middle of the study and counted in front of the camera. The background-corrected counts per milliliter are used to calculate volume units from counts in the left ventricle: LV unit = LV counts divided by counts per milliliter of blood sample. The reports have shown a good correlation between the radioactive volume units and the left ventricular volumes calculated from contrast ventriculography performed within 24 to 48 hours. The equation obtained from the regression line can be used to convert volume units into milliliters. The difference between radionuclide and angiographic volumes was significant.

Two methods have been proposed that consider attenuation. The theoretic advantage is avoiding the utilization of a regression equation that has the potential error of disparities between the reference population used to calculate the equation and subsequent patients. One of the methods developed at Johns Hopkins University utilizes an attenuation factor obtained through the calculation of the distance between the camera and the theoretic center of the left ventricle, based on the linear attenuation coefficient of water. The volume is then calculated from the formula:

$$LVEDV = \frac{\text{count rate from LV in end-diastole}/e^{-md}}{\text{count rate per milliliter of blood sample}}$$

The calculation of the distance (d) is relatively simple. A radioactive point source is positioned over the left ventricle in the 40 degree left anterior oblique projection and fixed on the chest. The left ventricle and the source are imaged in the posterior-anterior view. The calculation of $d = x$ divided by sin 40 degrees, where x is the frontal plane length. The correlation was similar whether considering attenuation factors or not. When estimating the distance from the camera to the left ventricle, a difference of 1 cm represented a 14% change in the calculated left ventricular volume. No correlation was found between the distance and the calculated volume, the body surface area, or body morphology that could improve the calculation.

The Seattle group has proposed correcting for attenuation by calculating the thickness of soft tissue between the left ventricle and the skin using an x-ray along the camera axis. The correction factor would be incorporated when imaging the blood sample at the same distance that the camera was from the chest and with the interposition of the same thickness of material with an attenuation similar to soft tissue.

THE LV VOLUME RESPONSE TO EXERCISE

The response of left ventricular volume to exercise remains controversial. At the University of California, San Diego, we made volume measurements during supine and erect exercise in the same individuals, but our results showed a wide scatter of the volume data. Part of this was due to the fact that our patients were first studied supine and then erect one hour later. Patients do not become basal within this time frame both because of sympathetic stimulation and because of fluid shifts out of the vascular space. However, much of the scatter is due to methodologic difficulties with the technique. From studies and a review of the literature, the following analysis seems reasonable. In the supine position, end-diastolic volume is close to maximal, particularly if the feet are elevated (i.e., up on bicycle pedals); thus, there will be little change in volume in response to exercise. However, if the feet are on the plane of the body or below, both ESV and EDV increase during exercise in patients with coronary disease. In the erect position, end-diastolic volume begins at its lowest possible value but increases with exercise as venous return increases. At near-maximal levels, end-diastolic volume plateaus and, can possibly even drop. It is hard to imagine that the ischemic ventricle becomes so dyskinetic that it bulges in such a manner that total left ventricular end-diastolic volume is increased but apparently it can. The increase in EDV indicates that the Frank-Starling mechanism is functioning during exercise. It appears that there is a variable response of end-diastolic volume during submaximal exercise in both positions, probably due to sympathetic tone and venous return. It is doubtful that changes in end-diastolic volume during exercise have much diagnostic value because of their great individual variability. However, maximal and postexercise changes may have more meaning.

REPRODUCIBILITY

To determine the individual reproducibility of radionuclide ventriculography over one year, Jensen et al. at UCSD studied 33 patients with stable coronary artery disease at rest and during three stages of exercise. The individual interstudy variability of ejection fraction (EF), end-diastolic volume (EDV), end-systolic volume (ESV), and cardiac output (Q) was determined by calculating the mean and standard deviation of the difference between the individual studies (initial-one year). Despite high correlations between EF measured at study one and study two of .96 at rest and .87 during maximal exercise, the individual interstudy difference was .01 ± .04 and − .02 ± .09, respectively. The correlation of percent change in EF from rest to maximal exercise was .51 (Fig 8–6), and the individual interstudy difference was − 1.2% ± 19%. Correlations of the EDV were .81 at rest and .72 during maximal exercise while the individual difference was .7 ml and − .8 ± 49 ml, respectively. Considering two standard deviations as the confidence limits for a true change, an EF change of 8 EF units (.08) at rest and 18 (.18) during exercise and EDV

FIG 8–6.
Correlation of the LVEF response to maximal supine bike exercise initially and then one year later in stable patients with coronary heart disease.

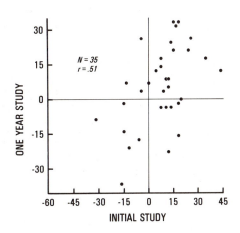

changes of approximately 100 ml are needed in an individual to state with confidence that the observed difference between two studies are true changes and not the result of technologic variability. Because of the large individual interstudy variability in EF and volume measurement, caution must be taken in assuming that any change over a year is due to more than technique variability.

Wackers et al. studied 83 patients twice within a five-day period at rest using equilibrium radionuclide ventriculography. In patients with a resting EF equal or greater than .55, the mean difference between the two studies was .06 ± .04, while those with resting EFs less than .55 had a significantly lower difference of .02 ± .02. When all 29 patients are analyzed together and the data are recalculated using a paired t-test (without absolute differences), a mean difference of .005 ± .06 was obtained. Similar results with slightly less variability were reported by these investigators when they studied 41 patients on two occasions within two hours.

Pfisterer and colleagues studied 16 patients with coronary artery disease twice within an average of 15 days using equilibrium radionuclide ventriculography at rest and during exercise. The authors concluded that to be 95% confident that the observed EF change in an individual is truly a significant change at rest and during exercise, the change must be at least .08 and .06, respectively.

Okada and colleagues studied observer agreement (called variance) by comparing radionuclide to contrast angiographic assessment of left ventricular wall motion and ejection fraction. They found similar or superior interobserver variance for wall motion by radionuclide than by contrast angiography, except for the septal wall motion in which contrast angiography was superior. In determining radionuclide gated blood pool ejection fraction both at exercise and rest, higher inter- and intraobserver variance of ejection fraction was noted, but they found it to be similar to contrast ventriculography.

Marshall and coworkers studied 12 patients with heart disease and 8 normals. Each patient was studied on three occasions separated by four days (range 1–12 days). They used the absolute differences in the statistical analysis. The mean variability of sequential EF measurements was .04 ± .04. Five of these patients (25%) had a greater than .10 EF change between the two studies despite no overt change in clinical status. The blood pressure and heart rate did not differ in those that had the large variation in EF when compared to those that did not. Upton et al. studied 10 normal volunteers both at rest and during exercise two days apart with first-pass radionuclide ventriculography. Using absolute differences, they reported a mean variability in rest EF, Q, and EDV of .04 ± .038, 1.24 ± 1.23 L/min, and 9.9 ± 5 ml, respectively. During exercise the variability in EF, Q, and EDV was .03 ± .025, 1.59 ± 0.67 L/min, and 9.8 ± 6.2 ml. When the EF data are reanalyzed using a paired t-test (without absolute differences), these results indicate the change in EF of .10 at rest and .07 during exercise should be seen to be 95% confident the change is significant and not due to technologic variability.

Hecht and coworkers contend that most studies of reproducibility failed to use the appropriate statistical tool in their data analysis. The measure of in-

TABLE 8–4.
Comparison of Interstudy Variability of Rest and Exercise Ejection Fraction With Other Investigations

CATEGORY	PRESENT STUDY	HECHT ET AL.	PFISTERER ET AL.	UPTON ET AL.
Technique	Equilibrium	Equilibrium	Equilibrium	First-pass
Subjects	33 CAD	18 CAD	16 CAD	10 normals
Study interval	1 year	14 days	1–66 days	2 days
Rest				
Mean (difference)	0.01	0.02	0.003	0.03
±1 SD (difference)	0.04	0.06	0.04	0.05
Exercise maximal EF				
Mean (difference)	0.02	0.01	0.02	0.004
±1 SD (difference)	0.09	0.07	0.03	0.04
%ΔEF				
Mean (difference)	−1.2	2.0	—	—
±1 SD (difference)	19	9.2	—	—

Mean (difference) = mean of the differences between the first and second studies; ±1 SD (difference) = standard deviation of the differences between the studies; CAD = coronary artery disease patients.

terstudy variability for individual patients should be represented by the mean and standard deviation of the difference between the initial and subsequent study using a paired t-test. In Hecht's study of 18 patients with coronary artery disease tested over a two-week period of time, the individual interstudy variability for rest and exercise EF were .02 ± .06 and .01 ± .07, respectively. For the group as a whole, values of 2.2 ± 1.4% and 1.2 ± 1.7%, respectively, were reported. They also reported a variability of 2.0 ± 9.2% for the percent change in EF from rest to exercise. The interstudy variability for two resting studies separated by only 30 minutes in the same population was only .01 ± .025 for individual patients and only 1.0 ± .006 for the entire group. This finding supports the hypothesis that reproducibility decreases as time between studies increases. Table 8–4 is a modified version of the review table presented by Hecht et al. with only the studies that reported rest and exercise data. Based on the variability of the EF measurement, two EF measurements performed on an individual patient would have to be different by greater than .12 during rest and greater than .15 during exercise to be real and not due to the variability of the technique.

The importance of differentiating between group and individual variability when assessing ventricular function changes over time was emphasized by McAnulty and coworkers. They studied 17 patients with cardiac disease (seven had coronary artery disease, seven had valvular disease, two had both, and one normal) on two successive days in the catheterization laboratory. When patients were evaluated as a group, no significant change in measurements of ventricular function was observed. However, when individual responses were analyzed, large variations occurred. The mean and standard deviation of the percent change from study one to study two for EF, EDV index, and ESV index was −.06 ± .16, −0.9 ± 23.1, and 10.2 ± 29.4. Despite the fairly high correlation (.80) of EF on day one compared to day two, there was still a great deal of individual variation. Thus, even the "gold standard," contrast ventriculography, by which radionuclide ventriculography is calibrated, is not as reproducible as one might wish.

Table 8–4 shows the variability of the EF at rest and during maximal exercise in four studies including Jensen. Based on the data in this table, it appears that at rest, the EF would have to change by approximately .08 following an intervention to be 95% confident that the change was due to an actual change rather than due to the variability of the technique. During exercise the data is less consistent, with the needed change in the EF between 0.07 and 0.18. It seems physiologically reasonable that there would be an increase in variability during exercise as compared to rest; we believe that an EF change of at least .15 is required in patients during exercise following an intervention.

Based on the results of our volume measurements, large changes are needed following an intervention to be confident that the changes are due to the intervention. Thus, EDV changes of at least 80 ml at rest and 100 ml during exercise are needed while changes of approximately 50 ml must be observed for ESV to be 95% confident that the observed changes are real.

Percent change in EF from rest to exercise was expected to be the most reproducible measurement. This was reasonable since it has been advocated to have great diagnostic value and because the errors in measurement due to positioning or technical differences seem to have a similar impact during temporally related measurements. However, as can be seen, the variability was great. The percent change from rest to exercise between the two studies had correlation coefficients of .39, .21, and .51 during the three stages of exercise, respectively. Though there was a small change, the standard deviation of the differences was 19%. This makes the percent change EF in response to exercise a poor means of assessing clinical changes in a patient.

Each laboratory should determine its own reproducibility. If this cannot be done, then the data in Table 8–4 provides information upon which to evaluate an individual patient. Only when these limits are exceeded can one have reasonable confidence that an intervention has actually had an effect or that a biological change has occurred.

CONCLUSION

Exercise thallium scintigraphy does not appear to offer as great an improvement in predictive accuracy over standard exercise testing as first thought. However, careful techniques using thallium may make it possible to quantify changes in myocardial ischemia brought about by interventions such as PTCA and exercise training much better than is possible with the exercise ECG.

Computer programs to improve the sensitivity of thallium scintigraphy have been developed, but most of these decrease specificity. Many of these are dependent upon assessment of slow washout, which is related to factors other than ischemia. A major problem in assessing the reported studies is the inclusion of patients who have had MIs and thus have defects on imaging. Also, approximately 25% of patients with ischemia and no scar still have defects at four hours and should be scanned again later.

The exact meaning of reverse redistribution is uncertain, but it may be related to incomplete subendocardial MIs. Additional criteria for an abnormal response have been proposed, including lung uptake of thallium and postexercise dilation of the images. All of these need careful investigation before they are applied clinically. Tomography has become popular, but reconstruction artifact appears to complicate these images.

The thallium exercise test can be of value in patients with chronotropic incompetence, poor exercise tolerance, abnormal resting ECGs, taking digoxin, or with false positive exercise ECGs. Another situation in which cold spot imaging has value is in patients who develop ventricular dysrhythmias during exercise without significant ST-segment depression. Since ventricular dysrhythmias have a poor predictive value for the diagnosis of coronary disease, a radionuclide study can help make a diagnostic decision in such patients. Patients with left bundle branch block can have septal fibrosis not due to coronary disease and thus have septal cold spots. However, reversible defects in other areas may indicate ischemia, and so thallium scintigraphy can be helpful in these patients.

Exercise radionuclide left ventricular function analysis can be performed using either the first-pass procedure or blood pooling agents that require gating. The first-pass procedure requires multiple injections for sequential studies, and regional wall motion analysis is best accomplished using a multicrystal camera. Gated blood pool studies have the advantage of enabling repeated analyses with one injection, but two minutes or longer are required for data gathering in order to obtain sufficient counts.

From the studies of patients post-MI, the radionuclide exercise techniques do not appear to offer a definite advantage over routine exercise testing. Resting ejection fraction is a more established measurement for patient management and prognostication. Certainly, the mixed results obtained using the nuclear techniques are not anywhere as extensive as the data reviewed for standard methods of exercise testing post-MI nor are they methodologically superior.

Measurements of left ventricular volume have little clinical value because of their poor reproducibility. The low specificity of the various criteria for an abnormal exercise ventriculography study makes it of little diagnostic value. However, it may have prognostic value. A surprising finding has been the poor correlation between the exercise test markers of ischemia (i.e., reversible thallium defects, EF response, and ST depression).

BIBLIOGRAPHY

Anderson JL, Wagner JM, Datz FL, et al: Comparative effects of diltiazem, propranolol, and placebo on exercise performance using radionuclide ventriculography in patients with symptomatic coronary artery disease: Results of a double-blind, randomized, crossover study. *Am Heart J* 1984;107:698–706.

Atwood JE, Jensen D, Froelicher VF, et al: Agreement in human interpretation of analog thallium myocardial perfusion images. *Circulation* 1981;64:601–609.

Ausubel K, Steingart RM, Shimshi M, et al: Maintenance of exercise stroke volume during ventricular versus atrial synchronous pacing: role of contractility. *Circulation* 1985; 72:1037–1043.

Bailey IK, Griffith LS, Rouleau J, et al: Thallium-201 myocardial perfusion imaging at rest and during exercise: Comparative sensitivity to electrocardiography in coronary artery disease. *Circulation* 1977;55:79.

Beller GA, Gibson RS, Watson DD: Radionuclide methods of identifying patients who may require coronary artery bypass surgery. *Circulation* 1985;72:V9.

Berger H, Matthay R, Loke J, et al: Assessment of cardiac performance with quantitative radionuclide angiography with right ventricular ejection fraction with reference to findings in chronic obstructive pulmonary disease. Am J Cardiol 1980;41:897.

Berger HJ, Zaret BL: Nuclear cardiology. N Engl J Med 1981;305:799.

Berman DS, Maddahi J: Which patients need exercise nuclear cardiology tests? A Bayesian approach. ACC Learning Center Highlights 1986;1:1–5.

Berman DS, Salel AF, Denardo GL, et al: Noninvasive detection of regional myocardial ischemia using rubidium-81 and the scintillation camera: Comparison with stress electrocardiography in patients with arteriographically documented coronary stenosis. Circulation 1979;60:1270.

Blood DK, McCarthy DM, Sciacca RR, et al: Comparison of single-dose and double-dose thallium-201 myocardial perfusion scintigraphy for the detection of coronary artery disease and prior myocardial infarction. Circulation 1978;58:777.

Bonow RO, Kent KM, Rosing DR, et al: Exercise-induced ischemia in mildly symptomatic patients with coronary-artery disease and preserved left ventricular function. N Engl J Med 1984;311:1339–1345.

Borer JS, Kent KM, Bacharach SL, et al: Sensitivity, specificity, and predictive accuracy of radionuclide cineangiography during exercise in patients with coronary artery disease. Circulation 1979;60:572.

Borer JS, Rosing DR, Miller RH, et al: Natural history of LVEF during one year after acute MI: comparison with clinical, ECG, and biochemical determinations. Am J Cardiol 1980;46:1–12.

Botvinick EH, Taradash MR, Shames DM, et al: Thallium-201 myocardial perfusion scintigraphy for the clinical clarification of normal, abnormal and equivocal electrocardiographic stress tests. Am J Cardiol 1978;41:43.

Boucher CA, Anderson MD, Schneider MS, et al: Left ventricular function before and after reaching the anaerobic threshold. Chest 1985;87:145–150.

Boucher CA, Brewster DC, Darling C, et al: Determination of cardiac risk by dipyridamole-thallium imaging before peripheral vascular surgery. N Engl J Med 1985;312:389–394.

Boucher CA, Kanarek DJ, Okada RD, et al: Exercise testing in aortic regurgitation: Comparison of radionuclide left ventricular ejection fraction with exercise performance at the anaerobic threshold and peak exercise. Am J Cardiol 1983;52:801–808.

Boucher CA, Okada RD: Thallium-201 myocardial perfusion imaging without exercise—rest and dipyridamole studies. Chest 1984;86:159–161.

Brown KA, McKay R, Heller GV, et al: Hemodynamic determinants of thallium-201 lung uptake in patients during atrial pacing stress. Am Heart J 1986;111:103.

Brown KA, Osbakken M, Boucher CA, et al: Positive exercise thallium-201 test responses in patients with less than 50% maximal coronary stenosis: Angiographic and clinical predictors. Am J Cardiol 1985;55:54–57.

Bulkley BH, Rouleau JR, Whitaker JQ, et al: The use of thallium-201 for myocardial perfusion imaging in sarcoid heart disease. Chest 1977;72:27.

Caldwell J, Stewart D, Dodge H, et al: Left ventricular volume during maximal supine exercise: A study using metallic epicardial markers. Circulation 1978;58:732.

Canhasi B, Dae M, Botvinick E, et al: Interaction of "supplementary" scintigraphic indicators of ischemia and stress electrocardiography in the diagnosis of multivessel coronary disease. J Am Coll Cardiol 1985;6:581–588.

Chaitman BR, Brevers G, Dupras G, et al: Diagnostic impact of thallium scintigraphy and cardiac fluoroscopy when the exercise ECG is strongly positive. Am Heart J 1984;108:260–265.

Corbett JR, Dehmer GJ, Lewis SE, et al: The prognostic value of submaximal exercise testing with radionuclide ventriculography before hospital discharge in patients with recent myocardial infarction. Circulation 1981;64:535–544.

Detrano R, Simpfendorfer C, Day K, et al: Comparison of stress digital ventriculography, stress thallium scintigraphy, and digital fluoroscopy in the diagnosis of coronary artery disease in subjects without prior myocardial infarction. Am J Cardiol 1985;56:434–440.

Dunn R, Freedman B, Bailey I, et al: Exercise thallium imaging: Location of perfusion abnormalities in single-vessel coronary disease. *J Nucl Med* 1980;21:717.

Dunn R, Wolff L, Wagner S, et al: The inconsistent pattern of thallium defects: A clue to the false positive perfusion scintigram. *Am J Cardiol* 1981;48:224.

Dymond DS, Foster C, Grenier RP, et al: Peak exercise and immediate post-exercise imaging for the detection of left ventricular functional abnormalities in coronary artery disease. *Am J Cardiol* 1984;53:1532–1537.

Follansbee WP, Curtiss EI, Medsger TA, et al: Myocardial function and perfusion in the CREST syndrome variant of progressive systemic sclerosis. *Am J Med* 1984;77:489–495.

Foster C, Anholm JD, Dymond DS, et al: Left ventricular function at rest, peak exercise, and postexercise. *Cardiology* 1982;69:224–230.

Foster C, Anholm JD, Hellman CK, et al: Left ventricular function during sudden strenuous exercise. *Circulation* 1981;63:592–596.

Foster C, Dymond DS, Anholm JD, et al: Effect of exercise protocol on the left ventricular response to exercise. *Am J Cardiol* 1983;51:859–864.

Gerson MC, Hurst JM, Hertzberg VS, et al: Cardiac prognosis in noncardiac geriatric surgery. *Ann Intern Med* 1985;103:832–837.

Gibbons RJ, Lee KL, Frederick RC, et al: Ejection fraction response to exercise in patients with chest pain, coronary artery disease and normal resting ventricular function. *Circulation* 1982;66:643–648.

Gibson RS: Prognostic value of exercise Thallium-201 scintigraphy after acute myocardial infarction. *J Cardiac Rehabil* 1985;5:28–39.

Gibson RS, Tayloer GJ, Watson DD, et al: Predicting the extent and location of coronary artery disease during the early post-infarction period by quantitative Thallium-201 scintigraphy. *Am J Cardiol* 1981;47:1010–1019.

Hecht H, Josephson M, Hopkins J, et al: Reproducibility of equilibrium radionuclide ventriculography in patients with coronary artery disease: response of left ventricular ejection fraction and regional wall motion to supine bicycle exercise. *Am Heart J* 1982;104:567–574.

Higginbotham MB, Morris KG, Coleman RE, et al: Sex-related differences in the normal cardiac response to upright exercise. *Circulation* 1984;70:357–366.

Hirzel HO, Senn M, Nuesch K, et al: Thallium-201 scintigraphy in complete left bundle branch block. *Am J Cardiol* 1984;53:764–769.

Hung J, Goris ML, Nash E, et al: Comparative value of maximal treadmill testing, exercise thallium myocardial perfusion scintigraphy and exercise radionuclide ventriculography for distinguishing high- and low-risk patients soon after acute myocardial infarction. *Am J Cardiol* 1984;53:1221–1227.

Iskandrain AS, Heo J: Radionuclide angiographic evaluation of left ventricular performance at rest and during exercise in patients with aortic regurgitation. *Am Heart J* 1986;111:1143–1148.

Iskandrian AS, Hakki A-H, Kotler MN, et al: Evaluation of patients with acute myocardial infarction: Which test, for whom, and why? *Am Heart J* 1985;109:391–394.

Iskandrian AS, Hakki AH, Goel IP, et al: The use of rest and exercise radionuclide ventriculography in risk stratification in patients with suspected coronary artery disease. *Prog Cardiol* 1985;110:864–871.

Iskandrian AS, Hakki AH, Goel IP, et al: The use of rest and exercise radionuclide ventriculography in risk stratification in patients with suspected coronary artery disease. *Am Heart J* 1985;110:864–878.

Iskandrian AS, Hakki AH, Segal BL, et al: Role of exercise thallium-201 imaging in decision making. *Arch Intern Med* 1986;146:1098–1100.

Jacobson HG, Silberstein EB: Value of computer analysis of exercise thallium images in the noninvasive detection of coronary artery disease. *JAMA* 1986;255:508–521.

Jengo JA, Freeman R, Brizendine M, et al: Detection of coronary artery disease: Comparison of exercise stress radionuclide angiocardiography and thallium stress perfusion scanning. *Am J Cardiol* 1980;45:535.

Johnson LL, McCarthy DM, Sciacca RR, et al: Right ventricular ejection fraction during exercise in patients with coronary artery disease. *Circulation* 1979;60:1284.

Kaul S, Boucher CA, Newell JB, et al: Determination of the quantitative thallium imaging variables that optimize detection of coronary artery disease. *J Am Coll Cardiol* 1986;7:527–537.

Kaul S, Chesler A, Pohost GM, et al: Influence of peak exercise heart rate on normal thallium-201 myocardial clearance. *J Nucl Med* 1986;27:26–30.

Kaul S, Kiess M, Liu P, et al: Comparison of exercise electrocardiography and quantitative thallium imaging for one-vessel coronary artery disease. *Am J Cardiol* 1985;56:257–261.

Lenaers A: Thallium-201 myocardial perfusion scintigraphy during rest and exercise. *Cardiovasc Radiol* 1979;2:195.

Liu P, Kiess MC, Okada RD, et al: The persistent defect on exercise thallium imaging and its fate after myocardial revascularization: Does it represent scar or ischemia? *Am Heart J* 1985;110:996–1001.

Maddahi J, Abdulla A, Garcia EV, et al: Noninvasive identification of left main and triple-vessel coronary artery disease: Improved accuracy using quantitative analysis of regional myocardial stress distribution and washout of thallium-201. *J Am Coll Cardiol* 1986;7:53–60.

Mann DL, Denenberg BS, Gash AK, et al: Effects of age on ventricular performance during graded supine exercise. *Am Heart J* 1986;111:108.

Marshall R, Wisenberg G, Schelbert H, et al: Effect of oral propranolol on rest, exercise, and postexercise left ventricular performance in normal subjects and patients with coronary artery disease. *Circulation* 1981;63:572–583.

Massie BM, Hollenberg M, Wisneski JA, et al: Scintigraphic quantification of myocardial ischemia: a new approach. *Circulation* 1983;68:747–755.

McGowan RL, Martin ND, Zaret BL, et al: Diagnostic accuracy of noninvasive myocardial imaging for coronary artery disease: An electrocardiographic and angiographic correlation. *Am J Cardiol* 1977;40:6.

Morris DD, Rozanski A, Berman DS, et al: Noninvasive prediction of the angiographic extent of coronary artery disease after myocardial infarction: Comparison of clinical bicycle exercise electrocardiographic and ventriculographic parameters. *Circulation* 1984;70:192–201.

Morris KG, Palmeri ST, Califf RM, et al: Value of radionuclide angiography for predicting specific cardiac events after acute myocardial infarction. *Am J Cardiol* 1985;55:318–324.

Newman G. Rerych S, Upton M, et al: Comparison of electrocardiographic and left ventricular functional changes during exercise. *Circulation* 1980;62:1204.

Norris SL, Slutsky FR, Gerber KH, et al: Sensitivity and specificity of nuclear phase analysis versus ejection fraction in coronary artery disease. *Am J Cardiol* 1984;53:1547–1552.

Nygaard TW, Gibson RS, Ryan JM, et al: Prevalence of high-risk thallium-201 scintigraphic findings in left main coronary artery stenosis: Comparison with patients with multiple-and single-vessel coronary artery disease. *Am J Cardiol* 1984;53:462–469.

Okada R, Kirschenbaum H, Kushner F, et al: Observer variance in the qualitative evaluation of left ventricular wall motion and the quantitation of left ventricular ejection fraction using rest and exercise multigated blood pool imaging. *Circulation* 1980;61:128.

Okada R, Pohost G, Kirschenbaum H, et al: Radionuclide-determined change in pulmonary blood volume with exercise improved sensitivity of multigated blood pool scanning in detecting coronary artery disease. *N Engl J Med* 1979;301:569.

Pasternack PF, Imparato AM, Riles TS, et al: The value of the radionuclide angiogram in the prediction of myocardial infarction in patients undergoing lower extremity revascularization procedures. *Peripheral Vasc Dis* 1985;72:II13–II17.

Pfisterer ME, Battler A, Zaret BL: Range of normal values for left and right ventricular ejection fraction at rest and during exercise assessed by radionuclide angiocardiography. *Eur Heart J* 1985;6:647–655.

Plotnick GD, Becker LC, Fisher ML: Value and limitations of exercise radionuclide angiography for detecting myocardial ischemia in healed myocardial infarction. *Am J Cardiol* 1985;56:1–7.

Poliner L, Dehmer G, Lewis S, et al: Left ventricular performance in normal subjects: A comparison of the responses to exercise in the upright and supine positions. *Circulation* 1980;62:528–534.

Poliner LR, Farber SH, Glaeser DH, et al: Alteration of diastolic filling rate during exercise radionuclide angiography: A highly sensitive technique for detecting of coronary artery disease. *Circulation* 1984;70:942–950.

Port S, Cobb F, Coleman R, et al: Effect of age on the response of the left ventricular ejection fraction to exercise. *N Engl J Med* 1980;303:1133.

Prigent F, Maddahi J, Garcia E, et al: Noninvasive quantification of the extent of jeopardized myocardium in patients with single-vessel coronary disease by stress thallium-201 single-photon emission computerized rotational tomography. *Am Heart J* 1986;111:578–586.

Pryor DB, Harrell FE, Lee KL, et al: Prognostic indicators from radionuclide angiography in medically treated patients with coronary artery disease. *Am J Cardiol* 1984;53:18–22.

Pulido JI, Doss J, Twieg D, et al: Submaximal exercise testing after acute myocardial infarction: Myocardial scintigraphic and electrocardiographic observations. *Am J Cardiol* 1978;42:19–28.

Rehn T, Griffith L, Auchuff S, et al: Exercise thallium-201 myocardial imaging in left main coronary artery disease: Sensitive but not specific. *Am J Cardiol* 1981;48:217.

Rerych SK, Scholz PM, Sabiston DC, et al: Effects of exercise training on left ventricular function in normal subjects: A longitudinal study by radionuclide angiography. *Am J Cardiol* 1980;45:244.

Rigo P, Bailey I, Griffith L, et al: Stress thallium-201 myocardial scintigraphy for the detection of individual coronary arterial lesions in patients with and without previous myocardial infarction. *Am J Cardiol* 1981;48:209.

Ritchie JL, Trobaugh GB, Hamilton GW, et al: Myocardial imaging with thallium-201 at rest and during exercise. *Circulation* 1977;56:66.

Ritchie JL, Zaret BL, Strauss HW, et al: Myocardial imaging with thallium-201: A multicenter study in patients with angina pectoris or acute myocardial infarction. *Am J Cardiol* 1978;42:345.

Rozanski A, Diamond GA, Berman D, et al: The declining specificity of exercise radionuclide ventriculography. *N Engl J Med* 1983;309:518–522.

Rozanski A, Diamond GA, Forrester JS, et al: Should the intent of testing influence its interpretation? *J Am Coll Cardiol* 1986;7:17–24.

Shen WF, Roubin GS, Hirasawa K, et al: Left ventricular volume and ejection fraction response to exercise in chronic congestive heart failure: Difference between dilated cardiomyopathy and previous myocardial infarction. *Am J Cardiol* 1985;55:1027–1031.

Silberstein EB, DeVries DF: Reverse redistribution phenomenon in thallium-201 stress tests: Angiographic correlation and clinical significance. *J Nucl Med* 1985;26:707–710.

Simoons ML, Reiber JHC: Nuclear imaging in clinical cardiology. Boston, Martinus Nijhoff Publishers, 1984, p 1–255.

Sorensen S, Ritchie J, Caldwell J, et al: Serial exercise radionuclide angiography-validation of count-derived changes in cardiac output and quantitation of maximal exercise ventricular volume change after nitroglycerin and propranolol in normal men. *Circulation* 1980;61:600.

Steingart RM, Wexler J, Slagle S, et al: Radionuclide ventriculographic responses to graded supine and upright exercise: Critical role of the Frank-Starling mechanism at submaximal exercise. *Am J Cardiol* 1984;53:1671–1677.

Tobrinick E, Schelbert H, Henning H, et al: Right ventricular ejection fraction in patients with acute anterior and inferior myocardial infarction. *Circulation* 1978;57:1078.

Trobaugh GB, Wackers FJ, Sokole EB, et al: Thallium-201 myocardial imaging: An inter-institutional study of observer variability. *J Nucl Med* 1978;19:359.

Turner JD, Schwartz KM, Logic JR, et al: Detection of residual jeopardized myocardium three weeks after MI by exercise testing with thallium scintigraphy. *Circulation* 1980;61:729–737.

Upton M, Rerych S, Newman G, et al: The reproducibility of radionuclide angiographic measurements of left ventricular function in normal subjects at rest and during exercise. *Circulation* 1980;62:126–132.

Upton MT, Rerych SK, Newman GE, et al: Detecting abnormalities in left ventricular function during exercise before angina and ST-segment depression. *Circulation* 1980;62:341.

van der Wall EE, Eenige van MJ, Visser FC, et al: Thallium-201 exercise testing in patients 6–8 weeks after myocardial infarction: Limited value for the detection of multivessel disease. *Eur Heart J* 1985;6:29–36.

Verani MS, Marcus ML, Razzak MA, et al: Sensitivity and specificity of thallium-201 perfusion scintigrams in the diagnosis of coronary artery disease. *J Nucl Med* 1978;19:773.

Verani MS, Marcus ML, Spoto G, et al: Thallium-201 myocardial perfusion scintigrams in the evaluation of aorto-coronary saphenous bypass surgery. *J Nucl Med* 1978;19:765.

Wahl JM, Hakki AH, Iskandrian AS: Prognostic implications of normal exercise thallium 201 images. *Arch Intern Med* 1985;145:253–256.

Wasserman AG, Katz RJ, Cleary P, et al: Noninvasive detection of multivessel disease after myocardial infarction by exercise radionuclide ventriculography. *Am J Cardiol* 1982; 50:1242–1247.

Wasserman AG, Katz RJ, Varghese PJ, et al: Exercise radionuclide ventriculographic responses in hypertensive patients with chest pain. *N Engl J Med* 1984;311:1276–1280.

Weintraub WS, Barr-Alderfer VA, Seelaus PA, et al: A sequential approach to the diagnosis of coronary artery disease using multivariate analysis. *Am Heart J* 1985;109:999–1005.

Weiss RJ, Morise AP, Raabe DS, et al: Prediction of single versus multivessel disease following myocardial infarction using 201 Thallium scintigraphy and electrocardiographic stress testing. *Clin Cardiol* 1983;6:519–526.

Weiss TA, Maddahi J, Lew AS, et al: Reverse redistribution of thallium-201: A sign of nontransmural myocardial infarction with patency of the infarct-related coronary artery. *J Am Coll Cardiol* 1986;7:61–67.

Weishammer S, Delagardelle C, Sigel HA, et al: Limitations of radionuclide ventriculography in the noninvasive diagnosis of coronary artery disease: A correlation with right heart hemodynamic values during exercise. *Br Heart J* 1985;53:603–610.

Wilson RA, Sullivan PJ, Okada RD, et al: The effect of eating on thallium myocardial imaging. *Chest* 1986;89:195–198.

Yoshida A, Kadota K, Kambara H, et al: Left ventricular responses to supine bicycle exercise assessed by radionuclide angiocardiography and swan-ganz catheter. *Jpn Circ J* 1985;49:661–671.

Zaret BL, Stenson RE, Martin ND, et al: Potassium-43 myocardial perfusion scanning for the noninvasive evaluation of patients with false-positive exercise tests. *Circulation* 1973;48:1234.

9 THE CARDIOVASCULAR EFFECTS OF CHRONIC EXERCISE

Exercise training and physical conditioning are terms used for chronic exercise or an exercise program. Exercise training can be defined as maintaining a regular habit of exercise at levels greater than those usually performed. An exercise program can be designed for increasing muscular strength, muscular endurance, or dynamic performance. Isometric exercise results in an increase in muscular strength. It involves developing muscular tension against resistance without much movement. Though this results in an increase in muscular mass along with strength, such exercises do not benefit the cardiovascular system. They cause a pressure load on the heart rather than a flow load because mean pressure is elevated, but not cardiac output. Flow cannot be increased much because of increased pressure within the active muscle groups. Dynamic exercise, also called isotonic, involves the rhythmic movement of large groups of muscles and requires an increase in cardiac output, ventilation, and oxygen consumption. Such exercise is also called aerobic because it must be performed with sufficient oxygen present. This is the type of exercise that results in the cardiovascular changes that will be described.

The features of an aerobic exercise program that must be considered include the mode, duration, intensity, and frequency of the exercise. In general, the mode of exercise must involve movement of large muscle groups such as is required by bicycling, walking, running, skating, cross country skiing, and swimming. The exercise should be carried out in at least three sessions a week and should be spread out through the week. Duration should be 30 to 60 minutes. Intensity should be at least 50% of the maximal oxygen consumption and involve at least 300 kilocalories of energy expenditure per session. The percentage of maximal oxygen consumption being performed can be approximated by heart rate or by the level of perceived exertion.

The results of such an aerobic exercise program include hemodynamic, morphologic, and metabolic changes. The hemodynamic consequences of an exercise program include a decrease in resting heart rate, a decrease in the heart rate and systolic blood pressure at any matched submaximal work load, an increase in work capacity and maximal oxygen consumption, and a faster recovery from a bout of exercise. It is debatable whether these changes are due to peripheral or to cardiac adaptations, but they are probably due to both.

Peripheral adaptations are more important in older individuals and in patients with heart or lung disease, while cardiac adaptations are more of a factor in younger individuals. Cardiac hemodynamic changes that have been observed in some instances include enhanced cardiac function and cardiac output.

The morphologic changes that occur with an exercise program are age-related. These changes occur most definitely in younger individuals and may not occur in older individuals. The exact age at which the response to chronic exercise is altered is uncertain, but it appears to be in the early 30s. Morphologic changes include an increase in myocardial mass and left ventricular end-diastolic volume. Paralleling these changes are increases in coronary artery size and the myocardial capillary to fiber ratio. These changes are clearly beneficial, making it possible for the heart to function more efficiently and to have greater perfusion during any stress. In older individuals, there can be a decrease in myocardial mass resulting in an improvement in capillary to muscle fiber ratio, but no change in coronary artery size. No studies have shown an exercise program to decrease atherosclerotic plaques once they are present. However, a monkey study has shown that exercise can offset the impact of an atherogenic diet by increases in coronary artery size.

The metabolic alterations secondary to an aerobic exercise program are summarized below. Total serum cholesterol level is not affected, but high-density lipoproteins (which remove cholesterol from the body) are increased particularly when weight loss accompanies the exercise. Serum triglyceride and fasting glucose levels are decreased. In addition, it appears that there are favorable alterations in insulin and glucagon responses. Diabetics need less insulin if they maintain a regular exercise program. Also, after an exercise program, blood catecholamine levels are lower in response to any stress. The fibrinolytic system seems to be enhanced, and since coronary thrombosis is no longer a misnomer, this seems to be beneficial in preventing myocardial infarction.

Although it is said that exercise enhances psychologic well-being and can even produce the "runner's high," few convincing studies have been performed in this area. It seems that exercise does have a tranquilizing effect and increases pain tolerance, which may be beneficial in some individuals. This chapter presents the studies that have investigated the effects of chronic exercise on the heart; specifically regarding animals as well as human studies of hemodynamics, the echocardiogram, and the electrocardiographic response to exercise testing.

ANIMAL STUDIES OF THE EFFECTS OF CHRONIC EXERCISE

Animal studies provide some of the strongest evidence for the health benefits of regular exercise. The many effects listed in Table 9–1 have been demonstrated in various studies, and a review of some of these follows.

TABLE 9–1.

Results of Animal Studies Investigating the Effects of Chronic Exercise

Age-dependent myocardial hypertrophy
Myocardial microcirculatory changes (increased ratio of capillaries to muscle fibers)
Proportional increase in coronary artery size
Mixed results when studying changes in coronary collateral circulation
Improved cardiac mechanical and metabolic performance
Favorable changes in skeletal muscle mitochondria and respiratory enzymes
Mixed results with myocardial mitochondria and enzyme changes
Little effect on established atherosclerotic lesions or risk factors
Improved peripheral blood flow during exercise

Note: These results are strong support for the exercise hypothesis. Perhaps if people were as "compliant" as animals, the benefits of exercise to humans would be more apparent.

Myocardial Hypertrophy.   Numerous studies have demonstrated that vigorous exercise can induce cardiac hypertrophy in animals. Heart/body ratios are invariably larger in wild animals as compared with the domestic form of an animal species. Cardiac hypertrophy can result from chronic exercise in young rats; in older rats, exercise can cause a decline in heart weight due to a loss of myocardial fibers or a decrease in fiber mass.

The cellular morphologic mechanism of exercise cardiac hypertrophy has not been determined. There is even controversy regarding pathologic cardiac hypertrophy, which has been investigated more extensively in animal experiments. In exercise hypertrophy, the increased cardiac weight could be due to myocardial fiber hyperplasia, fiber hypertrophy, or both. The classical belief has been that myocardial fiber hyperplasia does not occur beyond the immediate postnatal period. Several studies involving rat and human myocardial tissue, however, support the concept that myocardial fiber hyperplasia occurs beyond this time. Also, an increase in fiber length has been demonstrated in biventricular hypertrophy secondary to pulmonary artery banding.

Hyperplasia and fiber lengthening, which could result in increased cardiac mass without fiber thickening, are advantageous compared to fiber thickening which occurs with pathologic cardiac hypertrophy. Maintenance of normal fiber diameter is important, since the diffusion distance from surrounding capillaries to central myofibrils is not increased. Exercise studies have shown a constant myocardial fiber diameter, favoring hyperplasia or fiber lengthening as the cellular morphologic mechanism of exercise-induced hypertrophy.

Myocardial Microcirculatory Changes.   In comparing tame with wild animals (i.e., tame rabbit to hare, domesticated rat to wild rat), the density of muscle cells and capillaries was found to be much greater in the more active wild animals. In an experiment utilizing surgical constriction of the aorta, there was a 35% increase in heart weight in one-month-old rabbits and in adult rabbits. In the young rabbits, the hypertrophied hearts showed a normal capillary density; in the adult rabbits, it was decreased. From these observations, Poupa hypothesized that in young animals, cardiac hypertrophy is secondary to fiber hyperplasia; in older animals, it is secondary to cellular hypertrophy. Also, he hypothesized that the capillary bed responds to growth stimuli most markedly if applied at an early age.

Tomanek studied the age-related response of the ventricular capillary bed and myocardial fiber width in male albino rats to chronic exercise. Eighty male rats, aged 40 days (young), 130 days (adult), or 575 days (old), were assigned to experimental or to control groups. The exercised rats ran on a treadmill six days a week for approximately 40 minutes for 12 weeks. The rats developed a resting bradycardia with this exercise program. At autopsy, the myocardial fiber width was constant; the capillary-fiber ratio increased in the exercised rats over the controls in all age groups. The capillary density decreased with age and was increased over the controls only in the young exercised rats.

Leon and Bloor performed rat experiments to study the effects of chronic exercise on the heart at different ages. Male rats aged 1 to 12 months were divided into three age groups equivalent to teen years, the 20s to 40s, and the 50s to 70s in humans. Each of these age groups was subdivided into a control group, a group that swam for one hour daily, and a group that swam for an hour two days a week. After ten weeks, the animals were sacrificed. They concluded that although the response of the rat heart to chronic exercise varies with age, the capillary-fiber ratio increases at all ages. Their data regarding capillary changes are in agreement with the findings of Tomanek.

The only studies of the effects of an experimental program of exercise on myocardial capillary density using a species other than the rat have been those of Petren and associates and of Hakkila. Both used guinea pigs, but Petren's study showed an increase in capillary density while Hakkila found a decrease.

After injecting radioactive thymidine in rats exercised by swimming, Ljunggvist and Unge studied capillary proliferation in the heart and skeletal muscle by radioautography. Swimming led to hypertrophy of the myocardium and muscle fibers of the limbs. They found new formation of myocardial capillaries in swimming-induced cardiac hypertrophy while there was little capillary neoformation in the hypertrophied skeletal muscles.

McElroy and colleagues reported an exercise-induced reduction in myocardial infarction size after coronary artery occlusion in the rat. Rats, forced to swim one hour a day, five days a week for five weeks, were sacrificed, and the myocardial capillary bed was perfused with carbon black. When compared with sedentary controls, the capillary to muscle fiber ratio was increased by 30% in exercised rats. This training effect occurred in the absence of hypertrophy or increased fiber diameter. An additional 27 exercised rats and 25 control rats underwent left coronary artery occlusion and were sacrificed 48 hours later. Myocardial infarct size was measured by planimetry of the left ventricle. In exercised rats, 22% of the left ventricle was infarcted compared to 31% in the control rats. Exercise training resulted in a 30% reduction of myocardial infarct size after coronary artery occlusion, which suggests an increased myocardial vascularity.

Wexler and Greenberg reported the effects of exercise on myocardial infarction in young versus old rats. Subcutaneous injections of isoproterenol were given to induce acute myocardial ischemia and infarction in both groups. Exercise improved the survival rates of the old rats. In addition, the exercised old rats manifested cardiac hypertrophy, reduced infarction enzyme levels, and less evidence of arrhythmias or extensive myocardial infarction on their electrocardiographic tracings.

Coronary Artery Size Changes.   Tepperman and Pearlman studied the effects of exercise on the coronary tree of rats by the corrosion-cast technique. One group of rats ran approximately one mile a day for 36 days, and another group swam for 30 minutes a day for 10 weeks. When the animals were killed, their hearts were weighed, then the coronary arteries were injected with vinyl acetate. The hearts were digested with potassium hydroxide and the casts of the coronary arteries were weighed alone. Compared with the controls, both groups had an increased heart to body weight ratio and an increased coronary tree cast weight to heart weight ratio.

Stevenson and coworkers used the same corrosion-cast technique to ascertain the effects of exercise of different types, frequency, and duration. Their conclusion was that in the rat, forced exercise caused an increase in the coronary tree size as compared with the cardiac weight, provided the exercise was not too strenuous or frequent.

Leon and Bloor demonstrated that swimming in rats resulted in an increased luminal cross-sectional area of the main coronary arteries in the animals that experienced an increase in ventricular weight; that is, only the young and strenuously exercised adult rats. These results are supported by the studies of Kerr and colleagues that demonstrated coronary artery enlargement in rats with cardiac hypertrophy induced by hypoxia, aortic constriction, and thyroxin. Also, it has been shown that the relation between total heart weight and the diameter of the coronary arteries and ostia is linear in humans up to the upper weight limit of physiologic hypertrophy.

Coronary Artery Vasomotor Tone.   Bove and Dewey studied the effects of exercise on large coronary artery vasoreactivity in eight dogs trained in treadmill running for eight weeks. Six nontrained dogs were controls. The trained group showed a reduction in heart rate during submaximal exercise when compared with the controls, and resting plasma levels of norepinephrine and epinephrine were reduced in the trained group. Epicardial coronary responses to intracoronary infusion of serotonin and phenylephrine were elevated by quantitative coronary angiography, and myocardial blood flow was measured with radioactive microspheres. Left ventricular/body weight ratio was similar in the trained and nontrained groups, and no differences were noted in resting myocardial oxygen consumption or coronary arteriovenous oxygen difference. The constriction of the proximal left anterior descending artery (LAD) in response to serotonin infusion was not different in the two groups, but the LAD and circumflex artery constrictor responses to phenylephrine were attenuated in the trained when compared with the nontrained dogs. Endurance exercise diminished the large epicardial coronary vasoconstrictor response to alpha-adrenergic stimulation, but not to serotonin.

The blunted constrictor response in the trained animals suggests that exercise may be useful in reducing epicardial coronary vasoconstriction, which is thought to be important in some patients with coronary artery disease.

Myocardial blood flow is the major determinant of oxygen delivery to the myocardium, since oxygen extraction by the myocardium is near maximum in the resting state. Regulation of flow during exercise depends on local metabolic factors and, to a small extent, on autonomic tone. Maximum flow of 5–6 times resting has been measured in reactive hyperemia experiments. In strenuous exercise, myocardial oxygen delivery appears to be adequate and flow reserve seems capable of handling the increased oxygen demand. No evidence of myocardial failure in normal hearts due to excess exercise has been presented. However, pulmonary hemorrhages found in horses after strenuous racing may be due to inadequate cardiac performance at maximal capacity. In humans, severe limitations to myocardial blood flow are imposed by coronary artery disease and by cardiac hypertrophy. In both cases, regional myocardial ischemia may occur during the increased oxygen demands imposed by strenuous exercise.

Coronary Collateral Circulation. Eckstein performed the classic study of the effect of exercise and coronary artery narrowing on coronary collateral circulation. He surgically induced a constriction in the circumflex artery of approximately 100 dogs. Various degrees of narrowing were induced, but only dogs that developed ECG changes were included in the study. After one week of rest, the dogs were divided into two groups. One group was exercised on a treadmill one hour a day, five days a week, for six to eight weeks. The other group remained at rest in cages. The extent of arterial anastomoses to the circumflex artery was then determined as follows. The animals were anesthetized, a second thoracotomy was performed, and their blood pressure was stabilized mechanically. The circumflex artery was isolated and divided beyond the surgical constriction. The flow rate through the constriction and the flow rate from the distal end of the artery were measured. The flow rate through the constriction was inversely related to the degree of constriction.

When these values were plotted against one another, it was shown that the less the antegrade flow (or the greater the constriction), the greater the retrograde or collateral flow (Fig 9–1). Also, the exercised dogs had a greater value for retrograde flow than did the rested dogs for any degree of constriction. Eckstein concluded that moderate and severe arterial narrowing results in collateral development proportional to the degree of narrowing and that exercise leads to even greater coronary anastomosis.

Burt and Jackson used similar methods to study the effects of exercise on the collateral vessels of normal dogs. Twenty dogs were used; 13 rested and 7 exercised. Prior constriction of a coronary artery was not performed, as was in Eckstein's experiment. After one month of treadmill exercise, surgery was performed and retrograde flow measured from the distal portion of the circumflex artery with its proximal end ligated. There was no difference found in retrograde flow between the two groups. The authors concluded that exercise alone in the absence of an ischemic lesion is not sufficient to stimulate coronary collateral growth.

Kaplinsky and coworkers studied the effects of physical training in dogs after coronary artery ligation. Forty dogs were surgically subjected to complete occlusion of the left anterior descending coronary artery. Twenty-six dogs survived and, after one week of rest, were divided into exercise and control groups. The exercised dogs were run on a treadmill for one hour, six days a week for five weeks, and then both groups were put to death. A training effect was demonstrated in the exercise group. Selective cineangiography and postmortem coronary injections demonstrated extensive collateral for-

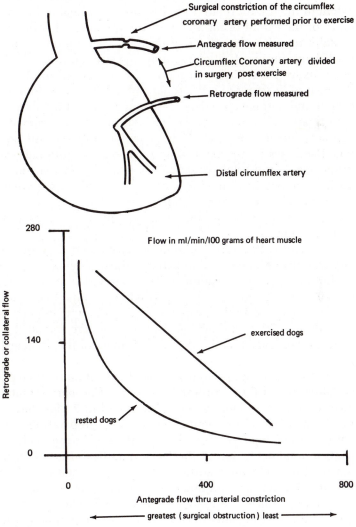

FIG 9–1.
Description of Eckstein's study showing the surgical procedure and the results.

mation, but there was no difference between the two groups. The authors concluded that exercise may not enhance collateralization when a large vessel is totally occluded.

Cobb and associates studied the effects of exercise on acute coronary occlusion in dogs with a prior partial occlusion. The anterior descending coronary artery was partially occluded (35% to 70%) in 50 dogs, and then they were divided into a control and an exercise group. The exercise consisted of treadmill running for 40 minutes a day for three months. Subsequently, a complete occlusion of the anterior descending artery was surgically produced. The animals were monitored for arrhythmias for six days, then sacrificed and their hearts removed. The coronary vessels were injected and the collateral vessels were quantitated radiographically. The two groups did not differ as to the extent of the infarct relative to the partial occlusion, the frequency of arrhythmias, or the extent of radiographically quantitated collaterals.

Malik reported the effects of exercise training on coronary blood flow and cardiac output in rats at rest and during stress induced by breathing a mixture of 5% oxygen and 95% nitrogen for five to seven minutes. Training decreased the resting heart rate and coronary blood flow and increased resting cardiac output and coronary vascular resistance. During hypoxic stress, arterial pressure, heart rate, and cardiac output fell in both the trained and sedentary rats; coronary blood flow also fell in sedentary rats but did not change in trained rats. Decreases in perfusion during hypoxia in both endocardium and epicardium were found solely in sedentary rats. The unchanged coronary blood flow during hypoxia in trained rats was associated with a greater decrease in coronary vascular resistance. Malik concluded that exercise training leads to greater coronary dilation during hemodynamic stresses and thereby maintains coronary flow.

Spear and colleagues studied coronary blood flow in exercised and sedentary rats using labeled microspheres during hypoxemic conditions designed to develop coronary dilatation. Rats trained for 12 to 18 weeks had a significantly greater flood flow than did sedentary rats. Even though cardiac hypertrophy was found in the trained rats, this increase in perfused mass accounted for only one third the increase in total coronary blood flow. Thus, there was a greater coronary blood flow per unit mass of the myocardium in the trained rats.

Bloor and colleagues reported the effects of endurance exercise on coronary collateral blood flow in miniature swine. Coronary collateral blood flow was measured in 10 sedentary control pigs and in 7 pigs that ran 20 miles a week for 10 months. Using acute, open chest preparations, radiolabeled microspheres were injected into the left atrium during each of three conditions: control, total occlusion of the left circumflex artery, and total occlusion plus mechanically elevated aortic pressure. Ten months of endurance exercise training did not have an effect on the development of coronary collaterals as assessed by microsphere blood flow measurements in the left ventricle of the pigs. These investigators have repeated this experiment after causing artificial partial occlusions in the coronary arteries of their pigs. With ischemia present, exercise enhanced myocardial perfusion.

Heaton and colleagues studied the effects of physical training on collateral blood flow in 14 dogs with chronic coronary occlusions. Regional blood flow was measured using injected radionuclide microspheres at rest and during exercise. One-half of the dogs subsequently trained for six weeks while the other half remained inactive in kennels. After six weeks, myocardial blood flow was not significantly changed in control animals. After training, however, myocardial blood flow to the underperfused endocardium of collateral-dependent zones was 39% greater than it was before training.

Scheel and colleagues studied 10 control beagles, 10 exercised beagles, 8 beagles with occluded circumflex arteries for five months, and 7 beagles similar to the last group but exercised. Using an isolated heart preparation, they found no increase in collaterals in the normal dogs, but doubled collateral conductance in the exercised ischemic dogs.

There is some question whether middle-aged patients with coronary artery disease can accomplish enough physical exertion to stimulate collateral development greater than the ischemia secondary to their disease. Neill and Oxedine studied the effects of exercise training on coronary collaterals developing in response to gradual coronary occlusion in dogs. Ameroid constrictors were used, which initially were nonobstructive but slowly absorbed body fluids and gradually expanded over two to three weeks. After placement of a constrictor on the proximal left circumflex coronary artery, 33 dogs were randomly assigned to exercise or to sedentary groups. After two months, the exercised dogs developed greater epicardial collateral connections to the occluded left circumflex as judged by higher blood flow and less distal pressure drop. However, no difference in collaterals was found angiographically. Injected microspheres demonstrated that exercised dogs were not better protected against subendocardial ischemia induced by increased heart rate in the myocardium supplied by the collaterals. These investigators concluded that exercise can promote coronary collateral development without improving perfusion of ischemic myocardium. These results raise an additional question: Even if collateral development does occur, does it significantly influence myocardial perfusion?

Cardiac Mechanical and Metabolic Performance.   Penpargkul and Scheuer reported that effect of physical training on the mechanical and metabolic performance of the isolated rat heart. Rats were exercised by swimming for 2½ hours a day, five days a week for two months. The exercised rats and controls were killed and their hearts isolated in a perfusion apparatus with cannulas inserted for life support, pressure and flow measurement, and metabolic analysis. When compared with sedentary controls, the hearts from conditioned rats had higher levels of cardiac work and output. Atrial pacing at increased rates caused greater differences in those parameters, and left ventricular pressures and dp/dt became higher in conditioned hearts. Atrial pacing also resulted in greater oxygen consumption in conditioned hearts; higher lactate and pyruvate concentrations occurred in sedentary hearts. Raising atrial filling pressures resulted in ventricular function curves that were superior in the conditioned hearts. Also, there were greater increments in oxygen consumption, a higher aerobic to anaerobic energy production ratio, and increased coronary artery flow. The authors concluded that in exercised rats, the function of the heart as a pump is improved and that this effect is at least partially due to improved oxygen delivery.

Crews and Aldinger presented data to support the concept that the exercise-hypertrophied heart is functionally superior to the normal heart. They randomly divided 30 female rats into control and exercise groups of 15 each. The exercised rats swam for six hours a day for approximately one month. Then a thoracotomy was performed and isometric systolic tension was measured while the animals were physiologically supported. This measurement was believed by the authors to reflect potential contractility and cardiac work. Measurements were also made of left ventricular pressure before and during aortic constriction. The animals were sacrificed and body weight, ventricular thickness, cardiac weight, and cardiac volume determined. All of these parameters were significantly increased in the exercise group compared to the controls. Aldinger reported a similar study involving a control and exercised group of rats receiving digitoxin. This study demonstrated that unlike the pathologic hypertrophy of disease, exercise hypertrophy and the increment in myocardial function concomitant with hypertrophy are not altered by digitoxin.

Tomoike and colleagues reported regional myocardial dynamics during brief strenuous bouts of running in 12 conscious dogs using telemetry before and after partial circumflex coronary artery obstruction. Regional myocardial dimensions were measured using surgically embedded ultrasonic crystals in a control segment and in a segment that would be made ischemic. In control exercise runs, heart rate, left ventricular systolic pressure, and dp/dt increased markedly. Also, segment length at end-diastole increased along with augmentation of regional myocardial performance. During circumflex constriction, exercise resulted in a similar heart rate, but left ventricular systolic pressure and dp/dt changes were significantly reduced. Shortening of the nonischemic segment did not change significantly, but ischemic segment power and stroke-work were depressed. In two dogs, ventricular fibrillation occurred during and immediately after running. Abnormal regional wall motion during and following exercise appeared to be a specific indicator of limited coronary reserve. This animal model could be used for evaluating changes secondary to training.

Carew and Covell reported indices of left ventricular function and diastolic compliance in 10 conscious, exercise-trained greyhounds with left ventricular hypertrophy. High-fidelity micromanometers and ultrasonic crystals were implanted; left ventricular contractility were measured and found to be similar to that measured previously in normal dogs. During volume loading, changes in contractility approximated those in normal dogs. Left ventricular diastolic stiffness did not differ from that of normal dogs. Left ventricular function in exercise-induced left ventricular hypertrophy was substantially normal arguing against the concept of the "athlete's heart" syndrome.

Bershon and Scheuer reported the effects of chronic exercise on the response of the rat heart to ischemia. Sedentary rats and those trained by swimming were sacrificed, and their hearts were perfused in an isolated working-heart apparatus under aerobic and ischemic perfusion conditions. During ischemia, coronary blood flow diminished by approximately 40%, and oxygen consumption was similar in the two groups. During oxygenated conditions, end-diastolic pressures and volumes were similar in exercised and sedentary rats. The hearts of the exercised rats had better responses of stroke volume and left ventricular systolic pressure to increases in atrial filling pressure. During ischemia, stroke volume was 30% greater in hearts of exercised rats than in sedentary controls, and left ventricular systolic pressure was also significantly higher. Relaxation was faster during aerobic and ischemic perfusion in hearts of exercised rats. The duration of diastole was increased in hearts of exercised rats under ischemic and aerobic conditions. Under these highly controlled loading conditions, hearts of chronically exercised rats continued to perform better during ischemia than did hearts of sedentary controls. This result did not seem to be due to altered diastolic pressure-volume relationships and may be related to an intrinsic improvement in myocardial function.

Wyatt and colleagues studied the influence of physical training on myocardial contractility in six cats. After training, right ventricular papillary muscles were studied in vitro, and adenylate cyclase activity was determined from ventricular muscle. Physical training did not alter the intrinsic contractile function or the contractile response to paired or frequency stimulation. However, training might have improved the catecholamine-induced enhancement of myocardial contractility and adenylate cyclase activity.

Stone reported the effects of exercise training on cardiac function in conscious dogs that are instrumented so that ascending aortic flow, left ventricular pressure, and left atrial pressure could be measured. A standardized submaximal test was performed before and after training. The heart rate in the trained animals was reduced by an average of 20 beats/min. The maximum derivative of left ventricular pressure increased in the trained animals. Ventricular function curves were lower in trained animals because of a reduction in heart rate response. These results indicate a reflex adaptation of the nervous system with training to improve cardiac function. The earliest changes found were in stroke volume and cardiac output. Later, changes occurred in the heart rate response to volume loading and the contractility of the left ventricle associated with the test. The early changes in stroke volume could be associated with change in ventricular end-diastolic volume, while changes in contractility and heart rate could be consistent with a change in the balance of autonomic innervation of the heart. Reflex changes in heart rate with volume loading indicate that there may have been some integrative changes in the central nervous system pathways associated with this reflex. In conscious dogs, the cardiac effect of exercise training tended to lower the submaximal energy requirements of the heart and to increase maximal pumping capacity of the heart.

Dowell and colleagues, using chronically instrumented dogs, studied myocardial contractility and adenosine triphosphatase (ATPase) activity of cardiac contractile proteins before and after exercise training. Before training, heart rate and the maximal rate of left ventricular pressure development were measured at rest and during submaximal exercise. Animals were then subjected to an 8- to 10-week treadmill running program. After training, maximal dp/dt was within normal limits at rest but significantly elevated by submaximal exercise. When maximal dp/dt was plotted as a function of heart rate, either at rest or during submaximal exercise, a marked elevation of maximal dp/dt at any given heart rate was observed following training. Myofibrillar protein content and ATPase activity of left ventricular myocardium were nearly identical before and after training. Although exercise training by treadmill running improved myocardial contractility in the unanesthetized dog, this response does not involve alterations in myofibrillar ATPase activity.

Bershon and Scheuer studied hemodynamics and ventricular performance in hearts from sedentary and swimming-trained rats. They used an isolated working-heart apparatus modified to measure end-diastolic volume by dye dilution. In addition, instantaneous aortic flow, left ventricular pressure, and oxygen consumption were measured. Heart rate and mean aortic pressure were kept constant, and atrial filling pressure was varied. Heart weights were equal and end-diastolic pressures and volumes were similar to all atrial pressures. However, ejection fraction and circumferential fiber work were both greater in hearts of conditioned rats. Maximal negative dp/dt was also greater at all three loads. Maximal oxygen consumption of trained rats increased in proportion to the increase in work. These results indicated that the improved pumping performance of trained hearts is due to a change in ventricular function. Faster cardiac relaxation is a prominent effect of physical training and may foster more complete filling at high heart rates.

Dowell and colleagues studied the functional responses of the rat heart to pressure overload in exercised and sedentary rats. The rats were trained with a moderate treadmill running program. Left ventricular RNA, DNA, and cytochrome C levels were unchanged. After training, when subjected to a pressure overload by sustained aortic constriction, exercised animals maintained or increased myocardial contractility. Exercised animals fully regained a normal cardiac output after the acute overload was relieved, but the cardiac output remained approximately 10% below control in sedentary animals. The improved ability of previously exercised animals to withstand pressure overload appears to be due to alterations in adaptation rather than augmentation of metabolism or function.

Ritzer and colleagues studied the effects of 10 weeks of treadmill exercise on left ventricular performance in nine dogs chronically instrumented with left ventricular pressure transducers. At similar exercise heart rates, the trained dogs had greater left contractility indices than the sedentary dogs.

Skeletal Muscle Mitochondria and Respiratory Enzyme Changes.   The changes that occur in chronically exercised skeletal muscles have been confirmed by numerous investigators, whose work has been reviewed by Holloszy. Mitochondria are increased in number, size, and the number of cristae. Amounts of mitochondrial protein and respiratory enzymes are also increased per gram of fresh muscle. There is an increased capacity for ATPase production and aerobic metabolism of many substrates. Myoglobin concentration is increased. This adaptation must partially account for the increased aerobic work capacity and for the decreased muscle blood flow at any level of submaximal exercise that occurs secondary to chronic exercise.

Tibbits and colleagues reported the results of 11 weeks of progressive treadmill exercise in rats. In the trained rats, gastrocnemius cytochrome C oxidase activity was 38% higher in the controls. They found that endurance training of this type did not necessarily increase myofibrillar ATPase activity or the time course of the isometric twitch of the rat papillary muscle. However, tension per unit area did increase and appeared to be due to a greater amount of calcium being made available to the contractile apparatus.

Myocardial Mitochondria and Respiratory Enzyme Changes. Arcos and colleagues studied female rats, using a protocol similar to that used by Aldinger. The rats were separated into a control group and three swimming groups, with total swimming time ranging from 60 to 500 hours. The rats who exceeded 300 hours of total swimming could not continue swimming six hours a day, so their daily time had to be decreased. The rats were sacrificed and their hearts analyzed by various methods. Mitochondrial mass was increased only in the rats that swam for approximately 160 hours. Electron microscopy showed increased size and number of mitochondria in this group; mitochondrial degeneration was noted in rats exercised for a longer time. No change in the respiratory rate of myocardial homogenates was found between the groups. The microscopic and histochemical sections showed evidence of myocardial degeneration in the exercised rat hearts. The authors suggested that the increase in mitochondrial mass is a compensatory response to exercise and that this increase brings about focal regions of hypoxia during periods of excessive exercise causing degenerative changes.

Aldinger and Sohal repeated the previous experiment but with the total swimming time increased to between 400 and 1,500 hours. Also, a control and an exercise group treated with digitoxin were included. Again, mitochondrial degenerative changes were seen in the myocardium of the nontreated swimmers. However, the swimmers receiving digitoxin showed no degenerative changes. In fact, they had an increase in the size of the mitochondria and in the number of mitochondrial cristae. In addition, the following subcellular changes occurred in the myocardium of both swimming groups: (1) increased mitochondrial-myofibril ratio; (2) occasional areas of myocardial hemorrhage; (3) increased distance between nuclei; and (4) dilatation and vesicle formation within intercalated disks. The authors suggested that some of these changes did not appear beneficial, but concluded that the morphologic integrity of the myocardial mitochondria is better preserved in the swimming rat receiving digitoxin than in the untreated swimming rat.

Banister, Tomanek, and Cvorkov reported a study of the effects of chronic exercise on rat heart mitochondrial morphology using the electron microscope. Male rats were run to exhaustion on a motor-driven treadmill for one hour a day over a 65-day period. Throughout the training period, four animals were sacrificed on certain days. The four consisted of one control, one trained animal killed immediately after exercise, one killed 30 minutes after exercise, and one killed 24 hours after exercise. On the first training day, exhaustive running resulted in mitochondrial degeneration in the animal killed immediately and in the one killed 30 minutes after exercise. The rat killed 24 hours after exercise showed mitochondrial morphology similar to the unexercised control rat. The effects of training began to appear after 10 days. Fewer altered mitochondria were seen in the trained rats sacrificed at any period after exercise. This study demonstrated that with physical training, exhaustive exercise has a less damaging effect on myocardial mitochondria, suggesting that this organelle adapts to exercise.

Oscai, Mole, and Holloszy studied rats using various exercise protocols including the same swimming protocol used by Arcos and Aldinger. They could not confirm an increase in mitochondrial protein or respiratory enzymes in the myocardium of exercised rats. They suggested that the capacity for aerobic metabolism of normal, untrained rat myocardium is adequate to meet the increased demands for ATPase imposed by an exercise program without augmenting mitochondrial mass or respiratory capacity. They found that respiratory enzyme levels are approximately five times higher in the heart than in the gastrocnemius muscle of the sedentary rat. They also confirmed the interesting finding that exercise depresses the appetite of male rats and does not affect the appetite of female rats. Because of problems with growth differences secondary to this phenomenon between controls and exercised rats, some investigators have used only female rats.

Tibbits and colleagues found tension per unit area increased in the papillary muscle of exercised rats, but this effect appeared to be due to a greater amount of calcium being made available to the contractile apparatus. Scheuer and coworkers measured increased cardiac glycogen stores in conditioned rat hearts but found no increase in the concentration of high-energy phosphate compounds.

Effects of Atherosclerosis and Risk Factors.   McAllister and colleagues reported an experiment that demonstrated an accelerating effect of muscular exercise on experimental atherosclerosis. Ten mongrel dogs were placed on identical high-cholesterol diets of equal caloric value and 150 mg of thiouracil daily. The diet and the thyroid antagonist were used to shorten the time period of the study. The dogs were treated identically, except that five were trained to run five miles a day at five miles per hour on a treadmill. At the end of one year, angiograms were performed, the dogs were sacrificed, and their arteries were analyzed for the extent of atherosclerosis. During the course of the study period, the serum cholesterol progressively rose with the runners having higher values. The runners also showed more atherosclerosis than did the sedentary dogs in all vessels, including the coronaries.

Myasnikov reported the results of studies performed by himself and his colleagues in Russia. Ten rabbits were given a high-cholesterol diet, 25 rabbits received the same diet but were run to exhaustion daily on a treadmill, and 8 rabbits received no cholesterol but were exercised. The exercised rabbits on a high-cholesterol diet had lower serum cholesterols than did those not exercised. At the end of six months, the animals were sacrificed and visual estimation showed that the physical exercise reduced to some extent the development of atherosclerosis in the aorta and coronary arteries. However, for unknown reasons, there were more marked pathologic changes in the myocardium of the exercised rabbits receiving cholesterol than in either of the other groups.

Kobernick and coworkers reported the results of a similar study. Eighteen rabbits were fed high cholesterol diets and exercised 10 minutes a day, while a nonexercised matched group received the same diet. Serial serum cholesterol values did not differ between the groups. After 13 weeks, the rabbits were sacrificed and their aortas inspected visually for atherosclerosis and chemically analyzed for cholesterol. The exercised rabbits had greater muscle mass, less body fat deposits, and less aortic atherosclerotic involvement than the nonexercised rabbits.

Warnock and colleagues reported an exercise study using young male roosters. All of the birds were caged and fed an atherogenic diet. Ten remained caged while 14 were taken from the cage and forced to walk briskly for one hour a day (approximately four miles a week). Weekly serum cholesterol values were determined and found to be lower in the exercised birds. The food consumption was equal in both groups but the exercised birds were heavier. At the end of 14 weeks, the birds were sacrificed and the aorta, its main branches, and samples of brain and liver were assayed for cholesterol. The cholesterol content was lower in the assayed vessels and liver of the exercised birds than in the nonexercised birds. The coronary arteries were not studied.

Carlson reported the results of strenuous exercise on the serum cholesterol of old rats. The trained group ran three hours daily for one month. At the end of this period, the serum cholesterol averaged 186 mg/100 ml in the trained group and 250 mg/100 ml in controls. The extent of atherosclerotic involvement was not studied. Faris and his coworkers performed a similar study in young rats. Both the control and the exercised animals had serum cholesterol readings of about 45 mg/100 ml, and there was no statistical difference between the groups. Neither investigator discussed the diet fed their rats, but Carlson stated that lipid levels in rats increased with age, just as they do in humans.

The influence of training on resting blood pressure in rats who were normotensive, borderline hypertensive, genetically hypertensive, or hypertensive but receiving drugs was investigated. Training resulted in lower blood pressure in normal rats. In the borderline hypertensive and genetically hypertensive rats, exercise training appeared to delay the onset of hypertension as well as the magnitude of the systolic pressure, but exercise was unable to normalize the resting pressure.

Rasmussen and Hostmark studied cholesterol and triglycerides in two groups of rats with widely different levels of physical activity. Cholesterol and triglycerides were measured from the age of three to eight months in females and from three months to one year in males. A pronounced increase in lipids with age was observed in the active male rats. In the inactive male rats and in all females, there was no major change in lipid levels. The data for male rats showed an association between the inherited tendency to perform spontaneous high levels of physical activity and an age-related increase in plasma lipids. However, running did not have any influence on the level of cholesterol or triglycerides.

Pedersoli reported the effects of exercise and of an atherogenic diet of serum lipids in swine. Twenty-two pigs were exercised daily, and 22 pigs served as controls. All were fed an atherogenic diet. Exercise training alone did not produce any change in serum lipids.

Kramsch and colleagues randomly allocated 27 young adult male monkeys into three groups. Two groups were studied for 36 months and one group was studied for 42 months. Of the groups studied for 36 months, one was fed a vegetarian diet for the entire study while the other was fed the vegetarian diet for 12 months and then an isocaloric atherogenic diet for 24 months. Both were designated as sedentary because their physical activity was limited to a single cage. The third group was fed the vegetarian diet for 18 months and then the atherogenic diet for 24 months. This group exercised regularly on a treadmill for the entire 42 months. Because two of the monkeys on the atherogenic diet (one sedentary and one exercising) did not develop elevated serum cholesterol levels, they were excluded from the study. For three years the animals were observed for objective evidence to support the protective value of periodic and regular exercise. Total serum cholesterol remained the same but HDL cholesterol was higher in the exercise group. Ischemic electrocardiographic changes, angiographic coronary artery narrowing, and sudden death were observed only in the sedentary monkeys fed the atherogenic diet. In addition, postmortem examination revealed marked coronary atherosclerosis and stenosis in this group. Exercise was associated with substantially reduced overall atherogenic involvement, lesion size, and collagen accumulation. These results demonstrate that exercise in young adult monkeys increases heart size, left ventricular mass, and the diameter of coronary arteries. Also, the subsequent experimental atherosclerosis, induced by the atherogenic diet given for two years, was substantially reduced. Exercise before exposure to the atherogenic diet delayed the development of the manifestation of coronary heart disease. The important question this study raises is: At what point comparable to the human lifespan were these studies initiated and what percentage of that lifespan was represented by the three years of observation?

Tibbits and colleagues reported marked changes in the lipid composition of highly purified plasma membranes isolated from the hearts of rats who exercised daily. Compared to sedentary controls, sarcolemmal content of total phospholipid and phosphatidylserine in the trained group was increased 23% and 50%, respectively. This observation suggests a mechanism by which cardiac contractility may be enhanced by exercise through increased fluidity of the plasma membrane during excitation-contraction coupling.

Studies in rats and dogs have found increased resistance to ventricular fibrillation after regular running, possibly through mechanisms involving cyclic adenosine monophosphate and the slow calcium channel. This provides experimental support for linking exercise training with decreased sudden death.

Goodrick studied 140 rats who were maintained in either wheel-cage units or cage units for their entire lifespan. Body weight increment or growth rate was negatively related to longevity, while growth duration was positively related to longevity. Rats who performed wheel exercise had a significantly increased mean longevity compared with controls.

Changes in Peripheral Blood Flow in Response to Acute Exercise.   Fixler and colleagues studied the distribution of cardiac output in six dogs at rest and during mild and moderate exercise. Organ blood flows were measured using radioactive microspheres. The greatest change was in diaphragmatic flow, which increased by 275% with mild exercise and by 500% with moderate exercise. Flow to intercostal muscles increased by 160% and 269%, to the exercising gastrocnemius muscle by 153% and 224%, and to the cardiac muscle by 57% and 109%, all during mild and moderate exercise, respectively. Renal and cerebral flows did not change. Significant decreases in flow occurred in the small and large intestines during moderate exercise. These results demonstrate that the increase in cardiac output during submaximal exercise was redistributed in a manner that limited flow to brain, intestines, and kidneys, and increased flow to the diaphragm, heart, and limb muscles. This organ blood-flow measurement technique should be useful in studying the peripheral adaptations to exercise brought about by training.

Summary.   Animal studies have provided substantial evidence of the cardiovascular benefits of regular physical activity. Improved coronary circulation has been demonstrated in exercise-trained animals by increased coronary artery size, greater capillary density, reduced myocardial infarction size, and maintenance of coronary flow in response to hypoxia. In an evaluation of the experimental evidence, Scheel proposes that ischemia initiates the development of collaterals while mechanical factors, such as shear forces and intraluminal pressure, further stimulate vascular growth until these stress forces return to normal. Whether changes in myocardial collateral perfusion occurs remains controversial, but exercise probably improves this when ischemia is present. Studies utilizing various animal models have reported improvement in cardiac function secondary to exercise training. Improved intrinsic contractility, faster relaxation, enzymatic alterations, calcium availability, and enhanced autonomic and hormonal control of function have all been implicated. Studies in experimental animals that clearly demonstrate increased myocardial capillary growth and enlargement of extramural vessels in response to chronic physical exercise continue to stimulate the search for proof that exercise programs in man will increase myocardial vascularity and develop coronary collaterals. Perhaps the beneficial effects of exercise would be more apparent in humans if we were as compliant with an exercise program as animals.

Animal studies add considerable data to our knowledge of the effects of chronic exercise on the heart. They demonstrate that there are morphologic and metabolic changes that make the cardiovascular system better able to withstand stress, possibly even that imposed by atherosclerosis. These favorable adaptations are more marked in young animals than in older animals. The data regarding beneficial effects of chronic exercise on the atherosclerotic process or on serum cholesterol levels are only suggestive, however, and better studies are required to confirm this effect. The study by Kramsch and colleagues provides the strongest evidence for a favorable impact of exercise on the primary prevention of coronary disease. In this study, exercise lessened ischemic manifestations, but only diet stopped progression of coronary atherosclerosis. Nevertheless, the therapeutic and preventive use of exercise is supported by animal studies, but such efforts should be adjunctive to modification of the risk factors that have a well-demonstrated influence on the atherosclerotic process.

HEMODYNAMIC STUDIES OF THE EFFECTS OF AN EXERCISE PROGRAM

The effects of an exercise program can be studied by the cross-sectional approach, comparing athletes to normal people, and by the longitudinal approach, comparing individuals before and after a training program. Both of these approaches have limitations and difficulties. The cross-sectional approach is the easier of the two because the trouble and expense of organizing a training program can be avoided. However, athletes are endowed with biologic attributes and motivation that make them capable of superior performance. Also, they undergo long periods of physical training that usually begin at a young age when dimensional and morphologic changes are more apt to occur. This makes comparison with normal people questionable since most trained normal individuals cannot reach an athlete's level of cardiovascular function or performance. For these reasons, only longitudinal studies are reviewed here.

Besides the expense and difficulty in organizing and maintaining an exercise program, there are other problems encountered in longitudinal studies. Volunteers often are athletic and differ from randomly selected normal people. An exercise program can modify significant variables, such as body weight and smoking habits, and results can be biased by dropouts. In persons with coronary heart disease, a placebo effect on hemodynamics has been documented and a training program may select a healthier group.

In any training program, the end result depends on several factors. These factors include the level of fitness, physical endowment, previous physical training, age, sex, and health of the individual entering the program. The changes are greater in sedentary individuals, as compared with those somewhat physically fit, and greater in younger individuals than in older individuals. The most important of these variables will be evaluated in this review by including studies of normal trainees of different ages and of persons with coronary heart disease.

The structure of an exercise program is important. Intensity and duration of the work periods must be considered, as well as the overall time of exercise. Individuals with stable coronary heart disease must be selected. During training, they follow a less demanding exercise protocol because of the danger of exercise-induced sudden death. An exercise program can be aimed at improving or increasing muscle strength and anaerobic or aerobic performance. Only the latter effect is dependent on the improvement of the oxygen transporting system (i.e., blood, lungs, heart, and blood vessels) and comes about mainly because of an improvement in the overall capacity of the cardiovascular system.

Muscle strength can be improved by repetitious isotonic or isometric muscle contractions of a few seconds duration and against resistance. This type of exercise does not improve cardiovascular function, as shown by relatively normal-size hearts, normal resting and exercise heart rates, and unexceptional maximal oxygen intakes of athletes who only train in this manner. Anaerobic capacity is necessary for short activities of high intensity or for activities that require more energy than is available from the oxygen transport system. This energy is derived from high-energy phosphate compounds that result from breakdown of glycogen to lactic acid without oxygen utilization. Athletes such as sprinters who require relatively infrequent short bursts of high-intensity activity acquire this capacity and often do not improve their overall cardiovascular function. Training aimed at developing anaerobic capacity should consist of maximal work periods of short duration (10 to 60 sec). This type of training requires much motivation because it is difficult and painful.

Aerobic performance depends on an increase in the oxygen transport system, which is developed principally through adaptations in the cardiovascular system and the skeletal muscles. Large muscle masses are active, so the greatest demand for oxygen is made. Physical activity ranging from work periods of a few seconds repeated quickly to hours of continuous work may induce an improvement in aerobic performance. The following patterns are effective:

1. Dash exercise training—maximal effort (i.e., running full-speed, preferably uphill) for 30 to 60 sec and repeated 5 to 10 times with several minutes of low-level activity between each dash. This pattern also improves anaerobic performance.
2. Interval exercise training—slightly less effort than maximal (80% of dash effort), lasting three to seven minutes, repeated three to seven times with low-level activity periods of six to eight minutes between each interval.
3. Continuous exercise training—submaximal effort for 45 to 75 minutes. Heart rates should range from 130 to 170 beats/min with maximal rates achieved at certain times.

These exercise training patterns are applicable to walking, running, bicycling, swimming, or isotonic arm exercises. Isometric exercises such as weight lifting are not aerobic, and they can be dangerous for heart disease patients with dilated ventricles because of the excessive level of myocardial pressure work associated with them.

The exercise prescription for cardiovascular changes and fitness must consider the frequency, duration, and intensity of aerobic exercise. Three times a week for at least 30 minutes is recommended. Less exercise may be suitable for maintenance, and more exercise is associated with an increased incidence of injuries. For cardiac patients, a warm-up and a cool-down are important.

Starting slowly can usually be substituted for the stretching "ritual" in normal subjects. Intensity should be at 60% to 80% of maximal oxygen uptake. This level is most easily monitored by heart rate, which is linearly related to oxygen consumption. The Karvonen technique for determining training heart rate most closely approximates the appropriate exercise intensity. It is calculated by subtracting basal heart rate from maximal, multiplying by 75%, and adding the product to the basal value. Perceived exertion levels of 13 to 14 seem to approximate an exercise intensity for achieving a training effect (see Chapter 1). For cardiac patients on beta blockers or with symptoms or signs that are maximal endpoints, an exercise effect can be achieved by subtracting 5 to 10 beats from the heart rate at the endpoint (i.e., at angina) or using the Borg perceived exertion scale.

There are only a few reported studies that have evaluated the hemodynamic consequences of exercise training using arterial and venous catheterization during exercise testing, the Douglas bag technique for collection of expired air, accurate oxygen measurement, and the Fick or dye dilution technique for estimation of cardiac output. Cardiac catheterization is necessary for accurate pressure measurement and determination of cardiac output. Central aortic pressure is necessary for obtaining hemodynamic measurements to estimate myocardial oxygen consumption, but most studies have been performed with brachial artery catheters. The Fick technique is the standard of reference for determining cardiac output, but it requires right heart catheterization for sampling of mixed venous blood. The dye dilution technique is not as accurate as the Fick method, but it does not require blood gas analysis or right heart catheterization.

Radionuclide techniques are not as accurate as either of these techniques. Currently, paramagnetic oxygen measurement techniques are very accurate, though the older chemical methods (Haldane, Scholander) are still the standards of reference. Direct gas flowmeter measurement of airflow during exercise is not accurate enough to replace the Douglas bag technique. The validity of hemodynamic measurements during exercise with catheters has been established. Even if the cardiac output, maximal oxygen intake, and heart rate are reduced in the catheterized exercising subject, the effect is consistent, and influences results similarly after as well as before the exercise program.

Studies of Normal Subjects.   The Dallas study included five male subjects aged 19 to 21. Three were sedentary and two were active. The former had maximal oxygen uptakes of 33 to 45 ml/kg/min prior to training, and the latter 61 and 47 ml/kg/min. The training program lasted for 55 days with workouts held twice each weekday and once on Saturday. The workouts consisted principally of running and were either interval-patterned, with periods of maximal effort for two to five minutes repeated 4 to 10 times with two-minute periods of rest, or continuous training, with running at a constant pace until exhaustion for longer than 10 minutes. Before and after training, hemodynamic measurements were determined at rest and during exercise with catheters in a peripheral arm vein and in the brachial artery. Both treadmill and supine bicycle ergometer testing were performed with maximal oxygen uptake measured. The previously sedentary trainees had the greatest measured changes.

The Stockholm study included eight sedentary male subjects aged 19 to 27. Maximal oxygen uptakes prior to training ranged from 36 to 50 ml/kg/min. The training program lasted for 120 days and consisted of cross-country running three times a week in dash, interval, and continuous patterning. Before and after training, hemodynamics were measured. Testing was done with the subject sitting on a bicycle ergometer and exerting maximal effort at work loads calculated to 25%, 50%, and 75% of the maximal oxygen uptake measured prior to training.

Tabkin and colleagues at the University of Vermont studied nine members of the university cross-country team before and after three months of daily training in preparation for competition. Training consisted of daily warm-up exercises, sprints, and five miles of running. The radial artery and a peripheral vein were catheterized. Measurements were made at rest and while walking on a treadmill at three miles per hour on the level and at 4%, 8%, 12%, and 14% elevation. No changes were noted other than a lowering of the cardiac output at the two lowest levels of exercise. The fact that the subjects were well-trained athletes explained this lack of significant change.

Frick and colleagues studied 14 men aged 19 to 26 before and after "hard" basic military training. The exact nature of this training was not described. Oxygen consumption was not measured, and cardiac output was estimated with Evans blue by a dye dilution technique using earlobe density changes. Physical work capacity was significantly increased after training. Hemodynamic measurements were made via a brachial artery catheter during supine bicycle exercise at 400 kpm/min for six minutes.

The Stockholm-Gothenburg Study was designed to evaluate the effects of an exercise program on middle-aged men. Sixty-eight employees of an insurance company who considered themselves healthy but who were judged to be inactive by their response to a questionnaire were asked to participate in a 10-week physical training program. The program consisted of two miles of intermittent or continuous running two to three times a week for a total time of about 18 hours and 55 miles of running. Twenty percent of the subjects dropped out for medical or other reasons. Of those who completed the program, half had significant orthopedic problems. Forty-two of the group had noninvasive studies performed, and 15 had venous and arterial catheterization. Maximal effort and multiple predetermined levels of submaximal exercise were performed sitting on a bicycle ergometer.

Hanson and colleagues studied the hemodynamic response of 25 normal men aged 40 to 49. Ten of these men could not perform a three-minute walk at three miles per hour and 14% elevation, and had a similar response to the treadmill test. They exhibited high resting oxygen consumption and stroke volume, then raised cardiac output excessively with level walking and maintained it throughout higher work loads. They demonstrated an initial overshoot and subsequent poor adaptation to exercise. The investigators assumed this response was due to prolonged physical inactivity. Seven of the 10 men completed three hourly sessions a week of competitive paddleball for 29 weeks. Catheterization was repeated and hemodynamic measurements made while walking on a treadmill at 3 mph level and at elevations of 4, 8, 12, and 14 degrees. Maximal work capacity and maximal oxygen consumption were increased following training.

Rerych and colleagues studied 18 athletes before and after six months of training for competitive swimming. They were studied during erect bicycle exercise using the first-pass technique and a multicrystal camera. Total blood volume increased after training, as did end-diastolic volume. Cardiac output at maximal exercise increased because of an increased diastolic volume with the same heart rate and ejection fraction. The reliability of this technique is questionable, particularly since one athlete reached a maximal cardiac output of 56.6 L/min. It appears, however, that exercise training in this group of healthy young college athletes resulted in no change in cardiac function but did induce an increase in left ventricular end-diastolic volume.

Studies of Coronary Heart Disease Patients.   Varnauskas and colleagues at the University of Gothenburg studied the hemodynamics of five patients with coronary heart disease before physical conditioning, after one month, and then after six months of physical conditioning. Coronary heart disease was diagnosed by clinical evaluation and coronary angiograms. The patients were exercised on a bicycle ergometer for 30 minutes three times a week, with the work load gradually increased according to individual tolerance and heart rate response. Measurements were made via catheters in the brachial artery and subclavian vein with the trainees sitting on a bicycle at rest and at 5 and 25 minutes while pedaling against an individualized work load. The dye dilution technique was used to estimate cardiac output and AV O_2 difference was calculated from the oxygen consumption and cardiac output. Plasma volume measured with ^{131}I-tagged albumin, total blood volume, and red cell mass calculated from the hematocrit all increased with training. The hemodynamic changes were more significant after six months of training than after one month. Cardiac output decreased at the submaximal level, and the AV O_2 difference increased. This favors a peripheral circulatory mechanism rather than a direct cardiac mechanism as the explanation for the increased work capacity in persons with coronary heart disease after training. However, Hanson and others have demonstrated this overshoot phenomenon in deconditioned persons. The exaggerated cardiac output and narrowed AV O_2 difference are returned to normal by an exercise program, just as they are in persons with vasoregulatory asthenia.

Frick and Katila studied six men aged 37 to 55 before and after an exercise program that began two to four months after a documented myocardial infarction. The exercise program consisted of pedaling a bicycle ergometer three times a week at progressive work loads. Each session consisted of 15 minutes of exercise at a heart rate of 100 bpm and then for 15 minutes at a heart rate of 150 bpm or until chest pain. Hemodynamic measurements were made while pedaling a bicycle ergometer in the supine position for six minutes at one or two individualized submaximal work loads. The resting mean heart volume did not change for the group, but two trainees with enlarged hearts had significant decreases in heart volume. Most of the subjects had abnormal hemodynamic measurements in response to acute exercise before and after the training program. This agrees with the criteria of Donald and Reeves for cardiac output and pulmonary wedge pressure response to supine exercise. All subjects increased their exercise capacity, and those with angina increased their angina-free work capacity.

Clausen and Trap-Jensen reported the effects of physical conditioning on hemodynamic measurements including hepatic and muscle blood flow during exercise in nine men with coronary heart disease. The men were aged 36 to 57 and had either a myocardial infarction or angina. The aim of the study was to determine the role of peripheral circulatory changes. The authors had demonstrated that in normal subjects, abdominal viscera perfusion was less reduced during exercise in trained subjects compared to untrained subjects and that muscle blood flow was reduced during exercise after training. The exercise program consisted of pedaling a bicycle ergometer in an intermittent pattern for 30 minutes, five days a week for 4 to 10 weeks. The work load was individualized, but progressively increased. For testing, catheters were placed in the brachial artery, superior vena cava, and right hepatic vein. Testing was performed sitting on a bicycle ergometer pedaling at work loads initially at 60% of and then equal to the pretraining maximal work load. Hepatic blood flow was estimated using indocyanine green and blood gas analysis, cardiac output was estimated using ^{131}I-tagged iodohippuric acid, and the blood flow in the vastus lateralis muscle was measured using the Xe133 local clearance technique. The cardiac output at the lowest exercise level clearly demonstrated the overshoot phenomenon, and this hyperkinetic response was normalized after training. At the higher submaximal exercise level, there was no change in cardiac output. Muscle blood flow was reduced at submaximal loads, and hepatic blood flow was less reduced during submaximal exercise after the training program.

Detry and colleagues collaborated on a study of patients from the University of Washington, Seattle, and the University of Louvain, Belgium. Six men with angina pectoris and six men with healed MI underwent right heart catheterization and brachial artery cannulation before and after three months of exercise. Their ages ranged from 34 to 68 years, with a mean of 48 years. The exercise program consisted of 45-minute sessions three times a week utilizing various submaximal exercises including walking and running. Maximal exercise was done on a bicycle ergometer or treadmill prior to the hemodynamic studies. Hemodynamic measurements were made while sitting on a bicycle ergometer at rest and during seven-minute exercise periods with work loads equal to 45% and then 75% of the pretraining maximal oxygen consumption. Surprisingly, arterial oxygen content was higher after training, indicating the possibility that improved oxygenation rather than improvements in the peripheral circulation made possible the increased AV O_2 difference. All of the trainees subjectively improved, and two previously limited by symptoms of angina pectoris were no longer symptomatic at any exercise level. These results favor the hypothesis of a peripheral mechanism for improved work tolerance of persons with coronary heart disease.

Bruce and colleagues performed invasive hemodynamic studies in coronary patients who had been in a long-term exercise program. Although all patients had improvement in exercise capacity and were able to perform at an exercise level satisfactory to themselves, some of the patients exhibited deterioration of cardiac function.

Ferguson and colleagues studied the effects of six months of bicycle ergometry training on coronary sinus blood flow and left ventricular oxygen consumption in 10 patients with exertional angina pectoris. After training, the patients increased physical work capacity by 18% at the same submaximal heart rate of approximately 114 beats/min. Coronary blood flow, myocardial oxygen consumption, and the rate-pressure product were not significantly different despite this increase in work load. Symptom-limited maximal exercise capacity increased 43% with training. The increase in exercise capacity in patients with angina pectoris did not depend on an augmented myocardial oxygen delivery but was related to a reduction in coronary flow requirement for a work load.

Sim and Neill studied eight patients with exertional angina pectoris before and after a four-month exercise program. The double product for angina was determined for upright bicycle exercise and for atrial pacing. This rate-pressure product at the exercise angina threshold was higher after conditioning, suggesting that conditioning increased the maximal myocardial oxygen supply during exercise. However, when the angina was induced by atrial pacing, heart rate, arterial blood pressure, coronary blood flow, myocardial oxygen consumption and the angina threshold were the same before and after conditioning. Myocardial lactate extraction was still abnormal during pacing, and there were no changes in coronary obstruction or collaterals as judged by coronary angiograms. The increase in anginal threshold during exercise appears to be due to functional adaptation either in myocardial oxygen supply or in the relation between hemodynamic work and myocardial oxygen consumption. The adaptation was limited to exercise and did not occur during atrial pacing. The effects of conditioning appear to be due to functional adaptation in either delivery or utilization of oxygen in the myocardium rather than to a static alteration in the coronary circulation. This study demonstrated an increase in the maximal rate-pressure product at the anginal threshold during exercise after training, but there was no change after atrial pacing. Hemodynamics at rest, left ventricular volume, and ejection fraction remained unchanged as did the coronary angiogram. These findings constitute a strong argument against a training effect on maximal coronary flow, but it is possible that coronary flow during exercise did increase. An alternate explanation is that changes affecting determinants of myocardial oxygen demand occurred that are not accounted for by the rate-pressure product (e.g., catecholamine levels, less prominent increase in contractile state during exercise) and that can explain the increased capacity after the exercise program.

Lee and colleagues studied the hemodynamic effects of physical training on coronary heart disease patients with impaired ventricular function. Eighteen coronary heart disease patients with an ejection fraction of 40% or less were entered into an exercise training program. Maximal symptom-limited exercise testing and cardiac catheterization were performed initially and at 12 to 14 months after exercise training. Exercise capacity improved, and resting and submaximal heart rates were significantly lowered; however, there was no significant change in pulmonary artery or left ventricular end-diastolic pressure, cardiac index, stroke index, left ventricular end-diastolic volume, or ejection fraction. An increase in work capacity was not correlated with improvement in ventricular function, and exercise training did not cause deterioration of ventricular function. They concluded that exercise training can be beneficial even for patients with impaired ventricular function.

Carter and Amundsen compared infarct size estimated from serum creatine kinase elevations with the functional exercise capacity for 22 myocardial infarction patients. The patients were studied 2.5 to 4.5 months after acute myocardial infarction. Eleven of the 22 entered an exercise program for four months and were subsequently retested on a bicycle. Prior to this exercise training, a significant correlation was demonstrated between aerobic capacity and estimated infarct size (r = −.68), but the correlation was higher (r = −.84) after training. Infarct size was not a predictor of the capacity of a patient to obtain a training effect. These results suggest that more accurate comparisons of training responses may be made when both infarct size and the time after infarction are considered.

DeBusk and colleagues studied the cardiovascular effects of exercise training very early after a clinically uncomplicated myocardial infarction. At 3 to 11 weeks after infarction, 28 men underwent gymnasium training, 12 trained at home, and 30 were followed as controls. Patients with ventricular gallops and other evidence of heart failure were avoided, and they were highly selected. Patients were "randomized" to the training programs only after stratification. If they had ST-segment depression or angina pectoris, they were only assigned to gymnasium training or to no training. By the 11th week, functional capacity increased significantly in all three groups: gymnasium training 66%, home training 41%, and controls 34%. Aerobic capacity at 11 weeks was 11 METs, 10.3 METs, and 9.4 METs, respectively, in the three groups. Exercise capacity increased more in the gymnasium-trained group than in the no-training group, but this difference was significant only in patients without exercise-induced ST-segment depression or angina. All three groups lowered their heart rate response to submaximal work. These authors concluded that (1) symptom-limited treadmill testing is safe and provides useful guidelines for cardiac rehabilitation, (2) patients who demonstrate nonischemic responses to treadmill testing soon after infarction may safely undergo unsupervised exercise training at home, and (3) supervised training may not be required to restore exercise capacity to near-normal values soon after a myocardial infarction in selected patients. This study may be the "way of the future," since exercise has traditionally commenced no sooner than six to eight weeks after MI. Sample size and careful patient selection, however, make it difficult to form convincing conclusions. Also, the control subjects did a considerable amount of walking on their own.

Nolewajka and colleagues studied 20 male patients three to six months post MI. One-half of the patients were randomly assigned to an exercise program.

The exercise program was maintained five days a week at 60% to 70% of maximal heart rate obtained during a bicycle test. They were considered to have a training effect if their heart rate dropped at least 10 bpm at an oxygen consumption of 1.2 L/min. Both groups underwent coronary angiography, invasive resting left ventricular function studies and intracoronary artery injection of radionuclide microspheres before and after a seven-month period. No differences were found to suggest an improvement in disease progression, resting myocardial perfusion or function, or myocardial collateralization.

Paterson and colleagues studied 79 patients under 54 years of age 3 to 12 months post MI, with CO_2 rebreathing during submaximal bicycle exercise both before and after 6 and 12 months of exercise training. Thirty-seven were randomized to a low-intensity activity as controls. Over the year of training, only predicted maximal oxygen consumption of the high-intensity training group increased. At six months, their heart rates were significantly reduced at each work load, with a widened AV O_2 difference, but there was no change in stroke volume. By the end of the year, their stroke volume had increased by 10%. These observations suggest that only peripheral changes occur in such patients after six months of high-intensity training, while longer periods can result in an increase in myocardial contractility.

Discussion.   Consistent hemodynamic results of a regular exercise program include a resting bradycardia, a decrease in heart rate and systolic blood pressure at any matched submaximal work load, an increase in maximal oxygen consumption and maximal cardiac output, and a more rapid return toward normal in recovery. It is somewhat controversial whether exercise can lower maximal heart rate. It appears that younger individuals who develop cardiomegaly with an increase in left ventricular end-diastolic volume and in mass may well lower their maximal heart rate, but this is not a consistent finding.

From the submaximal testing results, it is apparent that peripheral adaptations during acute exercise secondary to an exercise program are important. Lactic acid concentration during submaximal exercise decreases in spite of an unchanged or decreased cardiac output. Adaptations in the peripheral circulation were demonstrated by a decrease in active skeletal muscle blood flow and by a smaller decrease in liver blood flow. These changes in perfusion and aerobic metabolism are partially explained by morphologic and enzymatic adaptations in skeletal muscle.

The peripheral response to training is important for another reason. Clausen and Trap-Jensen have demonstrated that the training bradycardia is operative only when using trained skeletal muscles. They trained two groups of men using similar bicycle ergometer protocols; one group used their arms, the other used their legs. When tested with alternating arm and leg exercises after training, the trainees demonstrated a lower heart rate during exercise only when using the trained limbs. These investigators also trained individuals with fixed-rate ventricular pacemakers. These subjects responded to training with an increased work capacity in spite of a fixed ventricular rate. The atrial rate decreased after training in response to a similar submaximal work load.

Frick has demonstrated that individuals with congenital bradycardia respond to training by increasing stroke volume. These findings suggest that an exercise program induces a neural signal or a vascular response in the periphery that modifies the chronotropic and inotropic control of the heart during acute exercise.

The AV O_2 difference was either increased or unchanged in normal subjects during submaximal exercise after training. In coronary heart disease patients, Detry and Varnauskas demonstrated an increase in the AV O_2 difference whereas Frick found no change. Clausen did not measure AV O_2, but his data suggest that there was no change. Some investigators have suggested that the increase in AV O_2 difference supports the concept that peripheral changes rather than changes in cardiac function are of primary importance for the increased work capacity of trained coronary heart disease patients. It is conceivable that some hearts are so badly damaged that they cannot be modified by training. In such cases, peripheral circulatory changes and enzymatic and morphologic changes in skeletal muscle would be of primary importance. However, Frick and Paterson demonstrated improvement in cardiac function in coronary heart disease patients after an exercise program. Frick's data include changes in left ventricular stroke work versus pulmonary capillary wedge pressure during submaximal exercise (Sarnoff function curves), as well as increases in cardiac output for a given oxygen consumption in response to supine exercise. Thus, there appears to be evidence that an exercise program can improve ventricular function in selected patients with coronary heart disease.

In normal subjects, the cardiovascular response to acute exercise involves the integrated effects on the myocardium of tachycardia, sympathetic stimulation, and the Frank-Starling mechanism. The effects of an exercise program on these responses, as well as on the morphology of the heart, require delineation in humans. Along with exercise-induced ventricular hypertrophy, an increase in sympathetic tone could also explain an increase in contractility with training. Evidence for an increase in contractility secondary to an exercise program in humans is limited; however, the mean rate of systolic ejection increases, as does the dp/dt in the brachial artery, and in some cases, also the ejection fraction. Venous return could be facilitated by an exercise program, the end-diastolic volume for a given work load increased, and thus ventricular function improved.

Cardiac output was unchanged at identical submaximal work loads by an exercise program in normal subjects, except in the study by Hanson. However, this group of older normal individuals demonstrated a cardiac output overshoot phenomenon that was hypothesized to be secondary to prolonged physical inactivity. Approximately half of the coronary heart disease trainees had a similar overshoot phenomenon and lowered their cardiac output response to submaximal exercise, while the others did not. The correction of the exaggerated cardiac output and narrowed AV O_2 difference by an exercise program was similar to its effects on the abnormal hemodynamics of vasoregulatory asthenia. The lowering of cardiac output and widening of the AV O_2 difference in response to submaximal exercise are not the major effects of an exercise program, since this does not occur in all individuals who experience an increase in work capacity.

Measurement of myocardial oxygen consumption is technically difficult at rest, and there are many problems with its measurement during exercise. However, estimations can be made by blood pressure, heart rate, and ejection time. Blood pressure and ejection time can be lessened to some extent by an exercise program, but the major change is a lowering of heart rate. Because of lowered heart rate, hemodynamic values approximating changes in myocardial oxygen consumption will decrease after training. However, there is evidence that cardiac function improves with training, even in coronary heart disease patients. An increase in the contractile state of the myocardium or an increase in end-diastolic volume (Frank-Starling mechanism) would increase myocardial oxygen consumption and invalidate approximations using hemodynamic calculations. Myocardial work is a determinant of myocardial oxygen consumption; however, it is not sufficient to estimate this value alone. For instance, although calculated work might increase or not change if stroke volume increased and blood pressure decreased, myocardial oxygen consumption would decrease. This effect is due to myocardial flow work requiring less oxygen than does pressure work. However, even if myocardial oxygen consumption is not decreased by an exercise program, the training bradycardia is an important physiologic benefit. The concomitant increase in diastolic time increases the time available for myocardial perfusion. Myocardial changes brought about by an exercise program most likely are subtle and will only be apparent during a stress such as exercise.

ECHOCARDIOGRAPHIC STUDIES OF THE EFFECTS OF AN EXERCISE PROGRAM

The echocardiogram is an ultrasonic device that can be used to evaluate the effects of an exercise program on the heart since it noninvasively measures chamber size, wall thickness, and function. Echocardiographic studies have demonstrated morphologic and functional cardiac changes secondary to aerobic exercise training. These changes appear beneficial, so most of the studies appear to support the exercise hypothesis. Some of the cross-sectional and longitudinal studies of exercise training using echocardiography are summarized here.

Cross-Sectional Studies Comparing Echocardiographic Measurements of Normals and of Athletes (Table 9–2). Gilbert and colleagues at Emory University compared M-mode echocardiographic measurements of 20 endurance runners with 26 young sedentary subjects. A modest degree of right and left ventricular chamber enlargement and left ventricular hypertrophy was observed in endurance runners. There were no significant differences, unless differences in body size were accounted for with the use of indices based on body surface area. There was no significant difference in

TABLE 9–2.
Cross-Sectional Echocardiographic Studies Comparing
Athletes to Controls

Emory University Echocardiographic Study

	CONTROLS	ATHLETES
LVPWT	9.8	10.9
LVVIED	62	72
VO$_2$	43	71
EF	72%	68%
Resting HR	62	51

University of Missouri Echocardiographic Study

	CONTROLS	ATHLETES
LVPWT	9	11
LVEDD	52	57
LVESD	37	34
VO$_2$	47	74
EF	64%	78%
Resting HR	61	50
MVCFS	0.9	1.2

National Institutes of Health Echocardiographic Study

	AEROBIC ATHLETES	ISOMETRIC ATHLETES	NORMALS
LVPWT	11	13.7	10
Septum	10.8	13	10.3
LVEDD	55	48	46

University of California, San Diego, Echocardiographic Study

	CONTROLS	ATHLETES
RVEDD	13	21
Septum	13	14
LVPWT	10	11
LVEDD	50	54
LVESD	31	32
EF	76%	79%
MVCFS	1.13	1.18

LVPWT = left ventricular posterior wall thickness; LVVIED = left ventricular volume index at end diastole in ml; VO$_2$ = maximal oxygen consumption; EF = ejection fraction; HR = heart rate; LVESD = left ventricular end-systolic dimension; MVCFS = mean ventricular circumferential fiber shortening; LV or RVEDD = ventricular end-diastolic dimension. All dimensions are in millimeters, HR in beats/minute, oxygen consumption in ml O$_2$/kg/min, and MVCFS in circ/sec.

resting measurements of ventricular performance. This study suggests that isotonic leg training results in adaptive changes in ventricular volume and mass, slower heart rates that may be associated with more efficient function (increased stroke volume), and insignificant alterations in resting ejection phase indices of left ventricular function.

Parker and colleagues at the University of Missouri compared 12 long-distance runners with 12 normal control subjects using multiple noninvasive techniques. The athletes showed a higher prevalence of third and fourth heart sounds and ECG abnormalities consistent with right and left ventricular hypertrophy. Echocardiographic examination of the athletes revealed an increase in wall thickness, left ventricular muscle mass, diastolic volume, and ventricular function.

Morganroth and colleagues at the National Institutes of Health studied 56 athletes 18 to 24 years of age with M-mode echocardiography. Mean left ventricular end-diastolic volume and mass increased in aerobic athletes (runners, swimmers) while isometric athletes (wrestlers) had increased wall thickness and mass. The former had changes suggestive of chronic volume overload and the latter had changes similar to those of chronic pressure overload.

Roeske and colleagues at the University of California, San Diego, studied 10 professional basketball players and 10 matched subjects. Right and left ventricular enlargement were often present in aerobically trained athletes, but left ventricular performance was normal at rest.

Cohen and Segal measured left ventricular dimensions by M-mode echocardiography in 10 distance runners and 10 wrestlers, and compared them to 10 sedentary controls at rest and during graded semisupine bicycle exercise. At rest, runners and wrestlers demonstrated greater left ventricular mass compared to controls. In wrestlers, this was due to increased left ventricular septal (14 mm) and posterior wall thickness (13 mm) compared to controls (9 and 10 mm, respectively). In runners, this was due to increased left ventricular end-diastolic dimension (56 mm) compared to controls (50 mm). During exercise, the different patterns noted at rest among the three groups in left ventricular dimensions and function persisted; runners maintained a higher end-diastolic dimension compared to wrestlers and controls and greater shortening dimension compared to wrestlers. Absolute changes in left ventricular parameters from rest to exercise were not significantly different among the three groups. It appears that (1) different patterns of left ventricular hypertrophy exist among different types of athletes, and (2) these differences observed at rest persisted during exercise and have direct functional significance, thereby emphasizing the differences found in cardiac dimensions among different types of athletes.

Structural Features of the Athlete Heart.   As reviewed by Maron, the morphologic concepts of the "athlete heart" have been enhanced and clarified over the last 10 years by M-mode echocardiographic studies performed on more than 1,000 competitive athletes. Long-term athletic training produces relatively mild but predictable alterations in cardiac structure that result in an increase in left ventricular mass. This increase in mass observed in athletes is due to a mild increase in either transverse end-diastolic dimension of the left ventricle or left ventricular wall thickness, or both. Cardiac dimensions in athletes compared with matched controls show increases of about 10% for left ventricular end-diastolic dimension, about 15% to 20% for wall thickness, and about 45% for calculated left ventricular mass. There is evidence that the modest degree of "physiologic" left ventricular hypertrophy (both the cavity dilation and wall thickening) observed in athletes is dynamic and dependent upon age. It may develop rapidly within weeks or months after the initiation of a vigorous exercise program and may be reversed in a similar time period after the cessation of training. Several echocardiographic studies also suggest that the precise alterations in cardiac structure associated with training may differ depending on the type of athletic activity undertaken (that is, whether training is primarily dynamic or isometric).

Although the ventricular septal to free wall thickness ratio is almost always within normal limits (<1.3), occasionally an athlete will show mild asymmetric thickening of the anterior basal septum (usually 13 to 15 mm). This may mimic nonobstructive hypertrophic cardiomyopathy.

Echocardiography Before and After an Exercise Program
(Table 9–3). Ehsani and coworkers at Washington University reported rapid changes in left ventricular dimensions and mass in response to physical conditioning and deconditioning. Two groups of healthy young subjects were studied. The training group consisted of eight competitive swimmers who were studied serially for nine weeks. Mean left ventricular end-diastolic dimension increased by 4.3 mm in the first week. A total of 3.3 mm increase from the pretraining value was demonstrated by the ninth week of training. Mean left ventricular posterior wall thickness increased 0.7 mm by the end of the training period. There was no change in ejection fraction. The deconditioned group consisted of six competitive runners who stopped training for three weeks. Left ventricular end-diastolic dimension decreased 4.7 mm and posterior wall thickness decreased 2.7 mm by the end of the three-week period. Deconditioning did not influence ejection fraction. The authors concluded that exercise training-induced adaptive changes in left ventricular dimensions occur rapidly and mimic the pattern of chronic volume overload, and that modest degrees of exercise-induced left ventricular enlargement are reversible after cessation of training. Surprisingly, changes in left ventricular dimension occurred early during endurance training, but there was no significant increase in measured left ventricular posterior wall thickness until the fifth week of training. Estimated left ventricular mass significantly increased after the first week of training. The rapidity of this change makes one doubt its validity.

DeMaria and colleagues at the University of California, Davis, reported the results of M-mode echocardiography in 24 young normals before and after 11 weeks of endurance exercise training. Training consisted of a walk-run program at 70% maximal heart rate for one hour four days a week. The subjects were participating in a program of endurance physical conditioning as part of training for the Sacramento Police Academy. The group, 15 men and 11 women, ranged in age from 20 to 34 years (mean 26 years). After training, they exhibited an increased left ventricular end-diastolic dimension, a decreased end-systolic dimension, and both an increased stroke volume and shortening fraction. An increase in mean fiber shortening velocity was observed, as were increases in left ventricular wall thickness, electrocardiographic voltage, and left ventricular mass. The increase in left ventricular

TABLE 9–3.

Serial Echocardiographic Studies (Longitudinal or Prospective) Evaluating the Cardiac Effects of Exercise Training

WASHINGTON UNIVERSITY STUDY (COLLEGE ATHLETES)	EIGHT SWIMMERS TRAINED FOR NINE WKS		THREE RUNNERS DETRAINED FOR THREE WKS	
	BEFORE TRAINING	AFTER TRAINING	BEFORE DETRAINING	AFTER DETRAINING
LVEDD	48.7	52	51	46.3
LVPWT	9.4	10.1	10.7	8.0
VO$_2$	52	60	62	57
Resting HR	70	63	57	64
EF	63%	63%	68%	63%

UCD STUDY (POLICEMEN)	BEFORE TRAINING	AFTER TRAINING
LVEDD	48	50
LVESD	30	29
LVPWT	9.1	10.1
Resting HR	69	63
VO$_2$	36	41
EF	75%	80%
MVCFS	1.21	1.28

SUNY DOWNSTATE MEDICAL CENTER STUDY	BEFORE TRAINING		AFTER TRAINING	
	rest	300 kpm	rest	300 kpm
LVEDD	47	46	50	50
LVESD	32	21	32	30
EF	70%	90%	73%	78%

MONTREAL HEART INSTITUTE (NORMAL MEN ≃ 40 YRS OLD)	BEFORE TRAINING	AFTER TRAINING
VO$_2$	34	41
Septum	12.5	12.7
LVPWT	10	9.8
LVEDD	47.8	48.2
LVESD	33	33

SALT LAKE CITY STUDY (25 MEN EXERCISED THREE MONTHS, MEAN AGE 22 YRS)	BEFORE TRAINING	AFTER TRAINING
Resting HR	63	54
VO$_2$	49	56
% Body fat	17.2	13.7
R$_{V5}$	1.7 mV	2.0 mV
LVEDD	45.8	49.6
EF	62%	66%
LVPWT	10.9	10.3
LVESD	32.3	33.5

WASHINGTON UNIVERSITY REHAB STUDY (9 POST-MI PATIENTS, ONE YR OF EXERCISE)	BEFORE TRAINING	AFTER TRAINING
LVEDD	51	56
LVPWT	9	10
VO$_2$	26	35
R$_{V5}$	1.7 mV	2.0 mV

LVEDD = left ventricular end-diastolic dimension; LVPWT = left ventricular posterior wall thickness; VO$_2$ = maximal oxygen consumption; HR = heart rate; EF = ejection fraction; LVESD = left ventricular end-systolic dimension; MVCFS = mean ventricular circumferential fiber shortening; mV = millivolts. All dimensions are in millimeters, HR in beats/minute, oxygen consumption in ml of O$_2$/kg/min, and MVCFS in circ/sec.

shortening fraction and calculated stroke volume suggests enhanced cardiac performance. However, other parameters of hemodynamic functions including cardiac output, blood pressure, and peripheral vascular resistance at rest were not altered following conditioning. Hemodynamics in the posttraining period were characterized by a maintenance of the same cardiac output at a reduced heart rate and an increased stroke volume that was accomplished by an augmented left ventricular diastolic volume, shortening fraction, and contraction velocity. There was no change in peripheral resistance.

Stein and colleagues at the State University of New York Downstate Medical Center studied the effects of exercise training on ventricular dimensions at rest and during supine submaximal exercise. Fourteen healthy students were studied using M-mode echocardiography at rest and in the third minute of 300 kp of supine bike exercise. They were studied before and after a 14-week training program that resulted in a 30% increase in maximal oxygen consumption. Eleven nontrained students acted as controls and showed no changes. Ejection fraction was calculated by the cube technique. The authors concluded that exercise training is associated with an increased stroke volume mediated by the Frank-Starling effect and enhanced contractility.

Parrault and colleagues at the Montreal Heart Institute studied 14 subjects (40 ± 3 years of age) with a chest x-ray, electrocardiogram, vectorcardiogram, and echocardiogram before and after five months of training. Maximal oxygen consumption increased 20%. There was a slight increase in left precordial voltage, but no change in heart size from the chest x-ray. The echocardiograms showed no significant changes, in contrast to the studies in younger subjects. Wolfe and colleagues performed a similar study in 12 men with a mean age of 37 who exhibited 14% and 18% increases in aerobic capacity after three and six months of training, respectively. They concluded that resting end-diastolic volume and stroke volume were increased, but that left ventricular structure and resting contractile status are not altered by six months of jogging in healthy, previously sedentary men.

Frick and colleagues studied the effects of moderate physical training on heart volume using biplane chest x-rays, on blood volume by ^{133}-I-tagged human albumin, and on left ventricular wall thickness by ultrasound. Twenty normal men (19 to 20 years of age) participated in a moderate physical training program for two months. This training increased physical working capacity by 13% and maximal oxygen consumption by 6%. Heart and blood volumes remained essentially unchanged. There was no significant change in left ventricular wall thickness. A study by Thompson and colleagues in young men failed to find any changes in cardiac dimensions after 11 weeks of aerobic training.

The Salt Lake City research group noninvasively studied the effects of an aerobic training program on the hearts of healthy college age men (25 experimental subjects and 11 controls with a mean age of 22 years). Echocardiographic, electrocardiographic, and oxygen consumption measurements were obtained before and after a three-month exercise program. The exercise program consisted of 50 minutes of jogging five days a week at 85% of maximal heart rate. Compared with the control group, echocardiography after training showed an increase in left ventricular end-diastolic dimension, but no change in wall thickness or in ejection fraction. Electrocardiographic measurements revealed a decrease in resting heart rate and an increase in R-wave voltage in leads V5 and V6. Measured oxygen consumption increased by 16%. Although there was no change in myocardial wall thickness, the increase in end-diastolic dimension resulted in a calculated increase in left ventricular mass.

Landry et al. studied the sensitivity of the myocardium to endurance training. To evaluate variability in adaptation, 20 sedentary subjects and 10 pairs of monozygotic twins were submitted to a 20-week endurance exercise program. Maximal oxygen uptake increased significantly in both groups: 30% in the sedentary group and 13% in the monozygotic twins. Statistically significant increases in left ventricular diameter, posterior wall and septal thicknesses, as well as left ventricular end-diastolic volume and left ventricular mass were observed in the sedentary subjects, but not in the monozygotic twins. After training, twin pairs differed more from each other than at the start. Concomitantly, within-pair resemblance was greater after training than before. Results indicate that cardiac dimensions are amenable to significant modifications under controlled endurance training conditions and that the extent and variability of the response of cardiac structures to training are perhaps genotype dependent.

Studies in Patients With CHD.   Ehsani and colleagues reported their results after 12 months of intense aerobic exercise training in a highly selected group of 10 patients with coronary heart disease. The patients, ranging in age from 44 to 63 years, were the first to complete 12 months in a high-level exercise program. Nine had sustained a single myocardial infarction, and one had severe three-vessel coronary artery disease. All 10 had asymptomatic exercise-induced ST-segment depression. Eight similar men were considered as controls. After three months of exercise training at a level of 50% to 70% of maximal oxygen consumption, the level of training increased to 70% to 80%, with two to three intervals at 80% to 90% interspersed throughout the exercise session. Patients exercised three times a week during the first three months and four to five times a week for the next nine months. The duration was initially 30 minutes and later increased to 60 minutes.

Since none of these men developed symptoms during exercise testing, a true maximal oxygen consumption could be measured. The maximal amount of reported ST-segment depression was .30 mV, but most had .20 mV of depression which was less at repeat testing one year later in spite of a higher double product, greater treadmill work load, and a 38% increase in maximal oxygen consumption. In addition, 0.1 mV of ST-segment depression occurred at a higher double product after the year of training. A weight loss from a mean of 79 kg to 74 kg occurred. The sum of SV1 and RV5 increased by 15%. Both left ventricular end-diastolic dimension and posterior wall thickness were significantly increased after training. This resulted in an increase in left ventricular mass from 93 to 135 gm/m squared BSA.

It is questionable that these results can be generalized. These 10 men are a highly select group, all with asymptomatic ST-segment depression and able to exercise at levels often difficult for younger men. If applied to most patients with coronary disease, this intensity certainly could lead to a high incidence of orthopedic and cardiac complications. Cardiac patients with exercise-induced ST depression who exceed standard exercise prescriptions are at increased risk of cardiac events.

Ditchey et al. obtained echocardiograms on 14 coronary patients before and after an average of seven months (range 3 to 14 months) of supervised arm and leg exercise. Each echocardiogram was interpreted jointly by two blinded observers, using three different measurement conventions and a semiautomated method of analysis to minimize errors of interpretation. Exercise training led to subjective improvement in all 14 patients and to an objective increase in exercise capacity in 13 of 14 patients, as evidenced by an increase in maximal oxygen consumption estimated from symptom-limited treadmill testing (9 and 11 METs before and after training, respectively, P < .01). However, this functional improvement was not accompanied by any significant change in left ventricular end-diastolic diameter, posterior wall thickness, or interventricular septal thickness. Likewise, left ventricular cross-sectional area (CSA), an index of left ventricular mass that corrects for altered ventricular volume and theoretically reflects directional changes in mass despite nonuniform wall thickness, did not change significantly after training by any measurement convention. The left ventricular cross-sectional area was 18.0 ± 6.5 and 17.6 ± 6.5 cm^2 before and after training, respectively, determined by American Society of Echocardiography measurement standards. These data suggest that improved exercise capacity after exercise training in patients with ischemic heart disease is not due to exercise-induced left ventricular hypertrophy.

Discussion. Despite technical and theoretic limitations related to transducer angulation, beam-width distortion, and endocardial surface recognition, echocardiographic measurements of left ventricular posterior wall thickness and internal dimensions closely correspond to similar measurements determined by left ventriculography. Several echocardiographic methods of estimating left ventricular mass have been demonstrated to accurately reflect true anatomic mass. The usefulness of left ventricular cross-sectional area in evaluating myocardial mass has been previously reported. Since this index is relatively independent of changes in ventricular volume, cross-sectional area is a more reliable means of assessing serial changes in left ventricular mass than is either interventricular septal or posterior wall thickness alone. Furthermore, while echocardiography estimates of absolute left ventricular mass would be of questionable accuracy in the presence of nonuniform wall thickness, directional changes in cross-sectional area remain theoretically valid indices of changes in actual mass if measurements are derived from an area that includes at least some viable myocardium and if myocardial hypertrophy is uniform in distribution. For example, in a patient with septal scarring due to prior infarction, any change in ventricular mass should be reflected in cross-sectional area by changes in posterior wall thickness (corrected for altered ventricular volume). Although such changes would not necessarily be quantitatively accurate (because any regional area of nonviable myocardium could potentially reduce the magnitude of change in cross-sectional area disproportionately, when compared with its influence on change in ventricular mass as a whole), directional changes in both cross-sectional area and total mass would remain concordant.

The subjective nature of echocardiographic interpretation presents a further problem in terms of quantitative analysis. Special precautions are necessary to minimize subjective errors of interpretation and to ensure reproducibility. Foremost among these precautions is the elimination of echocardiograms on which chamber dimensions and wall thickness are not clearly defined. Although echocardiograms performed in nearly all of the coronary patients reported by Ditchey who entered our cardiac rehabilitation program were considered adequate for clinical purposes, less than half had both pretraining and posttraining studies of sufficient quality to justify more detailed analysis. Although this yield is lower than usually reported, a relatively strict approach was taken in an attempt to reduce interpretative errors. In addition, joint interpretation by two observers and a semiautomated analysis system were utilized both to limit the individual subjectivity inherent in echocardiographic interpretation and to ensure accuracy in calibration and arithmetic manipulation. Furthermore, potential bias due to the use of a single, arbitrary measurement convention was excluded by demonstrating concordance among results obtained by three widely recommended conventions. Even so, our individual estimates of cross-sectional area were not perfectly reproducible. However, there was a good overall correlation between repeated measurements and directional changes in mean values before and after training were the same. Furthermore, the same conclusions were supposed by both sets of measurements. Two-dimensional (2-D) echocardiography has theoretical advantages, particularly in patients with regional disease, but endo- and epicardial measurements are even more tenuous. Perhaps digital enhancement of echocardiographic images will improve this situation.

EXERCISE ELECTROCARDIOGRAM

Since abnormal ST-segment shifts in coronary patients are most likely secondary to ischemia, lessening of such shifts would be consistent with improved myocardial perfusion. For purposes of comparison, only similar myocardial oxygen demands can be considered. Therefore, it is necessary only to compare ST segments at matched exercise heart rate-systolic blood pressure products. The product of heart rate times systolic blood pressure is the best noninvasive estimate of myocardial oxygen demand during exercise. The following describes the studies of the effect of an exercise program on the exercise electrocardiogram, and they are summarized in Table 9–4.

Costill and colleagues entered 24 men who demonstrated ST-segment depression in lead CM5 during treadmill testing three months into an exercise program. A second group of men with coronary heart disease and ST depression were reexamined at the same interval but were not trained. A third group

TABLE 9–4.
Studies Performed With Exercise Electrocardiographic Analysis Before and After an Exercise Program

PRINCIPAL INVESTIGATOR	NUMBER TRAINED	NUMBER OF CONTROLS	LENGTH OF EXERCISE PROGRAM	ECG LEAD(S) MONITORED	DESCRIPTION OF SUBJECTS	EXERCISE ECG RESULTS
Costill	24	—	3 mos	CM_5	Three groups (see text)	No change in ST-segment response
Salzman	100	None	33 mos	C_4V, CH_6	MI, angina, and/or abnormal exercise ECG	ST-segment changes correlated to changes in functional capacity
Kattus	13	15	5 mos	CA_5	Asymptomatic with abnormal exercise ECG	Similar ST-segment improvement rate in control subjects
Detry	14	None	3 mos	CB_5	MI and/or angina	No change in computerized ST-segment measurements at matched DP
Raffo	12	12	6 mos	CM_5	Angina with abnormal exercise ECG	Higher heart rate for same amount of ST depression
Watanabe	14	None	6 mos	XYZ	Mixed coronary disease	Changes only in spatial analysis
Ehsani	10	8	12 mos	V_{4-6}	9 post-MI > 4 mos; 1 with 3-VD; all with asymptomatic ST depression	Less ST-segment depression at matched DP and at maximal exercise; higher DP at ischemic ST threshold (0.1 mV flat)
PERFEXT	48	59	12 mos	XYZ	See Chapter 11	No significant difference at matched DP

MI = myocardial infarction; DP = double product (SBP × HR); VD = vessel disease; ECG = electrocardiogram.

of men with low physical fitness and no ST-segment depression were trained at the same relative intensity as the trained group with coronary disease. After 12 weeks of training, maximal oxygen consumption was increased by approximately 25% in the trained groups. Training produced a lowering of heart rate for all submaximal exercise levels, permitting the men to perform more work before the onset of angina or ST-segment depression (which occurred at the same heart rate before and after training) or both. Training had no effect on the amount of exercise-induced ST-segment depression.

Salzman and colleagues analyzed the exercise ECGs of 100 coronary patients with a mean age of 48 years before and after an average of 33 months of cardiac rehabilitation. The exercise ECG improved in 31 subjects, did not change in 41, and deteriorated in 28. Improvement in the exercise ECG was more likely to occur in the group who showed improvement in physical fitness; deterioration was more likely in the group that showed a worsening of physical fitness. Improvement in the exercise electrocardiogram occurred in 80% of subjects with initial borderline or abnormal exercise ECGs and who had an improvement in physical fitness. Deterioration of the exercise ECG occurred in 70% of the patients with initially normal exercise ECG who had a worsening of physical fitness. They concluded that improvement of the exercise ECG was directly related to improved physiologic function, but these findings could be due to selection.

Kattus and colleagues identified 30 subjects with abnormal ST-segment depression in response to exercise testing and without anginal pain in a screening study. All 30 of the abnormal responders were invited to enter a supervised exercise program. Two refused further participation and 15 found it impossible to participate in the training program but agreed to return for a repeat treadmill test in the future. Thirteen of the abnormal responders participated in a supervised exercise program that led to an increased exercise capacity. Four of these 13 subjects (13%) had reversion of their ST-segment depression to normal. Among those abnormal responders who did not train, there was no improvement of exercise capacity, yet two of the 15 (13%) subjects normalized their electrocardiographic patterns.

Detry and Bruce measured symptom-limited maximal oxygen uptake and electrocardiographic response to treadmill testing before and after three months of exercise training in 14 patients with coronary heart disease. ST-segment responses were measured by computer averaging of 100 beats/sample of lead CB5, which was recorded on magnetic tape during the last two minutes of each exercise level. ST measurements were made 50 to 70 msec after the nadir of the S-wave. There was less ST-segment depression at submaximal exercise, along with the lower double product. However, at maximal exercise, both depression and double product were greater. The quantitative relationship of ST-segment depression to exercise heart rate, to the product of heart rate and systolic blood pressure (double product), or to rate pressure product (heart rate times mean blood pressure) was unaffected by the exercise program. Maximal oxygen consumption increased by 21%, and the product of heart rate and systolic blood pressure at symptom-limited maximal exercise increased by 10% in the angina patients. Apparently, the only electrocardiographic changes were due to changes in the heart rate and blood pressure response to exercise rather than due to improved coronary circulation.

Raffo and colleagues studied 24 patients with stable angina and exercise-induced ST depression who were randomized into two groups. The 12 patients in group one followed the Canadian Air Force exercise program and the 12 patients in group two were controls. Exercise testing on a bicycle ergometer was performed at entry and six months later. Heart rate at the same level of ST-segment depression in CM5 and the duration of the test increased in those in the exercise program while heart rate at submaximal work loads decreased.

The findings of Ehsani and colleagues regarding exercise-induced ST-segment depression are described along with their other findings in the echocardiographic section.

As part of PERFEXT, 48 patients who exercised and 59 control patients had computerized exercise ECGs performed initially and one year later. ST-segment displacement was analyzed 60 milliseconds after the end of the QRS complex in the three-dimensional X, Y, and Z leads and utilizing the spatial amplitude derived from them. There were no significant differences between the groups except for less ST-segment displacement at a matched work load, but this could be explained by a lowered heart rate. Analysis of variance yielded some minor differences within clinical subgroups, particularly in the spatial analysis. Obvious changes in exercise-induced ST-segment depression could not be demonstrated in our heterogeneous group of selected volunteers with coronary artery disease secondary to an exercise program.

CONCLUSION

Animal studies strongly support the benefits of regular exercise on the heart. Myocardial ischemia is a necessary stimulus for the development of collateral vessels, but exercise appears to enhance their development. Exercise does not affect the atherosclerotic process, but lesions are less of a threat to myocardium supplied by coronary arteries enlarged by exercise.

M-mode echocardiography has been utilized to evaluate cardiac adaptations to exercise training in both cross-sectional and longitudinal studies. Reported cardiac changes secondary to endurance training in young subjects have included increased ventricular mass, wall thickness, volume, and function. The echocardiographic studies have failed to yield consistent and conclusive results, probably because of the subjective nature of echocardiographic measurements. However, increases in left ventricular mass may not occur in younger subjects unless higher levels of exercise are used and may never occur in older subjects.

An exercise program cannot be said to lessen exercise-induced ischemia as assessed indirectly by ST-segment depression in most cardiac patients. If cardiac patients are pushed to higher levels of exercise than usually accomplished or tolerated by middle-aged individuals, perhaps more dramatic cardiac changes can be induced. However, patients with exercise-induced ST-segment depression who exceed their usually prescribed exercise limits are known to be at higher risk of cardiac events during and immediately after bouts of exercise.

BIBLIOGRAPHY

Adams TD, Yanowitz FG, Fischer AG, et al: Noninvasive evaluation of exercise training in college-age men. *Circulation* 1981;64:958.

Aldinger EE, Sohal RS: Effects of digitoxin on the ultrastructural myocardial changes in the rat subjected to chronic exercise. *Am J Cardiol* 1970;26:369.

Anholm JD, Foster C, Carpenter J, et al: Effect of habitual exercise on left ventricular response to exercise. *J Appl Physiol: Respirat Environ Exerc Physiol* 1982;52:1648–1651.

Banister EW, Tomanek RJ, Cvorkov N: Ultrastructural modifications in rat heart-responses to exercise and training. *Am J Physiol* 1971;220:1935.

Barnard RJ, Duncan HW, Baldwin KM, et al: Effects of intensive exercise training on myocardial performance and coronary blood flow. *J Appl Physiol* 1980;49:444–449.

Bershon MM, Scheuer J: Effect of ischemia on the performance of hearts from physically trained rats. *Am J Physiol* 1978;234:H215.

Billman GE, Schwartz PJ, Gagnol JP, et al: Cardiac response to submaximal exercise in dogs susceptible to sudden cardiac death. *J Appl Physiol* 1985;59:890–897.

Billman GE, Schwartz PJ, Stone HL: The effects of daily exercise on susceptibility to sudden cardiac death. *Circulation* 1984;69:1182–1189.

Bloor CM, Pasyk S, Leon AS: Interaction of age and exercise on organ and cellular development. *Am J Pathol* 1970;58:185.

Bloor CM, White FC, Sanders TM: Effects of exercise on collateral development in myocardial ischemia in pigs. *J Appl Physiol: Respirat Environ Exerc Physiol* 1984;56:656–665.

Bove AA: Effects of strenuous exercise on myocardial blood flow. *Med Sci Sports Exerc* 1985;17:517–521.

Bove AA, Dewey JD: Proximal coronary vasomotor reactivity after exercise training in dogs. *Circulation* 1985;71:620–625.

Bradley LM, Galioto FM, Vaccaro P, et al: Effect of intense aerobic training on exercise performance in children after surgical repair of tetralogy of fallot or complete transposition of the great arteries. *Am J Cardiol* 1985;56:816–818.

Bruce RW, Kusumi F, Frederick R: Differences in cardiac function with prolonged physical training for cardiac rehabilitation. *Am J Cardiol* 1977;40:597.

Burt JJ, Jackson R: The effects of physical exercise on the coronary collateral circulation of dogs. *J Sports Med Phys Fitness* 1965;4:203.

Carew TE, Covell JW: Left ventricular function in exercise-induced hypertrophy in dogs. *Am J Cardiol* 1978;42:82.

Clausen JP, Trap-Jensen J: Effects of training on the distribution of cardiac output in patients with coronary artery disease. *Circulation* 1970;42:611.

Colan SD, Sanders SP, MacPherson D, et al: Left ventricular diastolic function in elite athletes with physiologic cardiac hypertrophy. *J Am Coll Cardiol* 1985;6:545–549.

Convertino VA, Goldwater DJ, Sandler H: VO_2 kinetics of constant-load exercise following bed-rest-induced deconditioning. *J Appl Physiol: Respirat Environ Exerc Physiol* 1984;57:1545–1550.

Convertino VA, Keil LC, Greenleaf JE: Plasma volume, renin, and vasopressive responses to graded exercise after training. *J Appl Physiol* 1983;54:508–514.

Costill DL, Branam GE, Moore JC, et al: Effects of physical training in men with coronary heart disease. *Med Sci Sports* 1974;6:95.

Coyle EF, Hemmert MK, Coggan AR: Effects of detraining on cardiovascular responses to exercise: role of blood volume. *J Appl Physiol* 1986;60:95–99.

Crews J, Aldinger EE: Effect of chronic exercise on myocardial function. *Am Heart J* 1967;74:536.

Davies KJA, Packer L, Brooks GA: Biochemical adaptation of mitrochondria, muscle, and whole-animal respiration to endurance training. *Arch Biochem Biophys* 1981;209:539–554.

DeBusk RF, Houston H, Haskell W, et al: Exercise training soon after myocardial infarction. *Am J Cardiol* 1979;44:1223.

DeMaria AN, Neumann A, Lee G, et al: Alterations in ventricular mass and performance induced by exercise training in man evaluated by echocardiography. *Circulation* 1978;57:237–244.

Detry J, Bruce RA: Effects of physical training on exertional ST segment depression in coronary heart disease. *Circulation* 1971;44:390–397.

Detry JR, Rousseau M, Vandenbroucke W, et al: Increased arteriovenous oxygen difference after physical training in coronary heart disease. *Circulation* 1971;44:109.

Ditchey RV, Watkins J, McKirnan MD, et al: Effects of exercise training on left ventricular mass in patients with ischemic heart disease. *Am Heart J* 1981;101:701–706.

Dowell RT, Cutilletta AF, Rudnik MA, et al: Heart functional responses to pressure overload in exercised and sedentary rats. *Am J Cardiol* 1976;230:199.

Dowell RT, Stone HL, Sordahl LA, et al: Contractile function and myofibrillar ATPase activity in the exercise-trained dog heart. *J Appl Physiol* 1977;43:977.

Eckstein RW: Effect of exercise and coronary artery narrowing on coronary collateral circulation. *Circ Res* 1957;5:230.

Ehsani AA, Hagberg JM, Hickson RC: Rapid changes in left ventricular dimensions and mass in response to physical conditioning and deconditioning. *Am J Cardiol* 1978;42:52.

Ehsani AA, Heath GW, Hagberg JM, et al: Noninvasive assessment of changes in left ventricular function induced by graded isometric exercise in healthy subjects. *Chest* 1981;80:51.

Ehsani AA, Heath GW, Hagberg JM, et al: Effects of 12 months of intense exercise training on ischemic ST-segment depression in patients with coronary artery disease. *Circulation* 1981;64:1116–1124.

Ehsani AA, Heath GW, Martin WH, et al: Effects of intense exercise training on plasma catecholamines in coronary patients. *J Appl Physiol* 1984;57:154–159.

Enger SC, Herbjornsen K, Erikssen J, et al: High density lipoproteins (HDL) and physical activity: The influence of physical exercise, age, and smoking on HDL-cholesterol and the HDL-/total cholesterol ratio. *Scand J Clin Invest* 1977;37:251–255.

Fagard R, Aubert A, Lysens R, et al: Noninvasive assessment of seasonal variations in cardiac structure and function in cyclists. *Circulation* 1983;67:896–901.

Fagard R, Aubert A, Staessen J, et al: Cardiac structure and function in cyclists and runners: Comparative echocardiographic study. *Br Heart J* 1984; 52:124–129.

Ferguson RJ, Petitclerc R, Choquette G, et al: Effect of physical training on treadmill exercise capacity, collateral circulation, and progression of coronary disease. *Am J Cardiol* 1974;34:764.

Frick MH, Katila M: Hemodynamic consequences of physical training after myocardial infarction. *Circulation* 1968;37:192.

Frick MH, Sjogren AL, Paraslo J, et al: Cardiovascular dimensions and moderate physical training in young men. *J Appl Physiol* 1970;29:452–459.

Froelicher VF: The hemodynamic effects of physical-conditioning in healthy young, and middle-aged individuals, and in coronary heart disease patients, in Naughton J, Hellerstein H, Mahler I (eds):*Exercise Testing and Exercise Training in Coronary Heart Disease* New York, Academic Press, 1973, p. 63.

Froelicher VF, Brown P: Exercise and coronary heart disease. *J Cardiac Rehabil* 1981; 4:277–284.

Gaffney FA, Nixon JV, Karlsson ES, et al: Cardiovascular deconditioning produced by 20 hours of bedrest with head-down tilt (− 5 degrees) in middle-aged healthy men. *Am J Cardiol* 1985;56:634–638.

Gilbert CA, Nutter DO, Felner JM, et al: Echocardiographic study of cardiac dimensions and function in the endurance-trained athlete. *Am J Cardiol* 1977;40:528.

Goodrick CL: Effects of long-term voluntary wheel exercise on male and female Wistar rats. *Gerontology* 1980;26:22.

Graettinger WF: The cardiovascular response to chronic physical exertion and exercise training: An echocardiographic review. *Am Heart J* 1984;108:1014–1018.

Greenen DL, Gilliam TB, Crowley D, et al: Echocardiographic measures in 6- to 7-year-old children after an eight-month exercise program. *Am J Cardiol* 1982;49:1990–1995.

Guski H: The effect of exercise on myocardial interstitium: An ultrastructural morphometric study. *Exp Mol Pathol* 1980;18:141.

Hagan RD, Laird WP, Gettman LR: The problems of per-surface area and per-weight standardization indices in the determination of cardiac hypertrophy in endurance-trained athletes. *J Cardiopulmonary Rehabil* 1985;5:554–560.

Hagberg JM, Ehsani AA, Holloszy JO: Effect of 12 months of intense exercise training on stroke volume in patients with coronary artery disease. *Circulation* 1983;67:1194–1198.

Hakkila J: Studies of the myocardial capillary concentration in cardiac hypertrophy due to training. *Ann Acad Sci Fenn* 1955;33:1.

Haller RG, Lewis SF: Pathophysiology of exercise performance in muscle disease. *Med Sci Sports Exerc* 1984;16:456–459.

Hanson JS, Tabakin BS, Levy AM: Comparative exercise: Cardiorespiratory performance of normal men in the third, fourth, and fifth decades of life. *Circulation* 1968;37:345.

Hanson JS, Tabakin BS, Levy AM, et al: Long-term physical training and cardiovascular dynamics in middle-aged men. *Circulation* 1968;38:783.

Hartley LH, Grimby G, Kilbom A, et al: Physical training in sedentary middle-aged and older men. *Scand J Clin Lab Invest* 1969;24:335.

Haslam RW, Cobb RB: Frequency of intensive, prolonged exercise as a determinant of relative coronary circumference index. *Int J Sports Med* 1982;3:118–121.

Hauser AM, Dressendorfer RH, Vos M, et al: Symmetric cardiac enlargement in highly trained endurance athletes: A two-dimensional echocardiographic study. *Am Heart J* 1985;109:1038–1044.

Heaton WH, Marr KC, Capurro NL, et al: Beneficial effect of physical training on blood flow to myocardium perfused by chronic collaterals in the exercising dog. *Circulation* 1978;57:575.

Holloszy JO, Smith EK, Vining M, et al: Effect of voluntary exercise on longevity of rats. *J Appl Physiol* 1985;59:826–831.

Huston TP, Puffer JC, Todney WM: The athletic heart syndrome. *N Engl J Med* 1985;313:24–31.

Kaplinsky E, Hood WB, McCarthy B, et al: Effects of physical training in dogs with coronary artery ligation. *Circulation* 1968;37:556.

Kasch FW, Wallace JP, Van Camp SP: Effects of 18 years of endurance exercise on the physical work capacity of older men. *J Cardiopulmonary Rehabil* 1985;5:308–312.

Kattus AA, Jorgensen CR, Worden RE, et al: ST-segment depression with near-maximal exercise: Its modification by physical conditioning. *Chest* 1972;62:678.

Kayar SR, Conley KE, Claassen H, et al: Capillarity and mitochondrial distribution in rat myocardium following exercise training. *J Exp Biol* 1986;120:189–199.

Kerr A, Bommer WJ, Pilato S: Coronary artery enlargement in experimental cardiac hypertrophy. *Am Heart J* 1968;75:144.

Kilbom A, Hartley LH, Saltin B, et al: Physical training in sedentary middle-aged and older men. *Scand J Clin Lab Invest* 1969;24:315.

Knight DR, Stone HL: Alteration of ischemic cardiac function in normal heart by daily exercise. *J Appl Physiol: Respirat Environ Exerc Physiol* 1983;55:52.

Kobernick SD, Niawayama G, Zuehlewski AC: Effect of physical activity on cholesterol atherosclerosis in rabbits. *Proc Soc Exp Biol Med* 1957;96:623.

Kramsch DM, Aspen AJ, Abramowitz BM, et al: Reduction of coronary atherosclerosis by moderate conditioning exercise in monkeys on an atherogenic diet. *N Engl J Med* 1981;305:1483–1489.

Laks MM, Morady F, Swan HJC: Myocardial hypertrophy produced by chronic infusion of subhypertensive doses of norepinephrine in the dog. *Chest* 1973;64:75–78.

Landry F, Bouchard C, Dumesnil J: Cardiac dimension changes with endurance training. *JAMA* 1985;254:77–80.

Laughlin MH: Effects of exercise training on coronary transport capacity. *J Appl Physiol* 1985;58:468–476.

Lee AP, Ice R, Blessey R, et al: Long-term effects of physical training on coronary patients with impaired ventricular function. *Circulation* 1979;60:1519.

Letac B, Cribier A, Desplances JF: A study of LV function in coronary patients before and after physical training. *Circulation* 1977;56:375.

Levine SN, Kinasewitz GT: Exercise conditioning increases rat myocardial calcium uptake. *J Appl Physiol* 1986;60:1673–1679.

Ljungqvist A, Unge G: Capillary proliferative activity in myocardium and skeletal muscle of exercised rats. *J Appl Physiol* 1978;43:306.

Longhurst JC, Kelly AR, Gonyea WJ, et al: Chronic training with static and dynamic exercise: Cardiovascular adaptation, and response to exercise. *Circ Res* 1981;48:171.

MacMahon SW, Wilcken DEL, Macdonald GJ: The effect of weight reduction on left ventricular mass. *N Engl J Med* 1986;314:334–339.

Mahler DA, Loke J: The physiology of endurance exercise. *Clin Chest Med* 1984;5:63–75.

Malik AB: Coronary vascular adjustments in exercise training. *Cardiovasc Med* 1977;2:1137.

Martin WH, Coyle EF, Bloomfield SA, et al: Effects of physical deconditioning after intense endurance training on left ventricular dimensions and stroke volume. *J Am Coll Cardiol* 1986;7:982–989.

McAllister FF, Bertsch R, Jacobson J, et al: The accelerating effect of muscular exercise on experimental atherosclerosis. *Arch Surg* 1959;80:54.

McElroy CL, Gissen SA, Fishbein MC: Exercise-induced reduction in myocardial infarction size after coronary artery occlusion in the rat. *Circulation* 1978;57:958.

Miller WT, Kertzer R, Bunk CL, et al: Normal variations in body surface electrocardiographic potential distributions during QRS: Effects of exercise and exercise training. *J Electrocardiology* 1985;18:239–250.

Morganroth J, Maron BJ, Henry WL, et al: Comparative left ventricular dimensions in trained athletes. *Ann Intern Med* 1975;82:521.

Moskowitz RM, Burns JJ, DiCarlo EF, et al: Cage size and exercise affects on infarct size in rats after coronary artery cauterization. *J Appl Physiol: Respirat Environ Exerc Physiol* 1979;47:393.

Neil A, Oxedine R: Do collaterals improve perfusion during exercise? *Circulation* 1979;60:1501.

Niemela KO, Palatsi IJ, Ikaheimo MJ, et al: Evidence of impaired left ventricular performance after an uninterrupted competitive 24-hour run. *Circulation* 1984;70:350–356.

Noakes TD, Higginson L, Opie LH: Physical training increases ventricular fibrillation thresholds of isolated rat hearts during normoxia, hypoxia, and regional ischemia. *Circulation* 1983;67:24–30.

Nolewajka AJ, Kostuk WJ, Rechnitzer PA, et al: Exercise and human collateralization: An angiographic and scintigraphic assessment. *Circulation* 1979;60:114.

Ong TC, Sothy SP: Exercise and cardiorespiratory fitness. *Ergonomics* 1986;29:273–280.

Osbakken M, Locko R: Scintigraphic determination of ventricular function and coronary perfusion in long-distance runners. *Am Heart J* 1984;108:296–303.

Oscai LB, Mole PA, Holloszy JO: Effects of exercise on cardiac weight and mitochondria in male and female rats. *Am J Physiol* 1971;220:1944.

Parker BM, Londeree BR, Cupp GV, et al: The noninvasive cardiac evaluation of long-distance runners. *Chest* 1978;73:376.

Parrault H, Peronnet F, Cleroux J, et al: Electro- and echocardiographic assessment of left ventricle before and after training in man. *Can J Appl Sports Sci* 1978;3:180.

Paterson DH, Shephard RK, Cunningham D: Effects of physical training on cardiovascular function following myocardial infarction. *J Appl Physiol* 1979;47:482.

Paulsen W, Boughner DR, Patrick KO, et al: Left ventricular function in marathon runners: echocardiographic assessment. *J Appl Physiol* 1981;51:881.

Pedersoli WM: Physical exercise, atherogenic diet, and serum lipids in swine. *Cur Therap Res* 1978;23:464.

Raffo JA, Luksic IY, Kappagoda CT, et al: Effects of physical training on myocardial ischemia in patients with coronary artery disease. *Br Heart J* 1980;43:262.

Rasmussen EW, Hostmark AT: Age-related changes in the concentration of plasma cholesterol and triglycerides in two groups of rats with inherited widely different levels of spontaneous physical activity. *Circ Res* 1978;42:598.

Rerych S, Scholz P, Sabiston D, et al: Effects of exercise training on left ventricular function in normal subjects: A longitudinal study by radionuclide angiography. *Am J Cardiol* 1980;45:244.

Ritzer TF, Bove AA, Care RA: Left ventricular performance characteristics in trained and sedentary dogs. *J Appl Physiol: Respirat Environ Exerc Physiol* 1980;48:130.

Sachs ML, Pargman D: Running addiction: An indepth interview examination. *J Sport Behavior* 1979;2:143–147.

Saltin B, Blomqvist G, Mitchell JH, et al: Response to exercise after bed rest and after training. *Circulation* 1968;38:1.

Saltin B, Hartley LH, Kilbom A, et al: Physical training in sedentary middle-aged and older men. *Scand J Clin Lab Invest* 1969;24:323.

Salzman SH, Hellerstein HK, Radke JD, et al: Quantitative effects of physical conditioning on the exercise electrocardiogram of middle-aged subjects with arteriosclerotic heart disease. *Measurements in Exercise ECG* 1969;388.

Sanders M, White FC, Peterson TM, et al: Effects of endurance exercise on coronary collateral blood flow in miniature swine. *Am J Physiol* 1978;234:H614.

Schaper W: Influence of physical exercise in coronary collateral blood flow in chronic experimental two-vessel occlusion. *Circulation* 1982;65:905–912.

Scheel K, Ingram L, Wilson J: Effects of exercise on the coronary and collateral vasculature of beagles with and without coronary occlusion. *Circ Res* 1981;48:523.

Scheel KW: The stimulus for coronary collateral growth: Ischemia or mechanical factors. *J Cardiac Rehabil* 1981;1:149–153.

Scheuer J: Effects of physical training on myocardial vascularity and perfusion. *Circulation* 1982;66:491–495.

Schieken RM, Clarke WR, Mahoney LT, et al: Measurement criteria for group echocardiographic studies. *Am J Epidemiol* 1979;110:504.

Seals DR, Hagberg JM, Hurley BF, et al: Effects of endurance training on glucose tolerance and plasma lipid levels in older men and women. *JAMA* 1984;252:645–649.

Seals DR, Hagberg JM, Hurley BF, et al: Endurance training in older men and women I. Cardiovascular responses to exercise. *J Appl Physiol: Respirat Environ Exerc Physiol* 1984;57:1024–1029.

Shephard RJ: Factors influencing the exercise behavior of patients. *Sports Med* 1985; 2:348–366.

Sidney KH, Shephard RJ: Training and electrocardiographic abnormalities in the elderly. *Br Heart J* 1977;39:1114.

Sim DN, Neill WA: Investigation of the physiological basis for increased exercise threshold for angina pectoris after physical conditioning. *J Clin Invest* 1974;54:763–770.

Sinyor SG, Schwartz SG, Peronnet F, et al: Aerobic fitness level and reactivity to psychosocial stress: Physiological, biochemical, and subjective measures. *Psychosom Med* 1983; 45:205–217.

Stamler J: Lifestyles, major risk factors, proof and public policy. *Circulation* 1978;58:3–19.

Stein RA, Michielli D, Fox EL, et al: Continuous ventricular dimensions in man during supine exercise and recovery. *Am J Cardiol* 1978;41:655.

Stevenson JA, Feleki V, Rechnitzer P, et al: Effect of exercise on coronary tree size i[...] Circ Res 1964;15:265.

Stone HL: Coronary flow, myocardial oxygen consumption and exercise training in d[...] Appl Physiol: Respirat Environ Exerc Physiol 1980;49:759.

Tabkin BS, Hanson JS, Levy AM: Effects of physical training on the cardiovascular and respiratory response to graded upright exercise in distance runners. Br Heart J 1965;27:205.

Taylor NAS, Wilkinson JG: Exercise-induced skeletal muscle growth hypertrophy or hyperplasia? Sports Med 1986;3:190–200.

Tepperman J, Pearlman D: Effects of exercise and anemia on coronary arteries of small animals as revealed by the corrosion-case technique. Circ Res 1961;9:576.

Tharp GD, Wagner CT: Chronic exercise and cardiac vascularization. Eur J Appl Physiol 1982;48:97–104.

Thompson P, Lewis S, Areskog N, et al: Generalized training effects without changes in cardiac performance. Med Sci Sports 1978;10:1–8.

Tibbits G, Barnard R, Baldwin K, et al: Influence of exercise on excitation-contraction coupling in rat myocardium. Am J Physiol 1981;240:H472.

Tibbits G, Nagatomo T, Saski M, et al: Cardiac sarcolemma: Compositional adaptation to exercise. Science 1981;213:1271–1273.

Tipton CM, Matthes RD, Callahan A, et al: The role of chronic exercise on resting blood pressure of normotensive and hypertensive rats. Med Sci Sports 1977;9:168.

Thomanek RJ, Tounton CA, Liskop KS: Relationship between age, chronic exercise, and connective tissue of the heart. J Gerontol 1972;27:33.

Tomoike H, Franklin D, McKown D, et al: Regional myocardial dysfunction and hemodynamic abnormalities during strenuous exercise in dogs with limited coronary flow. Circ Res 1978;42:487.

Upton MT, Rerych SK, Roeback JR, et al: Effect of brief and prolonged exercise on left ventricular function. Am J Cardiol 1980;45:1154–1159.

Vanhees L, Fagard R, Grauwels R, et al: Changes in systolic time intervals during physical training in patients with ischemic heart disease. Cardiology 1984;71:207–214.

Varnauskas E, Bjorntorp P, Fahlen M, et al: Effects of physical training on exercise blood flow and enzymatic activity in skeletal muscle. Cardiovasc Res 1970;4:418.

Warnock NH, Clarkson RB, Stevenson R: Effect of exercise on blood coagulation time and atherosclerosis of cholesterol-fed cockerels. Circ Res 1957;5:478.

Watanabe K, Bhargava B, Froelicher VF: A computerized approach to evaluating rest and exercise-induced ECG/VCG changes after cardiac rehabilitation. Clin Cardiol 1982;5:27–34.

Westheim A, Simonsen K, Schamaun O, et al: Effect of exercise training in patients with essential hypertension. J Hypertens 1985;3:S479–S481.

Wexler BC, Greenberg BP: Effect of exercise on myocardial infarction in young vs old male rats: Electrocardiographic changes. Am Heart J 1974;88:343.

Wilmore JH, Rody FB, Stanforth PR, et al: Ratings of perceived exertion, heart rate, and treadmill speed in the prediction of maximal oxygen uptake during submaximal treadmill exercise. J Cardiopulmonary Rehabil 1985;5:540–546.

Wolfe L, Cunningham D, Rechnitzer P, et al: Effects of endurance training on left ventricular dimensions in healthy men. J Appl Physiol: Respirat Environ Exerc Physiol 1979;47:207.

Wolfe LA, Martin RP, Watson DD, et al: Chronic exercise and left ventricular structure and function in healthy human subjects. J Appl Physiol 1985;58:409–415.

Wyatt HL, Chuck L, Rabinowitz B, et al: Enhanced cardiac response to catecholamines in physically trained cats. Am J Physiol 1978;234:H608.

10 EXERCISE IN THE PREVENTION OF CORONARY HEART DISEASE

Since most animal, clinical, and pathologic studies have not shown exercise to be directly related to the atherosclerotic process, it is reasonable to conclude that physical inactivity does not have a direct effect on atherosclerosis. Instead, the effects of regular exercise enable the body to better tolerate ischemia and lessen the manifestations of coronary heart disease. In addition, it can possibly alter other risk factors for atherosclerosis. The potential beneficial actions of regular exercise are multifactorial which makes physical inactivity a complex risk factor to assess. Some of the difficulties in studying physical inactivity as a risk factor will be discussed along with many of the studies that have been performed.

PHYSICAL FITNESS VERSUS PHYSICAL ACTIVITY

The question remains whether activity level or actual maximal oxygen uptake best predicts the risk for coronary heart disease. Leon has shown that in healthy men the results of resting measurements and a questionnaire correlate highly with treadmill time using a multivariate equation. In order to classify physical fitness for intervention studies, Leon and colleagues studied the relationship of physical characteristics and life habits to treadmill performance. One hundred seventy-five apparently healthy men were recruited. They completed questionnaires about habitual physical activity, smoking, beverage consumption, and sleep habits. Body mass index, heart rate and blood pressure at rest and during submaximal exercise, frequency of premature ventricular beats, handgrip strength, and serum cholesterol were measured. These characteristics were correlated with the duration of exercise using the Bruce protocol. Univariate analysis indicated that treadmill performance was significantly and positively correlated with leisure activity and reports of sweating and dyspnea occurring regularly during such physical activity. Performance was negatively correlated with age, body mass index, resting heart rate, cigarette smoking, and consumption of caffeine-containing beverages. An r value of .75 was found between treadmill performance and 11 of the above variables, and it was increased to .81 by adding heart rate during submaximal exercise.

Health-related physical fitness is defined by Wilmore as (1) the ability to perform strenuous physical activity with vigor and without excessive fatigue, and (2) a demonstration of physical activity traits and capacities that are consistent with minimal risk of developing diseases associated with physical inactivity. It includes the components of (1) cardiorespiratory endurance, (2) muscular strength and endurance, (3) body composition, and (4) flexibility. Previous tests of "physical fitness" include components of motor fitness, i.e., agility, power, speed, and balance. While these are important considerations for the growing child and the athlete, they should not be considered as a part of a health-related physical fitness test battery for the general population.

Muscular and strength endurance can be assessed directly, either by simple field tests such as the one-repetition maximum (weight lifting) or by using sophisticated equipment such as a Cybex II isokinetic device. A handgrip test was used in the Framingham Study and was considered an indirect marker of fitness. However, it is unlikely that isometric hand strength closely relates to cardiovascular health.

There is no universal agreement on what constitutes an adequate flexibility test battery. Flexibility is highly specific to the joints being tested. Testing should involve activities of normal daily life that create limitations when flexibility is limited, i.e., tying one's shoes. Its assessment is confounded by the effects of age, arthritis, obesity, injury, and congenital abnormalities.

Hydrostatic or underwater weighing is the gold standard for estimating percent body fat, but skinfold measurements are a reasonable alternative usually used. A minimum of six sites should be chosen and equations should be used, but the absolute measurements should also be recorded. Equations to estimate percent body fat from these measurements have a great deal of variability and poorly correlate or agree. It is well-known that training decreases the percent body fat. The finding that the percent body fat of children is directly related to the number of hours they watch television daily suggests that such an analysis might have some value to assess activity level since children are sedentary while watching TV. Also, the association of body habitus with the probability of becoming obese may support the use of some body composition measurements.

Does exercise protect from coronary artery disease rather than select out those with less disease who are better able to tolerate being physically active? Exercise can be related to other risk factors or risk markers, and many studies have not considered the selection of these factors. Particularly in a modern, mechanized society, there is usually only a small gradient of activity between different jobs. An important consideration is that people often leave active jobs with onset of the first symptoms of heart disease, even without realizing the cause of the symptoms. That is, there is a premorbid transfer from an active job to a less active job, biasing the relationship of inactivity to coronary heart disease. Also, individuals are often selected for active jobs or for lifestyles of physical activity. There are other difficulties in studying this question, including the uncertainty of what type and quantity of exercise is protective.

Although the most accurate way of assessing the physiologic effect of an activity level would be an exercise test, few studies have had this luxury. Job title or class has often been used and in some instances was accurate. However, consideration of off-the-job activity is important. Questionnaires have been used, but their reproducibility and accuracy are often doubtful. Parameters such as vital capacity, handgrip strength, and dietary assays have obvious limitations.

The methods of diagnosing coronary artery disease have included death certificates, rest and exercise electrocardiograms, medical records, medical evaluations, and autopsy. Even an autopsy has distinct limitations since it is usually not done using standardized methods. The death certificate is often coded with the most common cause of death in the community rather than an accurate description of the cause of death. Also, multiple causes of death result in misclassification. Physicians functioning as clinicians or pathologists do not feel the same need for accuracy and precision in completing these forms and records as do epidemiologists.

Many different types of populations have been used for epidemiologic studies. There are three basic types of epidemiologic studies: retrospective, prevalence, and prospective studies. Retrospective studies involve populations in which data have been obtained in the past not specifically for epidemiologic purposes. Prevalence, or cross-sectional, studies consist of screening a population for the current manifestations of a disease. Prospective, or longitudinal, studies involve a cohort of individuals specifically chosen and studied for the purpose of following them over a period of time for the development of disease.

RETROSPECTIVE STUDIES OF PHYSICAL INACTIVITY AS A RISK FACTOR

This group of retrospective studies includes three large population studies that have utilized death certificate and population data from an entire city, state, or country. Activity level was judged from the occupation listed on the death certificate, and the endpoint was coronary artery disease listed on death certificates.

Morris has presented the data from the occupational-mortality records in England and Wales, interpreting the information as support for the hypothesis that occupational physical inactivity is a risk factor for coronary heart disease. Social class as used in these studies was based on the grading of occupation by its level of skill and role in production, and its general standing in the community. Social class ranged from class 1, which includes professions such as physicians and stockbrokers, to class 5, which includes unskilled workers such as railroad porters and builders' helpers. The level of activity was based on the independent evaluation of the occupations by several industrial experts. The activity level of the last job held was found to be inversely related to the mortality from coronary artery disease, as determined from death certificates. Some of the limitations of this study include imprecise diagnostic criteria and bias due to the selection of the sick for less active jobs.

Stamler and associates analyzed the mortality statistics in Chicago for the years 1951 and 1953. Both the cause of death and occupation were obtained from the death certificates, and the occupations were broken down into five categories: (1) professional and semiprofessional workers, proprietors, managers, and officials, (2) clerical and sales people, (3) craftsmen, foremen, and operatives, (4) service workers, and (5) laborers. These categories were also combined as white collar workers (categories 1 and 2) and blue collar workers (categories 3, 4, and 5). The authors found no significant occupational group differences in age-specific coronary artery disease death rates for white males aged 45 to 64 years of age.

Breslow and Buell compared groups with similar general mortality to make apparent the protective effect of physical activity, in agreement with the previously mentioned British studies. They analyzed census and death certificate data in California from 1949 to 1951. They found inconsistencies, however, in the records as to whether the last, the usual, or longest held occupation were reported. Nonetheless, they felt that the data revealed a gradient of decreasing mortality from coronary heart disease with increasing physical activity, but only when occupational groups of similar general mortality were considered.

The following retrospective studies involved analysis of data from a specific population with activity level assessed by job classification, questionnaire, or both, and with coronary artery disease listed on the death certificate or reported symptoms of coronary artery disease used as endpoints.

Morris and coworkers presented data from a sequence of epidemiologic studies to support the hypothesis quoted here. "Men in physically active jobs have a lower incidence of coronary heart disease than men in physically inactive jobs. More important, the disease is not so severe in physically active workers, tending to present first in them as angina pectoris and other relatively benign forms and to have a smaller early case fatality and a lower early mortality rate." The first study dealt with the drivers and conductors of the London transport system. Thirty-one thousand white males, 35 to 64 years of age, were included for analysis over a period of 18 months from 1949 to 1950. The endpoints were coronary insufficiency, myocardial infarction, and angina as reported on sickleave records, and listing of coronary artery disease on death certificates. The age-adjusted total incidence was 1.5 times higher in the driver group as compared with the conductor group, and the sudden and three-month mortality was two times higher. These findings could be explained by differences in constitution, mental stress, or physical activity. The difference in physical activity was only inferred from knowing that one group drove the buses whereas the other group conducted on the double-decked vehicles. No attempt was made to quantitate the activity difference or to measure differences in off-the-job activity.

In their original study, Morris and colleagues did not investigate differences due to selection in the two groups, but proceeded to a similar study with postmen and clerks, which also resulted in numbers that agreed with their hypothesis. In 1956, Morris published a paper subtitled "The Epidemiology of Uniforms," which reported that the drivers had greater girth (i.e., larger uniform sizes were considered since weight was not recorded) than the conductors. In 1966, Morris also showed that the drivers had higher serum cholesterols and higher blood pressures than did the conductors. Also, a study by Oliver documented that for some unknown reason, even the recruits for the two jobs differed in lipid level and in weight. These differences put the drivers at increased risk to coronary artery disease for reasons other than an approximated difference in physical activity.

Zukel and colleagues analyzed data from a population of 106,000 individuals living in six counties in North Dakota. From the 20,000 men aged 35 years or more within this population, they found 228 men with coronary artery disease that became manifest during 1957. The data were obtained from reviewing death certificates, office visits, or hospital admissions reported by local doctors for acute myocardial infarctions, coronary ischemia, congestive heart failure due to coronary artery disease, or angina. Farmers had slightly less total coronary artery disease and one-half the infarctions and death from coronary artery disease. The authors did not relate this result directly to differences in physical activity since they were aware of socioeconomic and environmental differences between the two groups. Physical activity was related to coronary artery disease based on a questionnaire of physical activity administered to survivors of infarction and to matched controls. Unfortunately, interview information on physical activity is very unreliable. Dividing hours of heavy physical work into 0, 1 to 6, and 7 or more, only a 51% agreement was found for 273 men in whom replicate information was obtained. Moreover, there was a tendency for men to report less heavy physical work in their usual occupation after their heart attacks than before.

Brunner has surveyed Jews of European origin living in kibbutzim or collective settlements in Israel over the period of 1946 to 1961, with 5,279 men aged 40 to 69 years in the group as of 1961. Coronary heart disease was determined from medical records of myocardial infarction, angina pectoris, and sudden death due to coronary artery disease. Sedentary workers, defined as those who spent 80% or more of their time at work sitting, had 2.5 to 4.0 times the incidence of coronary artery disease as the nonsedentary workers (all others). This population is ideal for study because their mode of life eliminates socioeconomic differences, but no investigation of differences in risk factors was reported. Other characteristics of the sedentary group could account for differences in the incidence of coronary artery disease.

These next retrospective studies involve data obtained from specific occupational groups with the activity level assessed by the standardized job title and with coronary artery disease listed as the cause of death in the industrial records as the endpoint.

In a mortality study, Adelstein compared white South Africans working for South African railroads as officers (clerks, administrators, highly paid execu-

tives) with railroad employees (ranging from unskilled laborers to skilled artisans). Mortality among these employees, secondary to coronary disease during 1954 to 1959, when age adjusted, did not differ from the general
population. The categories of artisans, semiskilled, and others were analyzed
with the physical demand of work within each group determined on a scale
of one to five by four experienced industrial health inspectors, and mean ratings were used. Again, no significant differences were found in mortality from
coronary disease and level of physical activity.

Taylor and colleagues have reported on the mortality of white males employed by the United States railroad industry. The employees were separated
by job title into three groups representing three levels of physical activity.
Death certificates for the years 1955 and 1956 were analyzed by these group-
ings, and the following age-adjusted rates were obtained: (1) clerks, light activity, 5.7 deaths per 1,000 man-years; (2) switchmen, moderate activity, 3.9
deaths per 1,000 man-years; and (3) section men, heavy activity, 2.8 deaths
per 1,000 man-years. They concluded that the data were consistent with the
hypothesis that men in sedentary occupations have more coronary disease
than do those in occupations requiring moderate to heavy physical activity.

In planning a prospective study, the authors discovered a number of important points that pertained to their mortality study. They found that the groups
were not clearly separated by occupation as to the level of physical activity.
Work analyses and further questioning revealed that some clerks consumed
as many calories per day as did section men, who presumably were working
more vigorously. The most important finding was that men with coronary
disease withdrew from the ranks of switchmen at a greater rate than from the
ranks of sedentary clerks. It became apparent that this bias in job transfers
and in retirement could explain the difference in mortality between the
groups, rather than any protective influence exerted by physical activity.

Kahn gathered information from federal employee records to analyze mortality data on men who were appointed to positions in the Washington, D.C.,
post office from 1906 to 1940. Of 2,240 men so identified, 93% were determined as either dead or alive as of January, 1962. The mortality data of sedentary clerks were compared with active mail carriers. Kahn noted that the
records showed that the carriers transferred to clerk positions much more frequently than clerks switched jobs. He adjusted for this effect by considering a
subsample of men who did not change jobs. The data from this preselected
group suggested that the clerks had 1.4 to 1.9 times the mortality from coronary disease than the carriers.

The following retrospective studies represent specific populations in which
the activity level was assessed by occupation or questionnaire; diagnosis of
acute myocardial infarction served as the endpoint.

Frank and associates have studied 55,000 men aged 25 to 64 years enrolled
in the Health Insurance Plan of Greater New York (HIP). In this group, 301
men were identified as having had an initial myocardial infarction between
November 1, 1961, and April 30, 1963. An index for on-the-job and off-the-
job activities was obtained by patient completion of a questionnaire during a
personal interview after the infarction by the patients or by the wives of those

who had died. The men were divided into three categories: least active, intermediate, and most active. The authors concluded that inquiry about customary physical activities on and off the job permitted delineation of a group of least active men who were much more likely to experience a clinically severe episode and die within four weeks of its onset than were men who were relatively more active.

There are a number of inherent difficulties in this study. Many of the 301 men who provided incidence data on MI were ill prior to MI. Twenty-two percent had manifestations of coronary disease, 19% had HBP, and 10% were diabetic, and it would be expected that these people would be less active. Being both less active and at high risk for acute myocardial infarction, they represent a statistical bias for inactivity and subsequent MI as well as for the severity of the MI. Another difficulty was that the widows tended to underestimate the physical activity of their dead husbands.

Shanoff and colleagues studied a group of men with documented MI, randomly selected from the files of the Toronto Veterans Administration Hospital and matched to a group, also from the hospital files, of patients admitted with nonchronic illnesses. Within both groups, there were approximately 25 individuals for each decade from the fourth through seventh decades of life for a total of 100 individuals per group. The individuals were questioned as to lifelong activity, and physical activity in childhood, youth, and adult life was assessed. This type of questioning made available additional information because the two groups did not differ as to present activity or occupation, but did differ as to habitual activity. In this study, coronary disease was not associated with habitual physical inactivity.

Forssman and Lindegard organized a study in Malmo, a Swedish town of about 200,000 people. The city is served by one hospital, and the study group was comprised of all male survivors of an acute myocardial infarction admitted to the hospital from 1948 to 1955 and whose age at the time of the study examination in 1956 was 55 or less. This group included 66 men for whom healthy similarly aged controls were randomly selected from the town. Occupational physical activity was determined by knowledge of the job rather than by personal questioning. No difference in occupational physical activity between the controls and postinfarction group was determined.

PREVALENCE STUDIES OF PHYSICAL INACTIVITY AS A RISK FACTOR

The following three prevalence or cross-sectional studies represent a modification of the retrospective or case history approach. The main advantage is that the statistics on the studied disease are gathered at the time of the study. Thus, the endpoints can be well defined, and the methods for diagnosis standardized. Unfortunately, selection is a problem.

In 1958, 1,465 male employees of a utility company in Chicago were evaluated. Prevalence of coronary disease was determined by reviewing industrial health records for diagnostic electrocardiographic changes or for history consistent with coronary artery disease. There was little difference in major risk factors between the activity level groups. Prevalence of coronary artery disease was lower in the blue collar workers than in the white collar workers, and in the nonsedentary than in the sedentary. These data were confounded by such factors as differential rates of retirement among blue and white collar workers, and shifts from blue collar to white collar jobs after a coronary disease episode.

From 1957 to 1959, 3,049 railroad men were randomly selected for study of the prevalence of risk factors in coronary disease. Active switchmen and sedentary clerks and executives were included to have two different activity groups for comparison. Extensive screening was performed, and the manifestations of coronary disease were well-defined. The data on the 1948 men that submitted to the evaluation suggested that the switchmen had less coronary disease. However, occupational mobility of the switchmen with coronary disease was greater than that of clerks. The majority of the factors affecting observed prevalence rates operated to exaggerate any true protective influences of physical activity.

In 1960, the population of Evans County, Georgia, was studied for the prevalence of coronary heart disease. Coronary artery disease was defined as angina pectoris, history of MI, or diagnostic ECG findings. The study group included 1,062 men consisting of almost equal numbers of high social class whites, low social class whites, and blacks. Within the study group there were 52 cases of coronary disease. Social class and occupational comparison among black males was not possible because they were predominantly of low social class and in physically active occupations. Among white males, distribution of coronary artery disease by occupation suggested that those with high activity had less prevalence of coronary artery disease. White males had three times the coronary artery disease as the black males, whereas high social class white males had two times as much disease as low social class white males, and five times as much as black males. Black males were believed to be more active by analysis of occupation and caloric consumption, but they also were thinner and had lower serum cholesterols. The authors concluded that physical activity appeared to be a major determinant of coronary artery disease prevalence. A seven-year prospective study in Evans County found the incidence of coronary artery disease to be lower among professionals (94/1,000) and highest among manual laborers and clerks (184/1,000). This contradictory result is interesting, especially since the two other prevalence studies were believed to be influenced by a bias that favored the physical activity hypothesis.

PROSPECTIVE STUDIES OF PHYSICAL INACTIVITY AS A RISK FACTOR

In 1958, Stamler and colleagues began a prospective study of 1,241 apparently healthy male employees of the Peoples Gas Company in Chicago. By 1965, there were 39 deaths due to coronary disease among the groups. They found that the coronary disease mortality was higher in blue collar workers (37 deaths per 1,000 men) who had an estimated higher habitual activity at work than in the white collar workers (20 deaths per 1,000). Stamler believed these findings were consistent with the hypothesis that groups of men with similar findings with respect to the cardinal risk factors (hypertension, hypercholesterolemia, cigarette smoking, and excessive weight) will experience similar incidence and mortality rates for coronary heart disease regardless of habitual physical activity at work. However, the population in general had a low level of physical activity, and lack of a gradient of physical activity limits the possibility of demonstrating an association of mortality and physical activity.

From 1956 to 1960, 687 healthy London busmen were examined for risk factors and coronary disease. In 1965, they were reexamined, and 47 cases of coronary disease were diagnosed, including sudden deaths, MI, ECG changes, and angina. Incidence rates per 100 men over five years were 4.7 for conductors and 8.5 for drivers. However, the drivers were found to have significantly higher blood pressure and serum cholesterol than the conductors. Furthermore, classifying the conductors as an activity-protected group was inconsistent because they had an incidence of coronary disease similar to sedentary London physicians.

Taylor studied the effects of occupational activity differences among railroad men. Thirty groups of men were randomly selected from a population of 3,049 men working for 20 northwestern railroads. Of this group, there were 860 sedentary clerks, 251 executives, and 837 active switchmen, 40 to 59 years of age, when first examined from 1957 to 1959. Energy expenditure was estimated by activity and dietary analysis. It was found that the switchmen expended 600 to 1,200 calories a day more than the sedentary groups. The groups did not differ by any of the major risk factors. After five years of follow-up, no difference in coronary incidence rates between the two different activity levels was found.

In 1957, 1,719 white men aged 40 to 55 years were randomly selected from the 20,000 employees of the Hawthorne Electric Works in Chicago. After eight years of follow-up, there were 24 deaths due to coronary disease, 53 MI, and 80 patients with angina pectoris. Activity off the job was assessed by a personal interview. Approximate differences in caloric expenditure and intensity of work were determined for shop workers and office workers, and also with special means for two different classes of shop workers. No difference was found in coronary disease among the different levels of activity.

In 1949, 1,403 healthy white men with a median age of 47 years were randomly chosen from 20,200 civil servants in Los Angeles. After an initial examination in 1951, periodic follow-up examinations and yearly questionnaires were completed. By 1962, a total of 177 new events of coronary disease as manifested by MI, sudden death, angina pectoris, or coronary insufficiency were diagnosed. No differences in the incidence of coronary disease were observed according to socioeconomic class or to level of physical activity as determined from job title.

The Western Electric collaborative group study was initiated in 1961 with emphasis on psychologic patterns. Annual follow-up studies were obtained through 1965 on 3,182 men, initially aged 35 to 59 years and healthy at the onset. New coronary disease as manifested by symptomatic MI, angina, and electrocardiographic changes was observed in 133 individuals. The customary exercise habits of each participant were determined by personal interview. Nine hundred sixty subjects were classified as exercising with reasonable regularity, i.e., daily or almost daily they performed some calisthenics, walking exercise, athletics, or equivalent physical activity. The remaining 2,222 subjects admitted to only occasionally engaging in some form of physical activity. No differences in age or risk factors in these two groups were apparent, except that the exercising group had slightly lower triglyceride and cholesterol measurements. After 4½ years of follow-up, the annual incidence of coronary heart disease was 10/1,000 for men without regular exercise habits, compared with 7.4/1,000 in men with such habits. This difference was due to symptomatic MI, since no difference was observed in the incidence of silent infarction, angina, or in recurring MI. Fatal myocardial infarction occurred in 2/1,000 men without regular exercise habits compared with 0.5/1,000 men with such habits.

The Seven Countries Coronary Artery Disease Study consists of collaborative groups from Japan, Yugoslavia, the United States, Finland, Italy, the Netherlands, and Greece. This study minimized self-selection rendering complete examination coverage to all men aged 40 to 59 years in the geographically defined areas. The examinations and definitions were rigidly standardized and coordinated at facilities at the University of Minnesota. Individuals were classified as sedentary, moderately active, or very active, as determined by a questionnaire for evaluating total physical activity. Data, from 200,000 man-years observed, showed no difference in coronary disease incidence between physically active and sedentary men.

In 1963, Werko and coworkers began a study on a cohort consisting of one-third of all men born in 1913 in the industrial Swedish town of Gothenburg. This cohort consisted of 834 males, 50 years of age, without signs or symptoms of coronary artery disease. Over the next four years, there were 23 acute myocardial infarctions, 18 individuals with angina pectoris, and 9 individuals with a MI by ECG. The symptomatic MI group was questioned to retrospectively assess activity level on and off the job one year prior to their MI. Activity levels were categorized as light, moderate, or heavy. A random sample of healthy men of a comparable age were questioned as to activity in a similar fashion, and in comparison, this sample group was more active than those with infarctions.

Epstein, Morris, and colleagues studied the relationship of vigorous exercise during leisure time to the resting ECG. From 1968 to 1970, approximately 17,000 middle-aged male executive civil servants on a randomly selected Monday morning recorded their leisure-time activities over the previous weekend. Their work was sedentary. In 1971, a sample of 509 of these men completed further questionnaires for medical, social, and smoking history; at that time, the 509 had a resting ECG, serum cholesterol, and other physiologic parameters recorded. Vigorous exercise in leisure time had previously been reported by 25% of the men. As a group, these active men had significantly fewer ECG abnormalities than the men not reporting vigorous exercise. The ECG abnormalities included changes consistent with myocardial ischemia, PVCs, and sinus tachycardia. This difference was maintained when all men with any history suggestive of cardiovascular disease were excluded from the analysis. Blood pressure, serum cholesterol, and smoking habits were examined along with vigorous exercise in relation to the ECG. The only relation found was increased ECG abnormalities with increasing BP. Even among men with higher blood pressures, those reporting vigorous exercise had fewer electrocardiographic abnormalities. An 8½-year follow-up of this population demonstrated a 50% lower incidence of coronary events in those maintaining rigorous activity on the weekend.

Morris and colleagues reported the results of following 337 healthy middle-aged Englishmen. During 1956 to 1966, these men participated in a seven-day dietary survey. By the end of 1976, 44 of them had developed clinical coronary disease that showed two relationships to diet. Men with a high-caloric intake, as assessed by diet, had a lower rate of disease. Independently of this fact, men with a high intake of dietary fiber from cereals also had a lower rate of disease. A high-caloric intake can be considered to be directly related to physical activity, supporting the exercise hypothesis.

Members of the Fellowship of Cycling Old-Timers (FCOT) were chosen arbitrarily and studied by means of a questionnaire. The club was formed in 1965 for cyclists over 50 years of age. There was a 90% response to 329 questionnaires sent to members living in England. The pattern of activity was 5,000 to 10,000 cycled miles per year, which declined to 2,000 miles as the member got older. At the time of the study, 75% of members were still cycling regularly throughout the year and 54% of those over 70 were cycling once a week or more throughout the year. A decrease in the incidence of MI and coronary disease was found in all cyclists, but the tenfold decrease in the incidence of all coronary disease in the over 75 age group was striking. Details of the cause of death were obtained from death certificates. The average age of death was high (79 years) due to the age restriction.

Costas and colleagues reported a prospective study involving 8,171 urban and rural men 45 to 64 years old participating in the Puerto Rico Heart Program. The 2½-year incidence of coronary disease was examined in relation to serum cholesterol, triglycerides, physical activity, and relative weight. A physical activity index was based on the number of hours spent at five different levels of physical activity as assessed by questionnaire. Endpoints included MI, death, and angina pectoris. A slight increase in risk was found in the least active group of urban men. The physical activity index was too crude, and the level of physical activity was not related to the incidence of coronary heart disease.

Investigations at the Aerobic Center in Dallas have used treadmill performance to quantitate physical fitness. In a cross-sectional study of 3,000 men, treadmill performance was found to be inversely related to body weight, percent body fat, lipids, glucose, and systolic blood pressure. In a longitudinal study, men who were treadmill tested both before and after an exercise program were analyzed to determine if their performance had improved. Those men who reached the upper quartile of improved aerobic fitness exhibited decreases in lipids, diastolic blood pressure, serum glucose, uric acid, and weight. Regular exercise resulting in increased aerobic capacity was associated with decreased risk factors.

Paffenbarger and colleagues have reported numerous analyses of epidemiologic data from the San Francisco longshoremen. Work on the waterfront has been performed at relatively high activity levels under conditions well-governed and documented by the longshoremen union. Longshoremen tend to enter the industry in youth and remain active in it for many years. Paffenbarger analyzed a 22-year follow-up of the longshoremen, from 1951 to 1972, for 59,401 man-years of energy expenditure on the job. One third of this experience was classified as high-energy work and the rest as low-energy work by analyzing the energy output for various longshoremen jobs. High energy jobs required 5 to 7 kcal/min (approximately 2 METs).

Multiphasic screening performed in 1951 assessed the men for obesity, smoking habits, blood pressure levels, and prior history of heart disease. Serum cholesterol was measured in 1961. An annual accounting was taken of job transfers so that the data on energy expenditures could be correlated to the occurrence of fatal MI. Deaths from MIs were assigned to the category in which the deceased had been employed six months prior to death to avoid selective bias due to premorbid job transfers (e.g., transfers to less active jobs secondary to illness). Age-adjusted frequencies of other risk factors among longshoremen were compared between the two energy expenditure groups, and little difference was found. Three parameters were associated with increased risk for fatal MI: low-energy work output, smoking cigarettes, and an elevated SBP. Each of these factors posed an approximate twice-normal risk. Potential reduction in rates of fatal MIs (theoretical effect of intervention), with the elimination of specific combinations of these risk factors, are listed in Table 10–1. Paffenbarger concluded that physical activity is protective and not selective (i.e., not an effect of premorbid job transfers or other biases). The threshold of 5 kcal/min seemed to hold for strenuous bursts rather than for sustained activity.

Paffenbarger performed another population study, one involving 36,000 Harvard University alumni who entered college between 1916 and 1950. Records of their physical activity were gathered from their student days and later

TABLE 10–1.
Potential Rate Reduction of Fatal Heart Attacks (the Theoretical Effect of Intervention With the Elimination of Specific Risk Factors or Combinations of Risk Factors)*

CATEGORY	REDUCTION
Increase physical activity	50%
Stop heavy smoking	30%
Lower systolic blood pressure	30%
Any two above	65%
All three	88%

*Study of longshoremen in San Francisco.

during middle age. Alumni offices and questionnaires were used to obtain information on adult exercise habits, morbidity, and mortality. A 6- to 10-year follow-up during the period of 1961 to 1972 totaled 117,680 man-years of observation after the first questionnaire, and apparently healthy men were classified with specific measures of energy expenditure. They remained under study until heart attack occurrence, death from any cause, age 75, or the end of observation in 1972. Weekly updating of death lists by the alumni office provided the means to obtain official death certificates. A physical activity index was devised to provide a composite estimate of total energy expenditure from stairs climbed, blocks walked, and sports played. This index was scaled in kcal/wk and was divided at 2,000 kcal/wk which produced a 60%–40% division of man-years of observation into low- and high-energy categories.

During the follow-up, 572 men had their first MI. Men with a physical activity index below 2,000 kcal/wk were at 64% higher risk than were classmates with a higher activity index. Varsity athletic status implied selective cardiovascular fitness, and such selection alone was insufficient to explain a lower heart attack risk in later adult years. Former varsity athletes retained a lower risk only if they maintained a high physical activity index as alumni.

Three high-risk characteristics were identified in this study: low physical activity index (less than 2,000 kcal/wk), cigarette smoking, and hypertension. Presence of any one characteristic was accompanied by a 50% increase in risk, and the presence of two characteristics tripled the risk. Maintenance of a high physical activity index could possibly have reduced heart attack risk by 26%. Innate or early acquired cardiovascular endowment may distinguish hardy from less vigorous individuals or the naturally more active from the less active. It would be an oversimplification to assume that early selection accounted for all the observed differences in MI risk.

In a second analysis of Harvard alumni, Paffenbarger and colleagues examined the physical activity and other life-style characteristics of 16,936 alumni, aged 35 to 74, for relations to rates of mortality from all causes and for influences on length of life. A total of 1,413 alumni died during 12 to 16 years to follow-up (1962 to 1978). Exercise reported as walking, stair climbing, and sports related inversely to total mortality, primarily to death due to cardiovascular or respiratory causes. Death rates declined steadily as energy expended on such activity increased from less than 500 to 3,500 kcal per week, beyond which rates increased slightly. Rates were one-quarter to one-third lower among alumni expending 2,000 or more kcal during exercise per week than among less active men. With or without consideration of hypertension, cigarette smoking, extremes or gains in body weight, or early parental death, alumni mortality rates were significantly lower among the physically active. Relative risks of death for individuals were highest among smokers and sedentary men. By the age of 80, the amount of additional life attributable to adequate exercise, as compared with sedentariness, was one to more than two years.

In Framingham, approximately 5,000 men and women, aged 30 to 62 years and free of clinical evidence of coronary disease at the onset, have been examined regularly since 1949. Coronary disease mortality was subsequently found to be higher in cohorts with indices or measurements consistent with a sedentary life-style. However, physical inactivity did not have the predictive power of the three cardinal risk factors. Kannel and Sorlie reanalyzed the Framingham data for the effects of physical activity on overall mortality and cardiovascular disease mortality. The effect on mortality of being sedentary was rather modest compared to the other risk factors but persisted when these other factors were taken into account. A low correlation was noted between physical activity level and the major risk factors.

Cady's prospective study suggests that poor physical work capacity, as measured by bicycle ergometry in apparently healthy, employed males is an important additional risk factor for MI. This study performed in L.A. County workers is one of the few studies to measure exercise capacity directly rather than to estimate activity level. An adjusted relative risk of 2.2 was found only in men with certain other risk factors present; namely, above-median cholesterol, smoking, above-median SBP, or a combination of these. Similar results were obtained in the Lipid Research Clinic Study using treadmill performance as the measure of exercise capacity related to mortality during follow-up.

POSTMORTEM STUDIES OF PHYSICAL INACTIVITY AS A RISK FACTOR

The results of 207 consecutive autopsies of otherwise healthy white men aged 30 to 60 years who died suddenly and unexpectedly from accident, homicide, or suicide were reported by Spain and Bradess. The autopsies were done in the medical examiner's office of Westchester County, New York. All major branches of the coronary arteries were examined in cross-section at 3-mm intervals. The estimated amount of reduction in luminal diameter by atherosclerotic lesions was used as the basic criterion for grading the degree of coronary atherosclerosis. The occupations of the individuals were determined from available information. All individuals who had a history or autopsy evidence of disease influencing atherosclerosis were excluded. They were separated by occupational title as active or sedentary, with approximately 100 in each group. The authors found no significant differences in the degree of coronary atherosclerosis between those engaged in sedentary occupations and those engaged in physically active occupations.

Mitrani and colleagues reported the results of consecutive specialized cardiovascular autopsies on 172 European-born Jews who were victims of traumatic death. According to personal documents and some information obtained from relatives, 93 had led a sedentary life and 79 were manual workers. Each coronary artery was cross-sectioned at 1-cm distances to measure internal and external diameters. The percentage of narrowing of the vessels was calculated using these measurements. There was no significant difference between the active and inactive groups.

Morris and Crawford sent out requests to approximately 200 British pathologists to complete a standard questionnaire on a series of autopsies performed on men aged 45 to 70 years of age. The pathologists were asked to give macroscopic estimates of the degree of coronary atheroma and fibrosis of the left ventricle and interventricular septum. The last occupation of the deceased was requested and estimated to involve light, active, or heavy physical activity on the basis of job title. In this manner, the results of 3,800 autopsies on individuals dying of causes other than coronary artery disease were gathered from 1954 to 1956. Ischemic myocardial fibrosis and complete coronary occlusion was more common in lighter work occupations, but coronary atheromas and diameter narrowing were of equally high prevalence in all occupational groups.

Measurements were made from radiographs of injected coronary arteries obtained from two necropsy studies at the Radcliff Infirmary, Oxford, England. Ninety-two cases without postmortem evidence of myocardial infarction were used as controls, while a group of 79 had evidence of acute or healed infarction. The right coronary artery was measured in a nondiseased segment, approximately one-half the distance between its origin and the right heart border, and was assumed to reflect the diameter of all the coronary arteries. The physical activity of the last occupation, as determined by job title, was described as light, active, or heavy. The diameter of the right coronary artery in normal subjects increased with age, but the infarction group showed a small diameter of the right coronary artery in each age group. Data were only suggestive that in normal subjects the right coronary artery diameter increased with activity of work, whereas in the infarction group it decreased with the activity of work. These differences were not statistically significant, and no determination of the degree of atherosclerosis was made.

OTHER STUDIES

Psychological Impact. Though frequent comments are made regarding exercise-enhanced psychological well-being and the "runner's high," few scientific studies have been performed in this area. However, it seems that exercise has a tranquilizing effect and increases pain tolerance which may be beneficial in some individuals. Perhaps behavioral scientists should help people become "addicted" to exercise. Exercise addiction has been defined as addiction, of a psychological and/or physiological nature, to a regular habit of exercise, characterized by withdrawal symptoms if not performed every one or two days. These withdrawal symptoms can include anxiety, restlessness, guilt, irritability, tension, bloatedness, muscle twitching, and discomfort. Such an addiction probably does not occur until after two years or more of running. A psychology study group from Montreal, applying stress adaptation models to young males, determined reactivity to psychosocial stressors and found significantly higher baseline prolactin levels, an earlier peak norepinephrine response, and a subjectively lower anxiety score among the trained individuals when evaluated in a contrived setting. Although aerobic fitness may indeed improve stress adaptation and coping behaviors, further work is needed to confirm this.

Recently, running addiction has been considered an analogue of anorexia nervosa. This is probably due to certain behavior similarities, but anorexia nervosa and bulimia are dangerous health problems while excessive exercise is usually self-limiting.

There are many reported psychological benefits of exercise. Few of these have been well-validated. Are those who exercise regularly less depressed or less likely to have drinking, drug dependency, or sleeping disturbances? Or is the personality who is addicted to exercise equally likely to be addicted to other less healthy behavior? Many individuals exercise as a means of relieving stress, and this can be a much healthier means of relieving stress than drinking or drugs. Another interesting consideration is whether exercise can be used to control antisocial behavior. Are aggressive and angry people made more tolerant of society by a regular exercise program? Can sports and exercise be promoted as a means to avoid gang behavior in the lower socioeconomic groups?

Risk Factors. High-density lipoprotein (HDL) cholesterol and HDL/total cholesterol ratio are significantly increased, while serum triglycerides are decreased, particularly if a weight loss occurs. Fasting glucose levels are decreased and it appears that there are favorable alterations in insulin and glucagon responses. Diabetics need less insulin if they maintain a regular exercise program. Also, after a training program, catecholamine levels are lower in response to any stress. The fibrinolytic system is enhanced, and since coronary thrombosis can precipitate ischemia, this seems beneficial in preventing MI.

Cross-sectional studies found runners to have higher levels of high-density lipoprotein (HDL) cholesterol, and prospective studies found high levels of HDL cholesterol to be protective from coronary disease. The main carriers of cholesterol in the blood are the beta lipoproteins (low-density lipoproteins or LDL) and the alpha lipoproteins (high-density lipoproteins). The low-density lipoproteins carry the majority of cholesterol, but HDL levels are important because HDL acts as a vehicle to transport cholesterol from the body. HDL appears to be important for transporting cholesterol from the intimal cells of arteries to the serum and eventually to the bile for excretion from the body. A person with a serum cholesterol of 240 mg% and HDL cholesterol of 90 mg% can have a low risk; if the HDL cholesterol is only 20 mg%, he can have a high risk for coronary disease. The ratio of total cholesterol to HDL cholesterol helps to estimate risk. There is an average risk with a ratio of 5, a high risk with a ratio of 10, and a low risk with a ratio of 3 or 4. Runners often exhibit a ratio of 3, but ratios below 2.5 are not physiologically possible.

There are two apoproteins in HDL, the A1 fraction and the A2 fraction. The A1 fraction, which is found in higher levels in runners, appears to be more important than the A2 in removing cholesterol from the intima of arteries. Leanness, high social status, and being female are also related to high HDL levels. Regular, moderate alcohol consumption may increase HDL levels. Using meta analysis to come to a consensus from over 200 studies evaluating the effect of exercise on blood lipids, Van Tray concluded that increases in HDL and decreases in total cholesterol only occurred when a weight loss was associated with the exercise program.

In a comprehensive review of the relationship between obesity and exercise, Thompson and colleagues pointed out methodological problems in past research including failure to convert levels of activity into caloric figures. As a result, the etiologic contribution of activity level to the development of obesity is unclear; however, exercise affects energy expenditure by altering caloric intake, metabolic rate, and body composition.

Though past studies looking at the effect of regular exercise on HBP have been disappointing, two recent ones have had encouraging results. Duncan et al. evaluated the effects of a 16-week aerobic exercise program on BP and plasma catecholamine levels in 56 patients with baseline diastolic BP of 90 to 140 mm Hg. The exercise group significantly improved their physical fitness and reduced systolic and diastolic blood pressures, compared with controls. To evaluate the relationship between exercise, blood pressure, and plasma catecholamine values, the exercise group was further divided into hyperadrenergic and normoadrenergic subgroups. Reductions in systolic pressures were 6, 10, and 1 for control, normoadrenergic, and hyperadrenergic groups, respectively. Diastolic changes were similar and also significant. Within the hyperadrenergic group, changes in blood pressures were associated with changes in values for plasma catecholamines following training. Their exercise program reduced blood pressure, which was partially mediated by changes in plasma catecholamine levels. Cade et al. studied 105 patients with established diastolic HBP enrolled in an exercise program to examine the effect of aerobic exercise on blood pressure. In four patients, the decrease in mean BP was less than 5 mm Hg; in all others, there was a significant decline. In 58 patients who were not taking drug medication in the preexercise period, mean blood pressure decreased by 15 mm Hg. Of 47 patients receiving drug therapy during the preexercise period, 24 were able to discontinue all medication. Mean BP in this group fell from 117 to 97. In patients still taking antihypertensive drugs, mean pressure decreased from 120 to 104 mm Hg after three months of exercise.

It has been hypothesized that those who maintain an active life-style are also more likely to modify other risk factors. Do those who exercise regularly have better nutritional habits, smoke less, have lower blood pressures, and optimal blood lipids? Do they more often turn to "quackery" and pseudo-health foods? Another important relationship has been that of obesity to exercise status. Do those who exercise regularly more easily control their weight? Does exercise turn out to be an effective means of weight control for many individuals or not? If exercise has "spinovers" into the other areas of healthy behavior modification, then it is something to be more strongly supported. We have all seen individuals who go on an exercise program and greatly alter their other risk factors. However, it is very difficult in the context of a cardiac rehabilitation program to modify other risk factors along with exercise capacity.

Marathon Hypothesis. Currens and White published the autopsy results of Clarence DeMar, a famous long-distance runner who died of rectal carcinoma. He was still actively involved in long-distance running until shortly before his death at age 70. His coronary arteries were found to be two to three times normal size, with some atherosclerotic involvement but no narrowing. Encouraged by this report and his own experience as a science fiction writer, pathologist, and runner, Thomas Bassler produced a series of over 40 "letters to the editor," often in prestigious journals promoting his theory that marathon running protected a person from death from heart disease. Belief in this irresponsible claim could be dangerous for individuals who choose to ignore symptoms of coronary heart disease and run.

DEATH AND OTHER COMPLICATIONS OF EXERCISE

Sudden death has been defined relative to onset of symptoms, i.e., instantaneous or within 1, 6, or 24 hours. Autopsy findings in people dying instantaneously and those dying after 24 hours are different. Deaths occurring within six hours of onset of symptoms include all electrical deaths, and are best defined as "sudden," since no anatomic change usually can be demonstrated. Most sudden deaths that occur during exertion do so within minutes of onset of symptoms. Sudden cardiac death is herein defined as "death occurring unexpectedly within six hours of onset of symptoms in a previously healthy person." The most frequent mode of death is sudden. The incidence of sudden death in the general population is high (15% to 30%) with the majority (80% to 90%) due to cardiovascular causes.

For the purpose of analyzing the relationship of death to physical activity, the types of physical activity can be divided into two: (1) jogging and/or marathon running and (2) other athletic activities, i.e., military training, all types of ball games, swimming, running, wrestling, mountain climbing, yachting.

Coronary Atherosclerosis in Joggers and Marathon Runners. Interest in causes of death in joggers and marathon runners was stimulated when claims were made that "marathon running provides complete immunity from coronary artery disease." Opie in 1975 first reported sudden death secondary to coronary heart disease in a long-distance runner. Since then, over 90 cases of death in joggers and marathon runners have been reported. The most common cause of death has been coronary atherosclerosis (75%). The other reported causes of death have been automobile accidents (9%), amyloidosis and tunnel coronary artery (2% each), and from myocarditis, congenital hypoplastic coronary arteries, heat stroke, floppy mitral valve, hypertrophic cardiomyopathy, and gastrointestinal hemorrhage (1% each). In 6% of cases, the cause of death was unknown.

Siscovik and colleagues reported a study of individuals who were reported by the paramedical immediate response system in Seattle to have had a sudden death. They were compared to a matched sample randomly chosen by a special telephone dialing device. To examine the risk of primary cardiac arrest during vigorous exercise, they interviewed the wives of 133 men without known prior heart disease. They were classified according to their time of cardiac arrest and the amount of their habitual vigorous activity. Among men with low levels of habitual activity, the relative risk of cardiac arrest during exercise compared with that at other times was 56. The risk during exercise among men at the highest level was also elevated but only 5× and their overall risk of cardiac arrest at any time was 40% that of sedentary men. Although the risk of primary cardiac arrest is transiently increased during vigorous exercise, regular exercise decreases the risk of this event.

Waller and Roberts have reported the autopsies of five conditioned runners aged 40 years and over, all with severe coronary atherosclerosis. The series by Thompson et al. described 18 joggers, with five "exercising regularly" for at least one year and nine exercising for three or more years. Fifteen of 18 died suddenly while jogging, and of them, 13 had coronary heart disease. Waller et al. described 10 patients over 30 years of age who ran 1 to 55 miles per week for 1 to 12 years. All had at least one artery severely narrowed by an atherosclerotic plaque and six had MIs.

Thompson and colleagues in California investigated the circumstances of death by considering the medical and activity histories of 18 individuals who died during or immediately after jogging and found coronary disease to be the most common cause. As a sequel to his study of jogging deaths in California, Thompson has focused on Rhode Island. From 1975 through 1980, 12 men died during jogging and the cause of death in 11 was coronary heart disease. From a telephone survey, he found that 7.4% of adult male Rhode Islanders jogged at least twice a week. Thompson et al. calculated the incidence of death during jogging for men between 30 and 64 years to be one per 7,620 joggers, or approximately one death per 396,000 man-hours of jogging. Although the death rate is seven times the estimated death rate from CHD during more sedentary activity, the numbers are too small to draw any conclusions, since only 12 deaths occurred in six years.

Vander and colleagues conducted a five-year retrospective survey of fatal and nonfatal cardiovascular events that occurred in community recreation centers. Fifty-eight facilities reported 30 nonfatal and 38 fatal events. There was one nonfatal and one fatal event every 1,124,200 and 887,526 hours of participation, respectively. Though exercise contributes to sudden death in susceptible persons, its rare occurrence demonstrates that the risk of exercise is small and suggests that routine screening is not justified. This is confirmed by the excellent review of this subject by McManus and colleagues.

What is the expected level of cardiovascular deaths among runners while running on the basis of chance alone? This is an important question because it is frequently assumed that exercise is the cause when a person dies of cardiovascular causes during recreational running. Koplan used data from the National Center of Health Statistics and found that approximately 100 cardiovascular deaths per year in runners in the United States can be predicted on a purely temporal basis. This is certainly higher than the number of deaths reported.

Morales and colleagues have reported three healthy individuals who died suddenly during strenuous exercise and were found to have a triad of pathological findings. There were two males aged 34 and 54 and one female 17 years of age. The pathological triad was muscle bridging of the left anterior descending coronary artery, poor circulation to the posterior surface of the heart, and septal fibrosis. The angiographic finding of a coronary artery that passes underneath a band of myocardium is not that unusual, and it has been debated whether it has functional significance. Some studies of coronary blood flow have suggested that the constriction of a coronary artery by this myocardial band during systole results in decreased flow; however, most of coronary flow takes place during diastole. In regard to the second finding, there is great variability in the coronary artery distribution on the posterior surface of the heart around the crux and the posterior margin of the septum. In the most common situation, the right coronary artery branches into a posterior descending artery that passes down the septum giving off septal perforators. Often though, there are normal variations where the left circumflex provides this branch or there are only small arteries in the area. Lastly, septal fibrosis could be due to chronic ischemia. These anatomic findings could be purely coincidental.

Noakes and colleagues presented four marathon runners with autopsy-proven coronary atherosclerosis. The first individual was a 44-year-old white male who, after 14 months of training, had completed seven marathons in under four hours. He suddenly dropped dead halfway through a marathon. At autopsy he was found to have an old anteroseptal myocardial infarction and 90% lesions of his left anterior descending and circumflex coronary arteries. The second was a 41-year-old male who, after two years of running, had a symptomatic myocardial infarction. After release from the hospital, he returned to training and ran in five marathons. He was hospitalized with unstable angina, and coronary angiography was performed. He was found to have severe triple-vessel coronary artery disease; while waiting for surgery, he died suddenly. The last two cases were 36- and 27-year-old athletes who had completed multiple marathons and were killed accidently. Both had left anterior descending coronary artery lesions at autopsy; the younger a 50% and the older a 90% lesion.

Virmani reported findings in 30 joggers or marathon runners who died non-traumatic deaths. Twenty-two men died with severe atherosclerosis; their ages ranged from 18 to 54 years (mean 36 years). The history of jogging was well-documented in 18 patients who ran 7 to 105 miles per week (mean 33) and had been running 1 to 28 years (mean 10). Three were marathon runners, and the other 12 had been jogging for at least six months. Review of records revealed a family history of heart disease in nine, systemic hypertension in nine, and a total cholesterol >200 mg% in seven. None were diabetic, and smoking history was uncertain. A history of CHD were present in eight (27%); of these, five were from a retrospective review of medical records. Nineteen died suddenly and three had a history of prolonged chest pain. In six patients, death occurred soon after jogging, and two were found dead in bed. At autopsy, the heart weight ranged from 345 to 600 gm (mean 432). In 16 patients, the heart weight was increased beyond the normal range. Twenty-two patients died of severe coronary atherosclerosis. Of the four major arteries examined for severe atherosclerosis, only one artery was involved in nine patients (41%), two coronary arteries in nine (41%), three and four coronary arteries in one each. Thrombi were noted in six (27%) patients. The most frequent single artery involved was the left anterior descending, and the most frequent combination was the left anterior descending and right coronary arteries.

Virmani et al. found that of a total of 70 coronary arteries examined in 20 joggers, 34 (49%) were severely narrowed, and the average number of coronary arteries greater than 75% narrowed was 1.65 per jogger. Those with a history of coronary heart disease had a similar extent of coronary atherosclerosis as those without such histories (1.7 versus 1.6 coronary arteries narrowed per patient). In 6 of the 22 with severe coronary atherosclerosis, an isolated healed MI was present; acute MI with or without healed MI was present in 8. A total of 14 (64%) of 22 who died of severe coronary atherosclerosis had MIs found at autopsy.

Virmani et al. studied another 11 male joggers with a mean age of 41 years (range 19–59 years). Sudden death occurred while jogging in 9 of 11 men. Available risk factor history was as follows: two had hypercholesterolemia, one had systemic hypertension, and one had family history of premature CHD. Only two had a history of prior cardiac disease: one had angina, and one had undergone left ventricular aneurysmectomy with coronary bypass surgery. A 43-year-old man had been jogging 50 miles per week for five to six years and had participated in several marathons. His heart weighed 600 gm, an acute MI was found, and there was a >75% atherosclerotic narrowing of the three major coronary arteries and also a thrombus in the left circumflex. Seven of the 11 had at least two vessels severely narrowed, one had one-vessel disease, and the other two had been described as having severe coronary atherosclerosis. Acute and/or healed MIs were present in 6 of 10.

Causes of Death During or Soon After Exercise Other Than Jogging or Marathon Running. Opie et al. reported sudden death in 21 athletes, 13 of whom took part in rugby or soccer. Eighteen were thought to be caused by CHD. The Squash Rackets Association estimated that there may be 2.5 million people in the United Kingdom playing squash once or more a month. The circumstances surrounding 60 sudden deaths associated with squash playing were described by Northcote and colleagues in Glasgow. The mean age of those who died was 46 years (range 22–66 years). They were able to gather a series of 89 sudden deaths associated with squash that occurred between October, 1976, and February, 1984, by examining press reports and by a prospective mail survey of sports centers and squash clubs throughout the United Kingdom. In 60 cases, we obtained sufficient information to investigate the death in detail.

Maron et al. reported sudden unexpected death in 29 highly conditioned, competitive athletes aged 13 to 30 years (mean 19) drawn from news media reports, the registry of the cardiovascular division of the Armed Forces Institute of Pathology and pathology branch of the NIH. All had been active, highly conditioned members of an organized athletic team for at least two years. The type of sport varied, but basketball and football were most common. In 28 of the 29 athletes, death occurred suddenly without warning, and was virtually instantaneous, occurring on the playing field in 13. One athlete survived 12 hours after collapse.

In 22 athletes, death occurred during or soon after severe exertion, in 2 after mild exertion, and in 5 during sedentary activities. Structural cardiovascular abnormalities were found in 28 athletes and were the cause of sudden death in 22. Of these, the most common anatomic abnormality was hypertrophic cardiomyopathy (HC), which was present in 14. HC was defined as asymmetric septal hypertrophy, with marked ventricular septal disorganization in another two. Four athletes had anomalous origin of the left coronary artery from the right sinus of Valsalva, including one patient with hypertrophic cardiomyopathy. Four athletes had concentric left ventricular hypertrophy, two with and two without disorganization. Three athletes (24 to 28 years of age) had severe coronary atherosclerosis. Two died of aortic rupture, both had evidence of cystic medial necrosis, and one had Marfan syndrome.

In six athletes, the cardiovascular abnormality was considered as probable evidence of cardiovascular disease: five had hypertrophied hearts (420–530 gm), one had mild prolapse of anterior and posterior mitral leaflets, one had normal heart weight with hypoplastic right coronary artery. Several died of coronary atherosclerosis, one after running a pass pattern in a professional football game. In this individual, they hypothesized that a blow to the chest while being tackled caused a hemorrhage into a plaque in the left anterior descending coronary artery. Several others had congenital anomalies of the coronary arteries.

All of these events were extremely unusual, and it would be difficult to screen for them. It is known that athletes frequently have abnormal ECGs and even echocardiographic hypertrophy. In addition, they have a higher prevalence of false positive exercise tests. However, screening for lipid abnormalities would be a wise public health measure regardless of a lack of specificity, and it would be advisable to obtain an echocardiogram on an athlete with symptoms or signs of a hypertrophic cardiomyopathy.

Vermani et al. reviewed records of 32 individuals who died suddenly while engaging in either military training (6) or in other sports activity: basketball (6), running (8), racketball (2), volleyball (2), tennis (2), swimming (2), football (2), and one each in gymnastics and bowling. Their ages ranged from 14 to 60 with a mean age of 28 years; 31 were males and one was female. The anatomic abnormalities were varied: coronary disease in eight, idiopathic myocarditis in four, congenital coronary abnormalities in three, hypertrophic cardiomyopathy in two, tunnel coronary artery in two, floppy mitral valve in two, intramural coronary thickening in two, and one each with rheumatic heart disease and aortic dissection. Four had left ventricular hypertrophy of unknown etiology (420- to 600-gm hearts) and were 17, 20, 21, and 32 years old. All died during exertion. Three had sickle cell trait, died while running, and were only 17, 20, and 22 years old.

The cause of death in Virmani's subjects is markedly different from Maron et al., probably because symptomatic individuals are excluded from military service and none was highly trained, whereas Maron's population included only highly trained athletes. Virmani's subjects had a wide age range with only 25 being 30 or younger, while Maron's athletes were 13 to 30 years, with a mean of 19 years. Prevalence of CHD is directly related to age. This has been confirmed in other studies of runners older than 40: CHD is their most common cause of death, and they usually have had symptoms of CHD prior to the event.

Effect of Environment. An important factor in sudden death among athletes and joggers is the climate in which exercise is being performed. Serious thermal injuries are preventable, and the American College of Sports Medicine recommends that long-distance races should not be conducted in temperatures that exceed 28°C (82.4°F).

The physiologic response to exercise is hyperthermia. The amount of heat generated is directly related to the intensity of exercise. The body is only 25% efficient in converting calories generated into external work, and the remaining 75% of energy is converted into heat. Therefore, a large amount of heat must be lost by the body to prevent raising the core temperature.

If no heat were being lost by the body, the core temperature would increase by 1°C every five minutes. It is the efficient mechanisms of thermoregulation of the body that prevent hypothermia. These mechanisms include sweating and heat loss by radiation and by conversion. The factors that prevent heat loss are high ambient temperature, high humidity, dehydration (which prevents cutaneous vasodilation), extremes of age, debilitation, excessive clothing and drugs that may impair thermoregulation.

The spectrum of heat injury includes three well-recognized syndromes: (1) heat cramps, (2) heat exhaustion, and (3) heat stroke. Heat cramps are painful spasms in the muscles in use, while heat exhaustion is characterized by fatigue, hyperventilation, headache, lightheadedness, nausea, and muscle cramps. Patients with heat exhaustion sweat and have chills in spite of the core temperature's being high.

Heat stroke, the most serious of thermal injuries, is characterized by an altered state of consciousness that may progress rapidly to unconsciousness and seizure activity. The heat stroke patient is hot, flushed, and has dry skin because sweating has stopped. Dehydration and circulatory collapse soon follow. Body temperature is usually above 41°C (106°F) and the laboratory tests show hemoconcentration, leukocytosis, azotemia, acidosis, and abnormal liver function tests and muscle enzymes. Treatment includes submersion in ice water and IV heparin to stop fibrinolysis.

At autopsy, the findings usually are nonspecific and consist of petechial hemorrhages in the skin, mucous membranes, brain, lung, and heart. The hemorrhages in the heart are most pronounced in the epicardial and endocardial region, especially on the left side of the ventricular septum. Damage to myocardial filaments and intercalated discs have been described by electron microscopy in patients with malignant hyperthermia induced by anesthetic agents.

Summary of Exercise Related Death in the Athlete.   Cardiovascular diseases responsible for sudden unexpected death in highly conditioned athletes are largely related to the age of the patient. In most young competitive athletes (<35 years of age), sudden death is due to congenital cardiovascular disease. Hypertrophic cardiomyopathy appears to be the most common cause of such deaths, accounting for about half of the sudden deaths in young athletes. Other cardiovascular abnormalities that appear to be less frequent in young athletes include congenital coronary artery anomalies, ruptured aorta (due to cystic medial necrosis), idiopathic left ventricular hypertrophy, and coronary atherosclerosis. Rare causes of sudden death include myocarditis, mitral valve prolapse, aortic valve stenosis, and sarcoidosis. Cardiovascular disease in young athletes is usually unsuspected during life, and most athletes who die suddenly have experienced no cardiac symptoms. In only about 25% of those competitive athletes who die suddenly is underlying cardiovascular disease detected or suspected before participation, and rarely is the correct clinical diagnosis made. In contrast, in older athletes (≥35 years of age), sudden death is usually due to coronary artery disease.

Noninvasive screening procedures are currently available that can detect many subjects at risk of sudden death but with an uncertain specificity. However, although some potentially lethal diseases can be excluded by a relatively simple screening program, other diseases require expensive procedures, such as echocardiography, exercise testing, and cardiac catheterization. This means that the sensitivity of detecting diseases leading to sudden death increases in proportion to the financial resources that can be applied to the screening program. Thus, when a screening program designed to identify all cardiac diseases that have the potential to cause sudden death is planned by a community, school, or nonprofessional athletic team, the costs will be prohibitive. The practicality of applying a community or school screening program can be questioned because of the very low incidence of sudden unexpected death in young healthy individuals. Comprehensive screening programs are confined to individuals or organizations with adequate financial resources. Less expensive, limited screening can be undertaken by individuals or groups to identify some subjects at risk of sudden death during athletic competition. An important consideration is the education of the team physician. Symptoms and family history of sudden death or syncope should not be overlooked. However, due to high vagal tone, young athletes often faint. In addition, ECG abnormalities, third heart sounds, and systolic murmurs are common.

The normal heart, even when subjected to vigorous forms of stress, is protected from lethal arrhythmias except in unusual conditions such as profound electrolyte derangement, thermal stress, or adverse drug reactions. Victims of sudden death almost always have underlying heart disease. Coronary artery disease is found in about 80% of victims of sudden cardiac death; other abnormalities, such as cardiomyopathy, valvular heart disease, or primary arrhythmic disorders, may also cause unexpected cardiac arrest. Although exertion-related death appears to be confined to patients with structural heart disease, a third of these individuals may be asymptomatic.

Mechanisms underlying sudden death in cardiac patients include ventricular fibrillation and myocardial ischemia. Ventricular fibrillation is the arrhythmia usually underlying the sudden cardiac death syndrome, particularly in exertion-related events. In following patients resuscitated from out-of-hospital ventricular fibrillation, Cobb recognized three major clinical settings in which ventricular fibrillation occurs: (1) as a complication of typical acute myocardial infarction; (2) as a manifestation of transient myocardial ischemia, especially during or after exertion; and (3) as an event unassociated with ischemia and occurring while sedentary. In the latter setting, ventricular fibrillation most often occurs in patients with prior myocardial infarction and left ventricular dysfunction.

Transient ischemia is a plausible cause for most episodes of exertion-related cardiac arrest in patients with coronary disease. In assessing resuscitated patients who collapsed during or after exertion, Cobb found that compared to persons with nonexertion-related cardiac arrest, these patients had less limitations and more often had no recognized preceding heart disease. In addition, warning symptoms were noted in only about 25%, and less than one-third had new Q-waves. These patients have few episodes of ventricular arrhythmia during ambulatory monitoring.

Although there has been no large, prospective assessment of the role of exertion in precipitating cardiac arrest, some relevant information is available. In patients treated by the paramedic system in Seattle, 36 (11%) of 316 consecutive victims had collapsed during or immediately after exertion or stress. This incidence is similar to that of 17% of 150 patients reported in Miami. In autopsy registries, the incidence of exertion-related cardiac arrest was reported to be 10% to 30% of all sudden deaths. In studies of unexpected sudden death in younger persons, cardiac arrest commonly was associated with physical activity.

In a prospective five-year survey by Hinkle involving approximately 270,000 men, 42% of the sudden coronary deaths occurred in persons without previously recognized coronary disease. About one-third of these deaths occurred within minutes of engaging in activities known to be associated with myocardial ischemia, or in the setting of suspected sympathetic nervous system stimulation. In a report from Cooper's Clinic of exercise in a predominantly normal population of middle-aged persons, one cardiac arrest occurred in 375,000 person-hours of exercise. In the Framingham Study, there was a significant association between the mode of death and activity; sudden death occurred more often in the setting of physical activity.

A recent report of 133 men who experienced cardiac arrest in Seattle estimated that the incidence of cardiac arrest was 5 to 56 times greater during high-intensity exercise than at other times. The persons considered in that study were aged 25 to 75 years and were without previously recognized cardiovascular disease. The estimated incidence of cardiac arrest during vigorous activity ranged from one case per 137,000 hours to one per 4.7 milli[   ] at risk.

These studies serve to point out that physical exertion may precipit[   ] diac arrest in the "normal" population and that prior recognition of [   ] tible individuals has not been possible. Exercise-induced cardiac arre[   ] real phenomenon, particularly in patients with known heart disease. However, the majority of sudden deaths are temporally associated with routine activities of daily life and not with exercise. Therefore, the number of deaths due to strenuous physical exertion is relatively modest. Exertion-related cardiac arrest is usually due to ventricular fibrillation or tachycardia, and exercise may increase its risk by 100 times.

COMPLICATIONS OTHER THAN DEATH

There are numerous risks for amateur and professional athletes. Heat stroke can be avoided by taking precautions for humid, hot environments including adequate oral replacement of dilute electrolyte solutions. There is no place for fluid restriction in order to limit sweating. Runners can have heat stroke and still be actively sweating, although it was once taught that heat stroke was always preceded by a cessation of sweating. Hematuria after a run can be due to bladder trauma, and proteinuria can even be normal. Diarrhea and other gastrointestinal complaints are fairly common in runners during and after events. Numerous episodes of anaphylaxis thought to be exercise-induced have been reported. Diagnosis by the findings of bronchospasm and urticaria is important because treatment with epinephrine and antihistamines can be lifesaving. This usually occurs in individuals that previously had an anaphylactic reaction to shellfish.

Orthopedic Injuries. The popular concern with fitness is responsible for both general practitioners and sports-medicine specialists noticing an increase in sports-related injuries among weekend and after-work athletes. Basketball and soccer leagues, ski vacations, evening runs, dance classes, and tennis games cause injuries once found chiefly among professional and college athletes.

The Center for Sports Medicine in San Francisco recently compiled statistics on over 10,000 injuries treated at the center. They found that nine activities—basketball, dance, football, gymnastics, running, skiing, tennis, soccer, and figure skating—accounted for nearly three-fourths of the injuries. More than two-thirds of the injuries were caused by overuse—problems such as shin splints and tendinitis that develop from a repetitive trauma to muscle and bone. Tennis, aerobic dance, and running frequently cause such problems. The remaining injuries were acute ones, incidents that happen instantly, such as a sprained ankle. These tend to occur in skiing, football, basketball, and soccer. Injuries to the knee cause the most visits, and skiers have the most knee problems. Aerobic dance causes more fractures than any other recreational activity. Many problems stem from acute injuries that occurred in the past. Unlike football injuries, most of the basketball injuries occur in participants over 25 years of age.

Education regarding how recreational injuries happen and how to treat them is an important step in prevention. Treatment may include weight lifting for rehabilitation, shoe inserts to correct irregularities in stride or foot strike, ultrasound and electrical stimulation for muscle tears and stiffness, and compression and icing to control swelling. Rest, ice, compression, and elevation is still the best treatment for all acute injuries. There has been a trend toward active rehabilitation. For instance, to treat a sprained ankle, a program that focuses on muscle strengthening is used because if ligaments do not heal well, a tear may become a persistent problem. Prolonged rest can cause a decrease in muscle mass around the ankle, resulting in a loss of strength. The muscles lose their ability to move quickly and stabilize the ankle. Instead, strengthening surrounding muscles will avoid atrophy. In many cases, the strengthened muscles will compensate for the deficient ligaments, making the joint stable for further activities.

Cardiac Enzyme Rises Postexercise.   Because of exercise-induced cardiac enzyme rises, it can be difficult to evaluate previously sedentary runners for symptoms suggestive of coronary artery disease as well as treating endurance athletes for overexertion syndrome. Abnormal levels of cardiac enzymes have been reported in people after prolonged strenuous exercise, which resemble patients with acute MI. Elevations in the MB-isoenzyme of creatine kinase (CK-MB), widely regarded as a sensitive and specific marker for acute myocardial damage, are quantitatively similar in asymptomatic marathon runners after competition to those in patients with Q-wave MI.

Studies confirm the presence of elevated cardiac enzyme levels, including CK-MB, in endurance-trained athletes after competition. The demonstration of elevated serum CK-MB levels is a sensitive and specific index of myocardial injury. A diagnostic dilemma exists when such athletes are seen with heat injury or circulatory collapse after competition. If the sensitivity and specificity of serum CK-MB levels are about 95%, it is worrisome that prolonged strenuous exercise leads to silent myocardial ischemia or infarction. When athletes in training are seen with cardiorespiratory symptoms unrelated to acute exertion, cardiac isoenzyme levels can remain chronically elevated similar to patients with myocardial injury. Concentrations of CK-MB in runners may exceed those used for diagnosis of MI. Data on serum CK-MB concentrations in asymptomatic runners lower the specificity of CK-MB for myocardial injury from 95% to less than 50%.

Siegal has performed thallium scintigraphy and cardiac enzyme determinations in marathon runners immediately after completion of a race. Since normal images are seen despite cumulative CK-MB levels similar to patients with Q-wave MI, this strongly suggests that the cardiac isoenzymes arise from a noncardiac source. Simon and Steinhaus have reported that skeletal muscle injured repeatedly by overuse is more likely to produce the CK isoenzyme that usually only comes from myocardial muscle.

Exercise-Induced Bronchospasm.   Patients with asthma develop exercise-induced bronchospasm (EIB) during exercise, but many mild asthmatics experience this phenomenon as the sole manifestation of asthma. Exercise-induced asthma is defined as a response to exercise in which there is a fall in the forced expiratory volume in the first second (FEV1) or peak expiratory flow rate of more than 10% from preexercise levels. The symptoms begin five to six minutes after beginning exercise. Complaints are chest tightness, shortness of breath, wheezing, and cough. The most severe symptoms usually occur within 15 minutes after completion of exercise. Cough can be more prominent and be the only manifestation of exercise-induced bronchospasm. Postexercise symptoms usually last from 30–60 minutes without treatment. EIB does not lead to status asthmaticus. There are several variations of typical EIB. One is the ability to "run through" exercise bronchospasm and the other is the so-called "refractory period." Experienced individuals with EIB learn that if they develop chest tightness after the first five to six minutes of exercise and they continue to exercise, at cessation of exercise, they will not experience typical bronchospastic symptoms. The refractory period is the development of a diminished response when exercise is repeated at intervals of less than two hours. Thus, preliminary calisthenics and light running can reduce or eliminate EIB. Unfortunately, a refractory period does not always occur. The type, intensity, and duration of physical activity influences EIB. Running causes more severe symptoms than does bicycling, swimming, or walking. Exercise that lasts less than two minutes, even if strenuous and intense, does not induce EIB, perhaps because of the release of endogenous catecholamines. Exercise that lasts approximately six minutes appears to cause maximum postexercise bronchospasm, while exercise lasting longer than 8–10 minutes does not increase the severity of EIB. The most important factor in determining the bronchospastic response produced by different types of physical exertion are the level of ventilation and the temperature and humidity of the environment. Strenuous exercise in a warm, humid environment produces the least amount of EIB, whereas that which takes place in a cold, dry environment produces the most. Swimming induces the least EIB while cross-country skiing causes the most. The increased ventilation caused by exercise increases the volume of air presented to the airways that must be warmed and humidified on inspiration. This results in increased respiratory heat and water loss that cools the airways and leads to hyperosmolarity in the airway mucosa. The resulting physiologic pulmonary function changes are identical to those occurring in spontaneous asthma. Expiratory flow rates are decreased and the airway resistance is increased. Measuring FEV1 after submaximal treadmill exercise is the best screening technique.

Management measures designed to decrease airway cooling and premedications can improve and even prevent EIB. The greatest protection is afforded by inhaled beta-adrenergic medications. Susceptible individuals should take two puffs of a beta agonist approximately 15 minutes before beginning exercise. Beta agonists have been shown to inhibit or totally prevent EIB in 90% of patients. The aerosolized route is the preferred method of administration because of the rapid onset of action as well as decreased systemic side effects such as muscle tremor. Cromolyn by the inhaled route is also effective in preventing EIB. Unlike beta agonists, Cromolyn is not a bronchodilator but appears to prevent the release of chemical mediators from mast cells or alter the response of airways to cooling and drying. Some individuals who do not respond to either medication alone may get better results with both drugs given in combination. Inhaled anticholinergic medications do not appear to consistently prevent bronchoconstriction induced by exercise and cold air. Acute administration of corticosteroid drugs by the inhaled route are of no proven benefit. Long-term administration of steroids via aerosol, however, may in part inhibit EIB. Calcium channel-blocking drugs appear to have some effect in EIB and are presently undergoing clinical trials. The following may help individuals with exercise-induced asthma: (1) take two puffs of a beta-adrenergic agonist 15 minutes before exercise. Cromolyn sodium may be used as an alternative, since certain medications are banned by athletic organizations; (2) briefly warm up with moderate exercise for one to two minutes before vigorous exercise; (3) if cough, wheezing, or chest tightness develops with exercise, an attempt should be made to "run through" the symptoms; (4) when exercising in cold, dry, environmental conditions, breathe through a scarf or mask; and (5) consider alternate forms of exercise in warm, humid environments such as swimming or other indoor sports during cold months.

NATIONAL EXERCISE HEALTH OBJECTIVES REGARDING EXERCISE

In 1980, the United States Public Health Service published a report titled, "Promoting Health/Preventing Disease: Objectives for the Nation." This document presented a series of goals and objectives formulated in each of 15 priority areas of concern for health promotion and disease prevention. These goals and objectives represent the consensus of opinion of more than 500 individuals and organizational representatives with expertise in the 15 areas. The areas addressed included: (1) high blood pressure; (2) family planning; (3) pregnancy and infant health; (4) immunization; (5) sexually transmitted diseases; (6) toxic agents and radiation; (7) occupational safety and health; (8) accidents and injuries; (9) dental health; (10) infectious diseases; (11) smoking; (12) alcohol and drugs; (13) improved nutrition; (14) physical fitness and exercise; and (15) control of stress and violent behavior.

For each of the fifteen priority areas, the report briefly outlines the nature and extent of the specific problem area, describes and evaluates available measures, and states national objectives. The objectives are categorized as: (1) improved health status; (2) reduced risk factors; (3) increased public or professional awareness; (4) improved services or protection; and (5) improved surveillance or evaluation systems. This last component was a directive to include a means to quantify the activity status of Americans.

In the establishment of the objectives in the areas of physical fitness and exercise, there were few data sets that provided accurate information on the existing fitness levels and exercise habits of the American population. National estimates of the physical fitness status of children and youths have been collected for more than 25 years, but there is no data on adults. Without a representative data base, it would be impossible to assess changes in the population as a result of various intervention strategies. To fill this void, the National Surveys (NHANES and NHIS) were requested to add a physical fitness and exercise component to their existing test batteries.

Specific objectives for the exercise and physical fitness priority area for 1990 included the following:

1. Improved health status: though increased levels of physical fitness may contribute to reduced disease rates, no specific objectives were developed.
2. Reduced risk factors: (a) the proportion of children and adolescents (ages 10–17) participating regularly in appropriate activities that can be carried into adulthood (sports other than baseball and football) should be greater than 90%; (b) greater than 60% should be participating in daily school physical education programs; (c) more that 60% of adults 18–65 should be participating regularly in vigorous exercise (in 1978, the estimate was 35%); (d) 50% of adults 65 years and older should be engaging in regular physical exercise (in 1975, about 36% took regular walks).
3. Increased public awareness: (a) more than 70% of adults should be able to identify the appropriate type of exercise needed; (b) more than 50% of primary care doctors should include an exercise history as part of their initial exam (the specific activity scale of Goldman or some similar tool).
4. Improved services/protection: (a) more than 25% of companies with more than 500 employees should offer sponsored physical fitness programs (in 1979, it was 2.5%).
5. Improved surveillance and evaluation services: (a) methodology for assessing physical fitness of 70% of our children; (b) data should be available to evaluate the health effects (positive and negative) of exercise programs; (c) data should be available to evaluate effects of job performance and health care costs; (d) data should be available for monitoring natural trends and patterns of participation in physical activity (random dialing, use of parks, tennis courts, and other surveys measuring the usage of exercise facilities).

Numerous questions remain regarding exercise and health. For instance, what is the relationship of activity status to other risk factors? Do those who exercise regularly have better nutritional habits, smoke less, have lower blood pressures and have lower lipids? How are exercise patterns related to alcohol ingestion and sleeping disorders? What knowledge, background, or factors motivate individuals to maintain a healthy life-style? Is activity related to educational and/or economic level? Does peer pressure to exercise or not exercise operate in the different socioeconomic groups? Is mental health better or worse in those who exercise? Are those who exercise less depressed? Is productivity greater in those who exercise regularly? Do they have less sick days? Do those who exercise at the job have a greater loyalty to their employers? Is usage of the health care system greater or less in those who exercise? Is the quality of life better for those who exercise? Is their dyadic adjustment and sexual activity better? Does a fear of exercise secondary to experiences or misconceptions affect exercise habits? Do parents encourage children to maintain an exercise program? Do those who exercise use the health care system more or less? Are they hypochondriacal? Do they turn more to quackery and "health foods?" All these questions could provide support for the exercise hypothesis and help find out why and how people comply with personal exercise programs and if there are adverse effects.

Health Care Utilization. It has been hypothesized that individuals who maintain a more active life-style utilize health care services much less than others. On the other hand, the increase in exercise-induced orthopedic injuries may have resulted in an "army of walking wounded' who stream into the offices of physicians. Where does the truth lie? Most likely somewhere in between. The neurotic weekend athlete is most likely an extreme; he or she may be a hypochondriacal individual who would be frequently consulting with a number of physicians even if he/she did not exercise.

CONCLUSION

Though many of us exercise and prescribe exercise for health reasons, there is no definitive evidence that this is effective in the prevention or management of coronary heart disease. The association between physical inactivity and the underlying atherosclerotic process is modest compared with other factors such as serum cholesterol, cigarette smoking, and hypertension. An inversely proportional association between the level of activity and degree of atherosclerosis has not been demonstrated. Physical inactivity does not necessarily precede the atherosclerotic process. However, most epidemiologic studies performed have found physical inactivity to be a risk factor. Sometimes physical inactivity has not been determined to be an independent risk factor because other risk factors and markers concentrated in the inactive group. The ability of physical inactivity or exercise capacity to predict coronary events has been reproducible when applied to different populations, but the consistency of the exercise hypothesis has not been documented in autopsy studies.

Studies point out that physical exertion may precipitate cardiac arrest in the "normal" population and that prior recognition of susceptible individuals has not been possible. Exercise-induced cardiac arrest is a real phenomenon, particularly in patients with known heart disease. However, the majority of sudden deaths are temporally associated with routine activities of daily life and not with exercise. Therefore, the number of deaths due to strenuous physical exertion is relatively modest. Exertion-related cardiac arrest is usually due to ventricular fibrillation or tachycardia, and exercise may increase its risk by 100 times in patients with underlying heart disease.

Recent studies of primary prevention support the life-style of regular physical activity. Regular exercise most likely decreases one's risk for coronary heart disease and helps to decrease other risk factors. The inclusion of regular moderate exercise in one's life-style makes good sense for many reasons. It can improve the quality of life by lessening fatigue and by increasing physical performance in those to whom such goals are important. The recommendation of a moderate exercise habit can help people pay attention to their health and make the changes necessary to lessen coronary risk factors. The most significant advances in public health have been in the prevention, not the treatment, of disease. The current public interest in physical fitness may be embarrassingly more effective than is the medical profession in making the public take responsibility for maintaining health.

BIBLIOGRAPHY

Adelstein AM: Some aspects of cardiovascular mortality in South Africa. *Br J Prev Soc Med* 1963;17:29.

Affairs of the Council for Science: Exercise programs for the elderly. *JAMA* 1984;252:544–546.

Anderson SD: Is there a unifying hypothesis for exercise-induced asthma? *J Allergy Clin Immunol* 1984;73:660–665.

Anderson SD: Exercise-induced asthma. *Chest* 1985;87:191S–194S.

Balady GJ, Cadigan JB, Ryan TJ: Electrocardiogram of the athlete: An analysis of 289 professional football players. *Am J Cardiol* 1984;53:1339–1343.

Ballantyne FC, Clark RS, Simpson HS, et al: The effect of moderate physical exercise on the plasma lipoprotein subfractions of male survivors of myocardial infarction. *Circulation* 1982;65:913–918.

Bar-Yishay E, Godfrey S: Exercise and hyperventilation induced asthma. *Clin Rev Allergy* 1985;3:441–461.

Barold SS, Hanss RJ, Falkoff MD, et al: Exercise-induced myocardial infarction due to coronary thrombosis. *Am Heart J* 1985;3:590–593.

Blackburn H, Taylor HL, Keys A: Coronary heart disease in seven countries. *Circulation* 1970;41:154.

Blair SN, Goodyear NN, Gibbons LW, et al: Physical fitness and incidence of hypertension in healthy normotensive men and women. *JAMA* 1984;252:487–490.

Blair SN, Haskell WL, Ho P, et al: Assessment of habitual physical activity by a seven-day recall in a community survey and controlled experiments. *Am J Epidemiol* 1985;122:794–804.

Blair SN, Wilbur CS, Crowder HJ: A public health intervention model for work-site health promotion. *JAMA* 1986;255:921–926.

Bleecker ER: Exercise-induced asthma. *Chest* 1984;5:109–119.

Blumenthal JA: Obligatory running and anorexia nervosa. *JAMA* 1985;253:979–980.

Blumenthal JA, Rose S, Chang JL: Anorexia nervosa and exercise implications from recent findings. *Sports Med* 1985;2:237–247.

Breslow L, Buell P: Mortality from coronary heart disease and physical activity of work in California. *J Chronic Dis* 1960;11:421.

Brunner D: The influence of physical activity on incidence and prognosis of ischemic heart disease. *Prev Ischemic Heart Dis* 1966;1.

Cade R, Mars D, Wagemaker H, et al: Effect of aerobic exercise training on patients with systemic arterial hypertension. *Am J Med* 1984;77:785–790.

Caldwell JE, Ahonen E, Mousiainen U: Differential effects of sauna-, diuretic-, and exercise-induced hypohydration. *J Appl Physiol: Respirat Environ Exerc Physiol* 1984;57:1018–1023.

Cantwell JD: Hypertrophic cardiomyopathy and the athlete. *Physician Sports Med* 1984;12:111–121.

Casale TB, Keahey TM, Kaliner M: Exercise-induced anaphylactic syndromes. *JAMA* 1986;255:2049–2053.

Chan KL, Davies RA, Chambers RJ: Coronary thrombosis and subsequent lysis after a marathon. *J Am Coll Cardiol* 1984;4:1322–1325.

Cobb LA, Weaver WD: Exercise: A risk for sudden death in patients with coronary heart disease. *J Am Coll Cardiol* 1986;7:215–219.

Coelho A, Pallileo E, Ashley W, et al: Tachyarrhythmias in young athletes. *J Am Coll Cardiol* 1986;7:237–243.

Costas R, Garcia-Palmieri MR, Nazario E, et al: Relation of lipids, weight and physical activity to incidence of coronary heart disease. *Am J Cardiol* 1978;42:653.

Coyle EF, Martin WH, Bloomfield SA, et al: Effects of detraining on responses to submaximal exercise. *J Appl Physiol* 1985;59:853–859.

Crouse SF, Hooper PL, Atterbom HA, et al: Zinc ingestion and lipoprotein values in sedentary and endurance-trained men. *JAMA* 1984;252:785–787.

Crow RS, Rautaharju PM, Prineas RJ, et al: Risk factors, exercise fitness and electrocardiographic response to exercise in 12,866 men at high risk of symptomatic coronary heart disease. *Am J Cardiol* 1986;57:1075–1082.

Currens JH, White PD: Half a century of running. *N Engl J Med* 1961;265:988.

Dressendorfer RH, Wade CE, Scaff JH: Renal function during short-term and prolonged strenuous exercise in coronary heart disease patients. *J Cardiac Rehabil* 1983;3:575–582.

Epstein L, Miller GJ, Stitt FW, et al: Vigorous exercise in leisure time, coronary risk factors, and resting electrocardiogram in middle-aged male civil servants. *Arch Intern Med* 1976;38:403.

Epstein SE, Maron BJ: Sudden death and the competitive athlete: Perspectives on preparticipation screening studies. *J Am Coll Cardiol* 1986;7:220–230.

Fiocchi R, Fagard R, Stassen J, et al: Atrioventricular block induced in an athlete by carotid baroreceptor stimulation. *Am Heart J* 1985;109:1102–1104.

Fogoros RN: Runner's trots: Gastrointestinal disturbances in runners. *JAMA* 1980;243:1743–1744.

Frank CW, Weinblatt E, Shapiro S, et al: Physical inactivity as a lethal factor in myocardial infarction among men. *Circulation* 1966;34:1022.

Frizzell RT, Lang GH, Lowance DC, et al: Hyponatremia and ultramarathon running. *JAMA* 1986;255:772–774.

Froelicher VF, Oberman A: Analysis of epidemiologic studies of physical inactivity as risk factor for coronary heart disease. *Prog Cardiovasc Dis* 1972;15:41.

Goff D, Dimsdale JE: The psychologic effects of exercise. *J Cardiopulmonary Rehabil* 1985;5:234–240.

Grossman A: Endorphins and exercise. *Clin Cardiol* 1984;7:255–260.

Gutin B, Alejandro D, Duni T, et al: Levels of serum sex hormones and risk factors for coronary heart disease in exercise-trained men. *Am J Med* 1985;79:79–84.

Hagberg JM, Hickson RC, McLane JA, et al: Disappearance of norepinephrine from the circulation following strenuous exercise. *J Am Physiol* 1979;47:1311–1314.

Hanson PG, Zimmerman SW: Exertional heatstroke in novice runners. *JAMA* 1979;242:154–157.

Hartung GH, Farge EJ, Mitchell RE: Effects of marathon running, jogging, and diet on coronary risk factors in middle-aged men. *Prev Med* 1981;10:316–323.

Hartung GH, Squires WC, Gotto AM: Effect of exercise training on plasma high-density lipoprotein cholesterol in coronary disease patients. *Am Heart J* 1981;101:181–184.

Haskell WL: Exercise-induced changes in plasma lipids and lipoproteins. *Prev Med* 1984;13:23–26.

Heath GW, Ehsani AA, Hagberg JM, et al: Exercise training improves lipoprotein lipid profiles in patients with coronary artery disease. *Am Heart J* 1983;105:889–894.

Herbert PN, Bernier DN, Cullinane EM, et al: High-density lipoprotein metabolism in runners and sedentary men. *JAMA* 1984;252:1034–1037.

Hinkle LE, Whitney LA, Lehman EW, et al: Occupation, education, and coronary heart disease. *Science* 1968;161:238

Huston TP, Puffer JC, Rodney WM: The athletic heart syndrome. *N Engl J Med* 1985;313:24–32.

Ingwall JS, Kramer MF, Fifer MA, et al: The creatine kinase system in normal and diseased human myocardium. *N Engl J Med* 1985;313:1050–1054.

Jaffe AS, Garfinkel BT, Ritter CS, et al: Plasma MB creatine kinase after vigorous exercise in professional athletes. *Am J Cardiol* 1984;53:856–858.

Jennings G, Nelson L, Nestel P, et al: The effects of changes in physical activity on major cardiovascular risk factors, hemodynamics, sympathetic function, and glucose utilization in man: A controlled study of four levels of activity. *Circulation* 1986;73:30–40.

Jeresaty RM: Mitral valve prolapse: Definition and implications in athletes. *J Am Coll Cardiol* 1986;7:231–236.

Kahn H: The relationship of reported coronary heart disease mortality to physical activity of work. *Am J Public Health* 1963;53:1058.

Kannel WB, Belanger A, D'Agostino R, et al: Physical activity and physical demand on the job and risk of CV disease and death: The Framingham Study. *Am Heart J* 1986;112:820–825.

Kannel WB, Sorlie P: Some health benefits of physical activity: The Framingham study. *Arch Intern Med* 1979;139:857–861.

Kaplan AA, Natbony SF, Tawil AP, et al: Exercise-induced anaphylaxis as a manifestation of cholinergic urticaria. *J Allergy Clin Immunol* 1981;68:319–325.

Kavanagh T, Shephard RJ, Lindley LJ, et al: Influence of exercise and life-style variables upon high density lipoprotein cholesterol after myocardial infarction. *Arteriosclerosis* 1983;3:249–259.

Keys A: Physical activity and the epidemiology of coronary heart disease. *Med Sports* 1970;4:255.

Koplan JP: Cardiovascular deaths while running. *JAMA* 1979;242:2578–2579.

Kottke TE, Caspersen CJ, Hill CS: Exercise in the management and rehabilitation of selected chronic diseases. *Prev Med* 1984;13:47–65.

Kupfer DJ, Sewitch DE, Epstein LH, et al: Exercise and subsequent sleep in male runners: Failure to support the slow wave sleep-mood-exercise hypothesis. *Neuropsychobiology* 1985;14:5–12.

Lane NE, Bloch DA, Jones HH, et al: Long-distance running, bone density, and osteoarthritis. *JAMA* 1986;255:1147–1151.

Leon AS, Jacobs DR, DeBacker G, et al: Relationship of physical characteristics of life habits to treadmill exercise capacity. *Am J Epidemiol* 1981;653–660.

Lilenfeld AM: Variation of mortality from heart disease. *Public Health Rep* 1956;71:545.

Loucks AB, Horvath SB: Athletic amenorrhea: A review. *Med Sci Sports Exerc* 1985;17:56–72.

Lowenthal DT, Kendrick ZV: Drug-exercise interactions. *Ann Rev Pharmacol Toxicol* 1985;25:275–305.

Marcus R, Cann C, Madvig P, et al: Menstrual function and bone mass in elite women distance runners. *Ann Intern Med* 1985;102:158–163.

Maron BJ: Structural features of the athlete heart as defined by echocardiography. *J Am Coll Cardiol* 1986;7:190–203.

Maron BJ, Epstein SE: Symposium on the athlete heart. *J Am Coll Cardiol* 1986;7:189–243.

Maron BJ, Epstein SE, Roberts WC: Causes of sudden death in competitive athletes. *J Am Coll Cardiol* 1986;7:204–214.

Martin WH, Coyle EF, Ehsani AA: Cardiovascular sensitivity to epinephrine in the trained and untrained states. *Am J Cardiol* 1984;54:1326–1330.

McDonagh AF: Sunlight-induced mutation of bilirubin in a long-distance runner. *N Engl J Med* 1986;314:121.

McDonough JR, Hames CG, Stulb SC, et al: Coronary heart disease among Negroes and whites in Evans County, Georgia. *J Chronic Dis* 1965;18:443.

McMahon LF, Ryan MJ, Larson D, et al: Occult gastrointestinal blood loss in marathon runners. *Ann Intern Med* 1984;100:846–847.

McManus BM, Waller BF, Graboys TB, et al: Exercise and sudden death, Part I and II. *Current Problems in Cardiology* 1982;6.

McMaster SB, Carney JM: Changes in drug sensitivity following acute and chronic exercise. *Pharmacol Biochem Behav* 1985;23:191–194.

Mitrani Y, Karplus H, Brunner D: Coronary atherosclerosis in cases of traumatic death. *Med Sports* 1970;4:241.

Morales AR, Romanelli R, Boucek RJ: The mural left anterior descending coronary artery: strenuous exercise and sudden death. *Circulation* 1980;62:230–237.

Moran BJ, Roberts WC, McAllister HA, et al: Sudden death in young athletes. *Circulation* 1980;62:218–225.

Morris HJN, Crawford MD: Coronary heart disease and physical activity of work. *Br Med J* 1958;2:1485.

Morris JN: *Uses of Epidemiology*. New York, Churchill Livingstone, Inc, 1975.

Morris NJ, Pollard R, Everitt MG, et al: Vigorous exercise in leisure-time: Protection against coronary heart disease. *Lancet* 1980;2:1207–1210.

Mueller JK, Gossard D, Adams FR, et al: Assessment of prescribed increases in physical activity: Application of a new method for microprocessor analysis of heart rate. *Am J Cardiol* 1986;57:441–445.

Noakes TD, Opie LH, Rose AG, et al: Autopsy-proved coronary atherosclerosis in marathon runners. *N Engl J Med* 1979;301:86–89.

Noakes TD, Rose AG: Exercise-related deaths in subjects with coexistent hypertrophic cardiomyopathy and coronary artery disease. *S Afr Med J* 1984;66:183–187.

Nomura G, Kumagai E, Midorikawa K, et al: Physical training in essential hypertension: Alone and in combination with dietary salt restriction. *J Cardiac Rehabil* 1984;4:469–475.

Oliver RM: Physique and serum lipids of young London busmen in relation to ischemic heart disease. *Br J Intern Med* 1967;24:181.

Paffenbarger R: Physical activity, mortality, and longevity. *N Engl J Med* 1986;314:606–613.

Paffenbarger RS, Brand RJ, Sholtz RI, et al: Energy expenditure, cigarette smoking, and blood pressure level as related to death from specific diseases. *Am J Epidemiol* 1978;108:12–20.

Paffenbarger RS, Hyde RT, Wing AL, et al: Physical activity, all-cause mortality, and longevity of college alumni. *N Engl J Med* 1986;314:605–613.

Paffenbarger RS, Hyde RT, Wing AL, et al: A natural history of athleticism and cardiovascular health. *JAMA* 1984;252:491–495.

Paffenbarger RS, Laughlin ME, Gima AS, et al: Work activity of longshoremen as related to death from coronary heart disease and stroke. *N Engl J Med* 1970;282:1109.

Paffenbarger RS, Jr, Wing AL, Hyde RT: Chronic disease in former college students: Physical activity as an index of heart attack risk in college alumni. *Am J Epidemiol* 1981;108(3):161–175.

Paffenberger RS, Wing AL, Hyde RT: Physical activity as an index of heart attack risk in college alumni. *Am J Epidemiol* 1978;108:161–167.

Palatini P, Maraglino G, Sperti G, et al: Prevalence and possible mechanisms of ventricular arrhythmias in athletes. *Am Heart J* 1985;110:560–567.

Panush RS, Schmidt C, Caldwell JR, et al: Is running associated with degenerative joint disease. *JAMA* 1986;255:1152–1154.

Pell S, D'Alonzo CA: A three-year study of myocardial infarction in a large employed population. *JAMA* 1961;175:463.

Pell S, D'Alonzo CA: Immediate mortality and five-year survival of employed men with a first myocardial infarction. *N Engl J Med* 1964;270:915.

Perloff JK, Child JS, Edwards JE: New guidelines for the clinical diagnosis of mitral valve prolapse. *Am J Cardiol* 1986;57:1124–1129.

Perper JA, Rozin L, Williams KE: Sudden unexpected death following exercise and congenital anomalies of coronary arteries. *Am J Forensic Med Pathol* 1985;6:289–292.

Peters RK, Cady LD, Bischoff DP, et al: Physical fitness and subsequent myocardial infarction in healthy workers. *JAMA* 1983;249:3052–3056.

Poortmans JR: Postexercise proteinuria in humans: Facts and mechanisms. *JAMA* 1985;253:236–240.

Posner JD, Gorman KM, Klein HS, et al: Exercise capacity in the elderly. *Am J Cardiol* 1986;57:52C–58C.

Powell KE, Spain KG, Christenson GM, et al: The status of the 1990 objectives for physical fitness and exercise. *Public Health Rep* 1986;101:15–22.

Priest JB, Oei TO, Moorehead WR: Exercise-induced changes in common laboratory tests. *Am J Clin Pathol* 1982;77:285–289.

Retchin SM, Fletcher RH, Earp J, et al: Mitral valve prolapse. Disease or illness? *Arch Intern Med* 1986;146:1081–1084.

Ribeiro JP, Hartley H, Sherwood J, et al: The effectiveness of a low lipid diet and exercise in the management of coronary artery disease. *Am Heart J* 1984;108:1183–1189.

Robertson HK: Heart disease in life-long cyclists. *Lancet* 1977;2:1635.

Rose G, Prineas RJ, Mitchell JR: Myocardial infarction and the intrinsic calibre of coronary arteries. *Br Heart J* 1967;29:548.

Sable DL, Brammell HL, Sheehan MW, et al: Attenuation of exercise conditioning by beta-adrenergic blockage. *Circulation* 1982;65:679–684.

Sawka MN, Francesconi RP, Young AJ, et al: Influence of hydration level and body fluids on exercise performance in the heat. *JAMA* 1984;252:1165–1169.

Serfass RC, Gerberich SG: Exercise for optimal health: Strategies and motivational considerations. *Prev Med* 1984;13:79–99.

Shanoff HM, Little JA: Studies of male survivors of myocardial infarction due to "essential" atherosclerosis: I. Characteristics of the patients. *Can Med Assoc J* 1961;84:519.

Sheffer AL, Austen KF: Exercise-induced anaphylaxis. *J Allergy Clin Immunology* 1984;73:699–703.

Shephard RJ, Kavanagh T, Tuck J, et al: Marathon jogging in post-myocardial infarction patients. *J Cardiac Rehabil* 1983;3:321–329.

Siegel AJ: Myocardial injury after exercise: A diagnostic dilemma. *J Cardiopulmonary Rehabil* 1985;5:415–420.

Siegel AJ, Silverman LM, Evans WJ: Elevated skeletal muscle creatine kinase MB isoenzyme levels in marathon runners. *JAMA* 1983;250:2835–2838.

Simon HB: The immunology of exercise. *JAMA* 1984;252:2735–2738.

Simon HB, Steinhaus DM: Creatine kinase levels after patients with cardiac disease. *Am J Med* 1984;77:497–500.

Simons AD, Epstein LH, McGowan CR, et al: Exercise as a treatment for depression: An update. *Clin Psychology Review* 1985;5:553–568.

Siscovick DS, Weiss NS, Fletcher RH, et al: The incidence of primary cardiac arrest during vigorous exercise. *N Engl J Med* 1984;311:874–877.

Siscovick DS, Weiss NS, Fletcher RH, et al: Habitual vigorous exercise and primary cardiac arrest: Effect of other risk factors on the relationship. *J Chron Dis* 1984;37:625–631.

Spain DM, Bradess V: Occupational physical activity and the degree of coronary atherosclerosis in "normal" men. *Circulation* 1960;22:239.

Stamler J: Lifestyles, major risk factors, proof and public policy. *Circulation* 1978;58:3.

Stamler J, Kjelsberg M, Hall Y: Epidemiologic studies on cardiovascular-renal diseases: I. Analysis of mortality by age-race-sex-occupation. *J Chronic Dis* 1960;12:440.

Status of the 1990 physical fitness and exercise objectives. *JAMA* 1985;254:1694–1697.

Steiner R: Commentary to renal function during exercise in coronary patients. *J Cardiac Rehabil* 1983;3:581–582.

Steward JG, Ahlquist DA, McGill DB, et al: Gastrointestinal blood loss and anemia in runners. *Ann Intern Med* 1984;100:843–845.

Symposium on endorphins. *Med Sci Sports Exerc* 1985;17:73–105.

Taylor HL, Blackburn H, Brozek J, et al: Railroad employees in the United States. *Acta Med Scand* 1966;460:55.

Taylor HL, Klepetar E, Keys A, et al: Death rates among physically active and sedentary employees of the railroad industry. *Am J Public Health* 1962;52:1697.

Thompson JK, Jarvie GJ, Lahey BB, et al: Exercise and obesity: Etiology, physiology, and intervention. *Psychol Bull* 1982;91:55–79.

Thompson PD: The cardiovascular risks of cardiac rehabilitation. *J Cardiopulmonary Rehabil* 1985;5:321–324.

Thompson PD, Cullinane EM, Eshleman R, et al: The effects of high-carbohydrate and high-fat diets on the serum lipid and lipoprotein concentrations of endurance athletes. *Metabolism* 1984;33:1003–1009.

Thompson PD, Cullinane EM, Eshleman R, et al: The effects of caloric restriction and exercise cessation on the serum lipid and lipoprotein concentrations of endurance athletes. *Metabolism* 1984;33:943–949.

Thompson PD, Funk EJ, Carleton RA, et al: Incidence of death during jogging in Rhode Island from 1975 through 1980. *JAMA* 1982;247:2535–2538.

Thompson PD, Stern MP, Williams P, et al: Death during jogging or running. *JAMA* 1979;242:1265.

Tomporowski PD, Ellis NR: Effects of exercise on cognitive processes: a review. *Psychol Bull* 1986;99:338–346.

Tran ZV, Weltman A: Differential effects of exercise serum lipid and lipoprotein levels seen with changes in body weight. *JAMA* 1985;254:919–924.

Van Camp SP: The Fixx tragedy: A cardiologist's perspective. *Physician Sports Med* 1984;12:153–157.

Vander L, Franklin B, Rubenfire M: Cardiovascular complications of recreational physical activity. *Physician Sports Med* 1982;10:89–98.

Virmani R, McAllister HA: Coronary heart disease at young age: A report of 187 autopsy patients who died of severe coronary atherosclerosis. *Cardiovasc Rev Rep* 1984;5:799–809.

Waller BF, Roberts WC: Sudden death while running in conditioned runners aged 40 years or over. *Am J Cardiol* 1980;45:1291.

Warnes CA, Roberts WC: Sudden coronary death: Relation of amount and distribution of coronary narrowing at necropsy to previous symptoms of myocardial ischemia, left ventricular scarring and heart weight. *Am J Cardiol* 1984;54:65–73.

Wilson PWF, Paffenbarger RS, Morris JN, et al: Assessment methods for physical activity and physical fitness in population studies: Report of a NHLBI workshop. *Am Heart J* 1986;111:77–92.

Zukel WJ, et al: A short-term community study of the epidemiology of coronary heart disease. *Am J Public Health* 1959;49:1630.

11

CARDIAC REHABILITATION

In the past, the patient who suffered a myocardial infarction (MI) was almost completely immobilized for six weeks or more and was even washed, shaved, and fed in order to keep the work that the heart had to do to a minimum. It was thought that this approach provided the heart with the opportunity to form a firm scar. Also, the patient was told not to expect to be able to return to a normal life. These were incorrect beliefs, particularly in the situation of an uncomplicated MI. Prolonged immobilization not only did not speed healing but exposed the patient to the additional risks of venous thrombosis, pulmonary embolism, muscle wasting, lung infections, and deconditioning. Equally serious was the psychological result of such an approach, often leading to psychological impairment. We now know that most patients can return to a normal life and most even have a normal life expectancy.

It is interesting to consider that following today's standard of care for the acute MI 20 years ago would have resulted in malpractice and vice versa. Today, the physician's approach to the acute MI has completely changed. A relatively brief period of time monitored by the high technology in the coronary care unit is followed by early mobilization, sitting at the bedside, carefully graduated exercise and, in the uncomplicated patient, discharge from the hospital within a week.

While this present policy has been shown by randomized trials to be safe from the point of view of cardiac complications, it has nevertheless generated problems for the physician, other health care personnel, and the entire health care system. It also puts a drain on already limited resources since modern health care must include mechanisms for safely prescribing exercise and for education and psychological rehabilitation. The shortened length of stay dictated by the DRG approach leaves little time for patient education and other rehabilitative services. Certainly all patients do not need all rehabilitation interventions, but exercise programs, educational sessions, group therapy, and psychological and vocational counseling should be available to those who need them.

Hospital admission for an acute MI is a stressful experience with a powerful impact. Hospital discharge, though less dramatic, can be equally stressful after relying on the highly protective hospital support systems. Discharge into an uncertain future and to a home and work setting in which one is considered

423

a helpless invalid can be as damaging to one's self-esteem as the acute event itself. The physician is faced with the difficult task not only of supervising the physical recovery of the patient but of maintaining morale, providing education, helping the family cope and provide support, and facilitating the return to a gratifying life-style. Cardiac rehabilitation can be considered the conservation of human life. Its goal is to restore the patient to optimal physiological, psychological, and vocational status.

THE PATHOPHYSIOLOGY OF AN ACUTE MYOCARDIAL INFARCTION

The pathophysiology of acute MI has become better understood. In the 1970s, we were taught not to call MI "coronary thrombosis." This was because a thrombosis was not found in the acute phase of a recent MI, but only in older infarctions. It was thought that the thrombosis was caused by the MI and did not precipitate it. However, studies utilizing coronary angiography at the time of infarction have shown that a thrombosis is usually seen acutely. This has led to attempts to lyse clots with streptokinase, urokinase, or thrombolysin plasminogen activator (TPA) or to remove them with catheters. Though in individual cases this has reportedly stopped progression of myocardial infarction, the randomized trials performed have not convincingly shown this procedure to alter morbidity and mortality. This is partially due to the difficulty of recognizing the preinfarction stage. It appears that thrombolysis is most effective in large anterior Q-wave infarcts or in MIs that are extending. But even when the thrombosis is lysed, the patient can proceed to infarct. The substrate (i.e., "dirty" plaque or critically narrowed artery) remains and another thrombosis quickly forms. This chemical debridement must be followed by more lasting interventions including percutaneous transluminal angioplasty (PTCA) or coronary artery bypass surgery (CABS) to abort an evolving infarction. Randomized trials using thrombolysis have demonstrated decreased mortality and less myocardial damage when the thrombolytic agents are given early. The time required for myocardial cell death appears to be three hours of ischemia, but this has considerable variability. Currently, there is no good indicator of irreversible cell death; even the electrocardiogram can be misleading. However, once this time has passed, intervention to restore blood flow does not appear to be warranted. There should be exciting advances in the next years as these techniques find their appropriate place in clinical practice.

Infarct Severity. Myocardial infarctions are divided basically into those that evolve Q-waves and result in transmural myocardial cell death and those that do not evolve Q-waves and result only in subendocardial cell death. Even though Q-wave infarcts are not always transmural and non-Q-wave infarcts can be transmural, the ECG pattern predicts the clinical course and outcome surprisingly well. Subendocardial MI cannot be localized while transmural MI can be roughly localized by the Q-wave pattern. Attempts have been made to judge MI severity or size electrocardiographically by Q-wave and R-wave scores and even by utilizing body surface mapping, but these methods provide only rough estimates. In general, the greater the number of areas with Q-waves and the greater the R-wave loss, the larger the MI. Non-Q-wave MIs are usually less associated with complications such as CHF or shock, but they can be complicated, particularly when prior MI has taken place. Their prognosis is particularly good if not associated with prior MIs and a decreased ejection fraction.

MI size can be judged by the creatinine kinase (CK) levels, particularly by the amount of MB band released. This enzyme has improved the laboratory diagnosis of myocardial infarction since it is highly specific for myocardium. In most laboratories, greater than 5% MB with a total score greater than 150 is associated with myocardial damage. Though careful sampling of CK over time has enabled construction of a MB-CK curve and the integrated area of the curve correlates with MI size, this has not been very helpful clinically. Unfortunately, many infarcts do not yield a smooth curve. In general, however, the higher the amount of MB released and the longer the CK stays elevated, the larger the infarction. Successful thrombolysis is characterized, however, with high CK values and arrhythmias. Elevations of the white count and sedimentation rate and pericarditis are also indicators of a relatively large MI.

A better understanding of the anatomic substrate of MI has occurred in recent years. An inferior Q-wave infarct is more likely to have associated multivessel disease than an anterior wall infarct. This is because occlusions of the right or left circumflex coronary arteries alone usually are "silent" because of the dual circulation to the posterior surface of the heart. Inferior infarcts usually occur only when both arteries are occluded and are more commonly associated with right ventricular infarction because of the common coronary artery supply. Inferior infarcts are usually smaller and less severe and less likely to be associated with shock or congestive heart failure. They are usually accompanied by bradycardia and sometimes temporary heart block. The associated pain is usually less severe and often imitates indigestion.

Anterior Q-wave MIs are usually larger than inferior infarcts and are more likely to be associated with congestive heart failure and cardiogenic shock. Anterior infarcts are more likely to cause aneurysms and a greater decrease in ejection fraction. Surprisingly, however, in follow-up they have a similar or not much poorer prognosis than inferior Q-wave MIs. Fifteen percent of patients with Q-wave MI lose their Q-waves over the following year but still have the same prognosis as those who do not lose their Q-waves.

Interventions. Much work has been done to try to limit myocardial infarction size. This is extremely important since prognosis after MI is largely predicted by the amount of remaining myocardium. Randomized trials suggest that pharmacological intervention can be applied in a logical fashion to possibly limit infarction size. An unresolved question is whether this then leaves the patient with relatively more jeopardized myocardium, ready for another myocardial infarction, or with angina pectoris. In most cases, nitrates and beta blockers can be useful in limiting MI size. Nitrates reduce preload and myocardial wall tension, which are important determinants of myocardial oxygen demand, and lessen coronary artery spasm which can occur during a MI. However, they can cause hypotension and headache.

Beta blockers must be used cautiously when congestive heart failure or heart block are present. However, when properly used, they rarely cause heart failure and definitely decrease myocardial oxygen consumption. Nitroprusside and nitroglycerin IV appear to be the choices for pre- and afterload reduction in patients with heart failure and hypertension. When a dropping systolic blood pressure is not due to hypovolemia, pressor agents can be helpful in shock, but the dismal prognosis in cardiogenic shock often necessitates artificial assisting devices, and intervention with PTCA or CABS. Neck vein distension, a sign of congestive heart failure, can also be caused by right ventricular infarction. This must be considered in patients with an inferior infarct with neck vein distension who do not have rales. Often intravenous fluids can help such patients. Calcium antagonists have been studied in randomized fashion and have not been found to be efficacious. In fact, they can cause hypotension and reduce coronary perfusion in the acute MI patient. There continues to be considerable debate over whether all patients should receive a continuous infusion of lidocaine in the acute phase of a myocardial infarction. On the one hand, lidocaine clearly decreases the incidence of ventricular tachycardia. However, its side effects can be detrimental to recovery; i.e., the mental obtundation and confusion can be upsetting to all patients, but particularly the elderly. Perhaps it should be used only when the risk of ventricular tachycardia is considered highly probable and when monitoring cannot be as intensive as it should be.

There is considerable experience with acute intervention with CABS and PTCA. Unfortunately, no randomized trial has been performed and certainly they should be considered only in high-risk MIs.

Risk Prediction.   It is well-known that morbidity and mortality in postinfarction patients who have complicated courses are much higher than in those with uncomplicated MIs. The criteria for a complicated MI are listed in Table 11–1. Early ambulation is not appropriate for the patient with a complicated infarct. The progressive ambulation program should be delayed until such individuals reach an uncomplicated status, and even then progressive ambulation should be slower.

TABLE 11–1.

Criteria for Classification of Complicated MI

Continued cardiac ischemia (pain, late enzyme rise)
Left ventricular failure (congestive heart failure, new murmurs, x-ray changes)
Shock (blood pressure drop, pallor, oliguria)
Important cardiac dysrhythmias (PVCs greater than 6/min, atrial fibrillation)
Conduction disturbances (bundle branch block, A-V block, hemiblock)
Severe pleurisy or pericarditis
Complicating illnesses
Marked creatinine kinase rise without a noncardiac explanation

There has been some controversy over the relative long-term risk of subendocardial versus transmural myocardial infarction. Some of this difficulty has been due to whether or not prior MIs occurred. An infarct with evolving Q-waves on the ECG is "transmural" and considered large, whereas an infarction with only ST and T-wave changes has been called "subendocardial" and considered small. Estimation of the severity of MI requires consideration of clinical findings and test results other than the ECG to judge a patient's risk and infarct size. The presence of Q-waves does not prove the occurrence of a transmural MI, and a transmural MI can occur with only ST and T-wave changes. The severity of an infarction should be judged by clinical findings, hemodynamic monitoring, the level of creatinine kinase elevation, and the presence of congestive heart failure or shock or both. The concept that a subendocardial infarction is "incomplete" and poses an increased postdischarge risk has not been substantiated; however, they are more likely to be associated with postinfarction angina. The Mayo Clinic study summarized in Chapter Six demonstrated that in the patient with a first MI, prognosis is much better in follow-up for a non-Q-wave MI than for a Q-wave MI. Patients with Q-wave MIs, particularly of the anterior wall infarcts, have a higher in-hospital morbidity and mortality, as do patients with a history of multiple MIs.

Clinical practice has evolved to the point that we now have the capability of recognizing the relative size of MI and the risk that it represents for subsequent morbidity and mortality. It is now possible to assess risk at different temporal points from presentation in the emergency room, through the coronary care unit and predischarge time, and during later follow-up. However, the clinical picture changes over time, and a low-risk patient can become a high-risk patient and vice versa. This changing risk is partially due to the vicissitudes of the atherosclerotic process, reformation of thrombus interventions, and disease-host interactions, For instance, a patient may present with premature ventricular contractions (PVCs), but then they can disappear or worsen, chest pain may come and go, the electrocardiographic pattern may change or the enzymes may have a late peak. This makes it difficult to strictly classify a patient as a high or low risk; it is only the patient's physician who can determine the relative risk, aided by the nursing staff. However, this can lead to a great deal of frustration for the patient and the nurses. Often, promises by the doctor of discharge from the coronary care unit or other changes signifying progress must be superceded by the day's findings. The progressive steps very often must be adjusted, sometimes even several times in a day. Table 11–2 lists the step therapy used at LBVAMC.

Early Ambulation.   Prior to 1960, patients with acute MI were thought to require prolonged restriction of physical activity. Patients were often kept at strict bed rest for two months with all activities performed by nursing personnel. The concern was that physical activity could lead to complications such as ventricular aneurysm formation, cardiac rupture, congestive heart failure, dysrhythmias, reinfarction, or sudden death (Table 11–3). Hospitalization could last for three to four months with limitations of activities for at least one year. Table 11–4 summarizes the recommendations

TABLE 11–2.
Post-Myocardial Infarction (MI) Protocol—Eight Levels of Activity*†

LEVEL	ACTIVITIES	NURSING	EXCEPTIONS
I CCU	Strict bed rest Commode vs. bedpan Feed self if set up	Complete bed bath (pt. may wash genitalia) *Exercises:* 5 × each BID: exercises 1–4 (see below)	Chest pain DOE Frequent PVCs HR greater than 100 Dizziness
< 2 METs			Diaphoresis

Teaching: simple explanations of equipment and procedures. Reassurance!

II CCU	Bed rest, up in chair 1 × vs. dangle Bedside commode	Bed bath; pt. may wash hands, face, genitalia *Exercises:* Passive ROM BID 5 × each BID: exercises 1–5	Chest pain, DOE Frequent PVCs HR greater than 100 Dizziness Diaphoresis
< 2 METs	Feed self		

Teaching: if diagnosis known—simple explanation, "You had a heart attack," and the role cardiac rehab
    team will play in education and increasing activity.

III CCU or Ward	Bed rest—up in chair 20 min TID Bedside commode Meals in chair	Bed bath—pt. may wash hands, face, genitalia *Exercises:* Active ROM all extremities 5 × each BID: Exercises 1–6	Chest pain, DOE Frequent PVCs HR greater than 100 Dizziness Diaphoresis
2 METs			

Teaching: restate diagnosis with healing time: three months. Activity progression to be slow and steady
    with attention to pacing convalescence.
Stress: report any cardiac symptoms—e.g., chest, neck, jaw, arm, or abdominal discomfort.

IV Ward	Bed rest—bathroom privileges Up in chair as desired Walk about room	Partial bath (in bed or at sink)—Pt. not to wash back, legs, or feet *Exercises:* Active ROM BID 10 × each BID: 1–6 Add 5 × each BID: 7	Chest pain, DOE HR greater than 110 Frequent PVCs Dizziness Diaphoresis
< 3 METs			

Teaching: rehabilitation group discussion—family invited.
1. Anatomy and physiology of heart in relation to MI.
2. Convalescent care, activity progression and risk factor management—HTN, diet, activity, smoking, stress
    reduction.
3. Diet class low sodium and low cholesterol.
Reexplain class information on one-to-one level. Begin medication teaching including use of nitroglycerin.

V Ward	Up in room Walk to TV room and back after warm-up exercises	Chair shower *Exercises:* Active ROM BID 10 × each BID 1–7 5 × each BID: exercise 8	Chest pain DOE HR greater than 110 Frequent PVCs Dizziness
4 METs	Up in chair		Diaphoresis

Teaching: taking pulse. Explain medications, beta blockers and digitalis (if applicable), action of meds.
    Reasons for slow, steady activity increase over three-month period. Report any problems noted as activity
    increases—e.g., (1) chest, neck, jaw, arm, abdominal pain, and/or pressure or discomfort; (2) shortness of
    breath.

VI Ward	Ward ambulation	Chair shower	Chest pain
	Work toward walking	*Exercises:*	DOE
	around floor square non-	10 × each BID: exercises 1–8	HR greater than 110
	stop (⅙ mile)		Frequent PVCs
	Start with 1 leg of square—		Dizziness
	gradually increase pace		Diaphoresis
	before distance (12 ×		
< 5 METs	around = mile)		

Teaching: reinforce activity progression. Do not leave ward unless pushed in a wheel chair (needs ward nurse knowledge to leave ward). No heart patient is to push another patient!

VII Ward	Ambulate off ward	Shower	Chest pain
	Walk up one flight of stairs	*Exercises:*	DOE
	with rehab team member	10 × each	Frequent PVCs
		BID: exercises 1–9	HR greater than 120
5 METs			Dizziness
			Diaphoresis

Teaching: review any questions.
Stress: treadmill test is not a pass/fail situation.

VIII	Submaximal Treadmill Test (5 MET) for discharge. If held in hospital for problems, return to
	level as indicated. If held in hospital for elective procedure (i.e., angiogram), stress the
	need to continue warm-up exercises and increase number of times around floor for
5 METs	training walk as in Level VI.

Exercises for Post-MI Protocols (numbers used above in "Nursing" column)
1. Foot circles
2. Ankle pumps
3. Toe flexion and extension
4. Neck exercises
    a. Head nod, chin on chest, then look to sky
    b. Head tilt: lean left ear to left shoulder, then right ear to right shoulder
    c. Head turn: look to left, then right with chin over shoulder
    d. Five complete head circles, both right and left
5. Quadriceps setting, thigh press with knee locked
6. Shoulder exercises
    a. Shrug both shoulders up toward ears
    b. Move each shoulder in a circle forward and then backward
    c. Lift arms straight up over head until elbow is straight; alternate arms
7. Bring alternate knee to chest
8. Straight leg lifts, alternate legs
9. Side bends

*Composite developed by Barbara Kellerman, RN, for use at LBVAMC.
†Primary physician is to draw a line down through levels, date, and initial order. Patient may be held at *any* level. MI Date_____Highest CK_____

for bed rest in the major text books of the times. This approach was based on pathological studies indicating that at least six weeks were required for necrotic myocardium to form a firm scar and on the increased prevalence of cardiac rupture reported among patients who infarcted in mental hospitals where bed rest could not be enforced.

Animal Experiments.   Hammerman designed a study to evaluate the effect of early exercise on late scar formation in an MI animal model. After occlusion of the proximal left coronary artery, infarct extent was

TABLE 11–3.

Hypothetical Risks of Early Ambulation After Acute Myocardial Infarction

Dysrhythmias
Congestive heart failure
Left ventricular aneurysm
Cardiac rupture
Reinfarction
Sudden death

TABLE 11–4.

A Review of Previous Recommendations for Bed Rest in Acute Myocardial Infarction

AUTHOR/TITLE	RECOMMENDATION
Lewis, T.: *Diseases of the Heart.* New York, Macmillan Publishing Co., 1937.	8 weeks of bed rest
White, P.D.: *Heart Disease,* ed. 3. New York, The Macmillan Company, 1945.	4 weeks of bed rest
Wood, P.: *Diseases of the Heart and Circulation,* ed. 2. London, Eyre and Spottiswoode, 1960.	3–6 weeks in bed
Friedberg, C.K.: *Diseases of the Heart,* ed. 3. Philadelphia, W.B. Saunders Co., 1966.	2–3 weeks minimum of bed rest
Wood, P.: *Diseases of the Heart and Circulation,* ed. 3. London, Erye and Spottiswoode, 1968.	2 weeks in bed

assessed 24 hours later by ECG criteria. The rats were divided into two groups: eight were subjected to daily graded swimming for up to 45 minutes a day for a week followed by two weeks of nonswimming; seven served as a control group. Twenty-two days after coronary occlusion, their hearts were excised and wall thickness determined histologically. A ratio for transmural infarcts was obtained from multiple measurements by dividing scar thickness by noninfarcted septal wall thickness. In the exercise group, there was marked scar thinning. Infarct extent was similar in both groups. They concluded that short-term swimming during the first week after an MI had affects on scar formation when assessed two weeks later. A similar study by Kloner and Kloner with rats forced to swim seven days post MI reported the same results. However, the relevance of rats forced to swim to the clinical situation is uncertain. Hochman and Healy performed similar experiments and found no signs in their rats of myocardial thinning or aneurysm formation.

Controlled clinical studies of early mobilization have not found a greater incidence of death or other complications in patients mobilized early compared to patients who remain at bed rest longer. The promising results of these studies led to recommendations of gradual mobilization during the early post-MI stages. In certain patients, the major cause of decreased exercise capacity is enforced bed rest. The exercise prescription for MI patients in the coronary care unit can avoid iatrogenically induced deconditioning.

Chair Treatment. A revolutionary approach to treatment occurred in the 1940s when Levine recommended "chair treatment" for the post-MI patient. This emphasized the benefits of the sitting versus the supine position for increasing peripheral venous pooling and reducing preload on the myocardium. Such a reduction should theoretically lead to a decrease in resting left ventricular wall tension and to a decrease in myocardial oxygen demand. This approach should also decrease the risk of thrombosis and pulmonary embolism.

Table 11–5 summarizes the potential complications of prolonged bed rest. Physiological studies have documented the hemodynamic alterations caused by deconditioning. After a prolonged bed rest, tachycardia and hypotension are common upon standing. This is most likely due to alterations in the baromotor reflexes and to hypovolemia that occurs with bed rest. Clearly, the disability secondary to most MIs is due both to bed rest and to myocardial dysfunction. The spontaneous hemodynamic improvement usually seen is due both to improving function (scar formation and possibly compensatory hypertrophy) and to a return to normal activities. An additional change was the use of a bedside commode, which is less of a hemodynamic stress than using a bedpan. The Valsalva maneuver, common when an individual is straining with a bowel movement, can lead to elevations of systolic blood pressure. However, in the sitting position, it is less forceful.

The Effects of Bed Rest Versus the Lack of Gravitational Stress.   There are definite hemodynamic alterations due to deconditioning and more noticeably with rest. Young men maintained at bed rest for three weeks demonstrated a 20% to 25% decrease in maximal oxygen consumption. Other than decreased functional capacity, prolonged bed rest results in orthostatic hypotension and venous thrombosis by a loss of blood volume, plasma loss exceeding red blood cell mass loss. Pulmonary function is decreased, and the patient can be in negative nitrogen and calcium balance.

The question has been raised as to whether the deleterious hemodynamic effects of bed rest, including decreased exercise capacity, are due to inactivity or to the loss of the upright exposure to gravity. There are at least four reasons supporting the concept that much of these alterations are due to loss of the upright exposure to gravity: (1) supine exercise does not prevent the deconditioning effects of being in bed; (2) there is both less of and a slower decline in maximal oxygen consumption with chair rest than with bed rest; (3) there is a greater decrease in the maximal oxygen consumption after a period of bed rest measured during upright exercise versus supine exercise; and, (4) a lower body positive pressure device decreases the deconditioning effect of bed rest. Perhaps intermittent exposure to gravitational stress during bed rest stage of

TABLE 11–5.
Potential Disadvantages of Prolonged Bed Rest

Orthostatic hypotension
Venous thrombosis
Reduced lung volume
Pulmonary emboli
Atelectasis; pneumonia
Metabolic alterations
Musculoskeletal problems

hospital convalescence from surgery or MI may obviate much of the deterioration in cardiovascular performance that can follow these events. Previous efforts to limit the decrease in capacity after myocardial infarction or surgery have emphasized low-level exercise training, but these data suggest that simple exposure to gravitational stress substantially accomplishes this purpose.

Progressive Activity.   In the early 1960s, reports were published using progressive activity for acute MI patients. Initially, this approach included an electrocardiogram and blood pressure monitoring for all activities. Early ambulation was not recommended for all patients, but for those who responded favorably. The Duke group improved this approach to early ambulation and discharge by separating patients into whether they had "complicated" or "uncomplicated" myocardial infarctions depending upon certain clinical findings. The features of a complicated myocardial infarction included: continued cardiac ischemia, left ventricular failure, shock, important cardiac dysrhythmias, conduction disturbances, severe pleurisy or pericarditis, complicating illnesses, and marked enzyme rises. If a patient had none of these clinical findings, he or she could be considered uncomplicated, rapidly progressed through an ambulation program, and discharged early.

The first approaches to early progressive ambulation included electrocardiographic and hemodynamic assessment at each stage. Serial small "exercise tests" were performed by the nursing staff to make sure that increasing levels of activity did no harm. However, this proved to be too time consuming for nurses, and so a day-by-day activity plan was generalized for all patients. It was up to the physician to individualize this plan according to his clinical assessment of the patient. Certainly the important variable of how the individual patient was responding to the exercise largely remained unknown except for the most serious symptoms. In addition, validation of the basis of symptoms was not obtained so that complaints based on anxiety alone were not recognized. There is much to be said for assessing the patient's response to exercise by measurement of the electrocardiogram, heart rate, and blood pressure.

A consideration often forgotten when dealing with an older patient or one with complicating illnesses is the level of activity that he or she maintained prior to MI. If a patient was physically limited prior to the event, the plan for progressive ambulation must be modified. It is generally inconceivable to expect a patient to be more physically active after an MI than before, unless previously limited by angina that disappeared later. It is important to assess the exercise capacity and activity level that existed prior to the myocardial infarction.

In addition to the oxygen cost and the heart rate achieved during activity, the duration of the activity must be considered. The effect of prolonged exercise on myocardial scar formation has not been carefully studied, but it is known that during prolonged steady-state dynamic exercise, heart rate increases, myocardial contractility declines, and left ventricular volume increases. It is apparent that even though certain oxygen cost levels can be achieved by a patient, they should not be maintained for long periods of time.

Probably the safest recommendation is to tell patients not to fatigue themselves and to limit the duration of exercise by their fatigue level and perceived exertion.

Postdischarge activity recommendations have had little basis for their enforcement. Return to work, driving, and sexual activity have been based on clinical judgments rather than physiological assessments. Because of this, physicians have left much of this up to their patients—allowing them to see how they respond symptomwise—rather than the older, very conservative approach that can foster invalidism. These decisions should be made considering the consequence of the coronary event (ischemia or symptoms of congestive failure, or dysrhythmias) and the nature of the activities (manual labor versus desk work, light driving versus congested freeway driving, sex with an established partner versus other relationships).

In 1961, Cain and colleagues reported the use of a progressive activity program for acute MI patients. They had difficulty having this report accepted for publication because the approach was considered dangerous. They reported 335 patients with an uncomplicated myocardial infarction who were at least 15 days postinfarction. The patients had been restricted to bed, chair, and commode. The electrocardiogram was monitored after the patient performed activities such as climbing stairs and walking up a grade.

In 1964, Torkelson reported his results in 10 patients with an uncomplicated MI. On the sixth week of his in-hospital rehabilitation program, a low-level treadmill test was performed using 1.7 mph at a 10% grade. He concluded that the treadmill test was a valuable procedure for the documentation of the specific exercise response of patients recovering from an acute MI.

Most later publications do not include ECG monitoring as part of progressive ambulation. Instead, generalized statements as to the activities on each postinfarct day are made for all patients, rather than individualized activity progression. Sivarajan, Bruce, and colleagues returned to the approach of Cain and Torkelson. They reported 12 patients with an acute MI whose symptoms, signs, and hemodynamic and ECG responses during and after three activities were assessed. These activities included sitting upright, walking to the toilet, and walking on a treadmill. Studies of these activities were done at 3, 6, and 10 days after infarction. They concluded that successful performance of these three activities provided useful criteria for discharge. If a patient has an abnormal response, such as a systolic blood pressure drop, severe chest pain, marked ST changes, or dysrhythmias, his or her progressive ambulation program and discharge from the hospital are delayed until the responses are acceptable. This approach constitutes optimal care of the postinfarct patient.

Hayes and colleagues studied 189 patients with an uncomplicated myocardial infarction selected at random for early or late mobilization and discharge from the hospital. Patients were admitted to the study after 48 hours in a coronary care unit if they were free of pain and showed no evidence of heart failure or significant dysrhythmias. One group of patients was mobilized immediately and discharged home after a total of nine days in the hospital, and the second group was mobilized on the ninth day and discharged on the 16th day. Outpatient assessment was carried out six weeks after admission. No significant differences were observed between the groups in terms of morbidity or mortality, as reflected by the incidence of recurrent chest pain or MI, heart failure, dysrhythmia, or venous thrombosis detected either clinically or by radionuclide scanning.

In a randomized study, Bloch and colleagues studied the effects of early mobilization after uncomplicated MI. One hundred fifty-four patients under 70 years of age who were hospitalized for an acute MI and had no complications on day one or day two were randomly assigned to two treatment groups. In the early mobilization group, patients were treated by a physiotherapist with a progressive activity program that began on day two or day three after infarction. In the control group, the patients underwent the traditional hospital regimen of strict bed rest for three or more weeks. The mean duration of hospitalization was 21 days for active patients and 33 days for the control group. The follow-up period ranged from 6 to 20 months, with an average of 11 months. There were no significant differences between the two groups with regard to hospital or follow-up mortality, to rates of reinfarction, dysrhythmias, heart failure, angina pectoris, ventricular aneurysm, or to the results of an exercise test. On follow-up examination, there was actually greater disability in the control than in the active group.

Sivarajan and colleagues have reported a study of the effects of early supervised exercises in preventing deconditioning after an acute MI. Eighty-four patients were randomized to a control group, 174 to an exercise group. The exercise program began at an average of 4.5 days after admission. The mean discharge was 10 days after admission for both groups. There were no differences between the two groups in the clinical, hemodynamic, or ECG responses to a low-level treadmill test performed on the day before hospital discharge. Nor was there any significant difference between the two groups for the incidence of complications or death. This well-designed and accomplished study was probably an anachronism. That is, by the time the study was funded, the standard of community medical care in Seattle included early ambulation and discharge. Therefore, the control group received treatment that was hardly different from that given the exercise group. Also, for safety reasons, the sicker patients who most needed rehabilitation were excluded from this study. Six patients needed cardiac surgery prior to discharge in the exercise group, but none required it in the control group, which can be explained by chance distribution (failure of randomization) rather than by the mild exercises employed.

These three randomized studies of patients with an uncomplicated infarction have demonstrated that the risks of early ambulation are minimal and that progressive mobilization during the early stages of an acute MI is recommended.

Medical Evaluation for Cardiac Rehabilitation. Certainly not all patients need cardiac rehabilitation, especially not all of its services, but most patients can benefit from it. It is rarely necessary to exclude patients. Patients can be in exercise programs with ejection fractions as low as 15%, with ventricular tachycardia, with left main disease, with exercise-induced drops in systolic blood pressure, and with an episode of cardiopulmonary resuscitation. Naturally, the exercise program needs to be individualized for patients with these problems. Algorithms of health care are difficult to develop since there is rarely a proven right or wrong way to practice medicine. The approach to each patient is individualized since each patient's reaction to problems and needs can be very different. Also, each test result only gives probabilities and does not absolutely predict an outcome. The following is one approach to assess patients prior to cardiac rehabilitation, placing them in a "niche" so one knows how to react to their symptoms, to them, and to their test results. Naturally, for every clinical situation, there are exceptions: there is the high-risk patient who outlives his physician, the patients with barely any myocardium left who can run a marathon, and the low-risk patient who dies. Biological systems are complex, and physicians continue to learn with each patient they treat.

The tools for assessment begin with the history and physical examination. These are especially important since this is the time during which the physician also establishes the patient's confidence and develops rapport. The electrocardiogram, chest x-ray, and exercise test are next in importance. Even though the exercise test can give confusing results, it is the key to prescribing exercise. Specialized tests including echocardiography, radionuclides, and cardiac catheterization confirm impressions or clarify incongruous clinical situations. They rarely yield surprises and the justification for their use must be separated from research and curiosity. Rarely is it justified to perform a test just in order "to know" if the knowing does not benefit the patient. It is best to understand these procedures so that they can be used when they are helpful.

The first step in evaluating patients for cardiac rehabilitation is to determine if their coronary heart disease is stable, and this is mainly determined by taking the patient's history. The manifestations of the disease that must be considered to be stable or not are myocardial ischemia, congestive heart failure, and dysrhythmias. Patients with ischemia can be symptomatic with classical angina pectoris, angina variants, or its equivalents (some forms of dyspnea on exertion or other pain radiations) or symptomatic. They can have normal resting ventricular function but have exercise-induced dysfunction. They can have myocardium in jeopardy of loss due to prolonged ischemia, but in general this does not appear to be as great a risk predictor as the amount of muscle already lost.

The hallmark symptom of ischemia is chest pain. Everyone has chest pain and usually ignores it. Once a person has been told he has heart disease, all the routine pains become very frightening, and it is important to separate nonischemic from ischemic chest pains. All chest pains should not be called angina pectoris. Angina classically comes on with increases in heart rate due to exercise or emotion. It is usually a substernal pressure, tightness, or pain that radiates up into the neck or down the left arm. It usually lasts no longer than 10 minutes and is relieved by rest and within two to three minutes by nitroglycerine sublingually. It can be exacerbated by cold weather and eating. One anginal variant is Prinzmetal angina due to spasm in normal coronary arteries or in arteries with partial occlusion. This occurs cyclically and usually at rest. It is associated with ST-segment elevation very often and with dysrhythmias, including ventricular tachycardia and heart block.

Another variant is unstable angina. Angina becomes unstable when it changes its pattern, occurring more frequently, at rest, or at lower work loads. The reason for the instability should be assessed. It is not as dangerous if due to emotional stress, stopping medications (i.e., because of side effects), increased activity, or increased cigarette smoking. True unstable angina has an increased risk and it should be treated promptly. The first step is to adjust medications. Beta blockers continue to be the first line of treatment. Since propranolol crosses the blood-brain barrier and causes more side effects, including fatigue and impotence, a common reason for instability is that a patient has stopped taking it. A patient can be switched to atenolol or Lopressor which have fewer side effects and can be taken only once a day. There is much less fatigue and impotence with these cardioselective drugs that are not lipophilic. Nitrates can be increased, but since long-acting nitrates have a questionable action, it is better to encourage a patient to take sublingual nitroglycerine as needed. If the angina attacks have taken on the characteristics of spasm, then calcium antagonists are the drugs of choice. Coronary artery bypass surgery is the best treatment for angina; if the patient is unhappy with his life-style, this procedure should be considered.

Increasing symptoms of congestive heart failure include sudden weight gain, edema in the lower extremities, dyspnea on exertion, and paroxysmal nocturnal dyspnea. Congestive heart failure should never be just accepted, but an explanation should be sought. Is it due to a large myocardial infarction, an aneurysm, valvular heart disease, a cardiomyopathy, or a ventricular septal defect? It is a frequent mistaken diagnosis made in older patients when they actually have pneumonia or lung disease. Signs include rales, an S3 gallop, signs of low output, weak carotids, increased neck vein distention, and a hepatojugular reflex. Treatment includes salt and fluid restriction, diuretics, and digoxin. Surgical treatment could include aneurysmectomy or mitral valve replacement. Aneurysmectomy is rarely helpful and the surgical removal of aneurysms is associated with a 10% or higher risk of death. It is not effective in relieving symptoms because aneurysms usually form a strong scar, and very often the surrounding muscle has poor function and total cardiac performance is not improved by removing the scar. Mitral valve replacement can be effective when the mitral leaflets are leaking due to papillary muscle rupture.

Combinations of both ischemia and congestive heart failure are difficult to manage. Patients with congestive heart failure often have too little muscle left to become very ischemic, and their chest pain is instead due to pulmonary artery hypertension. Also, ischemia can make a good ventricle fail temporarily, but the frequency of this is unknown.

Frequent premature ventricular contractions often indicate instability. However, they do not often indicate increased risk for sudden death. They can be due either to ischemia or to left ventricular dysfunction. The first line of treatment is to treat the ischemia or to lessen the left ventricular dysfunction. Surgery including aneurysmectomy, endocardial resection, and coronary artery bypass surgery have all had questionable results and are reserved for high-risk patients with sustained, refractory ventricular tachycardia. Though patients with refractory ventricular tachycardia have been treated by aneurysmectomy, in large series of patients, this has not been effective. Endocardial resection requires endocardial mapping, but it has a high mortality. Coronary artery bypass can perfuse ischemic tissue, but there are no good data to suggest that this stops the dysrhythmias. Pronestyl can be used for patients with high-risk PVCs, but it is difficult to stay on long-term because of joint aches. Quinidine and Norpace have their problems with Norpace causing congestive heart failure in damaged ventricles and both causing QT-interval prolongation. They can both be associated with sudden death, and many clinicians prefer to admit the patient to the hospital for initiating either agent. Beta blockers are an excellent choice, often very effective for controlling premature ventricular contractions. Newer drugs like flecainide and Ethmozine appear to be ideal for the patient with symptomatic PVCs causing palpitations. Amiodarone may be the only agent to improve survival in patients with refractory ventricular tachycardia.

If the patient is stable, further assessment can proceed. In general, coronary heart disease patients can be divided into those with limited myocardial reserve and those with myocardial ischemia or those with combinations of both. First, find the ischemic threshold as determined by the onset of angina pectoris or ST-segment depression at a particular heart rate, double product, or work load. Once this is clarified, the next evaluation is to determine the amount of mechanical reserve. Mechanical reserve relates to the amount of viable myocardium left after ischemic insults. Clinical clues that suggest the patient may not have much myocardial reserve include a history of congestive heart failure, cardiogenic shock, multiple prior MIs, a large anterior MI, cardiomegaly, a large creatinine kinase elevation, multiple Q-waves, underlying problems including cardiomyopathy or valvular heart disease. Patients with limited myocardial reserve have lost significant amounts of myocardium with their MI or may also have an underlying cardiomyopathy. The amount of myocardium lost is a strong prognostic feature of an infarct. Patients with large infarcts usually have large CK rises and extensive Q-wave patterns. They usually have had large anterior infarcts including the apex and lateral walls. Congestive heart failure (CHF) and cardiogenic shock indicate that a large amount of myocardium has been lost. Patients with multiple infarcts also usually have extensive myocardial damage. These patients must be watched for signs and symptoms of CHF while ischemic patients usually do not. They are limited by their maximal cardiac output which usually cannot be improved. However, afterload reduction with nitrates and Apresoline or captopril may be helpful in improving exercise capacity in some patients with poor myocardial reserve. Rather than chest pain, they are limited by fatigue and pulmonary symptoms. However, the symptoms of low output or CHF should never be left unexplained. In the infarct patients, they could be due to mitral valve insufficiency either due to papillary muscle dysfunction or rupture or due to a dilated mitral anulus. A rare explanation is a ventricular septal defect due to septal infarction. A second process could be having an effect such as a

cardiomyopathy or another valvular defect. Ischemia does not appear to predict risk as much as do signs of poor myocardial reserve, possibly because it
is difficult to quantify the amount of myocardium in jeopardy.

Exercise Testing Before Hospital Discharge.   The exercise test
early after an acute MI (from seven days to three weeks) has been shown to
be safe (see Chapter 6). This test has many benefits including clarification of
the response to exercise and the work capacity, determination of an exercise
prescription, and recognition of the need for medications or surgery. It appears to have a beneficial psychological impact on recovery and is an effective
part of rehabilitation.

Exercise Prescription.   In prescribing exercise, two basic
physiological principles should be considered. Myocardial oxygen consumption is the amount of oxygen required by the heart to maintain itself and do
the work of pumping blood to the other organs. It cannot be measured directly
without catheters but can be estimated by the product of systolic blood pressure and heart rate. The higher the product, the higher the myocardial oxygen
consumption, and the reverse is true. Patients usually have their angina at the
same double product, except for the impact of other factors such as catecholamine level, left ventricular end-diastolic volume, hemoglobin-oxygen disas-
sociation as affected by acid-base balance, and coronary artery spasm.

The second consideration is ventilatory oxygen consumption (VO_2), which
is the amount of oxygen taken in from inspired air by the body to maintain
itself and to do the work of muscular activity. Measuring this requires the
collection of expired air, gas analyzers, and skilled technical help. Presently,
there are no inexpensive devices that work with technical ease or accuracy to
make this important measurement. However, it can be estimated from knowing the work load of various activities. Since the body's mechanical efficiency
is relatively constant, measurements of the oxygen cost of an activity using
proper gas analysis can be applied between individuals. There are many tables giving the approximate oxygen cost of different activities. Since oxygen
consumption is equal to AV O_2 difference times cardiac output, and AV O_2
difference is roughly a constant at maximal exercise, maximal oxygen consumption can be an approximation of maximal cardiac output. However, patients with diseased hearts will often have a wider AV O_2 difference, a lower
cardiac output, and lower VO_2 than normal subjects performing the same submaximal work load.

Another important physiological concept of exercise is the type of work the
body is performing. Dynamic work (bicycling, running, jogging) requires the
movement of large muscle masses and requires a high blood flow and increased cardiac output. Since this movement is rhythmic, there is little resistance to flow and in fact, there is a "milking" action that returns blood to the
heart. The other type of muscular work is isometric work such as lifting a
weight or squeezing a ball. Isometric activities involve a constant muscular
contraction that limits blood flow. Instead of a cardiac response to increased
cardiac output and blood flow, as during dynamic exercise, blood pressure

must be increased in order to force blood into the active, contracting muscles. Pressure work is much more demanding of oxygen for the heart than is flow work. Also, since coronary artery blood flow depends upon cardiac output, the myocardial oxygen supply can become inadequate. Also, dynamic exercise is more easily controlled or graded so that myocardial oxygen consumption can be gradually increased, whereas isometric exercise can increase myocardial oxygen consumption needs very quickly. In addition, though isometric exercise is good for peripheral muscle tone and function, it does not result in the beneficial cardiac and hemodynamic effects of dynamic exercise.

Circuit Training. Kelemen and colleagues performed a prospective, randomized evaluation of the safety and efficacy of 10 weeks of circuit weight training in coronary disease patients, aged 35 to 70 years. Circuit weight training consisted of a series of weight-lifting exercises using a moderate load with frequent repetitions. Patients had participated in a supervised cardiac rehabilitation program for a minimum of three months before the study. Control patients (n = 20) continued with their regular exercise consisting of a walk/jog and volleyball program, while the experimental group (n = 20) substituted circuit weight training for volleyball. No sustained arrhythmias or cardiovascular problems occurred. The experimental group significantly increased treadmill time 12% while there was no change in the control patients. Circuit weight training was safe, and resulted in significant increases in aerobic endurance and musculoskeletal strength compared with traditional exercise used in cardiac rehabilitation programs.

Prognostic Indicators. Shephard analyzed the experience of the Ontario Multi-Center Exercise Trial to determine the recurrence of MI in an exercising population. The study followed 751 men post MI; comparison was made between the 50 participants who sustained a recurrence and the 701 participants who did not. Reinfarction was more likely with a history of multiple previous infarctions but was unrelated to such indicators of infarction severity as symptoms, electrocardiographic abnormalities, enzyme changes, cardiac arrest, dysrhythmias, or hypotension. Features noted on admission to the study suggesting an adverse prognosis included smoking history, disability, shortness of breath, and angina. The main physiologic warning sign was a low and decreasing cardiac output at submaximal work loads, with a widening of the AV O_2 difference. None of the adverse findings was of sufficient consistency to be of value when advising individual patients.

Kavanagh and colleagues evaluated prognostic indices in 610 patients, beginning eight months after MI and lasting three years, in a vigorous exercise-centered rehabilitation program. Over this period, 23 had fatal and 21 nonfatal recurrences of myocardial infarction. The most significant prognostic feature was noncompliance with the exercise program, but this was due to self-selection of those with symptoms or signs. Patients who dropped out of the exercise program had a reinfarction rate of approximately 50%, whereas those who stayed in the exercise program had a 2% recurrence rate. Risk ratios of 2 were observed for patients with persistent angina, aneurysm, enlarged heart, elevated serum cholesterol, and those who persisted in smoking cigarettes. ST-segment depression during the exercise test carried a risk ratio of greater than 3, whereas multiformed exercise-induced PVCs had a risk ratio of less than 2. There was a low yearly fatality rate of 1.2% in the 610 patients and of only 0.7% in those without exercise-induced ST-segment depression. A combination of ST-segment depression and high-serum cholesterol yielded a risk ratio of greater than 4. The prognosis for patients with these risk markers, however, remained at least as good as for comparable patients not receiving exercise training. Patients with the high-risk prognostic features had less lowering of their risk, but their prognosis remained more favorable than that of subjects who did not exercise. The high risk of being a dropout is most likely due to bias; i.e., the sickest could not tolerate the program.

A prospective study using risk indicators and an early exercise test was performed by Lindeval and colleagues to evaluate early mobilization and discharge of patients post-MI. One hundred eighty-four patients surviving after two days in a coronary care unit were divided into one rapidly and one conventionally mobilized group. Patients were not randomized, but selected on the basis of early risk indicators of electrical and mechanical instability. The five early risk indicators were sinus tachycardia or respiratory rate above 27 per minute, large enzyme rises, ventricular dysrhythmias, or heart blocks. A couple of days after selection, a submaximal bicycle test of 50 W was used, and 16% of the patients evaluated were excluded from the rapidly mobilized group. The late risk indicators included continued ischemia, dysrhythmias requiring treatment, a systolic time interval greater than .45, chest x-rays showing pulmonary congestion, heart rate greater than 125 beats per minute during the 50-W test, or if ST-segment elevation or depression, dysrhythmias, or angina occurred. The selected group was rapidly mobilized and discharged after a mean of nine days in contrast to a mean of 19 days for the group with risk indicators. No rapidly mobilized patient died in the hospital, and only one patient died during a six-month follow-up. In the conventionally mobilized group, 13% died in the hospital and an additional 25% died during the six-month follow-up. One-quarter of those patients that showed an abnormality during exercise were readmitted due to cardiac complications during the follow-up period. This study shows the ability of clinical parameters and exercise testing to stratify progressive ambulation and therapy in patients after a MI.

The prognostic implications of the ECG of an MI and the subsequent retention or disappearance of diagnostic Q-waves were examined in 4,524 patients. Those post-MI patients were followed for at least three years. Q-waves and infarction were classified as lateral, inferior, or anterior. Total mortality was not significantly different among patients with single infarct sites, while those with multiple infarct sites had a significantly higher mortality. Loss of a previously documented Q-wave occurred in 14% of the participants. However, mortality was not significantly different between those who lost the Q-wave versus those who had persistent Q-waves.

In 40 patients with coronary disease, Simoons and colleagues compared the heart rate levels and the incidence and types of premature ventricular complexes (PVCs) during exercise classes to those during 24-hour ambulatory monitoring and during a maximal exercise test. In six patients, peak heart rates during ambulatory monitoring exceeded those during exercise classes. Half of the patients reached higher heart rates during the exercise test. Twenty-three patients had significant PVCs during rehabilitation; nine had frequent, multiform, or repetitive PVCs. During the exercise test, 24 patients had PVCs, while during ambulatory monitoring, 34 did. Frequent, multiform, or repetitive PVCs occurred in eight patients during exercise testing and in 20 patients during monitoring. No relationship was found between either the incidence or the type of PVCs in individual patients under these three conditions. Thus, selection of patients with a high risk for dysrhythmias during cardiac rehabilitation is not feasible by either exercise testing or ambulatory recording.

Intervention Studies (Table 11–6).   Kallio and colleagues were part of a World Health Organization coordinated project to assess the effects of a comprehensive rehabilitation and secondary prevention program on morbidity, mortality, return to work, and various clinical, medical, and psychosocial factors after MI. The study included 375 consecutive patients under 65 years of age treated for acute MI from two urban areas in Finland between 1973 and 1975. General advice on rehabilitation and secondary preventive measures was given to all patients who were discharged from the hospital. On discharge, the patients were randomly allocated to an intervention or to a control group, both of which were followed for three years. Patients in the control goup were followed by their own doctors and were seen by the study team only once a year during the three-year follow-up. The program for the intervention group was started two weeks after hospital discharge. An exercise prescription was determined from a bicycle test; for most patients, the program was supervised.

After the three-year follow-up, the cumulative coronary mortality was significantly smaller in the intervention group than in the controls (18.6% versus 29.4%). This difference was mainly due to a reduction of sudden deaths in the intervention group (5.8% versus 14.4%). The reduction was greatest in the first six months after infarction. Of the intervention group and the controls, 18.1% and 11.2%, respectively, presented with nonfatal infarctions. Total mortality was 21.8% in the intervention group and 29.9% in the control group. Two weak points of this study are that more patients in the intervention group than in the control group took antihypertensives and beta blockers and that the exercise capacity measured at one, two, and three years after acute infarction was similar in both groups.

Kentala studied 298 consecutive males under 65 years of age admitted to the University of Helsinki Hospital in 1969 with a diagnosis of acute MI. They were divided by the year of birth; controls were from odd numbered years (n = 146) and exercisers were from even numbered years (n = 152). The average age was 53 years. Exclusions for controls included 10 with uncertain diagnosis, 24 who died in the hospital, 5 who refused or were not informed, 4 who had other severe disease, and 22 who lived too far away. Exclusions for the

TABLE 11–6.
Summary of the Randomized Trials of Cardiac Rehabilitation

| INVESTIGATOR | YEAR | POPULATION RANDOMIZED | | | | | MEAN NO. MONTHS ENTRY POST MI | MEAN AGE |
		TOTAL	CONTROLS	EXERCISED	EXCLUSIONS	% WOMEN		
Kentala	72	158	81	77	150		2	53
Palatsi	76	380	200	180	>65	19%	2.5	52
Wilhelmsen	77	313	157	158	27%, >57	10%	3	51
Kallio	79	375	187	183	>65	19%	3	55
NEHDP	81	651	328	323	280	0%	14	52
Ontario	82	733	354	379	28, >54	0%	6	48
Bengtsson	83	171	90	81	45, >65	0%	1.5	56
Carson	83	303	152	151	>70	0%	1.5	51
Vermeulen	83	98	51	47		0%	1.5	49
Roman	83	193	100	93		10%	2	55
Mayou	83	129	42	44	>60	0%	1	51
Froelicher	84	146	74	76		0%	4	53
Hedback	85	297	154	143	>65	15%	1.5	57
AVERAGES:								

exercise group included 12 with uncertain diagnosis, 21 who died in the hospital, 3 who were not informed, 3 who had other severe disease, and 36 who lived too far away. Eighty-one controls and 77 exercisers were accepted for the study. Of the 81 controls, 4 died, 3 were hospitalized, and 1 refused, leaving 73. Of the 77 randomized to exercises, 5 died, 3 were hospitalized and 1 refused, leaving 69 at one-year follow-up. Unless contraindicated, patients were kept on anticoagulation; beta blockers were avoided. Both groups made their own decisions on smoking, and diet information was given. The training group was also urged to increase home activities after the exercise program daily, especially walking.

There were two training sessions weekly, later increased to three a week, with 20-minute warm up, 20-minute exertion (bicycle, rowing, stairs), followed by a cool-down phase. The exercise HR was optimally set at 10 beats less than the maximal HR gotten from exercise testing. Attendance decreased to only 10 patients in the exercise group between the sixth and twelfth month. However, 16 trained on their own. Eleven controls were at a full training level after one year. There was no difference in morbidity or mortality between the groups. Both groups showed clear decreases in HR for given work loads, and both groups showed improved maximal work load, especially in those patients with greater than 70% attendance. Return to work was not influenced by training; 68% who worked before MI returned to work after one year.

Palatsi's study was a nonrandomized trial of 380 patients less than 65 years old recovering from MI. The patients were excluded if they had locomotive limitations, psychological problems, or congestive heart failure. The first 100 patients were allocated to an exercise program, and the second were the controls. The next 50 patients entered the exercise group, then 50 entered the control group. The final total included 180 patients for exercise including 37 women and 200 controls including 34 women. Patients with non-Q-wave MIs

| | DROPOUTS | | RETURN TO WORK | | RE-MI | | PERCENT MORTALITY | | | | | |
| | | | | | | | SUDDEN | | CARDIAC | | TOTAL | |
YEARS F-U	CNTRL	EX	CNTRL	EX	CNTRL	EX	CNTRL	EX	CNTRL	EX	CNTRL	EX
1			5%	8%							22%	17%
2.5		35%	33%	36%	15%	12%	3%	6%	14%	10%	14%	10%
4		46%					18%	16%			22%	18%
3					13%	20%	14%	6%	29%	19%	30%	22%
3	31%	23%			7%	5%			6%	4%	7%	5%
4	45%	46%			13%	14%					7%	10%
1			73%	75%	4%	2%					7%	10%
3.5	6%	17%	81%	81%	7%	7%					14%	8%
5					18%	9%			10%	4%	10%	4%
9	4%	4%			5%	4%	7%	4%	5%	3%	6%	4%
1.5	25%	25%	30%	57%								
1	14%	17%			1%	1%					0%	1%
1		45%	59%	66%	16.2%	5.4%			7.8%	8.4%	7.8%	9.1%
	21%	29%	47%	54%	10%	8%	11%	8%	12%	8%	12%	10%

were treated with bed rest for three days, allowed to sit for one week, were allowed to walk on the 10th day, and were discharged on the 12th day. Q-wave MI patients were at bed rest for seven days, sitting for one week, allowed to walk on the 14th day, and discharged on the 16th day.

Exercise training was begun 10 weeks after the MI and included breathing and relaxation exercises, calisthenics of all muscle groups, and walking which progressed to running in place. Heart rate was at least 70% of the maximum rate during 30-minute sessions. Patients were to do this at home every day. Once a month, the patients returned for progression of their exercise program. No effort was made to change smoking habits. The authors concluded that home training was not as efficient as continual supervised programs, but still accelerated recovery of aerobic capacity. Rehabilitation had no effect on the clinical condition of the trainees. There was no group difference in symptoms, smoking habits, serum cholesterol, or return to work.

Wilhelmsen's study included patients born in 1913 or later and hospitalized for an MI between 1968 and 1970 in Goteborg, Sweden. Patients were randomized to a control group (n = 157) or an exercise group (n = 158). Fifteen of the controls and 20 of the exercisers were females. The only criterion was an age of 60 years or older, but 27% of patients were excluded for cardiac complications. The two groups were comparable for hypertension, diabetes mellitus, treatment with digoxin, smoking status, CHF, and previous MI. The exercise group trained three times a week for 30 minutes a session. Calisthenics, cycling, and running were performed at 80% of the maximal age-predicted heart rate. All follow-up treatments were the same except for the exercise program. After one year the exercise group showed increased work capacity, lower blood pressure, but no difference in blood lipids. At one year, only 39% continued to come to the hospital to exercise, while 21% trained elsewhere. Initially, 81% of the training opportunities were utilized. At one year, only 63% of the sessions were utilized. Smoking after an MI was found to be a significant predictor of fatal recurrent MI. There was also an association between stopping smoking and attending the exercise program. No significant difference was seen with respect to cause of death, type of death, or place of death. They concluded that antismoking advise and treatment with beta blockers deserve higher priority than exercise training in the secondary prevention of MI.

NEHPD. The National Exercise and Heart Disease Project (NEHPD) included 651 men post-MI enrolled in five centers in the United States. It was a randomized three-year clinical trial of the effects of a prescribed supervised exercise program starting 2 to 36 months after an MI (80% were more than eight months postinfarction). In this study, 323 randomly selected patients performed exercise three times a week that was designed to increase their heart rate to 85% of their individual maximal heart rate achieved during treadmill testing, and 328 patients served as controls. This study was carefully designed by experts who took two years to complete the protocol. An initial low-level exercise session in both groups to exclude the faint of heart who would not comply with an exercise program was suprisingly effective in improving performance.

The three-year mortality rate was 7.3% (24 deaths) in the control group versus 4.6% (15 deaths) in the exercise group. Deaths from all cardiovascular causes (acute MI, sudden death, arrhythmias, congestive heart failure, cardiogenic shock, and stroke) for the three-year follow-up were 6.1% (20 deaths) in the control group versus 4.3% (14 deaths) in the exercise group. Neither difference was statistically significant. However, when deaths due to acute MI were considered as a separate category, the exercise group had a significantly lower rate: one acute fatal MI per three years (0.3%) in the exercise group versus eight fatal MIs (2.4%) in the control group (P <.05). The rate of all recurrent MI over three years, fatal and nonfatal, did not significantly differ between groups: 23 cases (7.0%) in the control versus 17 cases (5.3%) in the exercise group. The number of rehospitalizations for reasons other than MI were identical in the two groups (27.4% versus 28.5% per three years). The need for coronary artery surgery was also equal in both groups; 16 controls and 17 exercisers underwent surgery in the three-year period. This study suggests a beneficial effect of this cardiac rehabilitation program, but insufficient participants due to financial limitations and dropouts prevented a conclusion. Unfortunately, this study could not be definitive but instead demonstrated the feasibility of resolving this important issue. It is unfortunate that it was discontinued, especially since the results are so encouraging. Only 1,400 patients would be required to demonstrate a statistically significant reduction in mortality rate in the exercise group if the reported trend persisted. The patients in the exercise group who suffered a reinfarction had a lower mortality rate, suggesting that an exercise program increases an individual's ability to survive an MI.

The Ontario Study included seven Canadian centers that collaborated in this randomized perspective trial. Seven hundred thirty-three post-MI males underwent random stratified allocation to either a high-intensity group or a low-intensity exercise group. Patients were excluded for cardiac failure, insulin-dependent or uncontrolled diabetes, diastolic hypertension, orthopedic problems, and/or severe lung disease. The two groups were comparable for initial MI, angina, hypertension, type A personality, smokers, ex-smokers, and cholesterol level. Stratifying variables included (1) the presence or absence of hypertension, (2) blue versus white collar employment, (3) presence or absence of angina, and (4) type A and B personality. The high-intensity group trained by walking or jogging 65% to 85% of their maximal oxygen consumption twice a week for one hour each session. This continued for eight weeks, after which they trained four times a week on their own. The low-intensity group trained once a week with relaxation exercises, volleyball, bowling, or swimming for one hour. They attempted to keep their heart rate at less than 50% of their maximal oxygen consumption. Both groups were encouraged to stop smoking and control their weight. Less than 5% of the low-intensity group regularly exercised vigorously. The dropout rate was 47%. The rate of reinfarction in the high-intensity group was 14%, and 13% in the low-intensity group. They found that the high-intensity exercise program had similar results to one designed to produce a minimal training effect and did not reduce the risk of reinfarction.

Bengtsson reported 171 MI patients under the age of 65 who were randomized to a control and exercise group. Patients were excluded for congestive heart failure, post-MI syndrome, aortic insufficiency, hepatitis, polio, diabetes, new MI, thyroid disorders, stroke, or psychological problems. The rehabilitation program consisted of an outpatient exam, physical therapist-supervised exercise (large muscle group interval training by use of bicycles, calisthenics and jogging for 30 minutes, two days a week for three months at 90% of the maximal heart rate), and counseling. There was no reported difference between groups for age, sex, number of infarcts, highest enzyme, heart size, number of days in the hospital, number of admissions, angina, CHF arrhythmias, or depression or hypochondriasis on the MMPI.

The authors reported 100% compliance to the program. The exercisers showed lower mean SBP at rest and lower DBP at high work loads than controls. Equal percentages of the exercise group and of the controls (74%) returned to work. The exercisers performed 31% heavier work at the end of training and 63% at the end of follow-up. They concluded that at one year all patients were less physically and socially active than before their MI. They were more dependent on their relatives than before and they had a poor understanding of their illness. Their rehabilitation program (including exercise, information, counseling, and social measures during the first five months after an acute MI) did not change the outcome 8 to 19 months after the MI compared to controls when considering physical fitness, return to work, psychological factors and an understanding of their illness.

Carson et al. performed their 3½-year study in a population of 1,311 male MI patients. Of these, 12.5% died in the hospital, 4% died after discharge but prior to follow-up, and 4.8% failed to attend follow-up appointments. Thus, 70% of the original admissions remained. Patient exclusions included: greater than 70 years of age, CHF, cardiac enlargement, lung disease, hypertension, insulin, angina, orthopedic or medical problems, or personality disorders. After these exclusions, 442 patients were considered suitable; 139 of these declined, leaving 303. These patients accepted and were randomized to either a control or exercise group. There was no group difference with regard to site of MI, number of MIs, highest enzyme level, smoking habits, known diabetes, previous angina or MI, cholesterol levels, family history, LV failure, or occupation. The exercise group trained in a gym twice a week for 12 weeks at 85% of the exercise test determined maximal heart rate or until symptoms of angina, shortness of breath, or poor systolic blood pressure response. Isometric exercise was avoided. The dropout rate was 17% in the exercise group and 6% in the controls. Mean age at death was significantly different in the two groups: 50 in the exercise group and 57 in the control group. Return to work was 81% in both groups, and both groups showed a similar decrease in smoking after their MI. They concluded that the difference of fitness between the exercise and control patients after completion of the study was highly significant. There was no significant decrease in mortality for the exercise group except for those with an inferior wall MI.

Vermeulen described a prospective randomized trial with a five-year follow-up. Approximately one month after the MI, patients underwent a symptom-limited exercise test. There was no total population description, no training description, no dropout rate reported, and no return to work described. Both the control and exercise group received the same dietary advice. They found that rehabilitation did not influence smoking habits but lowered serum cholesterol. Their six-week rehabilitation program was associated with a 50% decrease in progressive CAD when compared to the control group. Mortality and morbidity was 50% lower in the rehabilitation group. The incidence of progression of CAD was significantly decreased in patients smoking less than 20 cigarettes a day. They concluded that cardiac rehabilitation is a safe procedure and of benefit to patients with MI due to direct effects on myocardial perfusion and to lowering of cholesterol levels.

Roman reported 139 patients including 19 females who entered into the cardiac rehabilitation study. A control and exercise group were comparable for age, sex, and MI location. The exercisers trained 30 minutes, three times a week, at 70% of maximum heart rate for an average of 42 months. At the nine-year follow-up, the control group had 24 cardiac deaths including 15 acute MIs, 7 sudden deaths, and congestive heart failure. The trained group had 13 deaths which included 7 acute MIs, 4 sudden deaths, and 2 patients with CHF. The mortality rate was 5.2% for the control group and 2.9% for the rehabilitation group. There were 23 recurrent MIs in the control group (4.9% per year) and 16 recurrent MIs in the rehabilitation group (3.6% per year). There was no difference in the incidence of myocardial ischemia, severe arrhythmias, or CVAs between the two groups. There was a significant decrease in angina in the exercise group. The overall attendance was 76%, and the dropout rate was 4.1% of the exercise group and 3.9% of the controls. The authors concluded that cardiac rehabilitation on a long-term basis seemed to lessen mortality and reduce the frequency of anginal pain.

Mayou and colleagues studied 129 men, 60 years of age or less, admitted with MI. They were sequentially allocated to either normal treatment, exercise training, or counseling groups. The control group received standard inpatient care, advice booklets, and one to two visits as outpatients. They had no other education, walking program, or instructions for exercise. The exercise group received the normal treatment plus eight sessions (two times a week) of circuit training in groups, written reminders, and reviews of their results. The "advice group" received normal treatment plus discussion groups, kept a daily activity diary, and had couples therapy and three to four follow-up sessions. The three groups were comparable socially, medically, and psychologically. Patients excluded were 13 who died and 1 with a stroke. Evaluation was performed after 12 weeks using exercise testing and standard tests of psychological state and social adjustment. There were no differences among the groups in psychological outcome, physical activity, or satisfaction with leisure or work. The exercise patients were more enthusiastic about their treatment and achieved higher work loads on exercise testing. At 18 months, the only significant findings were a better outcome in terms of overall satisfaction, hours of work, and frequency of sexual intercourse for the counseled group. The dropout rate was 25% overall. There was no difference in exercise capacity at 6 weeks, but at 12 weeks, there was a nonsignificant increase in the exercise group. The groups were similar for return to work, activities, sexual activity, and ratings of quality of life. There was no group difference with compliance to advice in smoking, diet, or exercise. They concluded that exercise training increased confidence during exercise in the early stages of convalescence, but that the exercise program had little value in regard to cardiac performance, daily function, or emotional state.

Hedback's study in Sweden was retrospective with a control group of 154 patients and an intervention group of 143 patients; 23 of the controls and 22 of the exercisers were women. There was no group difference regarding age, sex, risk factors for MI, rate of employment, income level, MI location or size, arrhythmias, medications, or discharge chest x-ray heart size. Exclusions for the training group included severe CHF, arthritis, and stroke. Thirty-one declined to enter the program. Seventy-eight of the 84 who began completed the training program. Both groups were treated the same during their acute hospitalization. Training began six weeks after MI following a bicycle test. Training was performed on a bicycle to a maximum HR of five beats below maximal HR as determined during the exercise test. If symptoms or signs occurred, HR was limited to 15 beats below maximal HR. Sessions were 25–30 minutes long. This was done for four weeks and then replaced by calisthenics and jogging plus a home program. Patients with a cholesterol level of 8 mmol/L were referred to the dietician. Beta blockers were administered to 60% of the patients. One year following the MI, there was no group difference in mortality, but the exercise group had a significantly lower rate of nonfatal reinfarction, fewer uncontrolled hypertensives, and fewer smokers.

May and colleagues have presented an excellent review of the long-term trials in secondary prevention after MI. Trials reported prior to November, 1981 were considered in which both intervention and follow-up were carried

TABLE 11–7.
Follow-up Randomized Intervention Trials After Myocardial Infarction Considered
Epidemiologically Valid*

INTERVENTION	NO. OF STUDIES (WITH SIGNIFICANT DIFFERENCE)	NO. OF PATIENTS RANDOMIZED	LENGTH OF FOLLOW-UP (RANGE OF MEANS)	% MORTALITY CONTROLS	% MORTALITY INTERVENTION	EFFECTIVENESS (% REDUCTION IN DEATHS)
Antidysrhythmics	6 (0)	1,675	4 mo.–2 yr	10.3	10.8	−4.6
Lipid lowering	9 (1)	19,834	21 mo.–11 yr	23.6	19.4	17.8
Anticoagulants	5 (0)	2,327	2–6 yr	17.7	13.7	22.6
Platelet active drugs	7 (0)	13,298	1–3 yr	10.5	9.7	7.6
Beta blockers	11 (4)	11,325	9 mo.–2 yr	11.5	8.8	23.5
Exercise	6 (1)	2,752	1–4.5 yr	14.7	11.9	19

*Adapted from May et al.

out beyond the time of hospital discharge. Random assignment and at least a total sample size of 100 were required. Total mortality was used whenever possible in order to minimize bias. All patients randomized were included in the mortality estimates to reduce the bias of differential withdrawal. Only the interventions listed in Table 11–7 have been properly evaluated. Interventions not yet properly studied include cigarette smoking, bypass surgery, percutaneous transluminal angioplasty, blood pressure reduction, fibrinolytic agents, calcium antagonist, inotropics, and afterload reduction. The number of studies presented are listed with parentheses around the ones that had a significant difference between the control and the intervention group. The effectiveness is calculated by considering the percent reduction in deaths that would have occurred if the intervention had been applied to the control group. Though few of the interventions resulted in a significant difference, all of them except for the antidysrhythmics show a trend toward efficacy. For those of us who recognize the clinical value of exercise and cardiac rehabilitation, the 19% effectiveness of the exercise programs is encouraging. It appears that exercise is as safe and effective as the other available means of secondary prevention. The relatively improved averages in Table 11–6 confirm the favorable outcome with cardiac rehabilitation.

COMPLICATIONS OF AN EXERCISE PROGRAM

There is a small but definite incidence of cardiac arrest associated with exercise testing of cardiac patients, particularly in the early minutes of recovery. A large multicenter survey of complications of exercise testing by Rochmis and Blackburn showed a combined mortality and morbidity rate of four events per 10,000 tests. In a retrospective review by Irving and Bruce of 10,751 symptom-limited exercise tests, five cardiac arrests were reported. All occurred in the first four minutes of recovery, and all five patients survived after defibrillation (one arrest per 2,000 tests). The relative risk of developing cardiac arrest with exercise testing (lasting 15 minutes) can be estimated to be one arrest per 538 hours of treadmill exercise, or 160 times greater than what might be expected to occur spontaneously (one death per 88,000 hours assuming a 10% yearly rate of sudden death).

Haskell surveyed 30 cardiac rehabilitation programs in North America using a questionnaire to assess major cardiovascular complications. This survey included approximately 14,000 patients for 1.6 million exercise-hours. Of 50 cardiopulmonary resuscitations (CPR), 8 resulted in death, and of 7 MIs, 2 resulted in death. Exercise programs resulted in four other fatalities occurring after hospitalization. Thus, there was one nonfatal event per 35,000 patient-hours and one fatal event per 160,000 patient-hours. The complication rates were lower in ECG-monitored programs. The current programs reported a 4% annual mortality during exercise, which is not different from that expected for such patients. Other programs have reported rates of cardiopulmonary resuscitations ranging from 1 in 6,000 to 1 in 25,000 man-hours of exercise. Such events are difficult to predict, can occur in patients with only single-vessel disease, and can occur at any time after being in a program.

A Seattle cardiac rehabilitation program (CAPRI) reported the highest rate of 1 CPR in 6,000 exercise hours. Of 15 patients requiring defibrillation, the CAPRI group successfully resuscitated all of them. Eleven had angiography, which showed single-vessel disease in four patients and multivessel disease in seven. Subsequently, the CAPRI record improved and they have had experience with defibrillating two patients simultaneously; on another occasion, a physician monitoring an exercise class was defibrillated. Of 2,464 patients observed during a 13-year period, 25 cardiac arrests occurred during 375,000 hours of supervised exercise, a rate of 1 arrest per 15,000 hours. The same incidence rate was reported in Toronto and in Atlanta where five arrests occurred in 75,000 hours of exercise, and a similar rate of one arrest per 12,000 hours (total of 36,000 gymnasium hours) was reported in Connecticut. In CAPRI, 12 of the 25 victims had been enrolled for 12 or more months. Fibrillation was recorded in 23 cases and ventricular tachycardia in 2. Prompt defibrillation was carried out and all patients survived. Each cardiac arrest was a "primary" arrhythmic event, and none was associated with acute MI. Eighteen of the 25 patients had ST-segment depression, and 5 had developed hypotension with prior exercise testing.

The incidence of exertion-related cardiac arrest in cardiac rehabilitation programs is small and, because of the availability of rapid defibrillation, death rarely occurs. Using an annual 10% incidence rate of sudden arrhythmic deaths (one per 88,000 man-hours) is one sixth that observed during participation in exercise programs. Using a more conservative 3 to 5% annual incidence rate of sudden death would increase the risk. In an earlier review of survival in the CAPRI population, 85% of cardiac arrests took place during exercise classes that the subjects attended for about three hours each week.

However, the majority of sudden deaths are temporally associated with routine activities of daily life and not with exercise. Therefore, the number of deaths due to strenuous physical exertion is relatively modest. Exertion-related cardiac arrest is usually due to ventricular fibrillation or tachycardia, and exercise may increase its risk by 100 times.

Fletcher and Cantwell reported five coronary disease patients resuscitated after ventricular fibrillation in an exercise program. Multivessel coronary disease that could be treated with bypass surgery was present in four of them. Resuscitation was required unexpectedly and at unpredictable times, occurring 2 to 48 months after being in the exercise program. These two experienced cardiologists are now reluctant to graduate patients to exercise without medical supervision. Shephard and Kavanagh also agree that the potential victim of a cardiac arrest during exercise training cannot be identified. Even trained patients should avoid excessive and unusual exertion, particularly when it is associated with competition and emotional excitement. Patients should also learn to recognize dysrhythmias and angina and should moderate their activity if they sense ischemic prodromes, tension, or depression.

Questionnaire.   To determine changes in American health care delivery over the past decade for patients with an uncomplicated MI, questionnaires were sent to 6,000 physicians in 1979. Responses were compared to a similar survey taken in 1970. Almost all physicians in 1979 reported the use of a coronary care unit with continuous electrocardiographic monitoring. The average hospital stay dropped from 21 days to 14 days. Patient education materials were used more frequently than in 1970. Exercise tests were more commonly used and usually at six weeks after infarction. Early ambulation and return to work were more common; most physicians recommended progressive physical activity after hospitalization.

Lipids.   To see if coronary patients can alter their lipids with exercise, Hartung and colleagues measured plasma high-density lipoprotein (HDL) cholesterol in 18 male patients. They found that HDL cholesterol was increased without changes in total cholesterol or body weight. Another study has shown a rise in HDL cholesterol in post-MI patients in an exercise program. Nineteen men were randomly allocated to an incremental exercise program and 23 to a control group for the six-month study. Though the exercise program altered plasma lipoproteins beneficially, there was no relationship between changes in lipoproteins and treadmill performance. Endurance exercise training in middle-aged males with coronary artery disease significantly lowered plasma cholesterol, low-density lipoprotein cholesterol, and triglycerides while increasing HDL cholesterol. These beneficial effects correlated best with increased VO_2 max after seven months of training.

Kavanagh and the Toronto group, in a multivariate analysis of post-MI patients for one year, found that modest increases in HDL cholesterol were apparently due to life-style alterations unless an exercise threshold of about 20 km per week was attained. Improvement of the lipid profile can be sustained by distance running.

Spontaneous Improvement Post-Myocardial Infarction.   To document spontaneous improvement in aerobic capacity, the Stanford group has measured VO_2 max within the first three months after an uncomplicated MI. Forty-six men underwent symptom-limited maximal treadmill tests 3 and 11 weeks after a MI. There was a significant increase between the two periods in heart rate, rate pressure product, and oxygen consumption during submaximal exercise. The mean maximal heart rate increased from 137 to 150 and VO_2 max from 21 to 27 cc O_2/kg/min. Maximal SBP, double product, and oxygen pulse also increased.

To evaluate hemodynamic changes after MI, Kelbaek and colleagues measured VO_2 max and performed invasive studies at rest and during two submaximal exercise levels. Thirty men were studied two, five, and eight months after an uncomplicated MI. Fourteen patients participated in an exercise program during the first three months of the study, while the other 16 patients attended the training during the second three-month period. An increase in VO_2 max occurred at the fifth month in both groups, 16% and 11%, respectively, along with an increase in cardiac index at the same relative submaximal work load. Later in the study, only slight increments in VO_2 max and no changes in hemodynamics were recorded within or between the two groups. They concluded that poor medical advice and pensions appeared to be the major factors responsible for unnecessary unemployment after an acute MI.

The UC Davis Group studied the effects of walking for 14 weeks on nine patients with coronary heart disease. Each patient was tested after training at the individually determined horizontal treadmill speed that induced ST-segment depression in the pretraining test. Although VO_2 max did not increase significantly with training, submaximal heart rate and the double product were reduced by 10% and 16%, respectively. Naturally, none of the patients had the same amount of ST-segment depression as in the first test. The patients became more efficient walkers with a 10% decrease in their oxygen consumption requirements. Though the authors proposed that this was due to the walking program, it has previously been shown that just serial treadmill testing results in improved efficiency.

Cardiac Changes in Coronary Heart Disease Patients.   Many favorable physiological changes have been documented in patients with coronary heart disease who have undertaken an aerobic exercise program. These include lower submaximal and resting heart rate, decreased symptoms, and increased maximal oxygen consumption. Peripheral adaptations are at least partially responsible for these changes, and controversy exists as to the effects of chronic exercise on the heart. In a review of the effects of exercise training on myocardial vascularity and perfusion, Scheurer concluded that in the normal animal heart, there is strong evidence that chronic training promotes myocardial capillary growth and enlargement of extramural vessels. However, it is unclear if these changes actually increase perfusion or protect the heart during ischemia. Controversy still remains as to whether exercise training can promote coronary collaterals in the animal model subjected to chronic ischemia even though Bloor's ischemic pig study supports this contention.

There have been several attempts to demonstrate the effects of exercise training on the hearts of patients with coronary heart disease. Ferguson and colleagues performed coronary angiography on 14 patients before and after 13 months of exercise. Despite a 25% increase in maximal oxygen uptake, collateral vessels were observed in only two coronary arteries, and 4 of 14 patients demonstrated progression of disease. Nolewajka and coworkers studied 10 male patients before and after seven months of exercise training. Neither the exercisers nor 10 control patients showed any changes in coronary angiograms, myocardial perfusion as assessed by intracoronary injection of radionuclides, or ejection fraction. Sim and Neill also failed to demonstrate cardiac changes in trained angina patients, including assessment of myocardial blood flow and oxygen consumption. Whether these negative findings can be explained by limitations in the techniques, patient selection, inadequate intensity, or length of training is uncertain.

Nuclear medicine procedures that noninvasively assess myocardial perfusion and performance have become important tools for the diagnosis of heart disease. They have also been used to evaluate the efficacy of CABS and PTCA. Scholl and coworkers studied 36 patients with exercise electrocardiography and thallium perfusion imaging before and after successful coronary angioplasty. The number of patients with an abnormal exercise ECG decreased from 20 before to 7 after angioplasty, while the number of abnormal thallium scans decreased from 21 to 6. Similar results have been reported by Berger and colleagues using thallium perfusion imaging to revaluate CABS in 22 patients. They reported that 37 of 48 (77%) thallium segments with stress-induced ischemia preoperatively reverted toward normal. Kent and colleagues reported that 17 of 23 patients who underwent CABS had significantly improved ejection fraction response to exercise postoperatively.

These techniques have been employed before and after exercise training in normals and cardiac patients. Verani and colleagues used radionuclide ventriculography and thallium scintigraphy to evaluate 16 coronary patients before and after 12 weeks of exercise training. Thirty patients entered the study, but only 16 completed it. Ten patients had a documented MI at least two months prior, and all but one of the others had angiographic documentation of coronary disease. Nine patients received propranolol throughout the exercise period. Both posttraining exercise studies were performed at the same double product as in the pretraining studies. For the ventriculography, a multicrystal camera was used and scintigraphy accomplished within 10 seconds of completion of exercise. After the training program, 15 of the 16 patients had improved exercise tolerance. Resting mean left ventricular ejection fraction increased from 52% to 57%, but no change was noted in exercise ejection fraction or regional wall motion abnormalities. The thallium studies were also unchanged.

The Duke group has reported the effects of six months of exercise training on treadmill and radionuclide ventriculography performance in 15 patients, all less than six months post-MI. A training effect was demonstrated by a lower heart rate at a submaximal work load and longer treadmill time in spite of a wide range of resting ventricular functions (ejection fractions from 17% to 67%). The mean ejection fraction, end-diastolic volume, and wall motion abnormalities during rest and at matched work loads and heart rates were not significantly different after training.

DeBusk and Hung randomized 11 coronary heart disease patients to a home exercise program and 10 to a control group three weeks post-MI. There was no significant difference in resting or exercise ejection fraction or thallium perfusion images between the two groups after eight weeks.

PERFEXT.   In 1979, a workshop on physical conditioning and rehabilitation was held at The National Heart, Lung and Blood Institute. It was concluded that there existed a need for continued research using small randomized studies to further clarify the value of physical training. Radionuclide techniques were suggested to have the potential to identify cardiac changes in such studies. Demonstration of such changes would be helpful in documenting the benefits of cardiac rehabilitation since larger trials utilizing morbidity and mortality endpoints have been inconclusive. Also, it might be possible to document which patients are likely to have cardiac benefits or adverse reactions to exercise therapy. In response to this, our group at the University of California, San Diego, proposed PERFEXT (PERFusion, PERFormance, EXercise Trial), which was subsequently funded.

The San Diego community was informed that we were recruiting male coronary heart disease patients between the ages of 35 and 65 for a free exercise program. The responding volunteers were a select group because they were highly motivated to be in an exercise program. They were encouraged to accept randomization by being promised that if randomized to the control group they could join the exercise classes after the one-year study was completed. Potential subjects were screened to determine if they: (1) had coronary heart disease; (2) were willing to be randomized and comply with either a low-level home walking program or a medically supervised exercise program at University Hospital; (3) could discontinue their medications for testing (digoxin for two weeks and beta blockers for three days); (4) had no complicating illnesses or locomotive limitations; (5) had not recently been in an exercise program; and, (6) had the approval of their physician. Patients with symptomatic congestive heart failure, unstable dysrhythmias, diabetes mellitus, significant symptomatic pulmonary disease, systemic hypertension of greater than 180 mm Hg systolic or 110 diastolic, severe claudication, or orthopedic problems were excluded. The patients were classified by the following criteria: (1) history of myocardial infarction; (2) stable exertional angina pectoris; or, (3) coronary artery bypass surgery. Disease stability was assured by careful history taking and by not allowing the patient to enter the study until at least four months after a cardiac event, a change in symptoms, or surgery. One hundred sixty-one patients were interviewed, signed consent forms, and agreed to randomization. The patients were then scheduled for three entry exercise tests done on separate days, usually within a two-week period. The thallium treadmill test was done first, for familiarization, followed by the maximal oxygen uptake treadmill test, and finally the supine bicycle radionuclide study. Of 146 patients randomized, 72 were in the training group and 74 in the control group.

A modified Balke-Ware protocol was used for both the thallium scintigraphy and maximal oxygen uptake procedures. The ECG data were digitized online using Marquette Electronics Data Loggers and later computer processed. The tests were maximal, except that the endpoint for the one-year thallium treadmill test was the maximal rate pressure product achieved at the initial thallium study. Perceived levels of exertion were recorded using the Borg scale. Oxygen uptake, carbon dioxide production, and minute ventilation were measured using the open circuit technique.

Two mCi of thallium-201 were introduced into an antecubital vein one minute prior to the maximal exercise endpoint. At one year, exactly the same camera angles were used, and an image with anatomic landmarks made during the initial test was used to ensure identical camera placement.

The thallium images were interpreted by three independent readers who had no pertinent patient information. The three views were each divided into three separate segments. The segments were graded using a previously published scoring system based on both the size and intensity of defects ranging from 1 for normal to 10 for the most severe. Three experienced observers scored them without knowledge as to name, group, or pre/post order, and the scores were averaged. A plus or a minus sign was assigned to the score after all images had been read to correspond with an improvement or worsening at one year. The form used is in Figure 11–1.

Radionuclide angiography was accomplished by the gated equilibrium technique with the subject in the supine position with the legs horizontal and not elevated. With the axis of the pedals at the same level as the body, the patient performed three stages of supine bicycle exercise each three minutes in duration. The work loads were set to approximate 40%, 80%, and 100% of the patient's maximal aerobic capacity as estimated by both a supine bicycle trial and a previous treadmill test. The ejection fraction was calculated from the formula: ejection fraction = EDC − ESC/EDC where EDC and ESC are ventricular counts at end-diastole and end-systole, respectively. Ventricular volumes at end-diastole and end-systole were estimated from EDC and ESC and the counts detected in 6 ml of blood taken during the corresponding rest and exercise periods.

The patients randomized to the exercise intervention group began training in a continuous electrocardiographic monitored class. The initial training intensity was set at a minimum of 60% of the estimated maximal oxygen uptake from the initial treadmill test. If the patient's physician wanted the patient to stay on beta blockers during training, a repeat test was done on the usual dosage for prescribing exercise. The intensity was usually progressively increased to 85% of the estimated maximal oxygen uptake by the eighth week of training. However, there was a considerable amount of variability since patients were not equally able or motivated to exercise. Aerobic training was carried out on arm, leg, and arm plus leg ergometers for 45 minutes three times per week. After completing eight weeks of ECG-monitored training, the

Patient Name: _____   Age: _____   Date: _____

Pretest Clinical History: MI ☐ ☐ (Yes No)   Hx Abnl TM ☐ ☐ (Yes No)   Chest Pain ☐ ☐ (Yes No)

Medications: Beta Blockers ☐ ☐ (Yes No)   Nitrates ☐ ☐ (Yes No)

Other _____

Max Effort ☐ ☐ (Yes No)   Angina ☐ ☐ (Yes No)   Test Endpoint: _____

Rest HR _____   Rest Blood Pressure _____   Maximum HR _____   Maximum Blood Pressure _____

Comments: _____

Background:

Lung Uptake	Normal ☐	Increased ☐
Visceral Uptake	Normal ☐	Increased ☐
Right Ventricle	Normal ☐	Increased ☐

Comments: _____

Heart:

Chamber Size	Normal	Small	Enlarged
Wall Thickness	Normal	Thin	Enlarged

Comments: _____

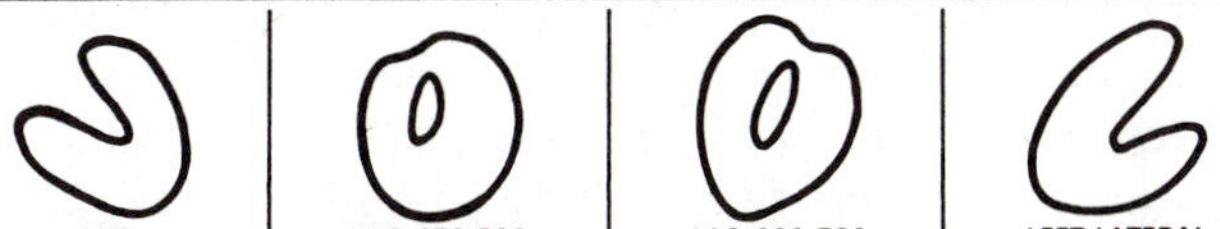

	ANT		LAO 45°-50°		LAO 60°-70°		LEFT LATERAL	
	Exercise	Delay	Exercise	Delay	Exercise	Delay	Exercise	Delay
Defect Size								
Defect Intensity								

Size: 1 = 10% of total myocardial area; 2 = 20%; 3 = 30%; 4 = 40%; 5 = 50%

Intensity: 1 = Normal; 2 = Just less than normal; 3 = Just greater than background; 4 = Background

Final Assessment:

FIG 11–1.
Form used for thallium scan scoring.

participant was considered for graduation to either our gymnasium or outdoor walk-run programs. There were no episodes of cardiac arrest or other major complications during exercise training sessions.

Patients randomized to the control group were offered a low-intensity walking program. The exercise intensity was set below 50% of the estimated maximal oxygen uptake for 30 minutes, three days per week. This careful follow-up detected two controls who crossed over to a level of exercise comparable to the intervention group. Nonetheless, their data were considered in the control group.

Differences between the control and exercise intervention groups were tested by standard statistical techniques such as the two-sample student t-test, analysis of variance (ANOVA), and analysis of covariance (ANACOVA). The appropriateness of these methods was checked by visual inspection of histograms, normal probability plots, and residual plots.

The decision to use ANOVA (which subsumes the t-test) or ANACOVA was based on the correlation between initial and one-year measurements in the control group. If this correlation was high, ANOVA was performed on the changes from initial measurement to one year. If the correlation was low, AN-

ACOVA was run using the one-year value as the dependent variable and the initial value as a covariate. Both methods of analysis attempted to adjust the one-year measurement with respect to the initial measurement.

Once randomized to control or intervention, a patient was always considered a member of that group regardless of his adherence to the protocol. There were 13 dropouts (six medical, seven motivational) in the exercise intervention group, and thus, one-year data were not available for these patients. To examine the possibility of a self-selection bias, the data were analyzed twice, and the results compared for consistency. In the first analysis, dropouts were not considered. In the second analysis, dropouts were included by considering their initial values to be their one-year values as well. This would tend to dilute any intervention effect if one existed but bolster conclusions based on significant results. There were no important differences between the two analyses. Unless otherwise indicated, the results presented are from analyses in which dropouts were not considered. The distribution of patients is illustrated in Figure 11–2.

Randomization was successful in equally distributing the clinical, treadmill, radionuclide ventriculography, and thallium imaging parameters between the two groups. The mean age was 53 (±8) years and the mean weight was 84 (±13) kilograms. Of the patients without bypass surgery who had

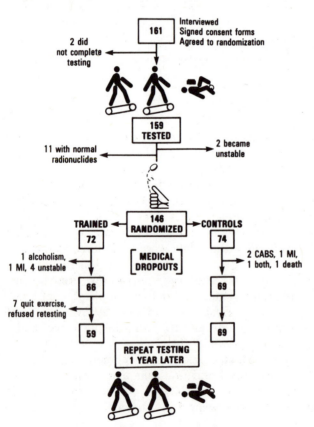

FIG 11–2.
Patient distribution and flow in the PERFEXT study.

coronary angiography (n = 43), 28% (12/43) had one-vessel disease, 40% (17/43) had two-vessel disease, 26% (11/43) had three-vessel disease, and 7% (3/43) had left main disease. Though nearly three-fourths had a history of angina pectoris at some time, only 35% had reproducible angina during initial treadmill testing. No statistically significant differences were found between the groups as shown in Tables 11–8 and 11–9.

During the course of the study year, there were five medical dropouts in the control group: two for coronary artery bypass surgery, one for MI, one with both myocardial infarction and coronary artery bypass surgery, and one death. There were six medical dropouts from the exercise intervention group: one for coronary artery bypass surgery, one for MI, one for alcoholism, and three who became unstable medically. One of these three had the only complication during testing. He required defibrillation for ventricular tachycardia during an extra treadmill test but suffered no sequellae. Of the 66 remaining in the exercise intervention group, seven dropped out of exercise classes because of job conflicts and/or lack of motivation and refused further testing. Repeat one-year testing was therefore performed on 59 of the 72 patients from the exercise intervention group and on 69 of the 74 controls.

Following completion of the study, the exercise records of the 59 exercise intervention patients who had one-year testing were extensively reviewed. Average intensities for the entire year were as follows: percent maximal estimated oxygen uptake and percent maximal heart rate by the Karvonen method was approximately 60% ± 10 (ranging from 40% to 100%). Percent of maximal heart rate and measured maximal oxygen uptake was approximately 80%. The average caloric expenditure per session was 319 ± 104 (130 to 719 calories). The mean attendance at exercise sessions was 76% ± 18 (23% to 97%).

Over the year of study, one control and one trained gained both abnormal

TABLE 11–8.
Distribution in Percentages of the Clinical Variables in the Two Groups After Randomization

CLINICAL VARIABLE	CONTROLS, % (N = 74)	EXERCISE-INTERVENTION GROUP, % (N = 72)
Currently smoking	8	14
Angina, documented by exercise testing	35	36
History of non-Q-wave myocardial infarction only	8	7
History of Q-wave myocardial infarction	68	68
Currently with		
Anterior Q-waves	22	28
Inferior Q-waves	39	30
Coronary artery bypass surgery	34	39
Medications taken before initial testing		
Digoxin	15	19
Beta blockers	57	42
Long-acting nitrates	43	31
Antidysrhythmics	15	14
Antihypertensives	9	17
History of congestive heart failure	9	10
Currently employed	65	56

TABLE 11–9.

Distribution of the Exercise Test Results in the Two Groups After Randomization

TEST	CONTROLS (N = 74)	EXERCISE-INTERVENTION GROUP (N = 72)
Maximal oxygen-uptake treadmill		
Heart rate, supine, beats/min	66 (9)	70 (12)
Blood pressure, supine, mm Hg	128 (13)/86 (9)	129 (16)/85 (9)
Heart rate, maximal, beats/min	154 (19)	156 (21)
Blood pressure, maximal, mm Hg	181 (26)/96 (10)	185 (29)/97 (11)
VO_2 estimated, mL/kg/min	33 (8)	33 (9)
VO_2 measured, mL/kg/min	26 (6)	26 (6)
Respiratory quotient	1.10 (.12)	1.13 (.11)
Maximal perceived exertion	17 (2)	17 (2)
% with abnormal ST depression	45 . . .	47 . . .
Radionuclide ventriculography		
Rest		
Ejection fraction	.52 (.13)	.52 (.15)
End-diastolic volume, mL	133 (61)	136 (60)
Stroke volume, mL	65 (28)	62 (21)
Cardiac output, L/min	4 (2)	4 (1)
Maximal exercise		
Heart rate, beats/min	139 (20)	137 (21)
Blood pressure, mm Hg	197 (26)/104 (11)	198 (30)/104 (13)
Ejection fraction	0.53 (0.15)	0.50 (0.16)
% change ejection fraction	1.5 (18)	−1.8 (16)
End-diastolic volume, mL	156 (59)	157 (68)
Stroke volume, mL	79 (30)	73 (26)
Cardiac output, L/min	9 (4)	8 (30)
Work load, kiloponds	769 (239)	739 (240)
Thallium 201 imaging		
% with fixed defects	71 . . .	68 . . .
Sum of ischemia scores		
4 hr minus immediate scores	3.4 (5)	4.5 (5)
Sum of immediate scores	16 (9)	16 (8)
% with reversible defects	50 . . .	51 . . .

treadmill-induced ST depression by visual interpretation and angina, one trained lost both, and three controls and one trained gained angina but lost criterion for abnormal ST depression. Nine controls and six trained lost abnormal ST depression, and four controls and three trained gained it. Ten trained and four controls lost or decreased treadmill-induced angina, and four controls and three trained gained it.

A significant training effect in the intervention group is evidenced by the decrease in their resting and submaximal heart rates, as well as the significant increase in the measured and estimated maximal oxygen uptake (Table 11–10). The control group showed a significant decrease in exercise capacity at least partially due to the lower maximal heart rate obtained at one year. There was also a small but significant decline in the submaximal heart rate and rate pressure product in the control group, probably due to habituation. No changes were observed in maximal perceived exertion, respiratory quotient, or systolic blood pressure between the two groups initially or at one year nor between the initial and one-year tests.

Analysis of variance testing confirmed that the training effect (including an increase in measured oxygen uptake) occurred in subgroups of the exercise intervention patients relative to controls. These subgroups included those with or without the following features: history of a Q-wave MI, treadmill test-induced angina, ejection fraction less than .40 or .50, abnormal exercise test-induced ST-segment depression, beta-blocker administration, or a dropping ejection fraction response. However, three-way analysis of variance revealed that those with angina but without a Q-wave MI in the intervention group did not increase their estimated oxygen uptake relative to controls.

Radionuclide ventriculography demonstrated a baseline increase in both

TABLE 11–10.
Initial and One-Year Measurements From the Maximal Treadmill Test Showing the Changes

TEST	CONTROL (N = 69)	EXERCISE-INTERVENTION GROUP (N = 59)
Heart rate, beats/min		
Supine		
Initial	66 (9)	69 (12)
1 year	69 (11)	65 (11)
Mean difference	2.2 (10)	−3.8 (10)†‡
Submaximal, 3.3 mph/5%		
Initial	125 (15)	126 (16)
1 year	121 (16)	118 (15)
Mean difference	−3.1 (11)†	−9.3 (12)†‡
Maximal		
Initial	154 (19)	156 (22)
1 year	149 (23)	154 (22)
Mean difference	−5.2 (13)†	−2.2 (11)
Rate pressure product§		
Submaximal, 3.3 mph/5%		
Initial	209 (44)	215 (47)
1 year	199 (49)	196 (42)
Mean difference	−8 (35)†	−19 (34)†
Maximal		
Initial	279 (57)	286 (59)
1 year	273 (60)	289 (67)
Mean difference	−6 (46)	3 (50)†
Maximal oxygen uptake		
Estimated, mL/kg/min		
Initial	33 (8)	33 (9)
1 year	32 (8)	37 (9)
Mean difference	1.3 (5)	4.7 (6)†‡
% change	−3 (18)	18 (24)†‡
Measured, L/min		
Initial	2.1 (.5)	2.2 (.6)
1 year	2.0 (.5)	2.3 (.6)
Mean difference	−.1 (.3)†	.1 (.3)†‡
% change	−4 (17)†	8.5 (17)†‡

† = significant change from rest; ‡ = significant difference between groups; § = HR × SBP.

end-systolic and end-diastolic volume in response to supine exercise. We examined the effect of training relative to controls, on the following variables: heart rate, ejection fraction, end-diastolic and end-systolic volumes, stroke volume, cardiac output at rest and at each of three stages, and percentage change of each from rest to each of three stages. The statistical method used was ANACOVA. The model employed the one-year value as the dependent variable, used the initial value as the covariate, and allowed for effects due to training, angina, and Q-wave MI. Differences due to angina and/or Q-wave MI alone are not reported.

Analysis of covariance revealed a differential effect of the intervention on stroke volume and cardiac output in patients with and without angina as shown in Table 11–11. For stroke volume, this was evident at stage 2 where rate pressure product was matched (p = .02) and at maximal exercise (p = .03), and suggested at rest (p = .06); and for cardiac output, only at maximal (p = .048). Exercise tended to increase stroke volume and cardiac output in patients without angina and to decrease them in patients with angina. Similar analysis for heart rate detected only a consistent exercise effect on all but maximal exercise. There was no significant difference at rest during the three stages of exercise or in the percentage change from rest to exercise between the control and trained group at one year in ejection fraction, end-diastolic volume, stroke volume, or cardiac output. However, Table 11–12 shows that the intervention group, relative to controls, had significantly lower percentage changes in end-systolic volume at all three work loads (p = .02, .04, and .05, respectively). The data suggested that the magnitude of the intervention effect differed in the MI and non-MI groups, though this was not statistically significant (p = .11, .09, and .12 at the three exercise stages, respectively); the intervention effect appeared consistently stronger in the non-MI group than in the MI group.

The sum of all the thallium defect scores on the immediate postexercise image are represented by the immediate score sum, while the difference between the total scores on the immediate and four-hour images is the ischemia score (Table 11–13). The effect of exercise on the immediate postexercise thallium scores was examined by ANOVA. The ANOVA model contained terms allowing for effects due to angina and Q-wave MI, as well as the intervention. The ANOVA results indicated a differential exercise effect, depending on the presence or absence of angina (p = .008). There was no indication of an ex-

TABLE 11–11.
Estimated Changes in Stroke Volume and Cardiac Output During Supine Bike Exercise After One Year

| CATEGORY | EXERCISE-INTERVENTION GROUP | | p VALUE |
	WITH ANGINA (N = 20)	WITHOUT ANGINA (N = 39)	
Resting supine stroke volume	−9.9 mL	7 mL	p = .06
Stroke volume, stage 2	−14.9 mL	11.9 mL	p = .02
Maximal stroke volume	−10.9 mL	10.3 mL	p = .03
Maximal cardiac output	−1.0 L/min	1.3 L/min	p = .048

TABLE 11–12.

Mean Values of Percent Change of Milliliters of End-Systolic Volume at One-Year Testing

| | | | | SUBGROUP WITHOUT Q-WAVE MI | | | |
| | TOTAL STUDY GROUP | | | WITH ANGINA | | WITHOUT ANGINA | |
% CESV*	CONTROL (N = 45)	EXERCISE INTERVENTION (N = 41)	p VALUE	CONTROL (N = 8)	EXERCISE INTERVENTION (N = 5)	CONTROL (N = 10)	EXERCISE INTERVENTION (N = 7)
Stage 1	8	−3	p = .02	6	−21	15	−2
Stage 2	12	2	p = .04	17	−12	24	−3
Maximal	28	16	p = .05	46	5	33	14

*% CESV indicates percent change end-systolic volume from rest to exercise. At a given exercise stage, the one-year means within the various subgroups are statistically adjusted by analysis of covariance to a common value of % CESV at randomization.

TABLE 11–13.

Initial and One-Year Measurements on Thallium Perfusion Images Using the Atwood Scores*

| | | | SUBGROUP WITH ANGINA | | | |
| | TOTAL STUDY GROUP | | MI‡ | | NO MI‡ | |
SCORES USED†	CONTROL (N = 59)	EXERCISE INTERVENTION (N = 59)	CONTROL (N = 13)	EXERCISE INTERVENTION (N = 11)	CONTROL (N = 10)	EXERCISE INTERVENTION (N = 9)
Sum of immediate scores						
Initial	16.1 (9)	16.6 (8)	20 (8)	21 (8)	16 (11)	15 (4)
1 year	16.4 (9)	15.0 (7)	22 (7)	16 (6)	16 (11)	12 (5)
Mean difference	.3 (4)	−1.3 (6)§	2.2 (4)	−4.6 (6)§	7 (4)	−3.0 (9)§
Sum of ischemia scores						
Initial	3.5 (4)	4.1 (4)	5 (8)	6 (5)	6 (6)	6 (5)
1 year	3.9 (5)	3.1 (4)	7 (6)	4 (4)	7 (8)	3 (4)
Mean difference	.4 (4)	−1.0 (4)§‖	1.5 (5)	−1.6 (4)§	1.5 (4)§	−2.6 (5)§

*All units are the Atwood scores described in the "Methods" section. Mean difference between initial and one-year study (1 year − initial).

†Column numbers and numbers in parentheses indicate mean (± 1 SD).

‡MI indicates myocardial infarction.

§Significant difference (P < .05) between exercise-trained and control groups.

‖Significant change (P < .05) from initial test to one-year test with a group.

ercise intervention effect in patients without angina relative to controls (p > .8; mean change of −.26 in controls, .05 in trained). There was a definite training effect relative to controls in patients with angina (p < .0005; with a mean change of 1.52 in controls, −3.90 in trained). The effect of exercise on the difference between the immediate and four-hour scores was also examined, using the same ANOVA model with terms for intervention, angina, and Q-wave myocardial infarctions. Again there was a differential effect of the intervention depending on the presence or absence of angina (p = .03). There was no indication of an exercise effect relative to controls in patients without angina (p > .8; mean change of − .20 in controls, − .47 in trained). There was an exercise effect relative to controls in patients with angina (p < .005; mean change of 1.48 in controls, − 2.05 in trained). Because of the relative concentration of changes in the radionuclide tests in the subgroup with angina, a careful analysis of maximal heart rate and rate pressure product was performed. There were no statistical differences found between the initial and one-year values with either test within those with angina with or without a history of a Q-wave MI.

When the immediate images were read side-by-side, blinded as to which was initial and final scan and group, no significant difference was noted between the control and trained group. Specifically, using the 0–3 scale previously explained, 105 patients (50 trained, 55 controls) had one-year scans with no change (average score of 0) from initial, 12 patients (six trained, six control) had a minor improvement (+ 1), two patients (one trained, one control) had a major improvement (+ 2). A minor worsening (− 1) was apparent at one year in four controls and five trained, while a major worsening (− 2) was seen in one control.

The one year of exercise training in our patients elicited the expected training response as seen in Table 11–10. The significant increase in estimated (18%) and measured (8.5%) VO_2 max is similar to most studies. We chose one year as the period of training because we were concerned that shorter periods might be inadequate in middle-aged cardiac patients. Peterson and colleagues found an improvement in exercise cardiac output at one year but not at six months in similar patients.

The PERFEXT exercise intervention group experienced a significant improvement in the exercise thallium images following the year using the Atwood scoring system. This scoring system was applied with the scans read independently, not in matched pairs. The scoring done with the images side-by-side paired for a given patient did not show a statistical difference though there was a trend to agree with the Atwood score. This may be explained by the greater gradations of the Atwood score from 1 to 10 while the side-by-side scoring only ranged from 0 to 3. Also, the Atwood score considered each area separately while the side-by-side score forced the readers to consider the entire scan. Thus, comparing thallium scans side-by-side which has been done effectively to evaluate surgical intervention was not successful in the clinical assessment of changes in myocardial perfusion caused by an exercise program. However, the improvement in the thallium scores, particularly in the angina patients, is consistent with animal studies suggesting that ischemia is the best inducer of collateral flow and that exercise can increase this stimulus. It was a disappointment that the ST-segment changes did not show an improvement or agree with the thallium changes.

One of the only changes in ventricular function or volume of a consistent nature was the significantly lower percentage change end-systolic volume in the exercise intervention patients. There were no significant differences in blood pressure at any stage of bicycle exercise, so there is no evidence that decreased afterload would explain this. It appears that the trained heart has to use the Frank Starling mechanism less than the untrained heart, probably due to lessened ischemia and/or improved contractility. This response may not have been seen had the patient's legs been elevated during supine exercise testing.

The other significant change was the effect of the intervention on stroke volume and maximal cardiac output. Training is known to increase both, but the differential effect due to angina was surprising. The decrease in stroke volume and cardiac output in the angina patients accompanies a lessening of ischemia and of the end-systolic volume increase in response to supine exercise. This suggests that absolute volume changes had to occur that could not be detected because of the variability of the volume technique. Future studies need to address the mechanism of this response.

In routine clinical practice, cardiac rehabilitation is begun as soon as possible after a cardiac event. However, given our study design and sample size limitation, we chose to deal only with patients with stable coronary heart disease. Studying patients recently post-MI is complicated by the degrees of severity and by the variable rate of spontaneous improvement. Our results may not be applicable to the cardiac population immediately postevent.

One criticism might be that our patients did not exercise hard enough and that if they had, more definite improvements might have been possible. However, even if we chose those who trained the most intensely or had the highest exercise class attendance, we did not find greater changes. Surprisingly, there was a poor correlation between the intensity or attendance and change in aerobic capacity or the radionuclide changes; and in fact, there was a poor correlation between the change in aerobic capacity and changes in the radionuclide tests. A paradox now exists regarding this. Ehsani and colleagues have reported impressive cardiac changes in a highly select group of cardiac patients with asymptomatic ST-segment depression exercised at very high levels. Hossack and Hartwick have reported an increased risk for exercise-induced events in similar patients. The question remains whether the usual cardiac patient can be exercised safely at higher levels than we utilized and, if so, whether more definite cardiac changes can be demonstrated.

The Effect of an Exercise Program on Anaerobic Threshold.   To document the benefits of chronic exercise during submaximal levels, investigators have considered the noninvasive measurement of the anaerobic threshold. The gas exchange anaerobic threshold (ATGE) has been defined as the oxygen uptake prior to the systematic increase in the ventilatory equivalent for oxygen (VE/VO_2) without a concomitant increase in the ventilatory equivalent for carbon dioxide (VE/VCO_2).

Following exercise training, an increase in the absolute oxygen uptake at which the ventilatory threshold occurs has been demonstrated in middle-aged men. In addition, Davis and colleagues reported a 15% increase in the ventilatory threshold expressed relative to peak oxygen uptake. The exercise programs utilized in these studies were both of high intensity, with 30- to 45-minute sessions, four to five times a week for nine weeks, at approximately 80% of peak oxygen uptake.

Although exercise programs for coronary heart disease patients are frequently at lower levels, improvements in both VO_2 max and submaximal heart rate response have been demonstrated. However, patients frequently have modest or no improvements in maximal oxygen uptake but are able to perform at higher work loads. One explanation for this would be an increase in ventilatory threshold. Therefore, the PERFEXT study results were looked at to evaluate the alterations in the ventilatory threshold before and after one year of moderate exercise training in patients with coronary heart disease. Forty-one coronary patients out of 156 had complete continuous gas exchange data.

Patients were tested on a calibrated treadmill using a modified Balke-Ware protocol consisting of an initial two-minute stage at 2.0 mph, 0% grade, a second stage at 3.3 mph, and then the grade was incremented by 5% every two minutes. This increment in work is approximately 150 kpm/min for an 80-kg man, which is less than the 180-kpm increment used by Ready and Quinney but somewhat higher than the 90 kpm used by Davis et al. All of the patients had previous treadmill experience and were not allowed to hold onto the handrails. Endpoints for testing were fatigue (exercise group 63%, control group 77%), moderately severe angina (exercise group 21%, control group 18%), and leg pain (two exercisers and one control). Gas samples were collected every minute through a low-resistance breathing valve into a series of evacuated weather balloons. Subjects had a nose clip in place throughout the gas collection period. A directional valve allowed for simultaneous collection, gas concentration analysis, and volume determination of three concurrent samples. Expired air concentration of oxygen and carbon dioxide were determined using an Applied Electrochemistry S-3A analyzer and a Gould Goddart MKII carbon dioxide analyzer. The gas analyzers were calibrated immediately before and after exercise using standard gas mixtures. Expired air volumes were determined on an American meter dry gas meter set at a flow rate of 160 L/min. The dry gas meter was calibrated in a range of 10–100 L at the flow rate of 160 L/min with 100 individual samples obtained from a tissot. The resultant regression equation was used to correct the volume obtained from the dry gas meter to that of the tissot. The flow rate of the gas meter was calibrated prior to each test.

The following variables were derived from the gas exchange data: (1) ventilation (VE L/min; ATPS, STPD, BTPS); (2) oxygen uptake (VO_2; L/min, ml/kg/min); (3) carbon dioxide production (VCO_2; L/min); (4) respiratory exchange ratio (R); (5) ventilatory equivalent for oxygen (VE/VO_2); and, (6) ventilatory equivalent for carbon dioxide (VE/VCO_2).

The ATGE was identified as the oxygen uptake prior to the systematic increase in VE/VO_2 without an increase in VE/VCO_5. Agreement by two of three independent, blinded observers was the criterion needed to determine the ATGE. This criterion was met in all but five tests, in which case the three observers collectively determined the ATGE.

A training effect was noted for supine rest and submaximal heart rates. The exercise group's peak VO_2 (L/min) increased only 1% which was significantly different from the controls largely due to the 7% decrease in peak VO_2 (L/min) in the control group. Although there was no statistically significant difference between groups with respect to change in peak VO_2 (ml/kg/min), there was a significant difference in total treadmill time (p < .01). With regard to the ATGE, there was no significant difference between groups when this variable was expressed in L/min, ml/kg/min, or as a percentage of peak VO_2. However, there was a trend in the control group to decrease these variables.

A significant correlation (r = .45; p < .05) between the absolute change in peak VO_2 (L/min) and the absolute change in ATGE VO_2 (L/min) was observed in the exercise group. In addition, there was a similar correlation (r = .46; p < .05) between the percent change in the ATGE VO_2 (L/min) and the estimated training intensity percent relative to the ATGE.

The expected alterations in gas exchange indices of exercise training did not occur. Although previous investigations in normal subjects utilizing high-intensity exercise programs have demonstrated increases in the ATGE, it was unknown whether the ATGE might increase following a lower-intensity program. In addition, the effect of exercise training on the ATGE in coronary heart disease patients has not been previously reported.

This study demonstrates that the level of exercise used was inadequate to cause an increase in the ATGE in patients with coronary heart disease. However, exercise counteracted the reduction in peak VO_2 and the ATGE VO_2 that occurred in the controls. Kinderman and colleagues suggested that to maintain a state of conditioning, exercise training should be performed in the range of the ATGE. Our study supports this contention since the mean ATGE is similar to the mean estimated training intensity when both are expressed as a percent of peak VO_2. Furthermore, it has been suggested that exercise training must occur at intensities above the ATGE to insure increases in cardiorespiratory variables such as peak VO_2 or the ATGE. The significant correlations between the training intensity relative to the ATGE or changes in peak VO_2 with respect to changes in the ATGE support this theory. Although these correlations appear weak, they represent all the patients randomized to the exercise group regardless of compliance. One can anticipate the observed variability in these relationships since attendance ranged from 25% to 97% with seven patients adhering to the exercise program less than two days a week.

Care must be taken in interpreting many of the studies evaluating the effect of chronic exercise in cardiac patients. Often initial testing is submaximal while follow-up tests are to a higher level because of increased patient and technician confidence and enthusiasm. This should be suspected when there are reported increases in maximal heart rate, blood pressure, respiratory exchange ratio, or perceived exertion. Our study did not show significant changes in these parameters because we had patients perform a maximal effort in their initial test. Also, if oxygen consumption is estimated from treadmill time rather than measured, the changes are very much exaggerated.

The present study demonstrates that in patients with coronary heart disease, exercising two to three times a week at an intensity approximately equal to their ATGE is adequate in altering the hemodynamic response to exercise and for maintaining a state of conditioning. Their improved exercise capacity (i.e., greater treadmill time) cannot be explained by an increase in their ATGE. It appears that when an increase in peak VO_2 or the ATGE is desired, the exercise intensity should be at a level above an individual's ATGE. However, in coronary disease patients, this exercise intensity may be contraindicated due to the signs or symptoms of their disease.

Changes in the Exercise ECG.   As part of PERFEXT, 48 patients who exercised and 59 control patients had computerized exercise ECGs performed initially and one year later. ST-segment displacement was analyzed 60 milliseconds after the end of the QRS complex in the three-dimensional X, Y, and Z leads and utilizing the spatial amplitude derived from them. There were no significant differences between the groups except for less ST-segment displacement at a matched work load, but this could be explained by a lowered heart rate. Analysis of variance yielded some minor differences within clinical subgroups, particularly in the spatial analysis. Obvious changes in exercise-induced ST-segment depression could not be demonstrated in our heterogeneous group of selected volunteers with coronary artery disease secondary to an exercise program.

The Effect of Beta Blockers on Exercise Training.   Randomized trials have demonstrated that beta blockers decrease mortality if taken during the first two years after myocardial infarction and that they are very effective in the treatment of both angina pectoris and hypertension. Both exercise training and beta blockade have at least one similar beneficial mechanism; they both lower the heart rate response to exercise. This allows ischemic patients to exercise to higher levels without exceeding their limitations for myocardial oxygen supply.

There is evidence that a functioning sympathetic nervous system may be necessary to achieve the beneficial hemodynamic alterations of training. In addition, the limitation in cardiac output due to beta blockade may result in fatigue and reduce the intensity of training or compliance to exercise. Also, if ischemia (the major stimulus for collateral development) is lessened by beta blockade, this potential benefit of training could also be impeded.

Beta-adrenergic blockade is widely used to treat patients with coronary heart disease, and aerobic exercise is also often prescribed particularly via cardiac rehabilitation programs. If beta-adrenergic stimulation is needed for the effects of exercise training to occur or if beta blockade lessens the ischemia necessary to promote collateralization, then beta blockade might be expected to interfere with the beneficial results of exercise. Beta-blockade could also increase perceived exertion and fatigue, thus lessening the tolerance for higher exercise levels and adherence to an exercise program. Therefore, a pharmacologically imposed limitation in heart rate and cardiac output during an exercise program may prohibit obtaining an optimal training effect. One of the beneficial hemodynamic effects of both regular exercise and beta blockade is that heart rate at rest and submaximal workloads are decreased. The mechanisms by which the hemodynamic changes occur secondary to regular exercise are poorly understood. High levels of sympathetic stimulation are present during aerobic exercise. It was concluded that regular intermittent infusions of dobutamine in dogs resulted in cardiovascular changes similar to those induced by an exercise program. However, the dogs did not get a true training effect. Other support for the importance of sympathetic stimulation for achieving the changes induced by exercise is that prolonged infusion of epinephrine has enhanced myocardial contractility in dogs and induced hypertrophy and that sympathectomy abolishes the increase in heart to body weight produced by exercise in rats. Hossack and colleagues found ventilatory changes during exercise in response to a single 40-mg oral dose of propranolol. They hypothesized that the changes were due to inhibited glucose metabolism that could impede the training effect, but this has not been substantiated. These observations suggest that repeated, sustained sympathetic stimulation might be an important factor in exercise training. If beta-adrenergic sympathetic stimulation is needed for an exercise effect to occur, then beta blockade might be expected to interfere with this process.

In 1974, Malmborg and colleagues first reported that a training effect could not be obtained in coronary patients with angina on beta blockers. However, their exercise program was only two times a week and 18 minutes long. Obma and colleagues reported a conflicting result in 1979. Their patients were limited by angina but demonstrated a significant increase in estimated oxygen consumption after an eight-week, 30–60 minutes, 5–7 days a week exercise program. Pratt and colleagues retrospectively studied 35 patients with coronary heart disease who underwent a three-month walk-jog cycle training program. Fourteen patients had received no beta blocker, 14 received propranolol 30–80 mg per day, and 7 patients received propranolol 120–240 mg per day at the discretion of their physicians. Training consisted of three one-hour periods per week at a heart rate 70% to 85% of maximal pretraining heart rate. Each group's estimated oxygen uptake assessed while on medications increased after training: by 27% in those not taking beta blockers, by 30% in those on a low dose, and by 46% in those on a high dose.

Vanhees and colleagues compared two groups of post-MI patients without angina pectoris, 15 receiving beta blockers and 15 not receiving them. Propranolol and metoprolol were the beta blockers most commonly used, at daily doses ranging from 30 to 120 and 75 to 200 mg, respectively. Exercise training was at an intensity of between 60% to 80% of their maximal capacity for three months. Both groups showed lower heart rates, systolic blood pressures, and rate pressure products after training, both at rest and at submaximal exercise. Testing was done while on beta blockers, but surprisingly, the maximal heart rate was only about 13 bpm higher in the group not on beta blockers. Heart rate decreases were significantly less in the group on beta blockade while systolic blood pressure decreases were less pronounced in the other group. Peak measured oxygen uptake increased an average of about 35% in both groups, but maximal heart rate and rate pressure product were also higher.

Controversy has even existed in the two studies of normals and the effects of beta blockade. Ewy and colleagues studied 27 healthy male adults (mean age 24) who first underwent two maximal treadmill tests. They were then randomly assigned to either a placebo group or to sotalol 320 mg per day. A third maximal treadmill test was performed one week after the administration of agent. Subjects then participated in a 13-week training program in which they exercised 45 minutes five times a week at a training heart rate equivalent to 75% of measured maximal oxygen uptake. A fourth maximal treadmill test was performed at conclusion of the training program while taking the agent; seven days after cessation of medication, a fifth maximal treadmill test was performed. Measured VO_2 max was increased following training in both groups; however, in the beta-blocked group, this was demonstrated only off beta blockers. These findings suggest that stroke volume had attained its maximal physiological capacity during beta-adrenergic blockade and reduction of maximal heart rate with beta blockade did not allow cardiac output to attain its potential for increase following training. These observations are supported by Tesch and Kaiser who observed markedly reduced VO_2 max in highly trained athletes after acute administration of propranolol.

Sable and colleagues studied normal young men before and after five weeks of aerobic training. In double-blind fashion, eight received placebo and nine propranolol throughout the period, while training at the same intensities. Maximal exercise tests were performed before starting drugs or training, and then were repeated three to five days after completing the exercise program when beta blockade was no longer present. The subjects who received propranolol had no increase in measured VO_2 max, while the placebo group changed from a mean of 44 to 53 cc O_2/kg/min. Maximal heart rate was unchanged in either group. High levels of propranolol were maintained by monitoring plasma levels with daily doses ranging from 160 to 640 mg. This certainly disagrees with what we and most others have found, possibly because of the high levels of beta blockade achieved. However, this same group just repeated this protocol using low doses of beta blockers and reported the same attenuation of changes in VO_2 max.

The following are possible explanations for the different results obtained in studies of the effects of beta blockers on training: (1) inadequate total time in training; (2) high initial levels of training or fitness; (3) differences in the percent of suppression of maximal heart rate by beta blockade; (4) only some studies have successfully blinded the subjects as to drug treatment; and (5) marked differences in the altitude at which training occurred.

Lester in 1968, Svendenhag in 1983, and Savin in 1984 performed studies on normals evaluating the effect of training while on beta blockade. The subjects were randomized to drug or placebo. Savin's study at Stanford has shown particularly interesting results. Beta blockade eliminated the echocardiographic changes in left ventricular posterior wall and septal thickening that was found in the placebo group who underwent training. Dressendorf, Laslett, and all of the other investigators who have done studies of cardiac patients have not randomized the patients to beta blockade, but have instead taken patients selected by their physicians to be on or off beta blockade.

In order to resolve these questions, we performed an analysis of patients in PERFEXT who exercised for one year and controls, all of whom were placed on beta blockers at the prerogative of their physicians. The patients' medical records were reviewed to see who had taken beta blockers prescribed by their physicians during the year of training for the exercise group and the year of observation for the controls. This information was then used to separate them into four groups: (1) controls on beta blockers; (2) controls not taking beta blockers; (3) trained on beta blockers; and (4) trained not taking beta blockers (Table 11–14).

More of the patients in the exercise group on beta blockers had exercise test-induced angina than those not on beta blockers (64% versus 16%, p<.01), and they tended to have more ST-segment depression and higher thallium ischemia scores. Also, there was a trend for a higher prevalence of prior by-pass surgery in those not on beta blockers. These differences are probably due to exercise training making limitations due to angina more obvious and leading to beta blocker administration.

Classification by beta blocker status during the year resulted in discrepancies with the status prior to initial testing since some patients in both groups had their beta-blocker status changed during the year of study. Some patients initially off beta blockers were put on and some on were taken off as judged necessary by their physicians. Only 82% and 91% of patients on beta blockers during the year were on them prior to testing. In Table 11–4, the patients off of beta blockers had a trend towards less exercise-induced ST depression but had significantly higher heart rates (and lower ejection fractions and stroke volumes) submaximally but no differences at maximal effort. To confirm that

TABLE 11–14.

Initial Clinical Characteristics of the PERFEXT Patients in Regard to Beta-Blocker Status

CATEGORY	CONTROL GROUP			EXERCISE GROUP		
	TOTAL (N = 69)	ON β BLOCKERS (N = 27) (% OF GROUP)	OFF β BLOCKERS (N = 42)	TOTAL (N = 59)	ON β BLOCKERS (N = 22) (% OF GROUP)	OFF β BLOCKERS (N = 37)
Angina (during exercise testing)	33	33	33	34	64	16*
History of non-Q-wave myocardial infarction only	9	7	10	5	9	3
History of Q-wave myocardial infarction	67	67	67	66	68	65
Current electrocardiogram with:						
Anterior Q-waves	23	26	21	22	18	24
Inferior Q-waves	36	30	40	29	27	30
Coronary artery bypass surgery	33	26	38	42	36	46
Medications before initial testing						
Digoxin	16	19	14	17	18	16
β Blockers	55	82	38	41	91	11
Long-acting nitrates	41	52	33	32	45	24
Antidysrhythmics	14	11	19	15	14	14
Antihypertensives	9	7	10	18	23	16
History of congestive heart failure	10	15	7	9	0	14
Currently employed	65	59	69	56	59	54

ECG = electrocardiogram; N = number of patients; * = significantly different.

this was due to being tapered off of beta blockers, the analysis was repeated by prior drug administration status and not by status during the year. Analysis confirmed a higher submaximal heart rate due to a rebound effect of being tapered off of beta blockers for testing (p<.03) despite a three-day washout period.

Sixty-four percent of the patients reached volitional fatigue during the initial treadmill test. Twenty-two percent were stopped due to moderately severe angina, 5% because of systolic blood pressure drop (usually accompanied by signs of ischemia), 4% because of leg pain (probably mild claudication), and one each because of shortness of breath due to lung disease, an excessive blood pressure rise, severe atypical chest pain, excessive ST depression, and frequent premature ventricular contractions.

The exercise records of the patients in the exercise group were reviewed. Average intensities for the year were as follows: percent maximal estimated oxygen uptake was 60% ± 12 (ranging from 40% to 100%), percent measured maximal oxygen uptake was 77% ± 14 (ranging from 42% to 100%), average calories expended per session were 323 ± 104 (ranging from 130 to 719). There were no significant differences between those on or off beta blockers. The mean values were 62% versus 59% for estimated, 74% versus 79% for measured maximal oxygen uptake, and 305 versus 335 calories, respectively. Attendance at exercise sessions was a mean of 76% ± 18 (ranging from 23% to 97%) with no difference between those on or off beta blockers. The mean attendance was 73% for those on beta blockers and 78% for those not taking them.

During the year, 18 of the controls and 15 of the exercisers were on Inderal (average dose 120 mg), five controls were on metoprolol, four controls and five exercisers were on tenormin (average dose 75 mg), and two exercisers were on nadolol (average dose 50 mg). There were no statistical differences between the exercisers and controls.

Changes in Treadmill Performance.   Two-way analysis of variance revealed highly significant changes in the treadmill parameters due to the exercise intervention. No interaction was detected due to beta-blocker status during the year. There was no correlation between beta-blocker dosage and the change in measured oxygen uptake in the exercise group. No other changes in treadmill parameters including maximal heart rate, blood pressure, perceived exertion, or respiratory quotient were detected. The changes in submaximal heart rate were significant despite the rebound effect of beta-blocker withdrawal.

Changes in Thallium Scintigrams.   Two-way analysis of variance considering the clinical classifications of angina, prior MI, and CABS only revealed significant (p<.01) improvement in the thallium scintigrams of the patients in the exercise progam with exercise test-induced angina. Therefore, three-way analysis of variance for angina, beta blockers, and intervention was performed. Although there was a trend for this improvement to be concentrated in angina patients not taking beta blockers (−6.7 and −5.2), this

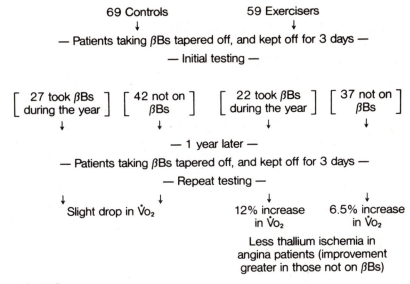

FIG 11–3.
Results of PERFEXT comparing those on or off beta blockers.

did not reach statistical significance (p = .08) because there were only six of these patients. The results of this study are summarized in Figure 11–3.

By design, our study demonstrated the effects of exercise training in patients selected by their physicians to be on or off of beta blockers. This clinical question is different from studying the effects of beta blockers on exercise training. However, this later question has not been resolved since conflicting results exist as to the effects of being randomized to beta blockade in normal subjects engaged in exercise training. In coronary patients selected for beta-blockade treatment by their physicians, the answer regarding the beneficial effects of exercise is more definitive. From previous studies, it has been demonstrated that the appropriate changes in oxygen uptake, submaximal heart rate, and exercise duration occur in patients who engage in exercise training. Our study supports this but also demonstrates no preferential difference between those patients trained on or off beta blockers. In addition, the present study has shown an increase in myocardial perfusion implied by improved thallium scintigrams in angina patients in an exercise program. Our findings and those summarized support the beneficial effects of exercise training in coronary patients taking beta blockers.

Exercise Programs for Patients Post-CABS.   Coronary artery bypass surgery (CABS) has been shown to prolong life and relieve angina in selected groups of patients with coronary artery disease. Advances in operative techniques, including cardioplegia, the use of the internal mammary artery, and more complete revascularization, have improved operative results. Attention must now be turned to other methods for further improvement of the functional result in these patients and for management of those with a less favorable result. Postoperative exercise programs are one means of optimizing the surgical result and helping those with inadequate revascularization.

Because of the large number of patients undergoing coronary artery bypass and their potential for rehabilitation, these patients have been included in exercise rehabilitation programs. However, less than 200 CABS patients in postoperative exercise programs in a total of seven studies have been reported. Previous studies have only considered patients with successful surgery that alleviated angina while our study group includes approximately a third with signs and/or symptoms of ischemia.

Adams and colleagues were the first to report a study of exercise training for coronary artery bypass patients. They entered four male CABS patients into a training program with 45 sedentary normal males and 11 men post-MI. After three months of walking and jogging at least three days a week, 40 minutes a day, at a heart rate of 75% to 85% of maximum, the bypass patients had exercise capacities equal to the trained postinfarction patients, and had shown an 11% increase in maximal oxygen uptake. As expected, the sedentary normal men outperformed both groups.

Oldridge and colleagues conducted a study of the effects of bypass surgery and an exercise program of 32 months duration. Twenty-one patients with angina were given maximal treadmill tests one week prior to CABS and again 16 weeks after surgery. Six of these patients then entered a program of 45 to 60 minutes of exercise, three times a week, at heart rates achieved at 65% to 75% of their postoperative functional capacity. A control group of six subjects from the remaining group of bypass patients was chosen. These men were matched "as closely as possible" to the exercising patients. The control group had only participated in sporadic physical activities such as tennis or walking since surgery. Treadmill tests were performed on the exercise subjects 32 months after training began, and 28 to 34 months after surgery in the control group. No significant change in resting heart rate or blood pressure was found in either group. Maximal oxygen uptake increased by 28% in the exercisers, with only a 3% increase observed in the controls. The exercise group had also been tested after four months of exercise, and by that time 90% of the total improvement in functional capacity observed at the end of 32 months had already occurred.

Soloff conducted a nonrandomized study of the effect of rehabilitation on mood and physical performance in 27 postbypass and 18 postinfarction patients. The postbypass patients significantly improved maximal oxygen uptake and maximum heart rate after an inpatient program of bedside exercise and early ambulation, followed by six weeks of monitored, three times weekly calisthenics and 20 minutes of bicycle ergometry.

In Ireland, Horgan and colleagues exercised 51 patients three times a week, in a program that began 8–10 weeks after coronary artery bypass surgery. These patients exercised 16 minutes each session at 85% of their maximal heart rate. After eight weeks of exercise, duration of exercise and maximum work load were increased. Similar results were seen in a group of postinfarction patients exercised simultaneously.

Hartung and Rangel reported their findings in 10 coronary artery bypass surgery patients who participated for three to six months in an exercise program. They exercised three times a week in 20- to 40-minute sessions of walking, jogging, or bicycle ergometry at an intensity of 70% to 85% of maximum heart rate beginning 10 months after surgery. Maximal oxygen uptake increased significantly at the conclusion of the study. Increased maximal oxygen uptake was also seen in 24 postinfarction patients and 16 high-risk asymptomatic individuals. No significant difference was found among the three groups in any of the variables evaluated.

Dornan et al. reported 210 men who were referred consecutively to a rehabilitation program following CABS. The program involved submaximal exercise testing at eight weeks with an intervening 12-week exercise program and a repeat exercise test. A retrospective analysis showed 50% of the patients to be on no medication throughout their rehabilitation while the others were on medication likely to affect cardiac performance. Age and the extent of revascularization did not appear to influence exercise tolerance. Following the 12-week exercise program, patients in both groups had improved significantly, but the initial and final performance of the cohort of patients requiring cardiac drugs was significantly poorer than those on no medication.

To assess the benefits of regular participation in a cardiac rehabilitation program, Fletcher studied retrospectively 22 patients who had undergone coronary artery bypass. Group I (mean age 53 years) was currently enrolled in the rehabilitation program. Group II (mean age 56 years) had begun but discontinued the program for nonmedical reasons. There was no difference in entry exercise tests and presurgical catheterization data between the groups. Group I had a higher maximal oxygen uptake (31 versus 24 ml/kg/min) and greater treadmill time (11 versus 8 minutes). Nine of 11 in group I were fully employed versus four in group II. One in group I had been rehospitalized versus five in group II. No one in group I smoked, while four of the 11 subjects in group II smoked. They concluded that the CABS patients in their program had greater maximal oxygen uptake, smoked less, were less often rehospitalized, and were more often fully employed than those who dropped out.

The effects of revascularization appear to be lasting with a recurrence rate of angina of 5% or less one year postsurgery. A randomized trial of aspirin and dipyridamole has demonstrated improved graft patency, and so efficacy could even be improved. The available studies, although limited by methodology, patient numbers, and highly variable details of the rehabilitation programs employed, demonstrate that exercise programs can improve the exercise capacity of patients who have undergone CABS.

PERFEXT CABS Patients.   Previous studies of cardiac rehabilitation in coronary bypass surgery patients have been hampered by lack of sufficient patient numbers, design problems, failure to consider patients with less successful surgery, and limitations in assessing results. Analysis of the CABS patients in our randomized exercise trial, who represented a third of the total study group of 159 patients, provides information not previously available. Fifty-three CABS patients were randomized, resulting in 28 in the exercise-intervention group and 25 in the control group.

The mean time from surgery until entry into the study was two years with a standard deviation of two years and a range of six months to nine years. Randomization was successful as clinical characteristics and treadmill responses were comparable. However, there was a trend for more markers of ischemia and angina in the exercise group. These patients could be considered surgical failures with inadequate or incomplete myocardial revascularization. Only patients with exercise test-induced classical angina pectoris are considered surgical "failures" and analyzed separately.

Dropouts. During the course of the study year, there were two medical dropouts in the control group: one died and the other had an MI. There were two medical dropouts from the exercise intervention group, one for increasing angina and the other for alcoholism. Of the 26 remaining in the exercise group, one dropped out of exercise classes because of a job conflict and refused testing. Repeat one-year testing was performed on 25 patients from the exercise group and on 23 controls.

All patients' exercise records were reviewed. Average intensities for the year were as follows: percent estimated VO_2 max and percent maximal heart rate by the Karvonen method was approximately 60% ± 10 (ranging from 40% to 100%). Percent maximal heart rate and measured oxygen uptake were approximately 80%. The average caloric expenditure per session was 330 ± 113

TABLE 11–15.
Clinical Characteristics of the Coronary Artery Bypass Patients in PERFEXT

CLINICAL VARIABLE	CONTROLS (N = 25)	EXERCISE-INTERVENTION GROUP (N = 28)
Age, yr (mean ± SD)	54 ± 7	53 ± 7
Weight, kg (mean ± SD)	82 ± 13	86 ± 12
Currently smoking, %	0	7
Angina during treadmill test, %	24	32
History of non-Q-wave myocardial infarction only, %	9	7
History of Q-wave myocardial infarction, %	64	54
Current electrocardiographic pattern, %		
Anterior Q-waves	16	29
Inferior Q-waves	36	39
Medications prior to initial testing, %		
Digoxin	16	25
β-Blockers	56	39
Long-acting nitrates	20	14
Antidysrhythmics	16	11
Antihypertensives	8	18
History of congestive heart failure, %	0	14
Currently employed, %	64	43
Cardiac catheterization results prior to surgery		
Ejection fraction (mean ± SD)	0.59 ± 0.15	0.58 ± 0.18
1-vessel disease, %	32	7
2-vessel disease, %	8	7
3-vessel disease, %	52	61
Left main coronary artery disease, %	8	25

TABLE 11–16.
Results of the Exercise Program in CABS Patients

MEASURE	CONTROLS			EXERCISE-INTERVENTION GROUP		
	ALL (N = 23) (MEAN ± SD)	NO ANGINA (N = 18)	ANGINA (N = 5)	ALL (N = 25) (MEAN ± SD)	NO ANGINA (N = 17)	ANGINA (N = 8)
Change in supine resting heart rate, beats/min	1.5 ± 13*	1	4	−5.8 ± 11*	−5	−11
Change in heart rate at 3.3 mph/5% grade, beats/min	−3 ± 8*	−1	−10†	−11 ± 14*	−7	−20†
% change in estimated maximal oxygen uptake	−5.7 ± 14*	−7	0	13 ± 22*	9	21
% change in measured maximal oxygen uptake	−2.9 ± 22*	−3	−1	7.1 ± 20*	8	6

*p<.01.
†p<.01 interaction due to angina from two-way analysis of variance.

(ranging from 172 to 719 calories). Attendance at exercise sessions was a mean of 82% ± 19 (ranging from 65% to 97%).

One trained patient developed treadmill-induced angina and abnormal ST-segment depression during the year. One control and three exercising patients lost abnormal ST depression, but the control still had angina and the others did not have angina. Two trained patients and two controls lost angina, while four trained and two controls gained or worsened their angina.

Changes in Hemodynamic Parameters.   The results of two-way analysis of variance considering intervention and angina are presented in Table 11–15. This was done in order to see if the intervention was effective in both those with and without successful revascularization. All of the hemodynamic improvements due to the intervention were statistically significant (p<.01). The exercisers had lower mean submaximal heart rates than the controls, but the nonexercisers with angina had as much change in submaximal heart rate as the exercisers without angina. This drop in heart rate during repeat testing is due to habituation. The decline in aerobic capacity in the controls was only significant for estimated uptake in those without angina.

Changes in Thallium Scintigraphy.   The results of two-way analysis of variance considering intervention and angina are presented in Table 11–16. Though in general the exercisers have greater negative values consistent with improved scans, statistical significance was not achieved. The most improvement was noted in the exercisers with angina (−1.6, −2.1 Atwood severity units) and this achieved a p = .08 level.

This study involved a small, highly select population, and the benefits might have been greater if the patients had entered training sooner after surgery. All of the hemodynamic benefits, including VO_2 max, were demonstrated in our bypass patients. Analysis of variance confirmed that the benefits also occurred in the patients still with angina.

Predicting Outcome in PERFEXT Patients.   Cardiac rehabilitation programs are expensive and carry a risk. If a patient's likelihood of improving work capacity could be predicted on the basis of initial data, much time and money could be saved. Considering VO_2 max and other indicators of a training effect, we asked the following questions: (1) Can clinical features prior to training predict whether or not beneficial changes occur with training? (2) Do initial treadmill and/or radionuclide measurements contribute information to improve this prediction? and (3) Does the intensity of training over the year predict beneficial changes?

Each of the parameters of change with training was regressed against the initial value of those parameters (i.e., resting heart rate, submaximal heart rate, estimated and measured VO_2 max, and thallium ischemia) as well as against age, amount of myocardial scar on the thallium scan, and the measures of intensity of training. All but two relationships showed correlation coefficients of less than 0.50. Correlation coefficients of greater than 0.25 were associated with p values of less than 0.05 and thus considered related by more than chance. Some of the plots are shown in Figure 11–4.

The initial thallium ischemia score showed a correlation coefficient of −0.56 with change in thallium ischemia. That is, those with initially the most ischemia showed the greatest decrease in ischemia with training. Similarly, those with the highest resting heart rates showed the greatest drop in resting heart rate with training (r = −0.56). For submaximal heart rate and estimated VO_2 max, patients with initial values consistent with the greatest deconditioning had the greatest improvement (r = −0.45 for submaximal heart rate and r = -0.26 for estimated VO_2 max). There were few significant interrelationships among the variables. High initial submaximal heart rate correlated with more of an increase in estimated oxygen consumption (r = 0.30). Low initial estimated oxygen consumption correlated with greater decrease in submaximal heart rate (r = 0.29).

There was no relationship between initial measured oxygen consumption and the change in oxygen consumption after the one-year period, or between the other parameters. The amount of scar present did not correlate with any of the measures of training. Older patients had less of an increase in measured oxygen uptake (r = −0.24) and less of a decrease in resting heart rate (r = 0.23), but neither of these relationships was statistically significant.

The markers of a training effect were also regressed on one another. The changes in measured and estimated VO_2 correlated significantly (r = 0.52) as did the changes in heart rate (r = −.43), but they did not correlate with each other nor with the change in thallium ischemia score. The measures of intensity of training showed poor correlations with outcome. Most correlation coefficients were less than 0.20, none achieved statistical significance, and trends were often conflicting. For instance, higher percent of maximal heart rate related to more of a drop in resting heart rate (r = −0.22) but less of a decrease in submaximal heart rate (r = 0.21).

To test whether presence of ischemia or scar related to a lack of training effect, t-tests were performed based on the presence or absence of: (1) markers of exercise-induced ischemia (drop in ejection fraction during the supine bicycle test, angina, or abnormal ST-segment depression during the treadmill test); (2) historical features (prior CABS, MI); and (3) features suggesting abnormal function. In no case was there a significant difference in any measure of training effect in those who had a given characteristic as compared to those who did not.

To test for the possibility that some patients who had an improved oxygen

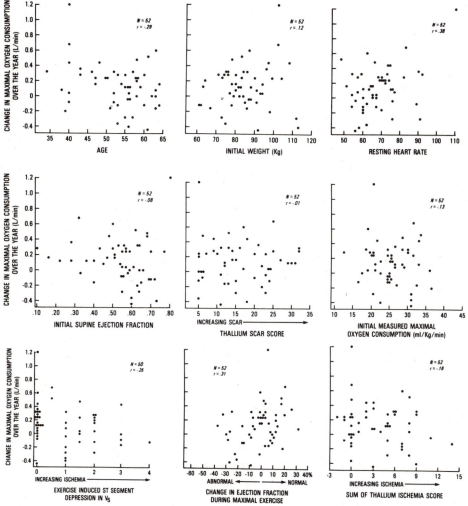

FIG 11–4.
Relationship of initial parameters to outcome of exercise program.

consumption in the second test were actually exerting more effort than in the initial test, correlations were performed between change in oxygen consumption after training and differences in respiratory quotient, maximal heart rate, ST-segment depression, and perceived exertion between the initial and final treadmill tests. These may represent differences in test endpoints. Significant correlations were demonstrated: 0.43 for increase in maximal heart rate, 0.36 for increase in perceived exertion, 0.28 for increase in ST depression, and 0.16 for increase in respiratory quotient.

Our major finding was that a patient's success or failure in improving aerobic capacity following a one-year aerobic exercise program was poorly predicted on the basis of initial clinical, treadmill, or radionuclide data. Correlations between initial parameters and outcome were poor. Training intensity had little to do with outcome. Those with ischemic markers (exercise test-induced angina, ST depression, or dropping ejection fraction) did not show a different degree of training effect than patients without ischemia; neither did those with markers of myocardial damage. History of CABS or MI had no bearing on whether a patient's work capacity would improve following the training period.

There was a trend for those who initially showed evidence of the poorest state of fitness (high resting or submaximal heart rate, low estimated oxygen consumption) or high thallium ischemia scores to have the most improvement in the same respective parameter. However, initial measured oxygen consumption, the best measure of aerobic capacity on entry, showed no relationship to any measure of training effect at the end of the year of training. Older patients showed only slightly less benefit than younger ones. Those with characteristics suggesting larger amounts of scar or ischemia did not have significantly different results from those with less. Multivariate analysis did not greatly improve the ability to predict outcome.

Previous studies have found that those with the lowest initial measured oxygen consumption often have the largest improvement with an exercise program. In our study, the correlation of initial measured oxygen consumption with any measure of training effect was always nonsignificant, and it was never selected by multivariate analyses.

The lack of correlation between training intensity and change in oxygen uptake over the year is difficult to explain. In healthy men, this relationship is good (r = 0.80); it is not clear from the present study why the correlations were so poor (r < 0.20). It may well be that setting exercise prescriptions using exercise tests limited by signs or symptoms gives too low of an exercise intensity.

The changes in test endpoints were moderately correlated to changes in oxygen uptake. This raises the question of what portion of the changes were due to the patients being encouraged to perform better on the one-year tests by those administering the tests or by their own faith in the exercise program. Even maximal testing appears of questionable reliability and argues for using a different technical staff for initial and final testing.

A detailed initial evaluation did not allow accurate prediction of who would train and who would not. Even those patients whose characteristics suggested they had the most ischemia or scar showed as much improvement from training as patients without such characteristics. Thus, for instance, using angina, a low-resting ejection fraction, ST-segment depression, or a dropping ejection fraction with exercise as a contraindication to an exercise program is unjustified. Since many of the benefits obtained from an exercise program are intangible, it seems inappropriate to eliminate any patient from an exercise program on the basis of clinical, treadmill, or radionuclide data.

BIBLIOGRAPHY

Abraham AS, Sever Y, Weinstein M, et al: Value of early ambulation in patients with and without complications after acute myocardial infarction. N Engl J Med 1975;292:719–722.

Adams WC, McHenry MM, Bernauer EM: Long-term physiologic adaptations to exercise with special reference to performance and cardiorespiratory function in health and disease. Am J Cardiol 1974;33:765–775.

AffairsCouncilScience: Physician-supervised exercise programs in rehabilitation of patients with coronary heart disease. JAMA 1981;245:1463–1466.

Almeida D, Wenger NK: Emotional responses of patients with acute myocardial infarction to their disease. Cardiology 1982;69:303–309.

Anderson JL, Marshall HW, Fray BE, et al: A randomized trial of intracoronary streptokinase in the treatment of acute myocardial infarction. N Engl J Med 1983;308:1312–1318.

Atwood JA, Nielsen DH: Scope of cardiac rehabilitation. J Am Phys Ther Assn 1985; 65:1812–1819.

Badke FR, O'Rourke RA: Vasodilator drug therapy in congestive heart failure. Current Problems in Cardiology 1982.

Baughman KL, Hutter AM, DeSanctis RW, et al: Early discharge following acute myocardial infarction: Long-term follow-up of randomized patients. Arch Intern Med 1982;142:875–878.

Bengtsson K: Rehabilitation after myocardial infarction. Scand J Rehabil Med 1983;15:1–9.

Blair SN, Piserchia PV, Wilbur CS, et al: A public health intervention model for work-site health promotion. JAMA 1986;255:921–926.

Bloch A, Maeder J, Haissly J, et al: Early mobilization after myocardial infarction: A controlled study. Am J Cardiol 1974;34:152–157.

Blumenthal JA: Psychologic assessment in cardiac rehabilitation. J Cardiopulmonary Rehabil 1985;5:208–215.

Bohlen JG, Held JP, Sanderson O, et al: Heart rate, rate-pressure product, and oxygen uptake during four sexual activities. Arch Intern Med 1984;144:1745–1748.

Boogaard AMD, Briody ME: Comparison of the rehabilitation of men and women post-myocardial infarction. J Cardiopulmonary Rehabil 1985;5:379–384.

Boone T, Frentz KL, Boyd NR: Carotid palpation at two exercise intensities. Med Sci Sports Exerc 1985;17:705–709.

Brown CF, Oldridge NB: Exercise-induced angina in the cold. Med Sci Sports Exerc 1985; 17:607–612.

Bruce EH, Frederick R, Bruce RA, et al: Comparison of active participants and dropouts in CAPRI cardiopulmonary rehabilitation programs. Am J Cardiol 1976;7:53–60.

Brush JE, Brand DA, Acampora D, et al: Use of the initial electrocardiogram to predict in-hospital complications of acute myocardial infarction. N Engl J Med 1985;312:1137–1141.

Cain HD, Frasher WG, Stivelman R: Graded activity program for safe return to self-care after myocardial infarction. JAMA 1961;177:111–120.

Carson P, Phillips R, Lloyd M, et al: Exercise after myocardial infarction: a controlled trial. *J R Coll Physicians Lond* 1982;16:147–151.

Caughey DE, Mercer CJ, Deeming LW, et al: Coronary prognostic index for predicting survival after recovery from acute myocardial infarction. *Lancet* 1970;2:485–488.

Celli BR, Rassulo J, Make BJ: Disynchronous breathing during arm but not leg exercise in patients with chronic airflow obstruction. *N Engl J Med* 1986;314:1485–1490.

Cintron GB, Hernandex E, Linares E, et al: Bedside recognition, incidence and clinical course of right ventricular infarction. *Am J Cardiol* 1981;47:224–227.

Cobb FR, Williams RS, McEwan P, et al: Effects of exercise training on ventricular function in patients with recent myocardial infarction. *Circulation* 1982;66:100–111.

Cohen M, Packer M, Gorlin R: Indications for left ventricular aneurysmectomy. *Circulation* 1983;65:717–722.

Connolly DC, Elveback LR: Coronary heart disease in residents of Rochester, Minnesota. VI. Hospital and posthospital course of patients with transmural and subendocardial myocardial infarction. *Mayo Clin Proc* 1985;60:375–381.

Convertino V, Hung J, Goldwater D, et al: Cardiovascular responses to exercise in middle-aged men after ten days of bedrest. *Circulation* 1982;66:134–140.

Convertino VA: Effect of orthostatic stress on exercise performance after bed rest: Relation to in-hospital rehabilitation. *J Cardiac Rehabil* 1983;3:660–663.

Corday E, Meerbaum S: Symposium on the present status of reperfusion of the acutely ischemic myocardium. *J Am Coll Cardiol* 1983;1:1031–1036.

CouncilSciAffairs: Physician-supervised exercise programs in rehabilitation of patients with coronary heart disease. *JAMA* 1981;245:1463–1466.

Davidson DM: Return to work after cardiac events: A review. *J Cardiac Rehabil* 1983;3:60–69.

DeBusk RF, Haskell WL, Miller NH, et al: Medically directed at-home rehabilitation soon after clinically uncomplicated acute myocardial infarction: A new model for patient care. *Am J Cardiol* 1985;55:251–257.

DeBusk RF, Hung J: Exercise conditioning soon after myocardial infarction: effects on myocardial perfusion and ventricular function. *Ann NY Acad Sci* 1982;382:343–351.

DeWood MA, Heit J, Spores J, et al: Anterior transmural myocardial infarction: Effects of surgical coronary reperfusion on global and regional left ventricular function. *J Am Coll Cardiol* 1983;1:1223–1234.

DeWood MA, Spores J, Notske R, et al: Prevalence of total coronary occlusion during the early hours of transmural myocardial infarction. *N Engl J Med* 1980;303:897–902.

Dimsdale JE, Hartley LH, Guiney T, et al: Postexercise peril: Plasma catecholamines and exercise. *JAMA* 1984;251:630–632.

Dornan J, Rolko AF, Greenfield C: Factors affecting rehabilitation following aortocoronary bypass procedures. *Can J Surg* 1982;25:677–680.

Dressendorfer RH, Smith JL, Amsterdam EA, et al: Reduction of submaximal exercise myocardial oxygen demand post-walk training program in coronary patients due to improved physical work efficiency. *Am Heart J* 1982;103:358–362.

Ehsani AA, Martin WH, Heath GW, et al: Cardiac effects of prolonged and intense exercise training in patients with coronary artery disease. *Am J Cardiol* 1982;50:246–254.

Epstein SE, Palmeri S, Patterson RE: Evaluation of patients after acute myocardial infarction: Indications for cardiac catheterization and surgical intervention. *N Engl J Med* 1982;307:1487–1492.

Ewart CK, Stewart KJ, Gillilan RE, et al: Usefulness of self-efficacy in predicting overexertion during programmed exercise in coronary artery disease. *Am J Cardiol* 1986;57:557–561.

Ewy GA, Wilmore JH, Morton AR, et al: The effect of beta-adrenergic blockade on obtaining a trained exercise state. *J Cardiac Rehabil* 1983;3(1):25–29.

Fagan ET, Wayne VS, McConachy DL: Serious ventricular arrhythmias in a cardiac rehabilitation program. *Med J Aust* 1984;141:421–424.

Ferguson RJ, Petitclerc R, Choquette G, et al: Effect of physical training on treadmill exercise capacity, collateral circulation and progression of coronary disease. *Am J Cardiol* 1974;34:764–772.

Froelicher V, Jensen D, Atwood JE, et al: Cardiac rehabilitation: Evidence for improvement in myocardial perfusion and function. *Arch Phys Med Rehabil* 1980;61:5117–5122.

Froelicher VF, Jensen D, Genter F, et al: A randomized trial of exercise training in patients with coronary heart disease. *JAMA* 1984;252:1291–1297.

Froelicher VF, Jensen D, Sullivan M: A randomized trial of the effects of exercise training after coronary artery bypass surgery. *Arch Intern Med* 1985;145:689–692.

Froelicher VF, Sullivan M, Myers J, et al: Can patients with coronary artery disease receiving beta blockers obtain a training effect? *Am J Cardiol* 1985;55:155D–161D.

Giese H, Schomer HH: Life-style changes and mood profile of cardiac patients after an exercise rehabilitation program. *J Cardiopulmonary Rehabil* 1986;6:30–37.

Gohlke H, Schnellbacher K, Samek L, et al: Long-term improvement of exercise tolerance and vocational rehabilitation after bypass surgery: A five-year follow-up. *J Cardiac Rehabil* 1982;2:531–540.

Gossard D, Haskell WL, Taylor B, et al: Effects of low- and high-intensity home-based exercise training on functional capacity in healthy middle-aged men. *Am J Cardiol* 1986;57:446–449.

Hagberg JM, Ehsani AA, Holloszy JO: Effect of 12 months of intense exercise training on stroke volume in patients with coronary artery disease. *Circulation* 1983;67:1194–1201.

Hammerman H, Schoen FJ, Kloner RA: Short-term exercise has a prolonged effect on scar formation after experimental acute myocardial infarction. *J Am Coll Cardiol* 1983;2:979–982.

Hammond KH, Kelly TL, Froelicher VF, et al: Use of clinical data in predicting improvement in exercise capacity after cardiac rehabilitation. *J Am Coll Cardiol* 1985;6:19–26.

Harri MNE: Physical training under the influence of beta-blockade in rats: II. Effects on vascular reactivity. *Eur J Appl Physiol* 1979;42:151–157.

Hartung GH, Rangel R: Exercise training in post-myocardial infarction patients: Comparison of results with high-risk coronary and post-bypass patients. *Arch Phys Med Rehabil* 1981;62:147–153.

Haskell WL: Cardiovascular complications during exercise training of cardiac patients. *Circulation* 1978;57(5):920–924.

Hayes MJ, Morris GK, Hampton JR: Comparison of mobilization after two and nine days in uncomplicated myocardial infarction. *Br Med J* 1974;3:10–13.

Hedback B, Perk J, Perski A: Effect of a post-myocardial infarction rehabilitation program on mortality, morbidity, and risk factors. *J Cardiopulmonary Rehabil* 1985;5:576–583.

Herlitz J, Elmfeldt D, Hjalmarson A, et al: Effects of metoprolol on indirect signs of the size and severity of acute myocardial infarction. *Am J Cardiol* 1983;51:1282–1288.

Hirsowitz GS, Lakier JB, Marks DS, et al: Comparison of radionuclide and enzymatic estimate of infarct size in patients with acute myocardial infarction. *J Am Coll Cardiol* 1983;1:1405–1412.

Hochman JS, Healy B: Effect of exercise on acute myocardial infarction in rats. *J Am Coll Cardiol* 1986;7:126–132.

Horgan JH, Teo KK, Murren KM, et al: The response to exercise training and vocational counseling in post-myocardial infarction and coronary artery bypass surgery patients. *Irish Med J* 1980;74:463–469.

Hossack KF, Bruce RA, Clarke LJ: Influence of propranolol on exercise prescription of training heart rates. *Cardiology* 1980;65:47–58.

Hossack KF, Bruce RA, Kusumi F: Altered exercise ventilatory responses by apparent propranolol-diminished glucose metabolism: Implications concerning impaired physical training benefit in coronary patients. *Am Heart J* 1981;102:378–382.

Hossack KF, Hartwig R: Cardiac arrest associated with supervised cardiac rehabilitation. *J Cardiac Rehabil* 1982;2:402–408.

Howard G, Till JS, Toole JF, et al: Factors influencing return to work following cerebral infarction. *JAMA* 1985;253:226–232.

Hung J, Gordon EP, Houston N, et al: Changes in rest and exercise myocardial perfusion and left ventricular function 3 to 26 weeks after clinically uncomplicated acute myocardial infarction: Effects of exercise training. *Am J Cardiol* 1984;54:943–950.

Jensen D, Atwood JE, Froelicher V, et al: Improvement in ventricular function during exercise studied with radionuclide ventriculography after cardiac rehabilitation. *Am J Cardiol* 1980;46:770–778.

Kallio V, Hamalainen H, Hakkila J, et al: Reduction in sudden deaths by a multifactorial intervention programme after acute myocardial infarction. *Lancet* 1979;2:1091–1094.

Kavanagh T, Shepard RS, Lindley LJ, et al: Influence of exercise and life-style variables upon HDL cholesterol and myocardial infarction. *Arteriosclerosis* 1983;3:249–259.

Kavanagh T, Shephard RJ, Chisholm AW, et al: Prognostic indexes for patients with ischemic heart disease enrolled in an exercise-centered rehabilitation program. *Am J Cardiol* 1979;44:1230–1240.

Kelbaek H, Eskildsen P, Hansen PF, et al: Spontaneous and or training-induced hemodynamic changes after myocardial infarction. *Int J Cardiol* 1981;1:205–213.

Kelemen MH, Steward KJ, Gillilan RE, et al: Circuit weight training in cardiac patients. *J Am Coll Cardiol* 1986;7:38–42.

Kentala E: Physical fitness and feasibility of physical rehabilitation after myocardial infarction in men of working age. *Ann Clin Res* 1972;4.

Khaja F, et al: Intracoronary fibrinolytic therapy in acute myocardial infarction: Report of a prospective randomized trial. *N Engl J Med* 1983;308:1305–1311.

King AR, Cairns FJ: Cardiac rupture: 30 consecutive cases from a series of medicolegal autopsies. *NZ Med J* 1978;88:436–438.

Kloner RA, Kloner JA: The effect of early exercise on myocardial infarct scar formation. *Am Heart J* 1983;106:1009–1014.

Knapp D, Blackwell B: Emotional and behavioral problems in cardiac rehabilitation patients. *J Cardiac Rehabil* 1985;5:112–123.

Kolman PB: The value of group psychotherapy after myocardial infarction: A critical review. *J Cardiac Rehabil* 1983;3:360–366.

Koppes GM, Beckmann CH, Jones FG: Propranolol therapy for ventricular arrhythmias two months after acute myocardial infarction. *Am J Cardiol* 1980;46:322–328.

Kottke TE, Caspersen CJ, Hill CS: Exercise in the management and rehabilitation of selected chronic diseases. *Prev Med* 1984;13:47–65.

Kupper W, Bleifeld W, Hanrath P, et al: Left ventricular hemodynamics and function in acute myocardial infarction: Studies during the acute phase, convalescence and late recovery. *Am J Cardiol* 1977;40:900–905.

La Rosa JC, Cleary P, Muesing RA, et al: Effects of long-term moderate physical exercise on plasma lipoproteins: The national exercise and heart disease project. *Arch Intern Med* 1983;142:2269–2274.

Leier CV, Huss P, Unverferth DV: Improved exercise capacity and differing arterial and venous tolerance during chronic isosorbide dinitrate therapy for congestive heart failure. *Circulation* 1983;67:817–822.

Leir CV, Huss P, Lewis RP, et al: Drug-induced conditioning in congestive heart failure. *Circulation* 1982;65:1382–1387.

Levine SA, Lown B: The "chair" treatment of acute coronary thrombosis. *Trans Assoc Am Physicians* 1951;64:316–319.

Liang C, Tuttle RR, Hood WB, et al: Conditioning effects of chronic infusions of dobutamine. *J Clin Invest* 1979;64:613–619.

Lindvall K, Erhardt LR, Lundman T, et al: Early mobilization and discharge of patients with acute myocardial infarction. A prospective study using risk indicators and early exercise tests. *Acta Med Scand* 1979;206:169–175.

Madsen EB, Gilpin E, Henning H: Evaluation of prognosis one year after myocardial infarction. *J Am Coll Cardiol* 1983;1:985–993.

Magder S, Linnarsson D, Gullstrand L: The effect of swimming on patients with ischemic heart disease. *Circulation* 1981;63:979–986.

Maisel AS, Ahnve S, Gilpin E, et al: Prognosis after extension of myocardial infarct: The role of Q-wave or non-Q-wave infarction. *Circulation* 1985;71:211–217.

Maisel AS, Gilpin E, Hoit B, et al: Survival after hospital discharge in matched populations with inferior or anterior myocardial infarction. *J Am Coll Cardiol* 1985;6:731–736.

Maisel AS, Scott N, Gilpin E, et al: Complex ventricular arrhythmias in patients with Q-wave versus non-Q-wave myocardial infarction. *Circulation* 1985;72:963–970.

Maresh CM, Harbrecht JJ, Blick BL, et al: Comparison of rehabilitation benefits after percutaneous transluminal coronary angioplasty and coronary artery bypass graft surgery. *J Cardiac Rehabil* 1985;5:124–130.

Marsh RC, Hiatt WR, Brammell HL, et al: Attenuation of exercise conditioning by low dose beta-adrenergic receptor blockade. *J Am Coll Cardiol* 1983;2:551–556.

Martinez MJ, Hill JC, Clarke JS: Long-term benefits of cardiac surgery in active duty patients. *Milit Med* 1985;150:447–450.

May GS, Eberlein KA, Furberg CD, et al: Secondary prevention after myocardial infarction: A review of long-term trials. *Prog Cardiovasc Dis* 1982;24:331–352.

Mayou R, MacMahon D, Sleight P, et al: Early rehabilitation after myocardial infarction. *Lancet* 1981;2:8260–8261.

Mayou RA: A controlled trial of early rehabilitation after myocardial infarction. *J Cardiac Rehabil* 1983;3:397–402.

Miller NH, Haskell WL, Berra K, et al: Home versus group exercise training for increasing functional capacity after myocardial infarction. *Circulation* 1984;70:645–649.

Mitchell M, Franklin B, Johnson S, et al: Exercise programs: Role of continuous electrocardiographic monitoring. *Arch Phys Med Rehabil* 1984;65(8):463–466.

Muller JE: Coronary artery thrombosis: Historical aspects. *J Am Coll Cardiol* 1983;1:893–896.

Myers J, Ahnve S, Froelicher V, et al: Spatial R-wave amplitude changes during exercise: Relation with left ventricular ischemia and function. *J Am Coll Cardiol* 1985;6:603–608.

Myers JH, Horwitz LD: Hemodynamic and metabolic response after abrupt withdrawal of long-term propranolol. *Circulation* 1978;58:196–201.

Neill WA, Branch LG, DeJong G, et al: The impact of coronary heart disease on patients' daily activities. *Arch Intern Med* 1985;145:1642.

Newton KM, Sivarajan ES, Clarke JL: Patient perceptions of risk factor changes and cardiac rehabilitation outcomes after myocardial infarction. *J Cardiac Rehabil* 1985;5:159–168.

Nolewajka AJ, Kostuk WJ, Rechnitzer PA, et al: Exercise and human collateralization: An angiographic and scintigraphic assessment. *Circulation* 1979;60:114–122.

Norris RM, Mercer CJ, Deeming LW, et al: Coronary prognostic index for predicting survival after recovery from acute myocardial infarction. *Lancet* 1970;2:485–488.

Obma RT, Wilson PK, Goebel ME, et al: Effect of a conditioning program in patients taking propranolol for angina pectoris. *Cardiology* 1979;64:365–371.

Oldridge NB, Nagle FJ, Balke B, et al: Aortocoronary bypass surgery: Effects of surgery and 32 months of physical conditioning on treadmill performance. *Arch Phys Med Rehabil* 1978;59(6):268–275.

Oldridge NB, Spencer J: Exercise habits and perceptions before and after graduation or dropout from supervised cardiac exercise rehabilitation. *J Cardiopulmonary Rehabil* 1985;5:313–319.

Ott CR, Sivarajan ES, Newton KM, et al: A controlled randomized study of early cardiac rehabilitation: The sickness impact profile as an assessment tool. *Heart Lung* 1983;12:162–170.

Palatsi I: Feasibility of physical training after myocardial infarction and its effect on return to work, morbidity, and mortality. *Acta Med Scand (Suppl)* 1976;599.

Parmley WW: President's page: Position report on cardiac rehabilitation. *J Am Coll Cardiol* 1986;7:451–453.

Passamani E: Nitroprusside in myocardial infarction. *N Engl J Med* 1982;306:1168–1170.

Paterson DH, Shephard RJ, Cunningham D, et al: Effects of physical training on cardiovascular function following myocardial infarction. *J Appl Physiol* 1979;47:482–489.

Patterson RP, Pearson J, Fisher SV: Work rest periods: Their effect on normal physiologic response to isometric and dynamic work. *Arch Phys Med Rehabil* 1985;66:348–352.

Phibbs B: Transmural versus subendocardial myocardial infarction: An electrocardiographic myth. *J Am Coll Cardiol* 1983;1:561–564.

Pratt CM, Francis MJ, Stone CL, et al: Transtelephonic electrocardiographic monitoring: Reliability in detecting the ischemic ST-segment response during exercise. *Am Heart J* 1984;108:967–973.

Pratt CM, Welton DE, Squired WG, et al: Demonstration of training effect during chronic beta-adrenergic blockade in patients with coronary artery disease. *Circulation* 1981;64:1125–1129.

Pyfer HR, Mead WF, Frederick RC: Exercise rehabilitation in coronary heart disease: Community program groups. *Arch Phys Med Rehabil* 1976;57(1):335.

Rahimtoola SH, Nunley D, Grunkeimeier G, et al: Ten-year survival after coronary bypass surgery for unstable angina. *N Engl J Med* 1983;308:676–681.

Rapaport E, Remedios P: The high-risk patient after recovery from myocardial infarction: Recognition and management. *J Am Coll Cardiol* 1983;1:391–400.

Rasmussen S, Leth A, Kjoller E, et al: Cardiac rupture in acute myocardial infarction. *Acta Med Scand* 1979;205:11–16.

Rechnitzer PA, Cunningham DA, Andrew GM, et al: Relation of exercise to the recurrence rate of myocardial infarction in men. *Am J Cardiol* 1983;51:65–69.

Rejeski WJ, Morley D, Sotile W: Cardiac rehabilitation: A conceptual framework for psychologic assessment. *J Cardiac Rehabil* 1985;5:172–180.

Ribeiro JP, Hartley H, Sherwood J, et al: The effectiveness of a low lipid diet in the management of coronary artery disease. *Am Heart J* 1984;108:1183–1189.

Robinson G, Froelicher VF, Utley JR: Rehabilitation of the coronary artery bypass graft surgery patient. *J Cardiac Rehabil* 1984;4:74–86.

Roman O, Gutierrez M, Luksic I, et al: Cardiac rehabilitation after acute myocardial infarction. *Cardiology* 1983;70:223–231.

Ruberman W, Weinblatt E, Goldberg JD, et al: Psychosocial influences on mortality after myocardial infarction. *N Engl J Med* 1984;311:552–559.

Rude RE, Muller JE, Braunwald E: Efforts to limit the size of myocardial infarcts. *Ann Intern Med* 1981;95:736–761.

Sable DL, Brammell HL, Shehan MV, et al: Attenuation of exercise conditioning by beta-adrenergic blockade. *Circulation* 1982;65:679–684.

Sanne H: Exercise tolerance and physical training of non-selected patients after myocardial infarction. *Acta Med Scand (Suppl)* 1973;551.

Sanz G, Castaner A, Betriu A, et al: Determinants of prognosis in survivors of myocardial infarction: A prospective clinical angiographic study. *N Engl J Med* 1982;306:1065–1070.

Savin WM, Haskell WL, Houston-Miller N, et al: Improvement in aerobic capacity soon after myocardial infarction. *J Cardiac Rehabil* 1981;1:337–342.

Scheuer J: Effects of physical training on myocardial vascularity and perfusion. *Circulation* 1982;66:491–495.

Schneider RM, Seaworth JF, Dohrmann ML, et al: Anatomic and prognostic implications of an early positive treadmill exercise test. *Am J Cardiol* 1982;50:682–688.

Shand DG, Wood AJ: Editorial. Propranolol withdrawal syndrome why? *Circulation* 1978;58:202–203.

Shaw LW: Effects of a prescribed supervised exercise program on mortality and cardiovascular morbidity in patients after a myocardial infarction. *Am J Cardiol* 1981;48:39–46.

Sheldahl LM, Wilke NA, Tristani FE: Exercise prescription to return to work. *J Cardiopulmonary Rehabil* 1985;5:567–575.

Sheldahl LM, Wilke NA, Tristani FE, et al: Continuing medical education response to repetitive static-dynamic exercise in patients with coronary artery disease. *J Cardiac Rehabil* 1985;5:139–145.

Shephard RJ: Post-coronary rehabilitation, body composition, and recurrent infarction: An analysis of data from the Ontario Exercise-Heart collaborative study. *Nutr Metab* 1980;24:383–395.

Shephard RJ: The value of exercise in ischemic heart disease: A cumulative analysis. *J Cardiac Rehabil* 1983;3:294–298.

Shephard RJ, Kavanagh T, Klavora P: Mood state during postcoronary cardiac rehabilitation. *J Cardiopulmonary Rehabil* 1985;5:480–484.

Shephard RJ, Kavanagh T, Tuck J, et al: Marathon jogging in post-myocardial infarction patients. *J Cardiac Rehabil* 1983;3:321–329.

Sikorski JM: Knowledge, concerns, and question of wives of convalescent coronary artery bypass graft surgery patients. *J Cardiac Rehabil* 1985;5:74–85.

Silvidi GI, Squires RW, Pollock ML, et al: Hemodynamic responses and medical problems associated with early exercise and ambulation in coronary artery bypass graft surgery patients. *J Cardiac Rehabil* 1982;2:355–362.

Sim DN, Neill WA: Investigation of the physiological basis for increased exercise threshold for angina pectoris after physical conditioning. *J Clin Invest* 1974;54:763–770.

Simoons M, Lap C, Pool J: Heart rate levels and ventricular ectopic activity during cardiac rehabilitation. *Am Heart J* 1980;100:9–14.

Sivarajan ES, Bruce RA, Aimes MJ, et al: In-hospital exercise after myocardial infarction does not improve treadmill performance. *N Engl J Med* 1981;305:357–362.

Sivarajan ES, Snydsman A, Smith B, et al: Low-level treadmill testing of 41 patients with acute myocardial infarction prior to discharge from the hospital. *Heart Lung* 1977;6:975–980.

Soloff PH: Medically and surgically treated coronary patients in cardiovascular rehabilitation: A comparative study. *Int J Psychiat Med* 1980;9:93–106.

Staniloff HM: Current concepts in cardiac rehabilitation. *Am J Surg* 1984;147(6):719–724.

Stevens R, Hanson P: Comparison of supervised and unsupervised exercise training after coronary bypass surgery. *Am J Cardiol* 1984;53:1524–1528.

Swan HJ: Duration of hospitalization in "uncomplicated" completed acute myocardial infarction. *Am J Cardiol* 1976;37:13–19.

Tesar GE, Hackett TP: Psychiatric management of the hospitalized cardiac patient. *J Cardiopulmonary Rehabil* 1985;5:219–225.

Tesch PA: Exercise performance and B-blockade: *Sports Med* 1985;2:389–412.

Tesch PA, Kaiser P: Effects of beta-adrenergic blockade on O_2 uptake during submaximal and maximal exercise. *J Appl Physiol: Respirat Environ Exerc Physiol* 1983;54:901–905.

Thompson PD: The cardiovascular risks of cardiac rehabilitation. *J Cardiopulmonary Rehabil* 1985;5:321–324.

Torkelson LO: Rehabilitation of the patient with acute myocardial infarction. *J Chron Dis* 1964;17:685–704.

Tucker HH, Carson PHM, Bass NM, et al: Results of early mobilization and discharge after myocardial infarction. *Br Med J* 1973;1:10–13.

Turi ZG, Braunwald E: The use of beta blockers after myocardial infarction. *JAMA* 1983;249:2512–2516.

Vanhees L, Fagard R, Amery A: Influence of beta-adrenergic blockage on effects of physical training in patients with ischemic heart diseae. *Br Heart J* 1982;48:33–38.

Vanhees L, Fagard R, Amery A: Influence of beta-adrenergic blockage on the hemodynamic effects of physical training in patients with ischemic heart disease. *Am Heart J* 1984;108:270.

Verani MS, Hartung GH, Harris-Hoepfel J, et al: Effects of exercise training on left ventricular performance and myocardial perfusion in patients with coronary artery disease. *Am J Cardiol* 1981;47:797–803.

Vermeulen A, Liew KI, Durrer D: Effects of cardiac rehabilitation after myocardial infarction: Changes in coronary risk factors and long-term prognosis. *Am Heart J* 1983;105:798–801.

Wasserman AG, Bren GB, Ross A, et al: Prognostic implications of diagnostic Q-waves after myocardial infarction. *Circulation* 1982;65:1451–1455.

Waters DD, Szlachcic J, Bonan R, et al: Comparative sensitivity of exercise, cold pressor and ergonovine testing in provoking attacks of variant angina in patients with active disease. *Circulation* 1983;67:310–315.

Watson F, Cornett S: Cardiac Rehabilitation: An Interdisciplinary Team Approach. New York, John Wiley & Sons, 1984.

Wenger NK, Cleeman JI, Herd JA, et al: Education of the patient with cardiac disease in the twenty-first century: An overview. *Am J Cardiol* 1986;57:1187–1189.

Wenger NK, Hellerstein HK, Blackburn H, et al: Uncomplicated myocardial infarction. *JAMA* 1973;224:511–514.

Wenger NK, Hellerstein HK, Blackburn H, et al: Physician practice in the management of patients with uncomplicated myocardial infarction: Changes in the past decade. *Circulation* 1982;65:421–427.

Wenger NK, Hurst JW: Coronary bypass surgery as a rehabilitative procedure. *Cardiac Rehabil Q* 1980;11:1–6.

West RR, Henderson AH: Randomized multicentre trial of early mobilization after uncomplicated myocardial infarction. *Br Heart J* 1979;42:381–385.

Wiklund I, Sanne H, Vedin A, et al: Determinants of return to work one year after a first myocardial infarction. *J Cardiac Rehabil* 1985;5:62–72.

Wilhelmsen L, Sanne H, Elmfeldt D, et al: A controlled trial of physical training after myocardial infarction. *Prev Med* 1975;4:491–508.

Wilke NA, Sheldahl LM, Tristani FE, et al: The safety of static-dynamic effort soon after myocardial infarction. *Am Heart J* 1985;110:542.

Williams MA, Maresh CM, Esterbrooks DJ, et al: Early exercise training in patients older than age 65 years compared with that in younger patients after acute myocardial infarction or coronary artery bypass grafting. *Am J Cardiol* 1985;55:263–266.

Williams PT, Wood PT, Haskell WL, et al: The effect of running mileage and duration on plasma lipoprotein levels. *JAMA* 1982;247:2674–2679.

Young SG, Abouantoun S, Savvides M, et al: Limitations of electrocardiographic scoring systems for estimation of left ventricular function. *J Am Coll Cardiol* 1983;1:1479–1488.

Zimmerman D, Parker BM: The pain of pulmonary hypertension. Fact or fancy? *JAMA* 1981;246:2345–2346.

APPENDIX A

In 1980, the American College of Cardiology and the American Heart Association formed a task force to assess cardiovascular procedures. The purpose of this task force was to examine the effect of developing technology on the practice and cost of medical care. Such analysis could potentially lower the cost of medical care without diminishing its effectiveness. The results of the task force were anticipated to have an impact on the reimbursement policies of Medicare, HCFA, and medical insurance companies. In the September 1986 issues of both *Circulation* and the *Journal of the American College of Cardiology*, the results of the subcommittee on exercise testing were published. The aims of the guidelines were:

1. To define the role of exercise testing in the diagnosis and management of patients with heart disease.
2. To address the contribution, uniqueness, sensitivity, specificity, indications, contraindications, and cost-efficacy of exercise testing.

The various uses of exercise testing were classified as:

> CLASS I—general consensus agreement that it is justified
> CLASS II—frequently used but divergence of opinion regarding justification
> CLASS III—general agreement regarding little or no value, or inappropriate to use exercise testing

The following is a summary of this special report.

CONTRAINDICATIONS FOR EXERCISE TESTING

Unstable angina prior to stabilization
Life-threatening arrhythmias
CHF, uncompensated
AV Block, advanced
Myocarditis
Critical aortic stenosis
Complicating illnesses

EXERCISE TESTING OF PATIENTS WITH SYMPTOMS/SIGNS SUGGESTIVE OF CORONARY ARTERY DISEASE (CAD) OR WITH KNOWN CAD

CLASS I (general agreement for use)
Diagnosis in male patients with atypical signs/symptoms of CAD
Assessment of functional capacity
Prognostication
Evaluation of patients with symptoms consistent with recurrent exercise-induced arrhythmias

CLASS II (divergent opinions regarding use)
Diagnosis in women with chest pain, angina
Diagnosis of CAD with digoxin being administered or RBBB present
Evaluation of functional capacity and response to therapy with drugs
    for patients with CAD or CHF
Evaluation of variant angina
Serial follow up (1 year or longer) of patients with CAD

CLASS III (agreement against use for CAD)
Evaluation of patients with single PVCs
Evaluation of patients serially in Rehab
Diagnosis of CAD in patients with WPW or LBBB

SCREENING OF APPARENTLY HEALTHY INDIVIDUALS

CLASS I (agreement)

CLASS II (divergent opinions)
Evaluation of asymptomatic males over 40
- in special occupations
- with two or more risk factors (cholesterol > 240, hypertension, cigarette smoking, diabetes mellitus, or a family history of CAD in individuals less than 55 years of age)
- who are sedentary and plan to enter a vigorous exercise program

CLASS III (not recommended)
Evaluation of asymptomatic men or women
- with no risk factors
- with chest discomfort not thought to be cardiac related

EXERCISE TESTING SOON AFTER MI

CLASS I (agreement for use)
Evaluation of prognosis and functional capacity in uncomplicated MIs

CLASS II (used but no agreement)
Evaluation of patients
- with baseline ECGs or medical problems that affect responses
- with complicated MIs

CLASS III (agreement against use)
Evaluation of patients
- with acute ischemia
- with instability or complicating illnesses

EXERCISE TESTING AFTER SPECIFIC PROCEDURES

CLASS I (agreement for use)
Evaluation after CABS, PTCA

CLASS II (used but with controversy)
Yearly follow up of asymptomatic patients with CABS or PTCA

EXERCISE TESTING IN PATIENTS WITH VALVULAR HEART DISEASE

CLASS I (agreement for use)
Not used

CLASS II (used but no agreement)
Evaluation of functional capacity

CLASS III (agreement against)
Evaluation of symptomatic critical aortic stenosis or obstructive cardiomyopathy

EXERCISE TESTING IN THE MANAGEMENT OF PATIENTS WITH HYPERTENSION (HBP) OR CARDIAC PACEMAKERS

CLASS I (agreement for use)
Not used

CLASS II (used but no agreement)
Evaluation of BP response in patients treated for HBP who wish to exercise vigorously

CLASS III (agreement against)
Evaluation of patients with severe HBP
Evaluation of HBP patients who do not plan to exercise
Evaluation of pacemaker function

CARDIAC REHABILITATION POSITION REPORT

In response to the Office of Health Care Technology, Department of Health and Human Services, the American College of Cardiology (ACC) appointed an Ad Hoc Task Force to develop a
position paper relative to cardiac rehabilitation. In response to a previous statement, Blue Cross
had stated that they would only pay for three outpatient visits after an MI under the category of
cardiac rehabilitation. Many individuals thought that this was inadequate and felt a new statement was needed. The following summarizes the position statement of ACC regarding Phase II
and III cardiac rehabilitation programs.

Contraindications. A number of contraindications to exercise and training have been identified
and can be categorized as being absolute or relative. Absolute contraindications are those known
or suspected conditions that eliminate the patient from participating in exercise programs. Some
of the absolute contraindications are unstable angina pectoris, dissecting aortic aneurysm, complete heart block, uncontrolled hypertension, CHF, or dysrhythmias, thrombophlebitis, and other
complicating illnesses. In some conditions, contraindications are relative; that is, the benefits
outweigh the risks involved if the patient exercises cautiously. The relative contraindications
include frequent PVCs, controlled dysrhythmias, intermittent claudication, metabolic disorders,
and moderate anemia or pulmonary disease.

In an aging population with a high prevalence of cardiovascular disorders, the demand for
cardiovascular rehabilitation programs is escalating at a time when dollar support is declining.
In response to efforts by Health Insurances to decrease payments for out of hospital programs,
the ACC has taken the following position. Since ECG monitoring is the most costly of the services
provided by these programs, it becomes imperative to redefine the role of the services provided.
To achieve the goals of post-hospital rehabilitation, programs can be formal or informal, supervised or unsupervised, ECG monitored or not ECG monitored. All patients should have access to
patient education with regard to risk factor modification, dietary and psychological counseling if
indicated.

The post-hospital rehabilitation program should be physician prescribed and can vary greatly from patient to patient. Most patients, following a cardiovascular event, will not require formal rehabilitation services to restore them to their previous level. Not all patients requiring rehabilitation services may have been hospitalized and rehabilitation services for these patients should begin at the discretion of the physician.

Entry Criteria. The following classification represents the categories of potential candidates for rehabilitation:
1. Coronary artery disease including patients who have or have had:
    a. myocardial infarction
    b. coronary bypass surgery
    c. coronary angioplasty
    d. stable angina
    e. silent myocardial ischemia
2. Those who have had other heart surgery, including transplantation
3. Patients with dilated cardiomyopathy, left ventricular dysfunction, or hypertensive cardiovascular disease
4. The elderly patient with heart disease. Rehabilitation services in this group may be the least expensive way to keep these patients out of more expensive care units

Only a percentage of patients will require supervised continuous ECG monitored exercise programs in addition to the counseling services. The major expense of rehabilitation programs is the supervised ECG monitored exercise portion which requires trained personnel and expensive equipment. However, programs can take various forms. The program could be informal, involving patient counseling by the primary physician with or without an exercise prescription by him to be carried out without supervision at home or in a health facility. It could involve patient counseling by a specialist in the absence of a primary physician, or if the physician were unable to provide this service, or at his request. Formal programs can include patient counseling by a primary physician or counseling services plus a supervised exercise prescription without continuous ECG monitoring, or they can include counseling plus supervised continuous ECG monitored exercise. The stratification of patients into these groups can be performed using the means described in the patient evaluation. Exercise training should be considered a dynamic rather than uniform prescription and may be subject to change during the course of the program.

Criteria for ECG monitoring during exercise program. In the event that the following patients are selected for an exercise program, ECG monitoring should be included:
    a. severely depressed left ventricular function (ejection fraction under 30)
    b. resting complex ventricular arrhythmia (Lown type 4 or 5)
    c. ventricular arrhythmias appearing or increasing with exercise
    d. decrease in systolic blood pressure with exercise
    e. survivors of sudden cardiac death
    f. patients following myocardial infarction complicated by congestive heart failure, cardiogenic shock, and/or serious ventricular arrhythmias
    g. patients with severe coronary artery disease and marked exercise-induced ischemia
    h. inability to self-monitor heart rate due to physical or intellectual impairment if monitoring heart rate is judged to be essential

REFERENCES

Exercise Testing Task Force Members: Guidelines for Exercise Testing. A Report of the American College of Cardiology/American Heart Association Task Force on Assessment of Cardiovascular Procedures (Subcommittee on Exercise Testing). JACC 1986;8(3):725–38.

Parmley, WW: President's Page: Position Report on Cardiac Rehabilitation. JACC 1986; 7(2):451–3.

APPENDIX B

PREDICTING SEVERITY OF LEFT MAIN CORONARY DISEASE: AN UPDATE

Since completing this book, two important papers regarding the prognostic implications of exercise testing were published. These two papers are summarized in the following pages.

PREDICTION OF LEFT MAIN CORONARY ARTERY DISEASE

Lee, Cook and Goldman have developed a strategy to identify patients with left main coronary artery disease (LMCAD). It is a simple model that could predict probability of LMCAD from a combination of clinical and exercise test variables and can be applied using a pocket calculator or graphs published in their paper. The model was derived from multivariate analysis of already published data obtained clinically without exercise testing and then from exercise test variables. They tested this model prospectively on a separate group of patients to confirm its ability to predict the probability of left main coronary artery disease. They found that the model using only three variables (age, angina, amount of ST depression) provided reasonably accurate perspective estimates of the prevalence of left main coronary artery disease in subsets of patients.

The model was developed using the Harvard University–Brigham coronary artery disease data bank containing over 900 items of clinical, angiographic, hemodynamic, surgical, and follow-up data from 947 patients. The patients underwent cardiac catheterization from 1977 to 1981 for suspected or known coronary artery disease but were free of valvular heart disease. The average age was 58 years and 74% were male. Of these patients, 477 underwent a Bruce test within six months before or several weeks after catheterization. Coronary artery disease was defined as a 70% luminal reduction except for the left main where 50% was considered significant. No significant coronary artery disease was found in 15% while 12% had LMCAD. Of the remaining patients, 40% had three-vessel disease, 22% had two-vessel disease, and 12% had one-vessel disease. They were divided into two groups: Group 1, which consisted of 508 patients whose clinical data were used to develop a model for predicting the probability of left main coronary artery disease; and Group 2, which consisted of 370 patients who had complete catheterization and exercise test data.

The clinical data in Group 1 were used to derive a model for predicting the results of coronary angiography. The historical, physical exam, and lab data that were considered included age, sex, chest pain characteristics, duration of symptoms, history of MI, unstable angina, history of smoking, diabetes, obesity, hyperlipidemia, cerebrovascular or peripheral vascular disease, hypertension, systolic blood pressure, serum cholesterol, diagnostic Q-waves and ST- and T-wave changes. A logistic regression model for predicting the probability of left main disease was constructed in a stepwise manner using variables listed above as candidates for the model. At each step of the logistic regression procedure, the variable that was most significantly associated with the presence of left main disease was selected, conditioning on all variables previously chosen. All variables that had significant incremental correlations with the presence of left main disease and that improved the overall accuracy of the model were included.

Having developed a simple model for predicting the pre-test probability of left main disease, a model was developed for predicting the post-exercise test probability using Bayes theorem. Likelihood ratios for left main disease could only be estimated for various degrees of ST-segment change, exercise duration and exertional hypotension by pooling results from published studies. Other reported markers had inadequate information regarding sensitivity and specificity. Various combinations of responses were suggested by investigators but none had been validated. A total of 4950 patients including 516 with left main disease were described in the 20 studies pooled.

By applying the logistic regression model derived from the patients in Group 1, a pre-exercise test probability of left main disease was calculated for each of the 370 patients in Group 2. The post-test probability of left main disease was calculated for each Group 2 patient using likelihood ratios based on the amount of ST change, the presence or absence of exertional hypotension and the duration of exercise. Thus, the post-exercise model was based on the assumption that exercise test findings were conditionally independent of the clinical factors in the pre-exercise test model. They also considered how the sequential use of more than one of these three exercise test factors should change the calculations of the post-test probability, assuming that the factors were not correlated with each other except by chance. Finally, a logistic regression analysis was performed on the validation set of patients (N = 370) to determine whether both the pre-exercise test probability and the information from the exercise test were significant independent predictors of left main coronary artery disease.

Multivariate logistic regression analysis of the clinical data from the patients in the training set showed that only 2 pre-exercise test factors—age and presence of typical angina—had statistically significant univariate and multivariate correlations with the presence of LMCAD. The information from the exercise test from the pooled studies reviewed revealed that the most sensitive predictor of left main disease was the presence of ST-segment depression but that the specificity was low. Exertional hypotension was fairly specific but not sensitive. In Group 2, 23% had less than 0.1 mV exercise-induced ST-segment depression, 22% had 0.1 to 0.2 mV, 29% had 0.2 to 0.3 mV, and 26% had greater than 0.3 mV depression. The prevalence of left main disease in these subgroups was 1%, 6%, 13%, and 19%, respectively. Also, in Group 2, percentages of duration on the treadmill were 19% for less than 3 minutes, 39% for 3 to 6 minutes and 43% for more than 6 minutes. The prevalence of left main disease in these subgroups was 15%, 13% and 6%. Of the 50 who had exertional hypotension, 16% had left main disease compared with 10% of those who did not. When ST change, exertional hypotension, and treadmill duration were used to modify the pre-exercise test probability in the validation set, ST-segment change was clearly the best of the three for predicting left main coronary disease. The best predictions were obtained from the post-test exercise test model that included three factors: age, presence of typical angina, and degree of ST-segment change. When the post-test probability with this model was lower than the pre-exercise test probability, 4% had left main disease. Conversely, when the post-test probability was higher than the pre-test probability, 16% had left main disease.

The key question in trying to identify patients with high risk coronary artery disease is: can those who are recognized have improved survival if they undergo coronary artery bypass surgery? In order to answer this question Weiner and the CASS group compared the survival of patients who underwent bypass surgery to those who received medical therapy in 5303 non-randomized patients from the CASS registry. Patients in the two treatment groups differed substantially with regard to important baseline variables. Analysis of 32 variables by the Cox regression model for survival revealed an independent beneficial effect of bypass surgery on survival. Patients were then stratified into subsets according to the results of exercise testing. Surgical benefit was greatest in the 789 patients who exhibited at least 0.1 mV of ST segment depression and who could exercise only into Stage 1 or less (5 METs or less). Among the 398 patients with three-vessel disease showing these characteristics, seven-year survival was 58% for the medical group and 81% for the surgical group. There was no difference in survival between the surgical and medical groups among the 1545 patients without ischemic ST-segment depression who were able to exercise into Stage 3 or greater (9 METs or more). Thus, in patients who demonstrate ST-segment depression on exercise testing and whose exercise capacity is limited, coronary artery bypass surgery appears to improve survival in comparison with medical therapy alone.

REFERENCES

Lee TH, Cook EF, Goldman L: Prospective evaluation: a clinical and exercise-test model for the prediction of left main coronary artery disease. *Medical Decision Making* 1986;6:136–144.

Weiner DA, Ryan TJ, McCabe CH, Chaitman BR, Sheffield LT, Fisher LD, Tristani F: Role of exercise testing in identifying patients with improved survival after coronary artery bypass surgery. *JACC* 1986;8:741–748.

INDEX